THE PROTEIN COUNTER

Did you know that a lunch of turkey, chicken or seafood can sharply increase alertness; or that foods high in tryptophan—bananas, dry-roasted sunflower seeds, pumpkin seeds, baked potatoes with their skins on, beans, peanuts, dates and even pizza—can calm you down?

Here is the essential information you need about protein, plus 15,000 entries—alphabetized for quick, easy reference—that show the portion sizes, calorie counts, and protein, carbohydrate and fat values for various foods. *THE PROTEIN COUNTER* also provides a clear explanation of the values listed on food labels so that you can make the best choices.

ANNETTE B. NATOW, Ph.D., R.D. and Jo-Ann Heslin, M.A., R.D., are the authors of twenty books on nutrition. Both are former faculty members of Adelphi University and the State University of New York, Downstate Medical Center. They are editors of the *Journal of Nutrition for the Elderly,* serve as editorial board members for the *Environmental Nutrition Newsletter,* and are frequent contributors to magazines and journals.

Books by Annette B. Natow and Jo-Ann Heslin

The Antioxidant Vitamin Counter
The Cholesterol Counter (Fourth edition)
The Diabetes Carbohydrate and Calorie Counter
The Fast Food Nutrition Counter
The Fat Attack Plan
The Fat Counter (Third edition)
The Iron Counter
Megadoses
No-Nonsense Nutrition for Kids
The Pocket Encyclopedia of Nutrition
The Pocket Fat Counter
The Pregnancy Nutrition Counter
The Protein Counter
The Sodium Counter
The Supermarket Nutrition Counter (Second edition)

Published by POCKET BOOKS

THE
PROTEIN
COUNTER

**Annette B. Natow, Ph.D., R.D.
and Jo-Ann Heslin, M.A., R.D.**

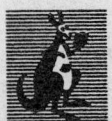

POCKET BOOKS
New York   London   Toronto   Sydney   Tokyo   Singapore

An *Original* Publication of POCKET BOOKS

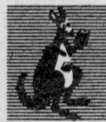

POCKET BOOKS, a division of Simon & Schuster Inc.
1230 Avenue of the Americas, New York, NY 10020

Copyright © 1997 by Jo-Ann Heslin and Annette Natow

ISBN: 0-671-00381-X

First Pocket Books printing March 1997

10 9 8 7 6 5 4

POCKET and colophon are registered trademarks of Simon & Schuster Inc.

Printed in the U.S.A.

To our families who support us through every project: Harry, Allen, Irene, Sarah, Meryl, Laura, Marty, George, Emily, Steven, Joe, Kristen and Karen

ACKNOWLEDGMENTS

———◇———

Without the tireless cooperation of Steven and Stephen, *The Protein Counter* would never have been completed. Our thanks to all the food manufacturers and processors who shared product information. A special thanks to our editor, Peter Wolverton, and our agent, Nancy Trichter.

"The fact that protein food is both a fuel and a building material makes its place in the diet confusing."

Mary Swartz Rose, Ph.D.
Feeding the Family
The Macmillan Company, 1919

SOURCES OF DATA

◇

Values in this counter have been obtained from the Composition of Foods, United States Department of Agriculture, Agricultural Handbooks: No. 8–1, Dairy and Egg Products; No. 8–2, Spices and Herbs; No. 8–3, Baby Foods; No. 8–4, Fats and Oils; No. 8–5, Poultry Products; No. 8–6, Soups, Sauces and Gravies; No. 8–7, Sausages and Luncheon Meats; No. 8–8, Breakfast Cereals; No. 8–9, Fruit and Fruit Juices; No. 8–10, Pork Products; No. 8–11, Vegetables and Vegetable Products; No. 8–12, Nut and Seed Products; No. 8–13, Beef Products; No. 8–14, Beverages; No. 8–15, Finfish and Shellfish Products; No. 8–16, Legumes and Legume Products; No. 8–17, Lamb, Veal and Game Products; No. 8–18, Baked Products; No. 8–19, Snacks and Sweets; No. 8–20, Cereal Grains and Pasta; No. 8–21, Fast Foods; Supplements 1989, 1990, 1991, 1992.

"Nutritive Value of Foods." United States Department of Agriculture, Home and Garden Bulletin No. 72.

J. Davies and J. Dickerson, *Nutrient Content of Food Portions.* Cambridge, UK: The Royal Society of Chemistry, 1991.

G. A. Leveille, M. E. Zabik, and K. J. Morgan, *Nutrients in Foods.* Cambridge, MA: The Nutrition Guild, 1983.

A. Moller, E. Saxholt, and B. E. Mikkelsen, *Food Composition Tables: Amino Acids, Carbohydrates and Fatty Acids in Danish Foods.* 1991.

Souci, Fachman, and Kraut, *Food Composition and Nutrition Tables.* Stuttgart: Wissenschaftliche Verlagsgesellschaft MbH, 1989.

Information from food labels, manufacturers and processors. The values are based on research conducted through the first half of 1996. Manufacturers' ingredients are subject to change, so current values may vary from those listed in the book. If the serving size on the package label is different from that listed in this counter, use the nutrition information provided as a guide. If the nutrition information listed in the Nutrition Facts panel is different from the information in this counter, assume that the product has been recently reformulated.

INTRODUCTION

———◇———

Every day your body loses millions of cells. They are used up, worn out, rubbed off and even cut off like your beard or fingernails. You need protein to replace these cells.

Except for water, there is more protein in your body than anything else. A 143-pound man has over 25 pounds of protein!

Protein is found in every cell, tissue and substance in the body except for urine and bile. Our bodies contain many thousands of specific proteins, each one different and designed to do its special job. Bones, teeth, muscles, enzymes, skin and blood all contain protein. Active tissues, like muscles and glands, are high in protein, while less active tissue, like fat, has less.

When you don't get enough protein to replace lost cells and maintain normal functions, your body will cannibalize its own tissues and begin to waste away. That's why it is so important to get enough protein. But you should realize, excess protein is of no benefit to the body. It is not stored. It is simply used up for energy or converted to fat and then stored. Converting the protein to energy or fat makes the liver and kidneys work overtime as they process the extra protein and get rid of the leftover waste.

Protein is very important because it is:

• Necessary for life.
• Necessary for growth.
• Part of every cell in your body.

- Needed to replace worn-out cells.
- Necessary to repair damaged tissue.
- A major part of the immune system.
- A major part of every enzyme.
- A source of energy.

You get protein from the food you eat. Foods like meat, milk, beans, vegetables and grains contain protein, which in turn supply *amino acids*. Your body uses amino acids as the building blocks to make the special proteins it needs. All body proteins are made from about twenty different amino acids. These amino acids combine in different ways to make distinct kinds of protein in the same way that different letters of the alphabet combine to form many different words.

AMINO ACIDS ARE VERY SPECIAL

Almost all foods contain protein, some more, some less. Fruits have little protein compared to meat, milk, cheese, beans, grains and vegetables. When you eat different foods, you get varying amounts of protein and varying amounts of the different amino acids they contain. Of the twenty different amino acids found in food, nine are essential. *These nine must be obtained directly in the food you eat.* The remaining eleven can be made in the body. This is one of the reasons why it is so important to eat a variety of protein foods. It guarantees you'll get all the different amino acids you need. For example, beans may be short in one of the essential amino acids, while rice and other grains have plenty of it. When you eat beans and rice together or even separately during the day, their amino acids pool together so that your body has a supply of all the amino acids needed to build its cells.

Protein and Amino Acid Supplements

Throughout history people have sought out ways to improve their physical ability. Meat was usually believed to be a good bet because it is animal muscle and was thought to build body muscle. There are reports that as early as the sixth century B.C. a dedicated Greek wrestler, Milo of Crotona, ate 20 pounds of meat every day to build up his body. Athletes today are still looking for ways to enhance their performance. Many believe, as Milo did, that extra meat or just more protein or even individual amino acids will increase their muscle size and strength. That simply isn't true. Eating more protein is not a shortcut to a strong, active body.

Extra protein, by itself, will not build muscles or improve athletic performance. In fact, the only thing that builds muscle is working the muscle. Although it is true that muscle is 22% protein, 8 grams of protein a day is all that is needed to build 5 pounds of muscle in a month! Because most Americans eat about twice as much protein as needed, we have more than enough to meet increased needs for muscle growth. Protein supplements are not needed. They are expensive, can have undesirable effects and may even be dangerous.

Your body does not store excess protein, so any extra is used for energy, if needed, or simply stored as fat. Excess protein builds body fat, not muscle, so when more protein calories are eaten than are needed, the body adds fat, not extra muscle. When you continuously make your body convert excess protein to fat or energy, you put a strain on the liver and kidneys, and this extra workload may damage these organs. Eliminating waste products formed from this conversion can lead to calcium loss, gout (painful joints) and dehydration.

What about protein supplements?

Protein supplements are made from food proteins, such as dried milk protein, egg white protein, soy protein or combinations of these. While there is no evidence that these supplements are of benefit to reasonably well nourished people, they can be used as a simple way to get low-fat protein when dieting or in training. Cheaper substitutes such as tuna packed in water, skim milk or skinless chicken breast work just as well. They're cheaper and you'll enjoy them more.

What about specific amino acid supplements?

Specific amino acids taken as supplements are one of the most popular ergogenic aids for endurance athletes and body builders. They are touted as being a legal replacement for anabolic androgenic steroids. Certain amino acids are billed as being able to build muscles, aid fat loss, provide energy and improve muscle repair.

Arginine and *ornithine* are taken to enhance growth hormone production. Arginine has been shown to increase growth hormone temporarily when taken at very high doses, but the increased hormone does not lead to an increase in muscle mass or strength.

Leucine has been shown to enhance protein production. Again, it does not seem to result in increased muscle mass or strength. Leucine, *isoleucine* and *valine*, a family of amino acids, are said to be the body's preferred energy source during endurance exercise. There is no evidence to support this claim.

Tryptophan is used by the body to make *serotonin*, a chemical that transmits nerve messages in the brain. Serotonin has a calming effect, and may make you feel sleepy and relieve pain. It also reduces appetite and the craving for carbohydrate in some people. Tryptophan is considered by some to be a natural tranquilizer. Prescription drugs that raise serotonin levels are used to treat depression and to promote weight loss.

In 1989 tryptophan supplements used to relieve insomnia caused a rare blood disorder and some deaths in persons taking them. As a result, the Food and Drug Administration recalled all tryptophan supplements at that time. They are now available and believed to be safe if manufactured properly. Athletes use tryptophan to calm their jitters and improve their performance. Meals high in carbohydrate, the body's most efficient energy source, also increase tryptophan (and serotonin) levels in the brain, causing the desired calming effect.

Lysine, another amino acid, is used by many to prevent and/or relieve canker sores, shingles, and herpes infections on the mouth and genitals. Scientific evidence does not support this.

There is no evidence that taking individual amino acids will be of any benefit to a well-nourished athlete. And there may be dangers. Taking individual amino acids can cause imbalances in the body that have caused toxic effects in animals.

Our bodies normally receive all the amino acids needed in the foods we eat. Foods are the best way for the body to get amino acids because then there is never a danger from imbalances caused by individual amino acids.

To sum up:

- Excess protein from protein powders or amino acid powders is not needed and may not be healthy.
- Converting excess protein to fat or using excess protein for energy may stress the liver and kidneys. This can have long-term negative effects on these organs.
- Protein breakdown products are excreted in the urine, pulling a good deal of water and minerals (electrolytes) from the body with the waste.
- Protein and amino acid supplements can cause excess weight gain, dehydration, gout and calcium loss, as well as possible liver and kidney damage.

Research shows that a meal high in protein helps to keep you awake and alert while a eating a meal high in carbohydrate tends to make you sleepy.

Growth and Protein

During times of rapid growth in infancy, childhood and adolescence and during pregnancy, protein needs are high. During the first six months of life, infants need more than twice as much protein in relation to their weight as adults. Premature infants need even more. Throughout childhood and adolescence, the protein need in relation to body weight gradually decreases until by age fifteen in females and nineteen in males, the recommended protein intake is at the adult level. During pregnancy, the protein needs reflect the growth rate of the baby. The need is greater in the second half of pregnancy. See the chart Your Daily Protein Factor, page xxiv.

NECESSARY NITROGEN

Protein is different from the other energy sources we eat like carbohydrate and fat because it contains nitrogen. The need for protein is really a need for nitrogen. We lose nitrogen each day in urine, feces, skin, hair, nails, perspiration and other secretions. The nitrogen is replaced in the protein we eat.

Repair and Protein

When the body is stressed in any way, physically or mentally, protein (nitrogen) is lost from the body. This increases the need for protein to restore the body to normal. When the environmental temperature is too hot or too cold, extra protein is needed. Heavy sweating calls for more protein to replace nitrogen lost in sweat. Exercise, fever and surgery all increase protein need as do recovering from injury, infection or broken bones. Even during emotional stress, like losing a job or taking an exam, extra nitrogen is lost from the body. Extra protein is needed to make up for the loss.

Athletes and Protein

Athletes need more protein. Although carbohydrate and fat are the major fuels used for energy, it is now accepted that during certain activities more protein may be used for energy too. That is why experts recommend an increased protein factor for athletes, with amounts ranging from 0.8 to 2.0, reflecting the level of energy used during their activity. Specific athletic protein factors can be found in the chart Your Daily Protein Factor, page xxiv.

Although you might not consider yourself an athlete, the number one public health message today is for all people to get more active. Experts recommend 30 minutes of activity for everyone every day.

Exercise helps keep the heart healthy, lowers cholesterol, strengthens immunity, improves balance, helps control weight, promotes mental health, enhances sexual desire and performance, helps relieve tension headaches, improves appearance and increases your sense of well-being. Exercise can also lower the risk of developing diabetes, osteoporosis and some cancers, In spite of all these benefits not many Americans have incorporated regular exercise into their lives. A survey in January, 1995 conducted by American Sports Data Inc. found that only 20% of responders exercise regularly, while 60% do nothing.

Sport Snacks

Athletic bars or energy bars are growing in popularity as athletes continue to look for a "quick fix" to improve their performance. The bars are a combination of grains, fruit, vitamins and minerals in a candy or cookie base. The benefit comes from the carbohydrate (and sometimes caffeine) they contain. Choose a bar that lists complex carbohydrate such as wheat, oats, rice or carbohydrate compounds, such as glucose polymer or malto-dextrin. Less desirable are bars loaded with simple sugars like white or brown sugar, corn syrup or glucose as their major ingredients. Simple sugars can cause your blood sugar to spike and then quickly fall, causing fatigue. The complex carbohydrates take longer to digest and give up their energy, keeping your blood sugar and energy more level.

Vegetarians and Protein

Who are vegetarians? Almost everyone! Some eat no animal products at all, others eat plant foods along with milk, or with eggs and milk, or eggs, milk and fish. Others eat all of these foods plus poultry but do not eat red meat. Some eat vegetarian choices some of the time but not all the time. Vegetarian eating has become part of the way we eat.

All of the diets that include some animal foods provide plenty of protein and other needed nutrients. Even a completely plant-based diet, when sufficient in calories and carefully planned, can provide adequate amounts of all needed nutrients including protein.

Standard protein recommendations may not be sufficient for normal growth and health in children who eat no animal foods at all. They may need extra protein, which can easily be found in foods like beans, soy milk, cereals and nuts.

Food Allergies

An allergy is an abnormal response of the immune system to an otherwise harmless food. It is usually a protein in the food that produces the allergic reaction. Hives, rashes, eczema, cramps, vomiting, diarrhea, breathing problems, wheezing and swelling or itching of the lips and tongue are usual symptoms of an allergic reaction. Severe reactions are less common but can be fatal.

Food intolerance is different from an allergy. Small amounts of the offending food can usually be eaten when there is an intolerance. With an allergy, you must completely avoid the food. Two percent of adults and up to 8% of children suffer from real food allergies. There is no treatment for food allergies: avoidance of the food is all that you can do.

Looking at Labels

The Nutrition Fact Panel on foods will give you information about the amount of protein in a single serving of the food. The amount of protein is given in grams and also as a percentage of the Daily Value (DV). The DV is based on the amount of protein recommended for a 2,000-calorie diet. This may be more or less than the amount of calories you usually eat. For example, the label of a can of solid white tuna in spring water shows that a 2-ounce serving (one-quarter cup) has 15 grams of protein, which is 27% of the DV. When you are counting your protein intake, the number of grams is a more useful figure so that you can see how the food fits into your personal protein recommendation for the day.

When you look at the ingredient list on a food, you may see some unfamiliar words. A can of chicken broth may show, in addition to chicken broth, *hydrolyzed protein, wheat gluten* and *monosodium glutamate*. These ingredients are actually protein and add to the total protein in the food. The following list gives some examples of protein ingredients.

THESE ARE PROTEIN TOO!

Casein	Hydrolyzed plant protein
Corn gluten	(HPP)
Egg whites	Hydrolyzed vegetable protein
Gelatin	(HVP)
Gluten	Isolated soy protein

Monosodium glutamate
(MSG)
Protein hydrolysates
Seitan (wheat gluten)
Skim milk powder
Soybean curd (tofu)
Soy flour

Soy milk
Soy protein concentrate
Textured vegetable protein
(TVP)
Tofu
Wheat gluten
Whey

YOUR DAILY PROTEIN FACTOR

Helps To Determine How Much Protein You Need Each Day

Age or Condition	Grams Protein per Kilogram of Target Weight
Teens	
Males	.9
Females	.8
Adults	.8
Mature adults	1.0
Recreational athlete	.8 to 1.0
Endurance athlete	1.2 to 1.8
Strength exercise	1.7 to 1.8
Strenuous exercise*	1.8 to 2.0
Mature athletes	1.0 to 1.5
Infections, fractures, fever, surgery	1.0 to 1.4
Severe trauma	1.5 to 2.5
Pregnancy	1.3 to 1.5
Breastfeeding	
1st six months	.8 + 15 grams
2nd six months	.8 + 12 grams

* Daily exercise program of one hour or more

Adapted from : Recommended Dietary Allowances, 10th edition, 1989, National Academy of Sciences, National Academy Press, Washington, DC; P.W.R. Lemon, Is Increased Dietary Protein Necessary or Benefical for Individuals with a Physically Active Lifestyle, *Nutrition Reviews*, 54(4, Part II):S169, 1996; G.A. Edwald, MD and C.R. McKenzie, MD, Eds., Manual of Medical Therapeutics, 28th Ed., Boston: Little Brown & Co., Pg. 31, 1995.

Figuring Your Daily Protein Requirement

1. Determine your daily protein factor.

Check the chart Your Daily Protein Factor, page xxiv to determine the category that is right for you.

Example: If you are a recreational athlete, your protein factor is 0.8 to 1.0 gram of protein.

YOUR DAILY PROTEIN FACTOR IS _____

2. Find your best, or target, weight.

Your protein requirement is based on your weight. Here is a simple way to determine your target weight.

Women

Give yourself 100 pounds for the first 5 feet of your height and add 5 pounds for each additional inch over 5 feet (or subtract 5 pounds for each inch under 5 feet).

Example: If you're 5 feet 6 inches tall:

100 pounds (for the first 5 feet)
+30 pounds (6 additional inches × 5 pounds each)

130 pounds Target weight

Men

Give yourself 106 pounds for the first 5 feet of your height and add 6 pounds for each additional inch over 5 feet.

Example: If you're 5 feet 9 inches tall:

106 pounds (for the first 5 feet)
+54 pounds (9 additional inches × 6 pounds each)

160 pounds Target weight

Add 10% for large body frame; subtract 10% for a small body frame. Not sure of your frame size—a large shoe size is a good predictor of a large frame.

_____ pounds (for the first 5 feet)
+ _____ pounds (_____ additional inches
× _____ pounds each)
_____ pounds Target weight

YOUR TARGET WEIGHT: _____

3. Convert your weight in pounds to kilograms.

To determine your weight in kilograms, divide your weight in pounds by 2.2.

_____ your weight (or target weight) ÷ 2.2 = _____
kilograms

The chart Converting Weight in Pounds to Kilograms (page xxvii) can be used to complete this step.

YOUR WEIGHT IN KILOGRAMS: _____

4. Setting your daily requirement for protein.

Multiply your protein factor (from Step 1) × your weight in kilograms (from Step 3).

Example: If you are a recreational athlete weighing 75 kilograms, your daily protein factor would be 0.8 to 1.0.

0.8 (protein factor) X 75 kilograms = 60 grams of protein/day

1.0 (protein factor) X 75 kilograms = 75 grams of protein/day

A recreational athlete weighing 75 kilograms should be eating a minimum of 60 to 75 grams of protein each day.

_____ your protein factor × _____ kilograms of weight
= _____ grams protein/day

YOUR DAILY PROTEIN REQUIREMENT IS _____ GRAMS

CONVERTING WEIGHT IN POUNDS TO KILOGRAMS

Weight in Pounds	Weight in Kilograms
85	39
90	41
95	42
100	45
105	48
110	50
115	52
120	54
125	57
130	59
135	61
140	64
145	66
150	68
155	70
160	73
165	75
170	77
175	79
180	82
185	84
190	86
195	88
200	91
210	93

Now that you know how many grams of protein your need each day, use *The Protein Counter* to select the best choices to meet your needs. If your situation changes, you become pregnant or you change your exercise program to a more vigorous schedule, simply use Steps 1 to 4 above to recalculate your daily protein requirement.

For example, if you are moderately active and weigh 150 pounds:

$$150 \times 15 \text{ calories a pound} = 2{,}250 \text{ calories per day}$$

Using the generally accepted daily recommendations of 15% protein calories, 55% carbohydrate calories and 30% fat calories, each day you should be eating

338 protein calories (2,250 calories × 15%)
1,238 carbohydrate calories (2,250 calories × 55%)
675 fat calories (2,250 × 30%)

Whether you want to track your protein intake for the day or you'd like to set up a complete eating plan that includes protein, fat and carbohydrate, *The Protein Counter* is the best guide you can use.

Caution: If you are thinking about increasing your daily protein by going to a high-protein diet, be sure to check with your doctor. Many medical experts feel very high protein diets are not for everyone. People with heart conditions or who are on medication for heart disease, high blood pressure or diabetes need medical supervision on a very high protein diet.

Want to Know More?

Americans get an average of 15 to 17% of their calories each day from protein. That leaves 83 to 85% calories remaining from fat and carbohydrate. The recommended intake of fat is 30%

or less of total calories, leaving 55 to 58% of daily calories as carbohydrate.

Your daily intake of protein, carbohydrate and fat calories should be

Protein	15%
Carbohydrate	55%
Fat	30%

You can individualize this, if you like, to decrease fat below 30% and increase protein or carbohydrate to meet your own needs. (See Caution on page xxviii if you are considering a very high protein diet.)

You may be wondering how to determine how many calories you need each day. Once you have figured your target weight, you can use this weight to get a good estimate of the amount of calories your need each day.

- If you are sedentary (do very little activity), you'll need 12 calories per pound of your target weight.
- If you are moderately active (get at least a half hour of activity a day), you'll need 15 calories per pound of your target weight.
- If you are very active (do daily vigorous exercise), you'll need 18 or more calories per pound of your target weight.

Eat well   Stay active   Be well!

Using Your Protein Counter

This book lists the protein values for over 15,000 foods. Now you can compare the protein in your favorite foods and choose substitutes for them before you go out to grocery shop or to eat. This will help you save time while making protein choices when you are deciding what to buy or eat.

The Protein Counter has foods listed alphabetically. For each category, you will find nonbranded (generic) foods are listed first in alphabetical order, followed by an alphabetical listing of brand name foods. The nonbranded listing will help you determine protein values for foods when you do not find your favorite brand listed. They also help you to evaluate generic and store brands. Large categories are divided into subcategories such as canned, fresh, frozen and ready-to-use to make it easier to find what you are looking for. Many categories have take-out and home recipe subcategories. Look there for foods you take out or order in a store or restaurant because these foods are not nutrition labeled.

Most foods are listed alphabetically. But in some cases, foods are grouped by category. For example, a tuna salad sandwich and tuna salad are found under the category TUNA DISHES. Other group categories include

DELI MEATS/COLD CUTS page 130
   Includes all sandwich meats except chicken,
   ham and turkey
DINNER page 136
   Includes all frozen dinners by brand name
ICE CREAM AND FROZEN DESSERTS page 208
   Includes all dairy and nondairy ice cream and
   frozen novelties
LIQUOR/LIQUEUR page 248
   Includes all alcoholic beverages except wine or beer
NUTRITIONAL SUPPLEMENTS page 278
   Includes all meal replacers, diet bars and diet drinks
ORIENTAL FOOD page 292
   Includes all Oriental-type foods
SPANISH FOOD page 461
   Includes all Spanish-type and Mexican foods

DEFINITIONS

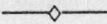

as prep (as prepared): refers to food that has been prepared according to package directions

home recipe: describes homemade dishes; those included can be used as a guide to the protein values of similar products you may prepare or takeout food you buy ready to eat

lean and fat: describes meat with some fat on its edges that is not cut away before cooking or poultry prepared with skin and fat as purchased

lean only: lean portion, trimmed of all visible fat

shelf stable: refers to prepared products found on the supermarket shelf that are ready to be heated and do not require refrigeration

take-out: describes prepared dishes that you purchase ready-to-eat; those included serve as a guide to the protein values of similar products you may purchase

trace (tr): value used when a food contains less than 1 gram of protein, carbohydrate or fat

ABBREVIATIONS

—◇—

avg	=	average
diam	=	diameter
fl	=	fluid
frzn	=	frozen
g	=	gram
in	=	inch
lb	=	pound
lg	=	large
med	=	medium
mg	=	milligram
oz	=	ounce
pkg	=	package
prep	=	prepared
pt	=	pint
qt	=	quart
reg	=	regular
serv	=	serving
sm	=	small
sq	=	square
tbsp	=	tablespoon
tr	=	trace
tsp	=	teaspoo
w/	=	with
w/o	=	without
<	=	less than

EQUIVALENT MEASURES

——◇——

1 tablespoon	=	3 teaspoons
4 tablespoons	=	¼ cup
8 tablespoons	=	½ cup
12 tablespoons	=	¾ cup
16 tablespoons	=	1 cup
1000 milligrams	=	1 gram
28 grams	=	1 ounce

Liquid Measurements

2 tablespoons	=	1 ounce
¼ cup	=	2 ounces
½ cup	=	4 ounces
¾ cup	=	6 ounces
1 cup	=	8 ounces
2 cups	=	1 pint
4 cups	=	1 quart

Dry Measurements

4 ounces	=	¼ pound
8 ounces	=	½ pound
12 ounces	=	¾ pound
16 ounces	=	1 pound

NOTES

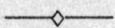

Protein, carbohydrate and fat values are given in grams (g).

A dash (—) indicates data not available.

Discrepancies in figures are due to rounding, product reformulation and reevaluation. Labeling law allows rounding of values. Most of the data are analysis data obtained directly from manufacturers, not from labels. In some cases, our values may not be exactly the same as label information because they have not been rounded.

THE
PROTEIN
COUNTER

FOOD	PORTION	CALS.	CARB.	FAT	PRO.
ABALONE					
fresh fried	3 oz	161	9	6	17
ACEROLA JUICE					
juice	1 cup	51	12	1	1
ADZUKI BEANS					
CANNED					
Eden					
Organic	½ cup (4.1 oz)	100	18	0	7
ALE					
(*see* BEER AND ALE, AND MALT)					
ALFALFA					
sprouts	1 tbsp	1	tr	tr	tr
ALLIGATOR					
tail cooked	3½ oz	143	1	3	29
ALMONDS					
almond butter honey & cinnamon	1 tbsp	96	4	8	3
almond butter w/ salt	1 tbsp	101	3	9	2
almond butter w/o salt	1 tbsp	101	3	10	2
almond meal	1 oz	116	8	5	11
dried blanched	1 oz	166	5	15	6
dried unblanched	1 oz	167	6	15	6
dry roasted unblanched	1 oz	167	7	15	5
dry roasted unblanched salted	1 oz	167	7	15	5
oil roasted blanched	1 oz	174	5	16	16
oil roasted blanched salted	1 oz	174	5	16	5
oil roasted unblanched	1 oz	176	5	16	6
toasted unblanched	1 oz	167	7	14	6
Beer Nuts					
Almonds	1 pkg (1 oz)	180	7	14	5
Dole					
Blanched Slivered	1 oz	170	5	14	6
Blanched Whole	1 oz	170	5	14	6
Chopped Natural	1 oz	170	5	14	6
Sliced Natural	1 oz	170	5	14	6
Whole Natural	1 oz	170	5	14	6
Erewhon					
Almond Butter	1 tbsp (16 g)	90	2	8	3
Hain					
Almond Butter Natural Raw	2 tbsp	190	3	18	8

FOOD	PORTION	CALS.	CARB.	FAT	PRO.
Hain (CONT.)					
Almond Butter Toasted	2 tbsp	220	3	19	8
Lance					
Smoked	1 pkg (0.7 oz)	120	3	11	6
Nutella					
Spread	1 tbsp (0.5 oz)	85	9	5	1
Planters					
Almonds	1 oz	170	5	15	6
Gold Measure Slivered	1 pkg (2 oz)	340	11	31	12
Honey Roasted	1 oz	160	7	14	5

AMARANTH
(*see also* CEREAL, COOKIES)

FOOD	PORTION	CALS.	CARB.	FAT	PRO.
cooked	½ cup	59	3	tr	1
Arrowhead					
Seeds	¼ cup (1.6 oz)	170	29	2	7
Health Valley					
Amaranth Cereal With Bananas	½ cup (1 oz)	110	20	2	4
Amaranth Crunch With Raisins	¼ cup (1 oz)	110	20	3	3
Amaranth Flakes 100% Organic	½ cup (1 oz)	90	21	tr	3
Fast Menu Amaranth With Garden Vegetables	7½ oz	140	16	3	8

ANASAZI BEANS
DRIED

FOOD	PORTION	CALS.	CARB.	FAT	PRO.
Bean Cuisine					
Dried	½ cup	115	—	1	8

ANCHOVY
CANNED

FOOD	PORTION	CALS.	CARB.	FAT	PRO.
in oil	5	42	0	2	6
in oil	1 can (1.6 oz)	95	0	4	13
FRESH					
fillets	3 (0.4 oz)	21	tr	1	2
raw	3 oz	62	0	4	17

ANTELOPE

FOOD	PORTION	CALS.	CARB.	FAT	PRO.
roasted	3 oz	127	0	2	25

APPLE
CANNED

FOOD	PORTION	CALS.	CARB.	FAT	PRO.
sliced sweetened	1 cup	136	34	1	tr

FOOD	PORTION	CALS.	CARB.	FAT	PRO.
DRIED					
cooked w/ sugar	½ cup	116	29	tr	tr
cooked w/o sugar	½ cup	172	20	tr	tr
rings	10	155	42	tr	1
FRESH					
apple	1	81	21	tr	tr
w/o skin sliced	1 cup	62	16	tr	tr
w/o skin sliced & cooked	1 cup	91	23	tr	tr
w/o skin sliced & microwaved	1 cup	96	25	tr	tr
FROZEN					
Mrs. Paul's					
Apple Fritters	2	270	35	9	4
Stouffer's					
Escalloped	1 cup (6 oz)	180	37	3	tr
APPLE JUICE					
frzn as prep	1 cup	111	28	tr	tr
frzn not prep	6 oz	349	87	1	1
juice	1 cup	116	29	tr	tr
After The Fall					
Organic	1 bottle (10 oz)	110	28	0	0
Vermont Harvest Moon Sparkling Apple Cider	8 fl oz	110	27	0	1
Apple & Eve					
Cider	6 fl oz	80	16	0	0
Minute Maid					
Box	8.45 fl oz	120	29	0	0
S&W					
100% Unsweetened	6 oz	85	20	0	0
Tree Top					
Unfiltered	6 oz	90	22	0	0
APPLESAUCE					
sweetened	½ cup	97	25	tr	tr
unsweetened	½ cup	53	14	tr	tr
Mott's					
Chunky	5 oz	110	26	0	0
Cinnamon	5 oz	120	29	0	0
Fruit Snacks Sweetened	4 oz	90	22	0	0
White House					
Natural Packed w/ Apple Juice	4 oz	60	14	0	0
APRICOT JUICE					
nectar	1 cup	141	36	tr	1

FOOD	PORTION	CALS.	CARB.	FAT	PRO.
APRICOTS					
CANNED					
halves heavy syrup pack w/ skin	1 cup (9.1 oz)	214	55	tr	1
halves water pack w/ skin	1 cup (8.5 oz)	65	16	tr	2
halves water pack w/o skin	1 cup (8 oz)	51	12	tr	2
heavy syrup w/ skin	3 halves	70	18	tr	tr
juice pack w/ skin	3 halves	40	10	tr	1
light syrup w/ skin	3 halves	54	14	tr	tr
puree juice pack w/ skin	1 cup (8.7 oz)	119	31	tr	2
puree from heavy syrup pack w/ skin	¾ cup (9.1 oz)	214	55	tr	1
puree from light pack w/ skin	¾ cup (8.9 oz)	160	42	tr	1
puree from water pack w/ skin	¾ cup (8.5 oz)	65	16	tr	2
water pack w/ skin	3 halves	22	5	tr	1
water pack w/o skin	4 halves	20	5	tr	1
DRIED					
halves	10	83	22	tr	1
halves cooked w/o sugar	½ cup	106	27	tr	2
FRESH					
apricots	3	51	12	tr	1
FROZEN					
sweetened	½ cup	119	30	tr	1
ARROWROOT					
flour	1 cup	457	113	tr	tr
ARTICHOKE					
CANNED					
S&W					
Hearts Marinated	½ cup	225	6	26	2
FRESH					
boiled	1 med (4 oz)	60	13	tr	4
hearts cooked	½ cup	42	9	tr	3
sunchoke raw sliced	½ cup	57	13	tr	2
FROZEN					
cooked	1 pkg (9 oz)	108	22	1	7
Birds Eye					
Hearts Deluxe	½ cup	30	7	0	2
ARUGULA					
raw	½ cup	2	tr	tr	tr

FOOD	PORTION	CALS.	CARB.	FAT	PRO.
ASPARAGUS					
CANNED					
spears	½ cup	24	3	1	3
FRESH					
cooked	4 spears	14	3	tr	2
cooked	½ cup	22	4	tr	2
raw	4 spears	14	3	tr	1
FROZEN					
cooked	4 spears	17	3	tr	2
AVOCADO					
FRESH					
avocado	1	324	15	31	4
puree	1 cup	370	17	35	5
BACON					
(see also BACON SUBSTITUTES*)*					
breakfast strips beef cooked	3 strips (34 g)	153	tr	12	11
cooked	3 strips	109	tr	9	6
grilled	2 slices (1.7 oz)	86	1	4	11
Hormel					
Bacon Bits	1 tsp (7 g)	30	0	2	3
Microwave cooked	2 slices (0.5 oz)	70	0	5	5
Oscar Mayer					
Thick Cut cooked	1 slice (0.4 oz)	50	0	4	4
BACON SUBSTITUTES					
bacon substitute	1 strip	25	1	2	1
Bac-Os					
Pieces	2 tsp (5 g)	25	2	1	2
Harvest Direct					
Bacon Bits	3.5 oz	320	24	15	40
Lightlife					
Fakin' Bacon	3 strips (2 oz)	79	6	3	9
Louis Rich					
Turkey Bacon	1 slice (0.5 oz)	30	0	3	2
McCormick					
Bac'n Pieces	2 tsp	20	1	tr	2
Morningstar Farms					
Breakfast Strips	3 (25 g)	80	4	6	3
Mr. Turkey					
Slice	1	25	0	2	3

FOOD	PORTION	CALS.	CARB.	FAT	PRO.
Worthington					
Stripples	4 strips (33 g)	120	6	9	4

BAGEL
(*see also* CRACKER)

FRESH

FOOD	PORTION	CALS.	CARB.	FAT	PRO.
cinnamon raisin	1 (3½ in)	194	39	1	7
cinnamon raisin toasted	1 (3½ in)	194	39	1	7
egg	1 (3½ in)	197	38	2	8
egg toasted	1 (3½ in)	197	38	2	8
oat bran	1 (3½ in)	181	38	1	8
oat bran toasted	1 (3½ in)	181	38	1	8
onion	1 (3½ in)	195	38	1	8
plain	1 (3½ in)	195	38	1	8
plain toasted	1 (3½ in)	195	38	1	8
poppy seed	1 (3½ in)	195	38	1	8
Alvarado St. Bakery					
Sprouted Wheat	1 (3.3 oz)	260	54	1	9
FROZEN					
Great Starts					
Ham & Cheese On A Bagel	3 oz	240	28	8	12
Lender's					
Cinnamon'N Raisin	1 (2.5 oz)	200	40	1	8
Sara Lee					
Egg	1 (3 oz)	250	48	2	9
Tree Of Life					
Sesame	1 (3 oz)	210	44	0	8
Weight Watchers					
Bagel Sandwich Ham And Cheese	1 (3 oz)	210	28	6	13

BAKING POWDER

FOOD	PORTION	CALS.	CARB.	FAT	PRO.
baking powder	1 tsp	2	1	0	0
low sodium	1 tsp	5	2	0	0

BAKING SODA

FOOD	PORTION	CALS.	CARB.	FAT	PRO.
baking soda	1 tsp	0	0	0	0

BAMBOO SHOOTS

CANNED

FOOD	PORTION	CALS.	CARB.	FAT	PRO.
sliced	1 cup	25	4	1	2
FRESH					
cooked	½ cup	15	2	tr	2
raw	½ cup	21	1	tr	2

FOOD	PORTION	CALS.	CARB.	FAT	PRO.
BANANA					
banana chips	1 oz	147	17	10	1
DRIED					
powder	1 tbsp	21	5	tr	tr
FRESH					
banana	1	105	27	tr	1
mashed	1 cup	207	53	1	2
BANANA JUICE					
Libby					
Nectar	1 can (11.5 fl oz)	190	47	0	0
BARBECUE SAUCE					
(*see also* SAUCE)					
barbecue	1 cup	188	32	5	5
BARLEY					
pearled cooked	½ cup	97	30	tr	2
pearled uncooked	½ cup	352	78	1	10
BASIL					
fresh chopped	2 tbsp	1	tr	tr	tr
leaves fresh	5	1	tr	tr	tr
BASS					
sea cooked	3 oz	105	0	2	20
striped baked	3 oz	105	0	3	19
BEAN SPROUTS					
(*see also* INDIVIDUAL BEAN NAMES)					
CANNED					
La Choy					
	⅔ cup	8	1	tr	1
BEANS					
(*see also* INDIVIDUAL NAMES)					
CANNED					
baked beans plain	½ cup	118	26	1	6
baked beans vegetarian	½ cup	118	26	1	6
baked beans w/ beef	½ cup	161	22	5	8
baked beans w/ franks	½ cup	182	20	8	9
baked beans w/ pork	½ cup	133	25	2	7
baked beans w/ pork & sweet sauce	½ cup	140	26	2	7
baked beans w/ pork & tomato sauce	½ cup	123	24	1	7
refried beans	½ cup	134	23	1	8
Green Giant					
Three Bean Salad	½ cup	70	18	tr	2

FOOD	PORTION	CALS.	CARB.	FAT	PRO.
Health Valley					
Fast Menu Honey Baked Organic Beans With Tofu Weiner	7½ oz	150	15	4	11
Vegetarian With Miso	7½ oz	180	38	1	8
Old El Paso					
Refried Fat Free	½ cup	90	17	0	6
Rosarita					
Refried With Green Chilies	4 oz	90	18	2	7
TAKE-OUT					
baked beans	½ cup	190	27	6	7
barbecue beans	3.5 oz	120	26	tr	4
refried beans	½ cup	43	5	2	2
three bean salad	¾ cup	230	31	11	5

BEAR

simmered	3 oz	220	0	11	28

BEAVER

roasted	3 oz	140	0	6	30
simmered	3 oz	141	0	5	23

BEECHNUTS

dried	1 oz	164	10	14	2

BEEF

(*see also* BEEF DISHES, VEAL)

(Beef is graded according to its marbling, the little flecks of fat in the muscle. Beef graded "Prime" has the highest percentage of fat, followed by "Choice" with less fat and "Select" with the least fat.)

FOOD	PORTION	CALS.	CARB.	FAT	PRO.
CANNED					
corned beef	3 oz	85	0	5	10
Armour					
Potted Meat	1 can (3 oz)	120	0	8	11
Roast Beef In Gravy	½ cup (4.6 oz)	150	3	4	25
Tripe	3 oz	90	0	2	18
Treet					
50% Less Fat	2 oz	120	4	8	6
Underwood					
Roast Beef Light	2.08 oz	90	2	6	9
DRIED					
Hormel					
Pillow Pack	10 slices (1 oz)	45	1	1	8

FOOD	PORTION	CALS.	CARB.	FAT	PRO.

FRESH

(Note that the values for cooked beef may differ slightly from values for raw beef. When meat is cooked some moisture and fat is lost, changing the nutrition value slightly. As a rule of thumb it can be assumed that a 4 oz raw portion will equal a 3 oz cooked portion of meat.)

FOOD	PORTION	CALS.	CARB.	FAT	PRO.
bottom round lean & fat trim 0 in Select braised	3 oz	171	0	6	27
bottom round lean & fat trim 0 in braised	3 oz	193	0	26	26
brisket flat half lean & fat trim 0 in braised	3 oz	183	0	8	26
brisket flat half lean & fat trim ¼ in braised	3 oz	309	0	24	21
chuck arm pot roast lean & fat trim 0 in braised	3 oz	238	0	14	25
chuck arm pot roast lean & fat trim ¼ in braised	3 oz	282	0	20	23
corned beef brisket cooked	3 oz	213	tr	16	15
eye of round lean & fat trim 0 in Choice roasted	3 oz	153	0	5	24
flank lean & fat trim 0 in broiled	3 oz	192	0	11	22
ground extra lean broiled medium	3 oz	217	0	14	22
ground extra lean broiled well done	3 oz	225	0	14	24
ground extra lean fried medium	3 oz	216	0	14	21
ground extra lean fried well done	3 oz	224	0	14	24
ground lean broiled medium	3 oz	231	0	16	21
ground lean broiled well done	3 oz	238	0	15	24
ground regular broiled medium	3 oz	246	0	18	20
ground regular broiled well done	3 oz	248	0	17	23
ground low-fat w/ carrageenan raw	4 oz	160	tr	7	20
porterhouse steak lean & fat trim ¼ in Choice broiled	3 oz	260	0	19	21

FOOD	PORTION	CALS.	CARB.	FAT	PRO.
rib eye small end lean & fat trim 0 in Choice broiled	3 oz	261	0	19	21
rib whole lean & fat trim ¼ in Choice roasted	3 oz	320	0	27	19
shank crosscut lean & fat trim ¼ in Choice simmered	3 oz	224	0	12	26
shortribs lean & fat Choice braised	3 oz	400	0	36	18
t-bone steak lean & fat trim ¼ in Choice broiled	3 oz	253	0	18	21
tenderloin lean & fat trim ¼ in Choice broiled	3 oz	259	0	19	21
tenderloin lean & fat trim ¼ in Choice roasted	3 oz	288	0	22	20
tenderloin lean & fat trim ¼ in Choice broiled	3 oz	208	0	12	23
top round lean & fat trim 0 in Choice braised	3 oz	184	0	6	30
top round lean & fat trim ¼ in Choice braised	3 oz	221	0	11	29
top sirloin lean & fat trim 0 in Select broiled	3 oz	166	0	6	25
top sirloin lean & fat trim ¼ in Choice broiled	3 oz	228	0	14	23
tripe raw	4 oz	111	0	4	16
FROZEN					
patties broiled medium	3 oz	240	0	17	21
READY-TO-USE					
Healthy Choice					
Deli-Thin Roast Beef	6 slices (2 oz)	60	1	2	11
Oscar Mayer					
Deli-Thin Roast Beef	4 slices (1.8 oz)	60	1	2	11
Weight Watchers					
Deli Thin Oven Roasted Cured	5 slices (⅓ oz)	10	tr	tr	2
TAKE-OUT					
roast beef medium	2 oz	70	0	2	12
roast beef rare	2 oz	70	0	2	12

BEEF DISHES
CANNED
corned beef hash	3 oz	155	9	10	10
Armour					
Roast Beef Hash	1 cup (8.4 oz)	400	23	25	20

BEEF DISHES · 11

FOOD	PORTION	CALS.	CARB.	FAT	PRO.
Armour (CONT.)					
Stew	1 cup (8.6 oz)	220	21	12	8
Dinty Moore					
American Classics Meatloaf With Mashed Potatoes	1 bowl (10 oz)	300	27	13	18
American Classics Salisbury Steak	1 bowl (10 oz)	310	22	14	23
Microwave Cup Beef Stew	1 cup (7.5 oz)	190	15	10	11
Microwave Cup Hearty Burger Stew	1 cup (7.5 oz)	240	19	13	12
Sliced Potatoes & Beef	1 can (7.5 oz)	230	28	9	10
Hormel					
Beef Goulash	1 can (7.5 oz)	230	19	11	13
Manwich					
Mexican as prep	1 sandwich	310	30	13	17
Sloppy Joe as prep	1 sandwich	310	31	13	17
Micro Cup Meals					
Beef Stew	1 cup (7.5 oz)	180	15	9	11
FROZEN					
Hot Pocket					
Stuffed Sandwich Barbecue	1 (4.5 oz)	340	45	12	13
Stuffed Sandwich Beef & Cheddar	1 (4.5 oz)	360	36	18	14
Stuffed Sandwich Beef Fajita	1 (4.5 oz)	360	39	17	14
Lean Pockets					
Stuffed Sandwich Beef & Broccoli	1 (4.5 oz)	250	37	7	9
Luigino's					
Creamed Sauce Shaved Cured Beef With Croutons	1 pkg (8 oz)	360	29	20	15
Egg Noodles Rich Gravy Swedish Meatballs	1 pkg (9 oz)	340	36	15	16
Ovenstuffs					
Beef/Cheddar Deli Melt	1 (4.75 oz)	390	28	22	18
Tyson					
Microwave BBQ Sandwich	1 sandwich	200	29	3	15
MIX					
Casbah					
Gyro as prep	1 patty (2 oz)	145	12	5	2

FOOD	PORTION	CALS.	CARB.	FAT	PRO.
Hamburger Helper					
Beef Noodle as prep	1 cup	330	29	15	20
Beef Romanoff as prep	1 cup	350	31	16	22
Beef Taco as prep	1 cup	330	33	14	19
Cheddar 'n Bacon as prep	1 cup	380	30	19	23
Cheeseburger Macaroni as prep	1 cup	370	28	19	21
Cheesy Italian as prep	1 cup	370	29	18	23
Chili Macaroni as prep	1 cup	330	32	14	19
Hamburger Hash as prep	1 cup	320	27	15	18
Hamburger Stew as prep	1 cup	300	26	14	18
Lasagne as prep	1 cup	340	33	14	20
Meat Loaf as prep	5 oz	360	14	22	27
Nacho Cheese as prep	1 cup	360	35	15	21
Pizza Dish as prep	1 cup	360	27	14	21
Pizzabake as prep	⅙ pkg (4.5 oz)	320	29	14	19
Potatoes Stroganoff as prep	1 cup	330	26	16	3
Potatoes Au Gratin as prep	1 cup	350	27	18	4
Rice Oriental as prep	1 cup	340	38	14	19
Sloppy Joe Bake as prep	5 oz	340	33	15	5
Spaghetti as prep	1 cup	340	32	14	21
Stroganoff as prep	1 cup	390	30	20	22
Tacobake as prep	⅙ pkg (5.75 oz)	320	31	15	17
Zesty Italian as prep	1 cup	340	35	13	21
Lipton					
Microeasy Hearty Beef Stew	¼ pkg	71	14	1	2
Microeasy Homestyle Meatloaf	¼ pkg	87	15	2	4
Manwich					
Seasoning Mix as prep	1 sandwich	320	31	13	17
SHELF-STABLE					
Lunch Bucket					
Beef Stew	1 pkg (7.5 oz)	180	13	11	8
TAKE-OUT					
bubble & squeak	5 oz	186	16	13	2
cornish pasty	1 (8 oz)	847	79	52	20
irish stew	1 cup (7 oz)	280	10	16	23
kebab indian	1 (5.4 oz)	553	2	40	47
kheena	6.7 oz	781	1	71	34
koftas	5	280	3	22	18

FOOD	PORTION	CALS.	CARB.	FAT	PRO.
roast beef sandwich plain	1	346	33	14	22
roast beef sandwich w/ cheese	1	402	27	18	32
roast beef submarine sandwich w/ tomato lettuce & mayonnaise	1	411	44	13	29
samosa	2 (4 oz)	652	20	62	6
shepherds pie	6 oz	196	15	10	13
steak & kidney pie w/ top crust	1 slice (5 oz)	400	23	26	21
steak sandwich w/ tomato lettuce salt & mayonnaise	1	459	52	14	30
stew	6 oz	208	6	13	17
stew w/ vegetables	1 cup	220	15	11	16
stroganoff	¾ cup	260	43	19	14
swiss steak	4.6 oz	214	10	9	23
toad in the hole	1 (4.7 oz)	383	23	29	10

BEEFALO
roasted	3 oz	160	0	5	26

BEER AND ALE
ale brown	10 oz	77	8	0	1
ale pale	10 oz	88	12	0	1
beer light	12 oz can	100	5	0	tr
beer regular	12 oz can	146	13	0	1
lager	10 oz	80	4	0	1
pilsener lager beer	7 fl oz	85	13	tr	1
stout	10 oz	102	6	0	1
Hamm's					
Nonalcoholic	12 oz	55	12	0	1
Pabst					
Nonalcoholic	12 oz	55	12	0	1
Spirit					
Nonalcoholic	12 oz	80	16	0	1

BEET JUICE
juice	3½ oz	36	8	0	1

BEETS
CANNED
harvard	½ cup	89	22	tr	1
pickled	½ cup	75	19	tr	1
sliced	½ cup	27	6	tr	1

FOOD	PORTION	CALS.	CARB.	FAT	PRO.
S&W					
Julienne French Style	½ cup	40	9	0	1
Seneca					
Diced	½ cup	35	9	0	0
Harvard	½ cup	90	21	0	1
Pickled With Onions	2 tbsp	20	6	0	0
FRESH					
greens cooked	½ cup	20	4	tr	2
sliced cooked	½ cup (3 oz)	38	9	tr	1
whole cooked	2 (3.5 oz)	44	10	tr	2

BEVERAGES

(*see* BEER AND ALE, CHAMPAGNE, COFFEE, DRINK MIXERS, FRUIT DRINKS, ICED TEA, MALT, MINERAL WATER/BOTTLED WATER, LIQUOR/LIQUEUR, SODA, TEA/HERBAL TEA, WINE, WINE COOLER)

BISCUIT

FOOD	PORTION	CALS.	CARB.	FAT	PRO.
FROZEN					
Great Starts					
Egg Canadian Bacon & Cheese	5.2 oz	420	37	22	16
Sausage	4.7 oz	410	36	22	14
Jimmy Dean					
Chicken Twin	2 (3.2 oz)	280	32	13	9
Sausage Twin	2 (3.4 oz)	330	25	21	10
Steak Twin	2 (3.2 oz)	270	26	13	10
Rudy's Farm					
Ham Twin	2 (3 oz)	160	23	3	10
Sausage & Cheese Twin	2 (3 oz)	290	22	18	9
Sausage Twin	2 (2.7 oz)	296	22	18	9
Weight Watchers					
Sausage Biscuit	3 oz	220	19	11	11
HOME RECIPE					
buttermilk	1 (2 oz)	212	27	10	4
oatcakes	2 (4 oz)	115	16	5	3
plain	1 (2 oz)	212	27	10	4
MIX					
buttermilk	1 (2 oz)	191	28	7	4
plain	1 (2 oz)	191	28	7	4
Arrowhead					
Biscuit Mix	¼ cup (1.2 oz)	120	23	1	5
Bisquick					
Mix	½ cup (2 oz)	240	37	8	4
Reduced Fat	½ cup (2 oz)	210	39	4	5

FOOD	PORTION	CALS.	CARB.	FAT	PRO.
Jiffy					
As prep	1	150	30	7	2
Buttermilk as prep	1	170	29	4	3
REFRIGERATED					
buttermilk	1 (1 oz)	98	14	4	2
plain	1 (1 oz)	98	14	4	2
1869 Brand					
Baking Powder	1	100	12	5	2
Buttermilk	1	100	12	5	2
Butter Tastin'	1	100	12	5	2
Ballard					
Ovenready	1	50	10	1	0
Ovenready Buttermilk	1	50	10	1	1
Big Country					
Southern Style	1	100	14	4	2
Hungry Jack					
Butter Tastin' Flaky	1	90	11	4	2
Buttermilk Flaky	1	90	12	4	2
Buttermilk Fluffy	1	90	12	4	2
Extra Rich Buttermilk	1	50	9	1	1
Flaky	1	80	12	4	2
Honey Tastin' Flaky	1	90	13	4	2
Pillsbury					
Big Country Butter Tastin'	1	100	14	4	2
Big Country Buttermilk	1	100	14	4	2
Butter	1	50	10	1	1
Buttermilk	1	50	10	1	1
Country	1	50	10	1	1
Deluxe Heat N' Eat Buttermilk	2	170	27	5	4
Good'N Buttery Fluffy	1	90	11	5	1
Hearty Grains Multi-Grain	1	80	15	2	2
Hearty Grains Oatmeal Raisin	1	90	16	2	2
Heat N' Eat Big Premium	2	280	32	15	5
Tender Layer Buttermilk	1	50	9	1	1
Roman Meal					
Biscuit	2 (2.4 oz)	180	34	4	4
Honey Nut Oat Bran	1 (1.5 oz)	131	21	5	2
TAKE-OUT					
buttermilk	1	127	17	6	2
plain	1 (35 g)	276	13	34	4

FOOD	PORTION	CALS.	CARB.	FAT	PRO.
w/ egg	1	315	24	20	11
w/ egg & bacon	1	457	29	31	17
w/ egg & sausage	1	582	41	39	19
w/ egg & steak	1	474	37	28	18
w/ egg cheese & bacon	1	477	33	31	16
w/ ham	1	387	44	18	13
w/ sausage	1	485	40	32	12
w/ steak	1	456	44	26	13

BISON
roasted	3 oz	122	0	2	24

BLACK BEANS
CANNED
Allen

Seasoned	½ cup (4.5 oz)	120	20	2	7

Eden

Organic	½ cup (4.3 oz)	100	17	0	7

Health Valley

Fast Menu Organic Black Beans With Tofu Weiners	7½ oz	150	20	1	14

Progresso

Black Beans	½ cup	90	19	1	9

Trappey

Seasoned	½ cup (4.5 oz)	120	20	2	7

DRIED

cooked	1 cup	227	41	1	15

MIX
Bean Cuisine

Black Turtle	½ cup	115	—	1	8
Pasta & Beans Black Beans With Fusilli	½ cup	174	27	4	6

Mahatma

Black Beans & Rice	1 cup	200	39	2	8

BLACKBERRIES
CANNED

in heavy syrup	½ cup	118	30	tr	2

FRESH

blackberries	½ cup	37	9	tr	1

FROZEN

unsweetened	1 cup	97	24	1	2

BLACKEYE PEAS
CANNED

w/pork	½ cup	199	40	4	7

FOOD	PORTION	CALS.	CARB.	FAT	PRO.
Allen					
Blackeye Peas	½ cup (4.5 oz)	110	18	1	7
Fresh Shell	½ cup (4.4 oz)	120	21	1	7
With Bacon	½ cup (4.5 oz)	105	20	2	7
With Snaps	½ cup (4.4 oz)	120	20	1	8
Dorman					
Fresh Shell	½ cup (4.4 oz)	120	21	1	7
East Texas Fair					
Blackeye Peas	½ cup (4.5 oz)	110	18	1	7
Fresh Shell	½ cup (4.4 oz)	120	21	1	7
With Snaps	½ cup (4.4 oz)	120	20	1	8
Homefolks					
Fresh Shell	½ cup (4.4 oz)	120	21	1	7
With Jalapeno	½ cup (4.4 oz)	120	20	1	7
With Snaps	½ cup (4.4 oz)	120	20	1	8
Sunshine					
With Bacon	½ cup (4.5 oz)	105	20	2	7
Trappey					
With Bacon	½ cup (4.5 oz)	120	19	2	7
With Bacon & Jalapeno	½ cup (4.4 oz)	110	19	2	6
DRIED					
cooked	1 cup	198	36	1	13
FROZEN					
Fresh Like	3.5 oz	138	24	1	10

BLINTZE
Empire					
Apple	2 (4.4 oz)	220	36	6	6
Blueberry	2 (4.4 oz)	190	36	4	4
Cheese	2 (4.4 oz)	200	29	6	11
Golden					
Cheese	1 (2.25 oz)	80	13	2	6
Cherry	1 (2.25 oz)	95	18	1	3
Potato	1 (2.25 oz)	90	15	4	3
TAKE-OUT					
cheese	2	186	18	6	13

BLUEBERRIES
CANNED					
in heavy sirup	1 cup	225	56	1	2
DRIED					
Sonoma					
Dried	¼ cup (1.3 oz)	140	33	0	1

FOOD	PORTION	CALS.	CARB.	FAT	PRO.
FRESH					
blueberries	1 cup	82	20	1	1
FROZEN					
unsweetened	1 cup	78	19	1	1
BLUEBERRY JUICE					
After The Fall					
Maine Coast	1 cup (8 oz)	90	25	0	0
BLUEFIN					
fillet baked	4.1 oz	186	0	6	30
BLUEFISH					
fresh baked	3 oz	135	0	5	22
BOAR					
wild roasted	3 oz	136	0	4	24
BOK CHOY					
Dole					
Shredded	½ cup	5	1	tr	1
BOYSENBERRIES					
in heavy sirup	1 cup	226	57	tr	3
unsweetened frzn	1 cup	66	16	tr	1
BOYSENBERRY JUICE					
Smucker's					
Juice	8 oz	120	30	0	0
Juice Sparkler	10 oz	130	31	tr	tr
BRAINS					
beef pan-fried	3 oz	167	0	13	11
beef simmered	3 oz	136	0	11	9
lamb braised	3 oz	124	0	9	11
lamb fried	3 oz	232	0	19	14
pork braised	3 oz	117	0	8	10
veal braised	3 oz	115	0	8	10
veal fried	3 oz	181	0	14	12
Armour					
Pork Brains In Milk Gravy	⅔ cup (5.5 oz)	150	10	5	16
BRAN					
corn	⅓ cup	56	21	tr	2
oat cooked	½ cup	44	13	tr	4
oat dry	½ cup	116	31	3	8
rice dry	⅓ cup	88	14	6	4
wheat dry	½ cup	65	19	1	5

FOOD	PORTION	CALS.	CARB.	FAT	PRO.
H-O					
Super Bran	⅓ cup	110	18	2	7
Health Valley					
Fast Menu Oat Bran Pilaf With Garden Vegetables	7½ oz	210	30	7	7
Kretschmer					
Toasted Wheat Bran	⅓ cup	57	15	2	6
Mother's					
Oat Bran	½ cup	150	24	3	8
Quaker					
Oat Bran	½ cup	150	24	3	8
Unprocessed	2 tbsp	8	4	tr	1
Stone-Buhr					
Oat	⅓ cup (1 oz)	90	20	2	4

BRAZIL NUTS

FOOD	PORTION	CALS.	CARB.	FAT	PRO.
dried unblanched	1 oz	186	4	19	4

BREAD

(*see also* BAGEL, BISCUIT, BREADSTICK, CROISSANT, ENGLISH MUFFIN, MUFFIN, ROLL, SCONE)

FOOD	PORTION	CALS.	CARB.	FAT	PRO.
CANNED					
B&M					
Brown Bread	½ in slice (⅛ oz)	92	21	0	2
Brown Bread Raisins	½ in slice (1.6 oz)	94	22	0	2
FROZEN					
Kineret					
Challah	⅛ loaf (2 oz)	150	25	4	5
HOME RECIPE					
banana	1 slice (2 oz)	195	33	6	3
cornbread as prep w/ 2% milk	1 piece (2.3 oz)	173	28	5	4
datenut	½ in slice	92	15	3	2
irish soda bread	1 slice (2 oz)	174	34	3	4
pumpkin	1 slice (1 oz)	94	15	4	1
white as prep w/ 2% milk	1 slice	81	14	2	2
whole wheat	1 slice	79	15	2	2
MIX					
Aunt Jemima					
Corn Bread Easy Mix	⅓ cup (1.3 oz)	150	26	4	2
Natural Ovens					
Cracked Wheat	2 slices (2.4 oz)	140	38	1	8
English Muffin Bread	2 slices (2.4 oz)	140	35	1	7
Executive Fitness Sunny Millet	2 slices (2.6 oz)	160	37	2	10

FOOD	PORTION	CALS.	CARB.	FAT	PRO.
Natural Ovens (CONT.)					
Garden Bread	1 oz	50	14	1	4
Glorious Cinnamon & Raisin Fat Free	2 slices (2.1 oz)	110	30	1	8
Honey 'N Flax	2 slices (2.5 oz)	140	30	1	6
Hunger Filler Bread	2 slices (2.1 oz)	110	28	2	6
Light Wheat	2 slices (2.2 oz)	84	30	1	7
Nutty Natural Wheat Bread	2 slices (2.5 oz)	140	32	2	7
Seven Grain Herb	2 slices (2.5 oz)	140	30	1	8
Soft Hearth Whole Wheat	2 slices (2 oz)	100	30	2	8
Soft Sandwich Very Low Fat	2 slices (2.3 oz)	110	26	1	6
Stay Slim	2 slices (2 oz)	100	20	2	10
READY-TO-EAT					
cracked wheat	1 slice	65	12	1	2
egg	1 slice (1.4 oz)	115	19	2	4
french	1 slice (1 oz)	78	15	1	3
gluten	1 slice	47	8	tr	2
italian	1 slice (1 oz)	81	15	1	3
navajo fry	1 (5 in diam)	296	48	9	6
oat bran	1 slice	71	12	1	3
oat bran reduced calorie	1 slice	46	10	1	2
oatmeal	1 slice	73	13	1	2
oatmeal reduced calorie	1 slice	48	10	1	2
pita	1 reg (2 oz)	165	33	1	5
pita	1 sm (1 oz)	78	16	tr	3
pita whole wheat	1 reg (2 oz)	170	35	2	6
pita whole wheat	1 sm (1 oz)	76	16	1	3
protein	1 slice	47	8	tr	2
pumpernickel	1 slice	80	15	1	3
raisin	1 slice	71	14	1	2
rice bran	1 slice	66	12	1	1
rye	1 slice	83	16	1	3
rye reduced calorie	1 slice	47	9	1	2
seven grain	1 slice	65	12	1	3
sourdough	1 slice (1 oz)	78	15	1	3
vienna	1 slice (1 oz)	78	15	1	3
wheat reduced calorie	1 slice	46	10	1	2
wheat berry	1 slice	65	12	1	3
wheat bran	1 slice	89	17	1	3
wheat germ	1 slice	74	14	1	3
white	1 slice	67	12	1	2

FOOD	PORTION	CALS.	CARB.	FAT	PRO.
white reduced calorie	1 slice	48	10	1	2
white toasted	1 slice	67	13	1	2
white cubed	1 cup	80	15	1	2
whole wheat	1 slice	70	13	1	3
Alvarado St. Bakery					
Barley	1 slice (1.2 oz)	70	15	1	3
California Style	1 slice (1.2 oz)	60	10	1	3
Multi-Grain	1 slice (1.2 oz)	60	11	1	3
Multi-Grain No-Salt	1 slice (1.2 oz)	60	11	1	3
Oat Berry	1 slice (1.2 oz)	70	13	1	3
Arnold					
12 Grain Natural	1 slice (0.8 oz)	60	10	0	2
Augusto Pan De Aqua	1 oz	80	14	1	3
Bran'nola Country Oat	1 slice (1.3 oz)	90	16	3	3
Bran'nola Dark Wheat	1 slice (1.3 oz)	90	15	3	4
Bran'nola Hearty Wheat	1 slice (1.3 oz)	100	15	3	3
Bran'nola Nutty Grains	1 slice (1.3 oz)	90	14	2	3
Bran'nola Original	1 slice (1.3 oz)	90	16	2	3
Cinnamon Chip	1 slice	80	13	2	2
Cinnamon Raisin	1 slice (0.9 oz)	70	13	1	2
Cranberry	1 slice (0.9 oz)	70	14	1	2
French Twin Loaves Franscisco	2 slices (2 oz)	150	27	2	5
French Stick Savoni	1 oz	80	15	tr	3
Italian Bakery Light	1 slice (0.7 oz)	40	7	tr	2
Oatmeal Bakery	1 slice	60	12	1	2
Oatmeal Bakery Light	1 slice	40	8	tr	2
Oatmeal Raisin	1 slice (0.9 oz)	60	12	tr	2
Pumpernickel	1 slice (1.1 oz)	70	15	1	3
Rye Bakery Soft Light	1 slice (1.1 oz)	40	7	tr	2
Rye Bakery Soft Seeded	1 slice (1.1 oz)	70	14	1	2
Rye Dill	1 slice (1.1 oz)	60	10	1	2
Rye Real Jewish Dijon	1 slice	70	15	tr	3
Rye Real Jewish Melba Thin	1 slice (0.7 oz)	40	9	tr	2
Rye Real Jewish With Caraway	1 slice	70	13	tr	3
Rye Real Jewish With Caraway	1 slice	80	16	tr	3
Wheat Brick Oven	1 slice (0.8 oz)	60	9	2	2
White Extra Fiber Brick Oven	1 slice (0.9 oz)	50	10	tr	2
White Premium Light	1 slice	40	7	tr	2
White Thin Sliced Brick Oven	1 slice	40	7	tr	1

FOOD	PORTION	CALS.	CARB.	FAT	PRO.
Arnold (CONT.)					
Whole Wheat 100% Light Brick Oven	1 slice (0.8 oz)	40	6	tr	2
Whole Wheat 100% Stoneground	1 slice (0.8 oz)	50	8	1	2
August Bros.					
Rye Onion	1 slice	80	14	1	3
Rye N' Pump	1 slice	90	18	1	3
Beefsteak					
Rye Soft	1 slice (1 oz)	70	13	1	3
White Robust	1 slice (1 oz)	70	13	1	3
Bread Du Jour					
French	3 in slice (1 oz)	130	26	1	6
Brownberry					
Bran'nola Country Oat	1 slice	90	18	2	4
Bran'nola Hearty Wheat	1 slice	88	17	2	4
Bran'nola Nutty Grains	1 slice	85	17	2	2
Bran'nola Original	1 slice	85	18	1	4
Health Nut	1 slice	71	12	3	2
Oatmeal Natural	1 slice	63	13	1	2
Oatmeal Soft	1 slice	48	10	1	2
Raisin Bran	1 slice	61	12	1	2
Raisin Cinnamon	1 slice	66	12	1	2
Raisin Walnut	1 slice	68	11	3	2
Wheat Apple Honey	1 slice	69	11	2	2
Wheat Soft	1 slice	74	12	2	2
Cedar's					
Mountain Bread Six Grain	1 piece (2.4 oz)	200	35	4	7
Damascus Bakeries					
Mountain Shepard Lahvash	⅓ loaf (2 oz)	135	28	0	5
Dicarlo's					
Foccaccia	⅛ bread (2 oz)	130	25	2	4
Freihofer's					
Country Potato	1 slice (1.3 oz)	100	19	1	3
Country White	1 slice (1.3 oz)	100	19	1	3
Home Pride					
Hearty Golden Honey Wheat	1 slice (1.3 oz)	90	18	2	5
Hearty Honey Oats & Cracked Wheat	1 slice (1.4 oz)	100	19	2	4
White	1 slice (0.9 oz)	70	13	1	2
White Light	3 slices (0.9 oz)	110	25	2	6

FOOD	PORTION	CALS.	CARB.	FAT	PRO.
Home Pride (CONT.)					
Whole Wheat Hearty 100% Stoneground	1 slice (1.4 oz)	90	18	2	5
Malsovit					
Bread	1 slice	66	12	1	3
Matthew's					
9 Grain & Nut	1 slice	80	9	3	3
Cinnamon	1 slice	70	13	1	3
Sodium Free	1 slice	70	12	2	3
Meditarranean Magic					
Focaccia	⅕ loaf (1.8 oz)	140	27	2	4
Monks' Bread					
Hi-Fibre	1 slice	50	13	1	3
Sunflower & Bran	1 slice	70	12	1	3
Parisian					
French Stick Extra Sour	2 oz	150	27	1	8
French Stick Sweet	2 oz	154	27	2	7
Pepperidge Farm					
Cracked Wheat	1 slice	70	13	1	2
Date Walnut	1 slice	90	14	3	2
French Fully Baked	2 oz	150	28	2	5
Honey Bran	1 slice	90	18	1	3
Italian Brown & Serve	1 oz	80	14	1	2
Rye Dijon	1 slice	50	9	1	2
Rye Party	4 slices	60	12	1	2
Sesame Wheat	2 slices	190	36	3	7
Sprouted Wheat	1 slice	70	11	2	3
Vienna Light	1 slice	45	10	0	2
Wheat Very Thin Sliced	1 slice	35	7	0	2
White Toasting	1 slice	90	17	1	3
White Very Thin Sliced	1 slice	40	8	0	1
Roman Meal					
Brown & Serve Mini Loaf	½ loaf (2 oz)	136	24	2	5
Hearty Wheat Light	1 slice (0.8 oz)	42	7	tr	2
Sandwich	1 slice (0.8 oz)	55	10	1	2
Sourdough Light	1 slice (0.8 oz)	41	7	tr	2
Sourdough Whole Grain Light	1 slice (0.8 oz)	40	7	tr	2
Sun Grain	1 slice (1 oz)	70	11	2	3
Twelve Grain	1 slice (1 oz)	70	11	2	3
Twelve Grain Light	1 slice (0.8 oz)	42	7	tr	2
Wheatberry Honey	1 slice (1 oz)	67	12	1	3
Wheatberry Light	1 slice (0.8 oz)	42	7	tr	2

FOOD	PORTION	CALS.	CARB.	FAT	PRO.
Sahara					
Pita White	½ pocket	78	16	1	3
Stroehmann					
White Whole Special Recipe Kids	1 slice	60	12	tr	2
Sunmaid					
Raisin	1 slice	70	13	tr	2
Tree Of Life					
100% Spelt	1 slice (1.8 oz)	130	22	3	4
Millet	1 slice (1.8 oz)	130	25	2	3
Rye Sour Dough	1 slice (1.8 oz)	110	24	0	3
Sprouted Seven Grain	1 slice (1.8 oz)	110	20	2	3
Weight Watchers					
Italian	1 slice (0.8 oz)	38	7	tr	2
Multi-Grain	1 slice (0.8 oz)	41	7	1	2
Oat	1 slice (0.8 oz)	42	7	1	2
Raisin	1 slice (0.9 oz)	55	11	tr	2
Rye	1 slice (0.8 oz)	38	7	tr	2
Wheat	1 slice (0.8 oz)	40	7	tr	2
White	1 slice (0.8 oz)	40	7	tr	2
Wonder					
Calcium Enriched	1 slice (1 oz)	70	12	1	3
Granola	1 slice (1.5 oz)	100	19	2	5
Kid	1 slice (0.9 oz)	70	13	1	2
Light Calcium Enriched	2 slices (1.6 oz)	80	18	1	5
Texas Toast	1 slice (1.4 oz)	100	19	1	3
Wheat Calcium Light	2 slices (1.6 oz)	80	18	1	5
White	1 slice (0.9 oz)	70	13	1	2
White Calcium	2 slices (1.6 oz)	100	20	1	4
White Calcium Light	2 slices (1.6 oz)	80	18	1	5
White Light	2 slices (1.6 oz)	80	18	1	5
REFRIGERATED					
Pillsbury					
Crusty French Loaf	1 in slice	60	11	tr	2
Pipin'Hot Wheat Loaf	1 in slice	70	12	2	2
Pipin'Hot White Loaf	1 in slice	70	12	2	3
Stefano's					
Stuffed Bread Broccoli & Cheese	½ bread (6 oz)	450	54	17	19
TAKE-OUT					
chapatis as prep w/ fat	1 (2½ oz)	230	34	9	6
chapatis as prep w/o fat	1 (2½ oz)	141	31	1	5
cornbread	2 in x 2 in (1.4 oz)	107	18	2	4
cornstick	1 (1.3 oz)	101	13	4	2

FOOD	PORTION	CALS.	CARB.	FAT	PRO.
focaccia onion	1 piece (4.6 oz)	282	43	10	6
focaccia rosemary	1 piece (3.5 oz)	251	40	7	6
focaccia tomato olive	1 piece (4.7 oz)	270	42	8	6
naan	1 (6 oz)	571	85	21	15
papadums fried	2 (1.5 oz)	81	9	4	4
paratha	1 (4.4 oz)	403	54	18	10

BREAD COATING
Golden Dipt

Breading Frying Mix	1 oz	90	20	0	3

Ka-Me

Tempura Batter Mix	1 oz	100	22	0	2

Shake 'N Bake

Original Barbecue For Chicken	¼ pkg (½ oz)	93	18	2	1
Original Country Mild	¼ pkg (½ oz)	76	10	4	1
Original For Chicken	¼ pkg (½ oz)	75	14	2	2

BREAD MACHINE MIX
Dromedary

Country White	½ in slice (2 oz)	140	28	1	4

Wanda's

Oregano Garlic	¼ cup mix per serv (1.2 oz)	130	25	1	5
Rosemary Basil	¼ cup mix per serv (1.2 oz)	130	26	0	4
Sourdough	¼ cup mix per serv (1.2 oz)	120	25	0	5
Wheat	¼ cup mix per serv (1.2 oz)	130	26	0	4

BREADCRUMBS

dry	1 cup	426	78	6	14
dry seasonsed	1 cup (4 oz)	441	85	3	17
fresh	⅔ cup	76	14	1	4

4C

Salt Free	1 tbsp (0.5 oz)	50	10	1	2

Jaclyn's

Organic Whole Wheat Plain	½ oz	28	13	1	4

BREADSTICKS
Angonoa

Garlic	6 (1 oz)	120	21	2	4
Italian Style Plain	5 (1 oz)	120	20	3	4
Sesame Mini	16 (1 oz)	130	19	4	4

FOOD	PORTION	CALS.	CARB.	FAT	PRO.
Angonoa (CONT.)					
Whole Wheat Mini	14 (1 oz)	130	19	4	4
Bread Du Jour					
Italian	1 (1.9 oz)	130	25	2	5
J.J. Cassone					
Garlic	1 (1.6 oz)	150	26	3	5
Lance					
Cheese	2	20	4	0	tr
Pillsbury					
Soft Bread Sticks	1	100	17	2	3
Stella D'Oro					
Garlic	1	35	6	1	1
Grissini Original Fat Free	3	60	12	0	2
Regular	1	40	7	1	1
Regular Sodium Free	2	80	14	2	2
Wheat	1	40	6	1	1

BREAKFAST BAR
(*see also* BREAKFAST DRINKS, NUTRITIONAL SUPPLEMENTS)

FOOD	PORTION	CALS.	CARB.	FAT	PRO.
Carnation					
Chewy Chocolate Chip	1 (1.26 oz)	150	22	6	2
Chewy Peanut Butter Chocolate Chip	1 (1.26 oz)	140	21	5	3
Glenny's					
Sunrise Bee Pollen	1 bar (1.5 oz)	190	22	8	5
Sunrise Ginseng	1 bar (1.5 oz)	160	24	7	1
Sunrise Spirulina	1 bar (1.5 oz)	140	21	5	3
Nutri-Grain					
Apple Cinnamon	1 (1.3 oz)	140	27	3	2
Blueberry	1 bar (1.3 oz)	140	27	3	2
Peach	1 (1.3 oz)	140	27	3	2
Raspberry	1 (1.3 oz)	140	27	3	2
Strawberry	1 (1.3 oz)	140	27	3	2

BREAKFAST DRINKS
(*see also* BREAKFAST BAR, NUTRITIONAL SUPPLEMENTS)

FOOD	PORTION	CALS.	CARB.	FAT	PRO.
orange drink powder	3 rounded tsp	93	24	0	0
orange drink powder as prep w/water	6 oz	86	22	0	0
Carnation					
Instant Breakfast Cafe Mocha	1 pkg + skim milk (9 fl oz)	220	39	1	12
Instant Breakfast Cafe Mocha	1 pkg	130	28	1	4
Instant Breakfast Cafe Mocha	1 can (10 fl oz) (9 fl oz)	220	35	3	12

FOOD	PORTION	CALS.	CARB.	FAT	PRO.
Carnation (CONT.)					
Instant Breakfast Classic Chocolate Malt	1 pkg + skim milk (9 fl oz)	220	39	1	12
Instant Breakfast Classic Chocolate Malt	1 pkg	130	26	2	4
Instant Breakfast Creamy Milk Chocolate	1 pkg + skim milk (9 fl oz)	220	39	1	12
Instant Breakfast Creamy Milk Chocolate	1 pkg	130	28	1	4
Instant Breakfast Creamy Milk Chocolate	8 fl oz	220	36	3	12
Instant Breakfast Creamy Milk Chocolate	1 can (10 fl oz)	220	37	3	12
Instant Breakfast French Vanilla	1 pkg	130	27	0	4
Instant Breakfast French Vanilla	1 pkg + skim milk	220	39	1	12
Instant Breakfast No Sugar Added Classic Chocolate	1 pkg	70	11	2	4
Instant Breakfast No Sugar Added Classic Chocolate	1 pkg + skim milk (9 fl oz)	160	24	2	12
Instant Breakfast No Sugar Added Creamy Milk Chocolate	1 pkg	70	12	1	4
Instant Breakfast No Sugar Added Creamy Milk Chocolate	1 pkg + skim milk (9 fl oz)	160	24	1	12
Instant Breakfast No Sugar Added French Vanilla	1 pkg + skim milk (9 fl oz)	150	24	1	12
Instant Breakfast No Sugar Added French Vanilla	1 pkg	70	12	0	4
Instant Breakfast No Sugar Added Strawberry Creme	1 pkg + skim milk (9 fl oz)	150	24	1	12
Instant Breakfast No Sugar Added Strawberry Creme	1 pkg	70	12	0	4

FOOD	PORTION	CALS.	CARB.	FAT	PRO.
Carnation (CONT.)					
Instant Breakfast Strawberry Creme	1 pkg + skim milk	220	39	1	12
Instant Breakfast Strawberry Creme	1 pkg	130	28	0	4
Pillsbury					
Instant Breakfast Chocolate Malt as prep w/ milk	1 serving	290	38	9	14
Instant Breakfast Chocolate as prep w/ milk	1 serving	290	38	9	14
Instant Breakfast Strawberry as prep w/ milk	1 serving	290	39	9	14
Instant Breakfast Vanilla as prep w/ whole milk	1 serving	300	41	9	14
BROAD BEANS					
canned	1 cup	183	**32**	1	14
dried cooked	1 cup	186	**33**	1	13
fresh cooked	3½ oz	56	**10**	tr	5
BROCCOLI					
FRESH					
chopped cooked	½ cup	22	4	tr	2
FROZEN					
chopped cooked	½ cup	25	5	tr	3
spears cooked	½ cup	25	5	tr	3
Big Valley					
Chopped	¾ cup (3 oz)	25	4	0	2
Birds Eye					
Baby Spears Deluxe	⅔ cup	30	5	0	3
Florets Deluxe	½ cup	25	5	0	3
Polybag Cuts	½ cup	25	4	0	3
With Cheese Sauce	½ pkg	110	9	5	5
Green Giant					
Harvest Fresh Spears	½ cup	20	4	0	2
In Butter Sauce	½ cup	40	6	2	2
In Cheese Sauce	½ cup	60	9	2	3
Valley Combinations Broccoli Fanfare	½ cup	80	14	2	3
Pepperidge Farm					
Broccoli With Cheese In Pastry	1	230	18	16	5

FOOD	PORTION	CALS.	CARB.	FAT	PRO.
BROWNIE					
FROZEN					
Weight Watchers					
Brownie Ala Mode	1	180	35	4	5
Chocolate Brownie	1 (1.25 oz)	100	16	3	3
HOME RECIPE					
plain	1 (0.8 oz)	112	12	7	2
w/nuts	1 (0.8 oz)	95	11	6	1
MIX					
plain	1 (1.2 oz)	139	20	7	1
plain low calorie	1 (0.8 oz)	84	16	2	1
Betty Crocker					
Brownie With Hot Fudge MicroRave Single	1	350	55	12	5
Frosted MicroRave	1	180	21	7	1
Supreme German Chocolate	1	160	24	7	1
Estee					
Lite	2	100	23	4	tr
Jiffy					
Fudge as prep	1	160	28	4	1
Pillsbury					
Deluxe Fudge Brownie With Walnuts	2 in sq	150	19	8	2
Fudge Microwave	1	190	25	9	2
READY-TO-EAT					
plain	1 lg (2 oz)	227	36	9	3
plain	1 sm (1 oz)	115	18	5	1
w/ nuts	1 (1 oz)	100	16	4	1
w/o nuts	1 (2 oz)	243	39	10	3
Greenfield					
Brownie HomeStyle	1 (1.4 oz)	120	29	0	2
Hostess					
Brownie Bites	5 (2 oz)	260	32	14	4
Brownie Bites Walnut	5 (2 oz)	270	31	15	4
Lance					
Brownie	1 pkg (78 g)	320	52	12	4
Little Debbie					
Fudge	1 pkg (2.1 oz)	270	39	13	2
Tastykake					
Brownie	1 (85 g)	340	53	14	4
BRUSSELS SPROUTS					
fresh	½ cup	30	7	tr	2

FOOD	PORTION	CALS.	CARB.	FAT	PRO.
FROZEN					
cooked	½ cup	33	6	tr	3
Green Giant					
In Butter Sauce	½ cup	40	8	1	3
BUCKWHEAT					
flour whole groat	1 cup	402	85	4	15
groats roasted cooked	½ cup	91	20	tr	3
groats roasted uncooked	½ cup	283	61	2	10
Wolff's					
Brown Groats Roasted	1 cup (8 oz)	900	188	4	16
Flour	1 cup (8 oz)	860	170	5	24
Kasha Coarse cooked	¼ cup (1.6 oz)	170	35	2	64
Kasha Fine cooked	¼ cup (1.6 oz)	170	35	2	64
Kasha Medium cooked	¼ cup (1.6 oz)	170	35	2	64
Kasha Whole cooked	¼ cup (1.6 oz)	170	35	2	64
White Grits	1 cup (8 oz)	840	173	3	24
BUFFALO					
water roasted	3 oz	111	0	2	23
BULGUR					
cooked	½ cup	76	17	tr	3
uncooked	½ cup	239	53	tr	9
Casbah					
Pilaf Mix as prep	1 cup	200	42	1	6
Salad Mix as prep	⅔ cup	90	20	tr	3
Good Shepard					
Bulgur	¼ cup (43 g)	150	33	1	4
Hodgson Mill					
Bulgur	¼ cup (1.4 oz)	120	24	1	6
BURDOCK ROOT					
cooked	1 cup	110	26	tr	3
BUTTER					
(*see also* BUTTER BLENDS, BUTTER SUBSTITUTES, MARGARINE)					
clarified butter	3½ oz	876	0	99	tr
stick	1 pat	36	tr	4	tr
stick	1 stick (4 oz)	813	tr	92	1
whipped	4 oz	542	tr	61	1
whipped	1 pat	27	tr	3	tr
BUTTER BEANS					
CANNED					
Allen					
Baby	½ cup (4.5 oz)	120	22	1	7

FOOD	PORTION	CALS.	CARB.	FAT	PRO.
Allen (CONT.)					
Large	½ cup (4.5 oz)	120	20	1	7
Trappey					
Baby White With Bacon	½ cup (4.5 oz)	130	21	2	8

BUTTER BLENDS
(see also BUTTER, BUTTER SUBSTITUTES, MARGARINE)

Country Morning					
Blend Light Stick	1 tbsp (0.5 oz)	50	0	6	0
Blend Light Tub	1 tbsp (0.5 oz)	50	0	6	0
Blend Tub	1 tbsp	100	0	11	0
Touch Of Butter					
Tub	1 tbsp (0.5 oz)	60	0	7	0

BUTTER SUBSTITUTES
(see also BUTTER BLENDS, MARGARINE)

Butter Buds					
Mix	1 tsp (2 g)	5	2	0	0
Sprinkles	1 tsp (2 g)	5	2	0	0
Molly McButter					
w/ Bacon	½ tsp (1 g)	4	1	tr	tr
w/ Cheese	½ tsp (0.9 g)	4	tr	tr	tr
w/ Sour Cream	½ tsp (1.1 g)	4	1	tr	tr
Watkins					
Butter Sprinkles	1 tsp (2 g)	5	1	0	0
Imitation Butter Flavored Mist	1 tbsp (0.5 oz)	120	0	14	0

BUTTERFISH

baked	3 oz	159	0	9	19

BUTTERNUTS

dried	1 oz	174	3	16	7

BUTTERSCOTCH
(see also CANDY)

Nestle					
Morsels	1 tbsp	80	10	4	0

CABBAGE
FRESH

chinese pak-choi raw shredded	½ cup	5	1	tr	1
chinese pak-choi shredded cooked	½ cup	10	2	tr	1

FOOD	PORTION	CALS.	CARB.	FAT	PRO.
chinese pe-tsai raw shredded	1 cup	12	2	tr	1
chinese pe-tsai shredded cooked	1 cup	16	3	tr	2
danish raw	1 head (2 lbs)	228	49	2	13
danish raw shredded	½ cup (1.2 oz)	9	2	tr	1
danish shredded cooked	½ cup (2.6 oz)	17	3	tr	1
green raw	1 head (2 lbs)	228	49	2	2
green raw shredded	½ cup (1.2 oz)	9	2	tr	1
green shredded cooked	½ cup (2.6 oz)	17	3	tr	1
red raw shredded	½ cup	10	2	tr	tr
red shredded cooked	½ cup	16	3	tr	1
savoy raw shredded	½ cup	10	2	tr	1
savoy shredded cooked	½ cup	18	4	tr	1
Dole					
Napa shredded	½ cup	6	1	tr	1
Fresh Express					
Cole Slaw	1½ cups (3 oz)	25	6	0	1
HOME RECIPE					
coleslaw w/ dressing	¾ cup	147	13	11	1
TAKE-OUT					
coleslaw w/ dressing	½ cup	42	7	2	1
stuffed cabbage	1 (6 oz)	373	18	22	25
sweet & sour red cabbage	4 oz	61	8	3	1
vinegar & oil coleslaw	3.5 oz	150	16	9	1

CAKE

(*see also* BROWNIE, COOKIE, DANISH PASTRY, DOUGHNUT, PIE)

FOOD	PORTION	CALS.	CARB.	FAT	PRO.
FROZEN					
Pepperidge Farm					
Butter Pound	1 slice (1 oz)	130	16	7	1
Chocolate Supreme	1 piece (2⅞ oz)	300	37	16	3
Sara Lee					
Carrot Light	1 (2.5 oz)	170	30	4	4
French Cheese	1 slice (2.9 oz)	250	23	16	4
Weight Watchers					
Chocolate Eclair	1 (2.1 oz)	120	19	4	2
HOME RECIPE					
angelfood	1/12 cake (1.9 oz)	142	32	tr	4
apple crisp	½ cup (5 oz)	230	46	5	37
boston cream pie	⅙ cake (3.3 oz)	293	43	12	4
cheesecake w/ cherry topping	1/12 cake (5 oz)	359	33	23	6
fruitcake	1/36 cake (2.9 oz)	302	54	10	3

FOOD	PORTION	CALS.	CARB.	FAT	PRO.
READY-TO-EAT					
angelfood	¹⁄₁₂ cake (1 oz)	73	16	tr	2
bakewell tart	1 slice (3 oz)	410	39	27	6
battenburg cake	1 slice (2 oz)	204	28	10	3
chocolate w/ chocolate frosting	¹⁄₈ cake (2.2 oz)	235	35	11	3
coffeecake cheese	¹⁄₆ cake (2.7 oz)	258	38	12	5
coffeecake crumb topped cheese	¹⁄₆ cake (2.7 oz)	258	38	12	5
coffeecake crumb topped cinnamon	¹⁄₉ cake (2.2 oz)	263	29	15	4
crumpets toasted	2 (4 oz)	119	26	1	4
panettone dal forno	¹⁄₉ cake (1.9 oz)	212	31	8	4
pound	¹⁄₁₀ cake (1 oz)	117	15	6	2
pound fat free	1 oz	80	17	tr	2
pound cake	1 slice (1 oz)	110	15	12	2
sponge	¹⁄₁₂ cake (1.3 oz)	110	23	1	2
strudel apple	1 piece (2½ oz)	195	29	8	2
tiramisu	1 piece (5.1 oz)	409	31	30	7
white w/ white frosting	¹⁄₁₆ cake	260	42	9	3
yellow w/ vanilla frosting	¹⁄₈ cake (2.2 oz)	239	38	9	2
yellow w/ chocolate frosting	¹⁄₈ cake (2.2 oz)	242	36	11	2
Dutch Mill					
Dessert Shells Chocolate Covered	1 (0.5 oz)	80	8	5	1
Entenmann's					
Cinnamon Buns	1 (2.1 oz)	230	31	10	4
Danish Ring	1 serving (1.5 oz)	180	18	10	3
Danish Ring Pecan	1 serving (1.5 oz)	190	19	12	3
Devil's Food Cake Fudge Iced	1 serving (1.2 oz)	130	19	5	2
Perugina					
Pannettone Au Beurre	¹⁄₆ cake (2.9 oz)	310	47	12	5
Sinbad					
Baklava	1 piece (2 oz)	337	44	20	5
Thomas'					
Date Nut Loaf	1 oz	90	18	2	1
REFRIGERATED					
Baby Watson					
Cheesecake	1 slice (3.8 oz)	390	23	30	6
Cheesecake Light	¹⁄₁₆ cake (3.9 oz)	280	24	16	8
Pillsbury					
Apple Turnovers	1	170	23	8	2

FOOD	PORTION	CALS.	CARB.	FAT	PRO.
Pillsbury (CONT.)					
Cherry Turnovers	1	170	23	8	2
SNACK					
Drake's					
Coffee Cake	1 (1.1 oz)	140	18	6	2
Coffee Cake Small	1 (2 oz)	220	33	9	3
Devil Dog	1 (1.5 oz)	160	24	6	2
Funny Bones	1 (1.25 oz)	150	18	8	3
Pound Cake	1	110	16	5	2
Ring Ding	1 (1.5 oz)	180	23	10	2
Sunny Doodle	1 (1 oz)	100	16	3	1
Yankee Doodle	1 (1 oz)	100	16	4	1
Yodel's	1 (1 oz)	150	16	9	2
Greenfield					
Blondie Apple Spice	1 (1.4 oz)	120	28	0	2
Blondie Chocolate Chip	1 (1.4 oz)	120	29	0	2
Hostess					
Crumb Cake	1 (1.9 oz)	210	33	8	2
Crumb Cake Light	1 (1.8 oz)	150	35	1	2
Cup Cakes Chocolate	1 (1.6 oz)	170	28	5	2
Cup Cakes Chocolate Light	1 (1.4 oz)	120	26	2	2
Ding Dongs	1 (1.3 oz)	160	21	9	1
Ho Ho's	1 (1 oz)	130	17	6	1
Sno Balls	1 (1.6 oz)	160	29	5	2
Twinkies	1 (1.4 oz)	140	25	4	1
Twinkies Devil Food	2 (2.7 oz)	300	47	12	3
Twinkies Lights	1 (1.4 oz)	120	24	2	2
Kellogg's					
Pop-Tarts Apple Cinnamon	1 (1.8 oz)	210	38	5	2
Pop-Tarts Brown Sugar Cinnamon	1 (1.8 oz)	220	32	9	3
Pop-Tarts Frosted Blueberry	1 (1.8 oz)	200	37	5	2
Pop-Tarts Frosted Chocolate Fudge	1 (1.8 oz)	200	37	5	3
Rice Krispies Treats	1 (0.8 oz)	90	18	2	1
Lance					
Dunking Sticks	1 (39 g)	190	22	10	2
Honey Buns	1 (85 g)	330	48	14	4
Little Debbie					
Banana Twins	1 pkg (2.2 oz)	250	40	10	15
Chocolate	1 pkg (3 oz)	360	52	17	2

FOOD	PORTION	CALS.	CARB.	FAT	PRO.
Little Debbie (CONT.)					
Chocolate Chip	1 pkg (2.4 oz)	290	42	15	2
Chocolate Twins	1 pkg (2.4 oz)	240	42	9	2
Coffee Cake Apple	1 pkg (1.9 oz)	220	36	7	2
Golden Cremes	1 pkg (3 oz)	330	50	15	3
Jelly Rolls	1 pkg (2.1 oz)	230	41	7	1
Nutty Bar	1 pkg (2 oz)	290	34	17	4
Spice	1 pkg (2.5 oz)	300	43	15	2
Swiss Rolls	1 pkg (2.1 oz)	250	38	12	1
Vanilla	1 pkg (3 oz)	370	53	18	2
Zebra Cakes	1 pkg (2.6 oz)	150	45	16	2
Pepperidge Farm					
Toaster Tart Cheese	1	190	22	10	5
Toaster Tart Strawberry	1	190	28	7	3
Rice Krispies					
Cereal Bar Chocolate Chip	1 (1 oz)	120	20	4	1
Sara Lee					
Chocolate Fudge Cake	1	190	24	10	2
Coffee Cake Apple Cinnamon	1	290	40	13	4
Coffee Cake Pecan	1	280	30	16	5
Sweet Rewards					
Fat Free Brownie	1 bar (1 oz)	90	21	0	2
Tastykake					
Butter Cream Cream Filled Cupcake	1 (32 g)	120	20	4	1
Honeybun Glazed	1 pkg (92 g)	360	42	20	6
Junior Chocolate	1 pkg (94 g)	340	57	12	4
Kandy Kake Chocolate	1 (19 g)	80	13	3	1
Kandy Kake Peanut Butter	1 (19 g)	90	11	4	2
Koffee Kake Cream Filled	1 (29 g)	110	18	4	1
Koffee Kake Junior	1 pkg (71 g)	260	44	8	3
Pastry Pocket Apple	1 (85 g)	320	38	18	4
Tasty Too Chocolate Cream Filled Cupcake	1 (32 g)	100	21	1	1
Tasty Too Vanilla Cream Filled Cupcake	1 (32 g)	100	21	1	1
Toast-R-Cakes					
Bran	1	103	18	3	2
Corn	1	120	19	4	2
Toastettes					
Frosted Cherry	1 (1.7 oz)	190	35	5	2

FOOD	PORTION	CALS.	CARB.	FAT	PRO.
Well-Bred Loaf					
Banana Bread	1 slice (3.5 oz)	330	52	11	4
Carrot	1 slice (4.3 oz)	480	64	24	6
Marble	1 slice (4.3 oz)	530	83	18	7
TAKE-OUT					
baklava	1 oz	126	10	9	2
trifle w/ cream	6 oz	291	34	16	4

CALZONE
TAKE-OUT

cheese	1 (12 oz)	1020	86	54	48

CANADIAN BACON
Jones

Slices	1	30	tr	1	3
Oscar Mayer					
Canadian Bacon	2 slices (1.6 oz)	50	0	2	9

CANDY
(*see also* MARSHMALLOW)

butterscotch	1 piece (6 g)	24	6	tr	0
candy corn	1 oz	105	27	0	tr
caramels	1 piece (8 g)	31	6	1	tr
caramels chocolate	1 piece (6 g)	22	6	tr	tr
carob bar	1 (3.1 oz)	453	42	28	11
crisped rice bar almond	1 bar (1 oz)	130	18	6	2
crisped rice bar chocolate chip	1 bar (1 oz)	115	21	4	4
dark chocolate	1 oz	150	16	10	1
fondant chocolate coated	1 lg (1.2 oz)	128	28	3	1
fondant mint	1 oz	105	27	0	tr
fruit pastilles	1 tube (1.4 oz)	101	25	0	2
gumdrops	10 sm (0.4 oz)	135	35	0	0
gumdrops	10 lg (3.8 oz)	420	108	0	0
hard candy	1 oz	106	28	0	0
jelly beans	10 sm (0.4 oz)	40	10	tr	0
jelly beans	10 lg (1 oz)	104	26	tr	0
lollipop	1 (6 g)	22	6	0	0
milk chocolate	1 bar (1.55 oz)	226	26	14	3
milk chocolate crisp	1 bar (1.45 oz)	203	28	11	3
milk chocolate w/ almonds	1 bar (1.45 oz)	215	22	14	4
nougat nut cream	3½ oz	342	58	31	4
peanut bar	1 (1.4 oz)	209	19	14	6
peanuts chocolate covered	10 (1.4 oz)	208	20	13	5
pretzels chocolate covered	1 (0.4 oz)	50	8	2	1

FOOD	PORTION	CALS.	CARB.	FAT	PRO.
sesame crunch	20 pieces (1.2 oz)	181	18	12	4
100 Grand					
Bar	1 bar (1.5 oz)	200	30	8	2
3 Musketeers					
Bar	1 (2.1 oz)	260	46	8	2
5th Avenue					
Bar	1 (2.1 oz)	290	39	13	5
After Eight					
Dark Chocolate Wafer Thin Mints	1	35	6	1	0
Almond Joy					
Bar	1 (1.76 oz)	250	28	14	3
Baby Ruth					
Bar	1 (2.1 oz)	280	38	12	4
Bar None					
Candy	1 (1.5 oz)	240	23	14	4
Bit-O-Honey					
Candy	1.7 oz	200	39	4	1
Bits O Brickle					
Candy	1 tbsp (0.5 oz)	80	9	5	0
Bonus					
Bar	1 bar (2.1 oz)	290	34	16	6
Breath Savers					
Sugar Free Peppermint	1 piece (2 g)	10	2	0	0
Brock					
Candy Corn	21 pieces (1.4 oz)	150	37	0	0
Gummy Bears	5 pieces (1.4 oz)	130	30	0	0
Lemon Drops	3 pieces (0.5 oz)	60	14	0	0
Orange Slices	4 pieces (1.5 oz)	140	36	0	0
Sour Balls	3 pieces (0.6 oz)	70	17	0	0
Spice Drops	12 pieces (1.4 oz)	130	33	0	0
Starlight Mints	3 pieces (0.6 oz)	60	16	0	0
Toffee	6 pieces (1.5 oz)	170	31	5	1
Butterfinger					
Bar	1 (2.1 oz)	280	41	11	4
Caramello					
Candy	1 (1.6 oz)	220	28	11	3
Cellas					
Chocolate Covered Cherries Milk Chocolate	2 pieces (1 oz)	110	18	4	tr
Certs					
Breath Mints	1 piece (1.67 g)	6	2	0	0
Sugar Free	1 piece (1.67 g)	7	2	0	0

FOOD	PORTION	CALS.	CARB.	FAT	PRO.
Chuckles					
Candy	4 pieces (1.4 oz)	140	34	0	0
Chunky					
Bar	1 (1.4 oz)	200	22	11	3
Clorets					
Mints	1 piece (1.67 g)	6	2	0	0
Crunch					
Fun Size	4 bars (1.5 oz)	200	25	10	2
Dove					
Dark Chocolate	1 bar (1.3 oz)	200	22	12	2
Milk Chocolate	1 bar (1.3 oz)	200	22	12	2
Truffles	3 (1.2 oz)	200	19	13	2
Estee					
Caramels Chocolate & Vanilla No Sugar Added	5 (1.3 oz)	150	26	5	1
Dark Chocolate	½ bar (1.4 oz)	200	23	14	2
Gum Drops Assorted Fruit Sugar Free	23 (1.4 oz)	140	36	0	0
Gum Drops Licorice	23 (1.4 oz)	140	36	0	0
Gummy Bears Sugar Free	16 (1.4 oz)	140	31	0	4
Hard Candies Assorted Fruit Sugar Free	5 (0.5 oz)	60	16	0	0
Hard Candies Assorted Mint Sugar Free	5 (0.5 oz)	60	16	0	0
Hard Candies Butterscotch Sugar Free	2 (0.4 oz)	50	12	0	0
Hard Candies Peppermint Swirls Sugar Free	3 (0.5 oz)	60	14	0	0
Hard Candies Tropical Fruit Sugar Free	5 (0.5 oz)	60	16	0	0
Lollipops Assorted Fruit Sugar Free	2 (0.5 oz)	60	16	0	0
Milk Chocolate	½ bar (1.4 oz)	230	17	17	4
Milk Chocolate With Almonds	½ bar (1.4 oz)	230	16	17	4
Milk Chocolate With Crisp Rice	1 bar (2.3 oz)	370	29	26	7
Milk Chocolate With Fruit & Nuts	½ bar (1.4 oz)	220	18	16	4
Mint Chocolate	½ bar (1.4 oz)	200	23	14	2

FOOD	PORTION	CALS.	CARB.	FAT	PRO.
Estee (CONT.)					
Peanut Brittle No Sugar Added	⅓ box (1.5 oz)	210	28	9	4r
Peanut Butter Cups	1 (0.3 oz)	40	3	3	1
Peanut Butter Cups	5 (1.3 oz)	200	19	12	5
Toffee Sugar Free	5 (0.5 oz)	60	16	0	0
Ferreo Rocher					
Candy	3 pieces (1.3 oz)	220	17	15	4
Candy	2 pieces (0.9 oz)	150	11	10	2
Franklin					
Crunch 'N Munch Candied	1.25 oz	170	28	7	2
Crunch 'N Munch Caramel	1.25 oz	160	28	5	2
Crunch 'N Munch Maple Walnut	1.25 oz	160	28	6	1
Crunch 'N Munch Toffee	1.25 oz	160	28	5	2
Glenny's					
Brown Rice Treat Raisin Bran	1 bar (1.75 oz)	170	38	1	2
Brown Rice Treats Carob & Mint With Oat Bran	1 bar (1.75 oz)	180	37	2	3
Brown Rice Treats Cinnamon & Raisin	1 bar (1.75 oz)	170	38	1	2
Brown Rice Treats Peanut & Raisin	1 bar (2 oz)	210	39	5	4
Brown Rice Treats Plain & Fancy	1 bar (1.25 oz)	120	28	1	1
Brown Rice Treats Toasted Almond With Oat Bran	1 bar (1.75 oz)	200	34	5	4
Fruit Drops Black Cherry	1	6	1	tr	tr
Fruit Drops Gentle Mint	1	6	1	tr	tr
Fruit Drops Mandarin Orange	1	6	1	tr	tr
Fruit Drops Mixed Fruit	1	6	1	tr	tr
Fruit Drops Twist Of Lemon	1	6	1	tr	tr
Hard Candies Fruit	1	19	4	tr	tr
Hard Candies Peppermint	1	19	4	tr	tr
Lollipops C Pops	1	35	8	tr	tr
Lollipops Fruit	1	21	5	tr	tr

FOOD	PORTION	CALS.	CARB.	FAT	PRO.
Glenny's (CONT.)					
Moist & Chewy Coconut Almondine Bar	1 bar (1.5 oz)	190	22	10	3
Moist & Chewy Oatmeal Raisin Bar	1 bar (1.5 oz)	160	30	3	3
Moist & Chewy Peanut Bar	1 bar (1.5 oz)	180	24	7	5
Moist & Chewy Sunflower Bar	1 bar (1.5 oz)	180	24	7	5
Snack Bar Fat-Free Apple-Cinnamon	1 (125 oz)	120	28	1	1
Snack Bar Fat-Free Caramel	1 (1.25 oz)	120	29	tr	1
Snack Bar Fat-Free Chocolate	1 (1.25 oz)	120	28	tr	1
Snack Bar Fat-Free Raspberry	1 (1.25 oz)	120	29	tr	1
Godiva					
Almond Butter Dome	3 pieces (1.5 oz)	240	19	17	4
Bouchee Au Chocolat	1 piece (1.5 oz)	210	25	11	3
Gold Ballotin	3 pieces (1.5 oz)	210	27	10	2
Truffle Amaretto Di Saronno	2 pieces (1.5 oz)	210	24	12	2
Golden Almond					
Bar	½ bar	260	20	17	5
Golden III					
Bar	½ bar	250	26	15	3
Goldenberg's					
Peanut Chews	3 pieces (1.3 oz)	180	22	9	4
Goobers					
Peanuts	1 pkg (1.38 oz)	210	19	13	5
Good & Fruity					
Candy	1 box (1.8 oz)	140	35	1	0
Good & Plenty					
Snacksize	3 boxes (1.5 oz)	140	34	0	1
Heath					
Bar	1 (1.4 oz)	210	25	13	2
Hershey					
Bar	1 (1.55 oz)	240	25	14	4
Bar With Almonds	1 (1.45 oz)	230	20	14	5
Kisses	9 pieces (1.46 oz)	220	23	13	3
Jolly Rancher					
Candies	3 pieces (0.6 oz)	60	14	0	0

FOOD	PORTION	CALS.	CARB.	FAT	PRO.
Joyva					
Halvah	1.5 oz	240	16	16	4
Halvah Chocolate Covered	1 bar (2 oz)	380	20	23	5
Jells Raspberry	3 pieces (1.6 oz)	200	25	3	0
Marshmallow Twists Chocolate Covered	2 (1.5 oz)	190	21	4	1
Twists Vanilla & Cherry	2 pieces (1.5 oz)	190	21	4	1
Juicefuls					
Candy	3 pieces (0.5 oz)	60	15	0	0
Kit Kat					
Bar	1 (1.625 oz)	250	29	13	3
Krackel					
Bar	1 (1.55 oz)	230	27	13	3
Kraft					
Peanut Brittle	5 pieces (1.3 oz)	170	29	5	3
Laffy Taffy					
Apple Chews	1 oz	110	26	1	0
Passion Punch Chews	1 oz	110	26	1	0
Watermelon Chews	1 oz	110	26	1	0
Lance					
Chocolaty Peanut Bar	1 (57 g)	320	29	18	9
Peanut Bar	1 pkg (50 g)	260	24	14	9
Popscotch	1 pkg (35 g)	160	24	6	3
Lifesavers					
Fruit Juicers Lollipops	1	40	10	0	0
Gummi Savers Five Flavor	1 roll (1.5 oz)	130	32	0	2
Holes Five Flavor	20 pieces (5 g)	20	5	0	0
Lollipops Fruit Flavors	1 (0.4 oz)	45	11	0	0
Roll Butter Rum	2 pieces (5 g)	20	5	0	0
Roll Cryst-O-Mint	2 pieces (5 g)	20	5	0	0
Roll Five Flavor	2 pieces (5 g)	20	5	0	0
Roll Fruits On Fire	2 pieces (5 g)	20	5	0	0
Roll Pep-O-Mint	3 pieces (5 g)	20	5	0	0
Roll Spear-O-Mint	3 pieces (5 g)	20	5	0	0
Roll Sunshine Fruits	2 pieces (5 g)	20	5	0	0
Roll Wint-O-Green	3 pieces (5 g)	20	5	0	0
Sugar Free Iced Mint	1 piece (2 g)	10	2	0	0
Sugar Free Vanilla Mint	1 piece (2 g)	10	2	0	0
M&M's					
Almond	1 pkg (1.3 oz)	200	21	11	3
Mint	1 pkg (1.7 oz)	230	34	10	2
Peanut	1 pkg (1.7 oz)	250	30	13	5

FOOD	PORTION	CALS.	CARB.	FAT	PRO.
M&M's (CONT.)					
Plain	1 pkg (1.7 oz)	230	34	10	2
Mars					
Almond Bar	1 bar (1.8 oz)	240	31	13	3
Milk Duds					
Pieces	1 box (1.8 oz)	230	38	8	1
Milkshake					
Bar	1 bar (1.8 oz)	220	38	7	2
Milky Way					
Bar	1 (2.1 oz)	280	43	11	2
Dark	1 bar (1.8 oz)	220	36	8	1
Mounds					
Bar	1 (1.9 oz)	260	31	14	2
Mr. Goodbar					
Candy	1 (1.75 oz)	290	23	19	7
Natural Touch					
Caroby Almond Bar	4 sections (28 g)	150	12	10	4
Caroby Milk Bar	4 sections (28 g)	150	13	9	4
Caroby Milk Free Bar	4 sections (28 g)	160	11	11	4
Caroby Mint Bar	4 sections (28 g)	150	13	9	4
Nestle					
Areo Bar	1 bar (1.45 oz)	210	26	13	<1
Buncha Crunch	1 pkg (1.4 oz)	90	26	10	2
Milk Chocolate	1 bar (1.45 oz)	220	23	13	4
Turtles Pecan Caramel Candy	2 pieces (1.2 oz)	160	20	9	2
Nips					
Butter Rum	2 pieces (0.5 oz)	60	12	2	0
Chocolate Parfait	2 pieces (0.5 oz)	60	11	2	tr
Ocean Spray					
Fruit Waves Assorted	3 pieces (0.3 oz)	35	9	0	0
Oh Henry!					
Bar	1 (1.8 oz)	230	32	9	6
PayDay					
Bar	1 (1.85 oz)	240	28	12	7
Pearson					
Licorice	2 pieces (0.5 oz)	60	12	2	0
Pez					
Candy	1 roll (0.3 oz)	30	8	0	0
Planters					
Original Peanut Bar	1 pkg (1.6 oz)	230	22	14	6
Raisinets					
Raisins	1 pkg (1.58 oz)	200	31	8	2

FOOD	PORTION	CALS.	CARB.	FAT	PRO.
Reese's					
Peanut Butter Cups	1 (1.8 oz)	280	26	17	6
Pieces	1.85 oz	260	32	11	8
Riesen					
Candy	5 pieces (1.4 oz)	180	29	7	3
Rolo					
Carmels In Milk Chocolate	8 pieces (1.93 oz)	270	37	12	3
Russell Stover					
Assorted Creams	3 pieces (1.4 oz)	180	29	7	1
Skittles					
Original	1 pkg (2.8 oz)	250	55	3	0
Skor					
Toffee Bar	1 (1.4 oz)	220	22	14	2
Snickers					
Bar	1 bar (2.1 oz)	280	36	14	4
Munch Bar	1 (1.4 oz)	230	17	15	6
Sno Caps					
Candies	1 pkg (2.3 oz)	300	48	13	2
Solitaires					
Candies	½ bag	260	20	17	6
Sour Punch					
Candy Straws Sour Apple	6 pieces (1.4 oz)	130	31	1	1
Spice Stix					
And Drops	14 pieces (1.6 oz)	140	35	0	0
Starburst					
California Fruits	8 pieces (1.4 oz)	160	33	3	0
Original Fruits	8 pieces (1.4 oz)	160	33	3	0
Strawberry Fruits	8 pieces (1.4 oz)	160	33	3	0
Tropical Fruits	1 stick (2.1 oz)	240	48	5	0
Swedish Red Fish					
Candy	19 pieces (1.4 oz)	150	35	1	0
Switzer					
Cherry Bites	12 pieces (1.6 oz)	50	11	0	1
Licorice Bites	12 pieces (1.6 oz)	46	11	0	0
Symphony					
Almond/ Butterchips	1 (1.4 oz)	220	20	14	4
Milk Chocolate	1 (1.4 oz)	220	22	13	3
Terry's					
Orange Milk Chocolate	5 pieces (1.5 oz)	240	26	14	3
Twix					
Caramel	1 pkg (2 oz)	280	37	14	3

FOOD	PORTION	CALS.	CARB.	FAT	PRO.
Twizzlers					
Candy	4 pieces (1.4 oz)	130	30	1	1
Pull-n-Peel Cherry	1 piece (1.1 oz)	110	23	0	1
Velamints					
Peppermint	1 piece (1.7 g)	5	2	0	0
Whatchamacallit					
Bar	1 (1.8 oz)	260	30	13	5
Whitman's					
Assorted	3 pieces (1.4 oz)	190	27	8	2
Pecan Roll	1 bar (2 oz)	300	26	20	3
Whoppers					
Candy	1 pkg (1.8 oz)	230	36	10	2
Y&S					
Bites Cherry	1 oz	100	23	1	1
York					
Peppermint Patty	1 snack size (0.5 oz)	57	11	1	tr
Peppermint Patty	1 (1.5 oz)	180	34	4	1
Zero					
Bar	2 pieces (1.4 oz)	170	28	6	2
CANTALOUPE					
FRESH					
cubed	1 cup	57	13	tr	1
half	½	94	22	1	2
FROZEN					
Big Valley					
Balls	¾ cup (4.9 oz)	40	10	0	1
CAPERS					
Reese					
Capers	1 tsp (5 g)	0	0	0	0
CARAMBOLA					
fresh	1	42	10	tr	1
CARIBOU					
roasted	3 oz	142	0	4	25
CAROB					
carob mix	3 tsp	45	11	0	tr
carob mix as prep w/ whole milk	9 oz	195	23	8	8
CARP					
fresh cooked	3 oz	138	0	6	19
fresh cooked	1 fillet (6 oz)	276	0	12	39

FOOD	PORTION	CALS.	CARB.	FAT	PRO.
CARROT JUICE					
canned	6 oz	73	17	tr	2
Hain					
Juice	6 fl oz	80	17	0	1
Hollywood					
Juice	6 fl oz	80	17	0	1
Odwalla					
Juice	8 fl oz	70	18	0	2
CARROTS					
CANNED					
slices	½ cup	17	4	tr	tr
slices low sodium	½ cup	17	4	tr	tr
S&W					
Whole Tiny Fancy	½ cup	30	7	0	1
FRESH					
baby raw	1 (½ oz)	6	1	tr	tr
raw	1 (2.5 oz)	31	7	tr	1
raw shredded	½ cup	24	6	tr	1
slices cooked	½ cup	35	8	tr	1
FROZEN					
slices cooked	½ cup	26	6	tr	1
Birds Eye					
Baby Whole Deluxe	½ cup	40	9	0	1
Polybag Sliced	¾ cup	35	8	0	1
CASABA					
cubed	1 cup	45	11	tr	2
fresh	1/10	43	10	tr	1
CASHEWS					
cashew butter w/o salt	1 tbsp	94	4	8	3
dry roasted	1 oz	163	9	13	4
dry roasted salted	1 oz	163	9	13	4
oil roasted	1 oz	163	8	14	5
oil roasted salted	1 oz	163	8	14	5
Eagle					
Honey Roasted	1 oz	170	9	12	4
Low Salt	1 oz	170	7	14	6
Hain					
Cashew Butter Raw	2 tbsp	190	8	15	6
Cashew Butter Raw Unsalted	2 tbsp	210	8	19	5
Cashew Butter Toasted	2 tbsp	210	7	17	7
CASSAVA					
raw	3½ oz	120	27	tr	3

FOOD	PORTION	CALS.	CARB.	FAT	PRO.
CATFISH					
channel breaded & fried	3 oz	194	7	11	15
CATSUP					
(*see* KETCHUP)					
CAULIFLOWER					
FRESH					
cooked	½ cup (2.2 oz)	14	3	tr	1
flowerets cooked	3 (2 oz)	12	2	tr	1
flowerets raw	3 (2 oz)	14	3	tr	1
green cooked	½ cup (2.2 oz)	20	4	tr	2
green raw	½ cup (1.8 oz)	16	3	tr	1
FROZEN					
cooked	½ cup	17	3	tr	1
Birds Eye					
With Cheese Sauce	½ pkg	90	8	5	5
Green Giant					
In Cheese Sauce	½ cup	60	10	2	2
JARRED					
Vlasic					
Hot & Spicy	1 oz	4	1	0	0
Sweet	1 oz	35	9	0	0
CAVIAR					
black granular	1 tbsp	40	1	3	4
red granular	1 tbsp	40	1	3	4
CELERIAC					
fresh cooked	3½ oz	25	6	tr	1
raw	½ cup	31	7	tr	1
CELERY					
FRESH					
diced cooked	½ cup	13	3	tr	1
raw	1 stalk (1.3 oz)	6	1	tr	tr
raw diced	½ cup	10	2	tr	tr
FROZEN					
Fresh Like					
Celery	3.5 oz	14	3	tr	1
CEREAL					
COOKED					
Arrowhead					
4 Grain + Flax	¼ cup (1.6 oz)	150	28	2	6
7 Grain	⅓ cup (1.4 oz)	140	25	2	6
Bear Mush	¼ cup (1.6 oz)	160	33	1	5

FOOD	PORTION	CALS.	CARB.	FAT	PRO.
Arrowhead (CONT.)					
Oat Flakes Rolled	⅓ cup (1.2 oz)	130	23	3	5
Oat Groats	¼ cup (1.5 oz)	160	29	3	6
Oatmeal Instant Original	1 oz	100	22	0	3
Rice & Shine	¼ cup (1.5 oz)	150	32	1	3
Wheat Flakes Rolled	⅓ cup (1.2 oz)	110	24	1	4
Aunt Jemima					
Enriched White Hominy Grits Regular	3 tbsp	101	22	tr	2
Erewhon					
Barley Plus	1 oz	110	22	1	3
Brown Rice Cream	1 oz	110	23	1	3
Oat Bran With Toasted Wheat Germ	1 oz	115	18	2	5
Oatmeal Instant Apple Cinnamon	1.25 oz	145	25	3	4
Oatmeal Instant Apple Raisin	1.3 oz	150	27	3	4
Oatmeal Instant Dates & Walnuts	1.2 oz	130	24	3	3
Oatmeal Instant Maple Spice	1.2 oz	140	24	3	4
Oatmeal Instant With Added Oat Bran	1.25 oz	125	23	3	6
Good Shepherd					
Spelt	1 oz	90	20	tr	4
H-O					
Farina Instant	1 pkg	110	22	0	3
Farina not prep	3 tbsp	120	26	0	3
Oatmeal Instant	1 pkg	110	18	2	4
Oatmeal Instant Apple Cinnamon	1 pkg	130	26	2	4
Oatmeal Instant Maple Brown Sugar	1 pkg	160	32	2	4
Oats 'n Fiber	1 pkg	110	18	2	5
Oats Quick	½ cup	130	22	2	5
Health Valley					
Oat Bran Natural Apples & Cinnamon	¼ cup (1 oz)	100	19	tr	3
Oat Bran Natural Raisins & Spice	¼ cup	100	19	tr	3
Kashi					
5-Bran	2½ oz	281	47	6	9
Cereal	2 oz	177	38	1	6

FOOD	PORTION	CALS.	CARB.	FAT	PRO.
Little Crow					
Coco Wheat	3 tbsp (36 g)	130	28	1	4
Maltex					
Cereal	1 oz	105	21	1	3
Maypo					
30 second	1 oz	100	19	1	4
Vermont Style	1 oz	105	20	1	4
McCann's					
Irish Oatmeal	1 oz	110	20	2	5
Mother's					
Oatmeal Instant	½ cup (1.4 oz)	150	27	3	5
Whole Wheat Natural	½ cup (1.4 oz)	130	30	1	5
Nabisco					
Cream Of Wheat Instant as prep	1 cup	120	25	0	3
Cream of Rice	1 oz	100	23	0	2
Cream of Wheat Quick as prep	1 cup	120	25	0	3
Cream of Wheat Regular as prep	1 cup	120	25	0	3
Mix'n Eat Cream Of Wheat Brown Sugar Cinnamon	1 pkg (1¼ oz)	130	29	0	2
Mix'n Eat Cream of Wheat Our Original	1 pkg (1¼ oz)	100	21	0	3
Pillsbury					
Farina	⅔ cup	80	17	tr	2
Quaker					
Enriched White Hominy Grits Quick	3 tbsp	101	22	tr	2
Enriched Yellow Hominy Quick Grits	3 tbsp	101	22	tr	2
Instant Grits White Hominy	1 pkg	79	18	tr	2
Multigrain	½ cup	130	29	2	5
Oatmeal Instant	1 pkg (1.2 oz)	130	22	3	5
Oatmeal Instant Cinnamon Spice	1 pkg (1.6 oz)	170	36	2	4
Oatmeal Instant Fruit & Cream Blueberry	1 pkg (1.2 oz)	130	27	3	3
Oatmeal Instant Honey Nut	1 pkg (1.2 oz)	130	25	3	3
Oatmeal Instant Maple Brown Sugar	1 pkg (1.5 oz)	160	33	2	4

FOOD	PORTION	CALS.	CARB.	FAT	PRO.
Quaker (CONT.)					
Oatmeal Instant Peaches & Cream	1 pkg (1.2 oz)	130	27	2	3
Oatmeal Instant Raisin Date Walnut	1 pkg (1.3 oz)	130	27	3	3
Oats Old Fashion	½ cup	150	27	3	5
Oats Quick	½ cup	150	27	3	5
Roman Meal					
Apple Cinnamon	1.2 oz	105	18	2	3
Cream Of Rye	1.3 oz	111	20	1	5
Oats Wheat Dates Raisins Almonds	1.3 oz	129	24	2	5
Oats Wheat Honey Coconuts Almonds	1.3 oz	155	22	5	4
Original	1 oz	83	15	1	4
Original With Oats	1.2 oz	108	19	1	5
Stone-Buhr					
4 Grain	⅓ cup (1.6 oz)	140	31	2	6
Cracked Wheat	¼ cup (2.4 oz)	210	48	1	8
Manna Golden	6 tsp (1.6 oz)	160	35	0	5
Rolled Oats Old Fashion	6 tsp (1.6 oz)	150	28	3	8
Scotch Oats	¼ cup (1.6 oz)	150	28	4	7
Uncle Roy's					
Muesli Swiss Style	½ cup (1.6 oz)	170	32	5	5
Wheatena					
Cereal	⅓ cup (1.4 oz)	150	32	1	5
READY-TO-EAT					
Arrowhead					
Amaranth Flakes	1 cup (1.2 oz)	130	25	2	4
Apple Corns	1 cup (1.5 oz)	150	35	2	3
Bran Flakes	1 cup (1 oz)	100	22	1	5
Kamut Flakes	1 cup (1.1 oz)	120	25	1	4
Maple Corns	1 cup (1.9 oz)	190	43	3	5
Multi Grain Flakes	1 cup (1.2 oz)	140	29	2	33
Nature O's	1 cup (1.1 oz)	130	24	2	4
Oat Bran Flakes	1 cup (1.2 oz)	110	22	2	6
Puffed Corn	1 cup (0.8 oz)	80	16	0	3
Puffed Kamut	1 cup (0.6 oz)	50	11	0	2
Puffed Millet	1 cup (0.9 oz)	90	19	1	3
Puffed Rice	1 cup (0.8 oz)	90	19	0	2
Puffed Wheat	1 cup (0.9)	90	20	1	3
Spelt Flakes	1 cup (1.1 oz)	100	22	1	5
Cap'n Crunch					
Original	¾ cup	113	24	2	2

FOOD	PORTION	CALS.	CARB.	FAT	PRO.
Chex					
Corn	1¼ cup (1 oz)	110	26	0	2
Wheat	¾ cup (1.8 oz)	190	41	1	5
Erewhon					
Aztec	1 oz	100	24	0	2
Crispy Brown Rice	1 oz	110	24	1	2
Fruit 'n Wheat	1 oz	100	21	1	2
Raisin Bran	1 oz	100	22	0	3
Super-O's	1 oz	110	24	0	3
Wheat Flakes	1 oz	100	22	0	3
Estee					
Corn Flakes	1 pkg (1 oz)	90	24	0	2
Raisin Bran	1 pkg (1 oz)	90	21	1	4
General Mills					
Basic 4	¾ cup	130	28	2	3
Cheerios	1¼ cup (1 oz)	110	20	2	4
Cheerios Apple Cinnamon	¾ cup (1 oz)	110	22	2	2
Cheerios Honey Nut	¾ cup (1 oz)	110	23	1	3
Cinnamon Toast Crunch	¾ cup (1 oz)	120	22	3	1
Cocoa Puffs	1 cup (1 oz)	110	25	1	1
Count Chocula	1 cup (1 oz)	110	24	1	2
Crispy Wheats 'N Raisins	¾ cup (1 oz)	100	23	1	2
Fiber One	½ cup (1 oz)	60	23	1	2
Golden Grahams	¾ cup (1 oz)	110	24	1	1
Kaboom	1 cup (1 oz)	110	23	1	2
Kix	1½ cup (1 oz)	110	24	1	2
Lucky Charms	1 cup (1 oz)	110	24	1	2
Raisin Nut Bran	½ cup (1 oz)	110	20	3	3
Total	1 cup (1 oz)	100	22	1	3
Total Corn Flakes	1 cup (1 oz)	110	24	tr	2
Total Raisin Bran	1 cup (1.5 oz)	140	33	1	3
Trix	1 cup (1 oz)	110	25	1	1
Wheaties	1 cup (1 oz)	100	23	1	3
Glenny's					
Maple Frosted Corn	1 oz	109	20	tr	4
Oat Mini Puffs	1 oz	108	22	tr	5
Oat Mini Puffs No Salt No Sugar	1 oz	108	22	tr	5
Rice Mini Puffs	1 oz	109	20	tr	4
Good Shepherd					
Millet Rice Flakes Wheat Free	1 oz	95	19	1	3

FOOD	PORTION	CALS.	CARB.	FAT	PRO.
Good Shepherd (CONT.)					
Spelt Flakes	1 oz	100	21	6	3
Grist Mill					
Apple Cinnamon Natural	½ cup (1.9 oz)	260	36	10	6
Bran	½ cup (1.9 oz)	250	37	8	7
Oat & Honey Natural	½ cup (1.9 oz)	270	34	12	7
Oat Honey & Raisin Natural	½ cup (1.9 oz)	260	35	10	6
Health Valley					
100% Natural Bran With Apples & Cinnamon	¼ cup (1 oz)	100	22	1	3
Blue Corn Flakes 100% Organic	½ cup (1 oz)	90	19	tr	3
Bran Cereal With Dates 100% Organic	¼ cup (1 oz)	100	20	1	4
Fiber 7 Flakes 100% Organic	½ cup (1 oz)	90	20	tr	3
Fruit & Fitness	1 cup (2 oz)	220	37	4	9
Fruit Lites Corn	½ cup (0.5 oz)	45	10	0	2
Fruit Lites Rice	½ cup (0.5 oz)	45	11	1	1
Fruit Lites Wheat	½ cup (0.5 oz)	45	11	1	1
Healthy Crunch Almond Date	¼ cup (1 oz)	110	18	3	4
Healthy Crunch Apple Cinnamon	¼ cup (1 oz)	110	18	3	4
Healthy O's 100% Organic	¾ cup (1 oz)	90	18	1	3
Lites Puffed Corn	½ cup (1 oz)	50	11	0	3
Lites Puffed Rice	½ cup (1 oz)	50	12	0	1
Lites Puffed Wheat	½ cup (1 oz)	50	11	0	2
Oat Bran Flakes 100% Organic	½ cup (1 oz)	100	20	tr	3
Oat Bran O'S 100% Organic	½ cup (1 oz)	110	20	tr	3
Orangeola Almonds & Dates	¼ cup	110	18	3	3
Raisin Bran Flakes 100% Organic	½ cup (1 oz)	100	21	tr	3
Real Oat Bran Almond Crunch	¼ cup (1 oz)	110	17	3	5
Rice Bran O's	½ cup	110	22	1	2
Sprouts 7 Bananas & Hawaiian Fruit	¼ cup (1 oz)	90	16	1	3
Sprouts 7 Raisin	¼ cup	90	16	1	4

FOOD	PORTION	CALS.	CARB.	FAT	PRO.
Health Valley (CONT.)					
Swiss Breakfast Raisin Nut	¼ cup (1 oz)	100	19	3	4
Healthy Choice					
Mulit-Grain Raisins & Almonds	1¼ cup (2 oz)	200	44	2	4
Multi-Grain Flakes	1 cup (1.1 oz)	100	26	0	3
Heartland					
Coconut	1 oz	130	18	5	3
Plain	1 oz	130	18	4	3
Raisin	1 oz	130	18	4	3
Kashi					
Brittles Sesame/Maple	3½ oz	473	65	19	10
Puffed	¾ oz	74	16	1	3
Kellogg's					
All-Bran	½ cup (1 oz)	80	22	1	4
Apple Jacks	1 cup (1 oz)	110	26	0	2
Bran Buds	⅓ cup (1 oz)	70	24	1	3
Cinnamon Mini Buns	¾ cup (1 oz)	120	27	1	1
Cocoa Krispies	¾ cup (1 oz)	120	27	1	2
Common Sense Oat Bran	¾ cup (1 oz)	110	23	1	4
Corn Flakes	1 cup (1 oz)	110	26	0	2
Corn Pops	1 cup (1 oz)	110	27	0	1
Cracklin' Oat Bran	¾ cup (1.9 oz)	230	40	8	4
Crispix	1 cup (1 oz)	110	26	0	2
Froot Loops	1 cup (1 oz)	120	26	1	1
Frosted Mini-Wheats	1 cup (1.9 oz)	190	45	1	5
Frosted Flakes	¾ cup (1 oz)	120	28	0	1
Mueslix Golden Crunch	¾ cup (1.9 oz)	210	40	5	6
Nut & Honey Crunch	1¼ cup (1.9 oz)	220	45	4	4
Product 19	1 cup (1 oz)	110	25	0	3
Raisin Bran	1 cup (1.9 oz)	170	43	1	5
Rice Krispies	1¼ cup (1 oz)	110	26	0	2
Special K	1 cup (1 oz)	110	21	0	6
Temptations French Vanilla Almond	¾ cup (1 oz)	120	24	2	2
Temptations Honey Roasted Pecan	1 cup (1 oz)	120	24	3	2
LaLoma					
Ruskets Biscuits	2 biscuits (30 g)	110	22	0	4
Life					
Cinnamon	⅔ cup	101	19	2	5
Original	⅔ cup	101	19	2	5

FOOD	PORTION	CALS.	CARB.	FAT	PRO.
Mueslix					
Crispy Blend	⅔ cup (1.9 oz)	200	42	2	4
Nabisco					
100% Bran	⅓ cup (1 oz)	70	21	2	3
Shredded Wheat Spoon Size	⅔ cup (1 oz)	90	23	1	3
Nutri-Grain					
Almond Raisin	1¼ cup (1.9 oz)	200	44	2	4
Golden Wheat	¾ cup (1 oz)	100	23	1	3
Post					
Alpha-Bits	1 cup (1 oz)	111	24	1	2
Cocoa Pebbles	⅞ cup (1 oz)	113	25	1	1
Fruit & Fibre Dates Raisins Walnuts With Oat Clusters	⅔ cup	120	27	2	3
Grape-Nuts	¼ cup (1 oz)	105	23	0	3
Grape-Nuts Raisin	¼ cup (1 oz)	102	23	0	3
Honey Bunches Of Oats Honey Roasted	⅔ cup (1 oz)	111	23	2	2
Honeycomb	1⅓ cups (1 oz)	110	26	0	2
Natural Bran Flakes	⅔ cup (1 oz)	88	23	0	3
Oat Flakes	⅔ cup (1 oz)	107	22	1	5
Post Toasties Corn Flakes	1¼ cup (1 oz)	111	24	0	2
Raisin Bran	⅔ cup (40 g)	122	32	1	3
Quaker					
100% Natural	¼ cup	127	18	6	3
King Vitaman	1½ cup	110	23	1	2
Puffed Rice	1 cup	54	13	tr	1
Puffed Wheat	1 cup	50	11	tr	2
Shredded Wheat	2 biscuits	132	32	1	4
Ralston					
Bran Flakes	¾ cup (1.1 oz)	110	24	1	3
Chex Multi-Bran	1¼ cup (2 oz)	220	46	2	5
Cocoa Crispy Rice	1 cup (1.8 oz)	200	45	1	3
Cookie Crisp	1 cup (1 oz)	120	25	2	1
Frosted Flakes	¾ cup (1.1 oz)	120	28	0	1
Muesli Blueberry	1 cup (1.9 oz)	200	41	3	5
Muesli Cranberry	¾ cup (1.9 oz)	200	40	3	5
Muesli Strawberry	1 cup (1.9 oz)	210	41	3	5
Raisin Bran	¾ cup (1.9 oz)	190	41	1	5
Tasteeos	1¼ cup (1.1 oz)	130	22	3	5
Smacks					
Cereal	¾ cup (1 oz)	110	26	1	2

FOOD	PORTION	CALS.	CARB.	FAT	PRO.
Stone-Buhr					
7 Grain	⅓ cup (1.6 oz)	140	31	2	6
Bran Flakes	¼ cup (0.6 oz)	64	14	0	2
Sunbelt					
Muesli	1.9 oz	210	44	2	4
Team					
Cereal	1 cup	110	24	1	2
US Mills					
Poppets	1 oz	110	24	1	2
Uncle Sam	1 oz	110	20	1	4
Weetabix					
Cereal	2 (1.3 oz)	142	31	1	4

CHAMPAGNE

FOOD	PORTION	CALS.	CARB.	FAT	PRO.
sekt german champagne	3.5 fl oz	84	5	0	tr
Andre					
Blush	1 fl oz	22	1	0	0
Brut	1 fl oz	21	1	0	0
Cold Duck	1 fl oz	25	2	0	0
Extra Dry	1 fl oz	23	1	0	0
Ballatore					
Spumante	1 fl oz	23	2	0	0
Eden Roc					
Brut	1 fl oz	21	1	0	0
Brut Rosé	1 fl oz	22	2	0	0
Extra Dry	1 fl oz	21	1	0	0
Tott's					
Blanc de Noir	1 fl oz	22	2	0	0
Brut	1 fl oz	20	tr	0	0
Extra Dry	1 fl oz	21	1	0	0

CHAYOTE

FOOD	PORTION	CALS.	CARB.	FAT	PRO.
fresh cooked	1 cup	38	8	1	1
raw cut up	1 cup	32	7	tr	1

CHEESE

(*see also* CHEESE DISHES, CHEESE SUBSTITUTES, COTTAGE CHEESE, CREAM CHEESE)

NATURAL

FOOD	PORTION	CALS.	CARB.	FAT	PRO.
bel paese	3½ oz	391	0	30	25
blue	1 oz	100	1	8	6
blue crumbled	1 cup	477	3	39	29
brick	1 oz	105	1	8	7
brie	1 oz	95	tr	8	8
cacio di roma sheep's milk cheese	1 oz	130	0	10	8

FOOD	PORTION	CALS.	CARB.	FAT	PRO.
caerphilly	1.4 oz	150	0	13	9
camembert	1 oz	85	tr	7	6
camembert	1 wedge (1 ⅓ oz)	114	tr	9	8
caraway	1 oz	107	1	8	7
cheddar	1 oz	114	tr	9	7
cheddar low fat	1 oz	49	1	2	9
cheddar low sodium	1 oz	113	1	9	7
cheddar reduced fat	1.4 oz	104	0	6	13
cheddar shredded	1 cup	455	1	37	28
cheshire	1 oz	110	1	9	7
cheshire reduced fat	1.4 oz	108	tr	6	13
colby	1 oz	112	1	9	7
colby low fat	1 oz	49	1	2	9
colby low sodium	1 oz	113	1	9	7
derby	1.4 oz	161	0	14	10
edam	1 oz	101	tr	8	7
edam reduced fat	1.4 oz	92	tr	4	13
emmentaler	3½ oz	403	tr	30	29
feta	1 oz	75	1	6	4
fontina	1 oz	110	tr	9	7
fromage frais	1.6 oz	51	3	3	3
gjetost	1 oz	132	12	8	3
gloucester double	1.4 oz	162	0	14	10
goat hard	1 oz	128	1	10	9
goat semi-soft	1 oz	103	1	8	6
goat soft	1 oz	76	tr	6	5
gorgonzola	3½ oz	376	1	31	19
gouda	1 oz	101	1	8	7
gruyere	1 oz	117	tr	9	8
lancashire	1.4 oz	149	0	12	9
leicester	1.4 oz	160	0	14	10
limburger	1 oz	93	tr	8	6
lymeswold	1.4 oz	170	tr	16	6
monterey	1 oz	106	tr	9	7
mozzarella	1 lb	1276	10	98	88
mozzarella	1 oz	80	1	6	6
mozzarella low moisture	1 oz	90	1	7	6
mozzarella low moisture part skim	1 oz	79	1	5	8
mozzarella part skim	1 oz	72	1	5	7
muenster	1 oz	104	tr	9	7
parmesan grated	1 oz	129	1	9	12
parmesan grated	1 tbsp	23	tr	2	2
parmesan hard	1 oz	111	1	7	10

FOOD	PORTION	CALS.	CARB.	FAT	PRO.
port du salut	1 oz	100	tr	8	7
provolone	1 oz	100	1	8	7
quark 20% fat	3½ oz	116	3	5	13
quark 40% fat	3½ oz	167	3	11	11
quark made w/ skim milk	3½ oz	78	4	tr	14
queso anego	1 oz	106	1	9	6
queso asadero	1 oz	101	1	8	6
queso chichuahua	1 oz	106	2	8	6
ricotta	1 cup	428	7	32	28
ricotta	½ cup	216	4	16	14
ricotta part skim	1 cup	340	13	19	28
ricotta part skim	½ cup	171	6	10	14
romadur 40% fat	3½ oz	289	tr	20	23
romano	1 oz	110	1	8	9
roquefort	1 oz	105	1	9	6
stilton blue	1.4 oz	164	0	14	9
stilton white	1.4 oz	145	0	13	8
swiss	1 oz	107	1	8	8
tilsit	1 oz	96	1	7	7
wensleydale	1.4 oz	151	0	13	9
whey cheese	3.5 oz	440	33	27	15
Alouette					
Brie Baby With Herbs	1 oz	110	2	9	5
Alpine Lace					
Cheddar Reduced Fat	1 piece (1 oz)	80	1	5	9
Colby Reduced Fat	1 piece (1 oz)	80	1	5	9
Feta Reduced Fat	1 piece (1 oz)	60	1	4	5
Muenster Reduced Sodium	1 piece (1 oz)	100	1	9	7
Provolone Smoked Reduced Fat	1 piece (1 oz)	70	1	5	9
Swiss Reduced Fat	1 piece (1 oz)	90	1	6	8
Armour					
Cheddar Lower Salt	1 oz	110	—	9	7
Monterey Jack Lower Salt	1 oz	110	—	9	7
BabyBel					
Mini Light	1 (0.7 oz)	45	0	3	6
Bongrain					
Montrachet	1 oz	70	tr	6	4
Bresse					
Brie Light	1 oz	70	1	4	8
Brier Run					
Cherve	1 oz	61	—	5	3

FOOD	PORTION	CALS.	CARB.	FAT	PRO.
Cabot					
Vitalait	1 oz	70	1	4	8
Di Giorno					
Parmesan Grated	2 tsp (5 g)	20	0	2	2
Romano Grated	2 tsp (5 g)	25	0	2	2
Dorman					
Provolone Reduced Fat Low Sodium	1 oz	80	1	4	9
Swiss No Salt Added	1 oz	100	tr	8	8
Swiss Reduced Fat Low Sodium	1 oz	90	tr	5	10
Friendship					
Farmer	2 tbsp (1 oz)	50	0	3	5
Farmer No Salt Added	2 tbsp (1 oz)	50	0	3	5
Hoop	2 tbsp (1 oz)	20	0	0	5
Frigo					
Asiago	1 oz	110	1	9	7
Feta	1 oz	100	1	8	6
Parmesan & Romano Dry Grated	1 oz	130	1	9	12
Pizza Shredded	1 oz	65	1	3	9
Ricotta Low Fat Low Salt	1 oz	30	1	1	3
Ricotta Part Skim	1 oz	40	1	3	3
Ricotta Whole Milk	1 oz	60	1	5	3
String	1 oz	80	1	5	7
String Lite	1 oz	60	1	2	9
Taco Shredded	1 oz	110	1	9	7
Healthy Choice					
Cheddar Fancy Shreds	¼ cup (1 oz)	45	2	0	9
Mozzarella Fancy Shreds	¼ cup (1 oz)	45	2	0	9
Pizza Fancy Shreds	¼ cup (1 oz)	45	2	0	9
Heluva Good Cheese					
Cheddar Mild White	1 oz	110	1	9	7
Cheddar Sharp	1 oz	110	1	9	7
Washed Curd Cheese	1 oz	110	1	9	7
Hollow Road Farms					
Sheep's Milk	1 oz	45	1	3	3
Keller's					
Chub	2 tbsp (1 oz)	100	1	10	2
Kraft					
Blue Crumbles	1 oz	100	tr	8	6
Brick	1 oz	110	0	9	6
Cheddar Nacho Blend With Peppers	1 oz	110	0	9	7

FOOD	PORTION	CALS.	CARB.	FAT	PRO.
Kraft (CONT.)					
Havarti	1 oz	120	0	11	6
Italian Blend Grated	2 tsp (0.2 oz)	25	0	2	3
Mozzarella Fat Free Shredded	¼ cup (1 oz)	50	2	0	9
Provolone Smoke Flavor	1 oz	100	tr	7	7
Shredded	¼ cup (1 oz)	120	tr	10	7
String With Jalapeno Peppers	1 oz	80	1	5	8
Swiss	1 oz	110	0	9	8
Swiss Shredded	¼ cup (1 oz)	80	0	9	8
Taco Cheddar & Monterey Jack Shredded	¼ cup (0.9 oz)	100	tr	8	6
Land O'Lakes					
Baby Swiss	1 oz	110	0	8	7
Brick	1 oz	100	tr	8	7
Chedarella	1 oz	100	0	8	7
Mozzarella	1 oz	80	tr	6	7
Laughing Cow					
Babybel	1 oz	90	0	7	7
Babybel Mini	1 (0.7 oz)	70	0	6	5
Bonbel	1 oz	100	0	8	6
Bonbel Mini	1 (0.7 oz)	70	0	6	5
Gouda Mini	1 (0.7 oz)	80	0	6	5
Marin French Cheese					
Breakfast	1 oz	86	1	7	5
Brie	1 oz	86	1	7	5
Camembert	1 oz	86	1	7	5
Schloss	1 oz	86	1	7	5
New Holland					
Havarti Lower Fat Garden Vegetable	1 oz	80	0	6	6
Polly-O					
Mozzarella Free	1 oz	35	tr	0	7
Mozzarella Lite	1 oz	60	tr	3	7
Mozzarella Part Skim	1 oz	70	tr	5	6
Mozzarella Shredded Lite	¼ cup	60	1	3	8
Mozzarella Whole Milk	1 oz	80	tr	6	6
Ricotta Free	¼ cup	50	2	0	10
Ricotta Lite	¼ cup	70	3	3	8
Ricotta Part Skim	¼ cup	90	2	6	8
Ricotta Whole Milk	¼ cup	110	2	8	7

FOOD	PORTION	CALS.	CARB.	FAT	PRO.
Polly-O (CONT.)					
String	1 oz	80	1	6	7
Sargento					
4 Cheese Mexican Recipe Blend Shredded	¼ cup (1 oz)	110	tr	9	6
Jarlsberg	1 slice (1.2 oz)	120	1	9	9
MooTown Snacker Cheese & Sticks	1 pkg (1 oz)	100	13	4	3
MooTown Snacker String	1 piece (0.8 oz)	70	tr	5	6
MooTown Snackers Cheddar	1 piece (0.8 oz)	100	1	8	5
MooTown Snackers Cheddar Mild Light	1 piece (0.8 oz)	60	tr	4	7
MooTown Snackers Cheese & Pretzels	1 pkg (1 oz)	90	12	3	3
MooTown Snackers Colby-Jack	1 piece (0.8 oz)	90	tr	8	5
MooTown Snackers Pizza Cheese & Sticks	1 pkg (1 oz)	100	13	4	3
MooTown Snackers String Light	1 piece (0.8 oz)	60	tr	3	7
Treasure Cave					
Blue Crumbled	1 oz	110	tr	9	6
Tree Of Life					
Cheddar 33% Reduced Fat Organic Milk	1 oz	90	1	6	8
Cheddar Low Sodium Raw Milk	1 oz	110	0	9	7
Colby Organic Milk	1 oz	120	1	10	7
Colby Raw Milk	1 oz	110	1	9	7
Farmer Part-Skim Organic Milk	1 oz	90	1	6	7
Jalapeno Jack Organic Milk	1 oz	110	1	9	6
Jalapeno Jack Semi-Soft Organic Milk	1 oz	110	0	9	7
Monterey Jack 35% Reduced Fat Organic Milk	1 oz	80	1	5	8
Monterey Jack Organic Milk	1 oz	100	1	8	6
Monterey Jack Semi-Soft Raw Milk	1 oz	110	0	9	7

FOOD	PORTION	CALS.	CARB.	FAT	PRO.
Tree Of Life (CONT.)					
Mozzarella Low Moisture Part Skim Organic Milk	1 oz	80	1	5	8
Muenster Organic Milk	1 oz	100	1	8	6
Muenster Semi-Soft Raw Milk	1 oz	100	0	9	7
Swiss Raw Milk	1 oz	110	1	8	8
Weight Watchers					
Cheddar Sharp White	1 oz	80	1	5	8
Cheddar Sharp Yellow	1 oz	80	1	5	8
PROCESSED					
american	1 oz	93	2	7	6
Alouette					
French Onion	2 tbsp (0.8 oz)	70	1	7	2
Garlic	2 tbsp (0.8 oz)	70	1	7	1
Light Garlic	2 tbsp (0.8 oz)	50	1	4	2
Alpine Lace					
American	1 slice (0.66 oz)	50	1	3	4
American Fat Free	1 piece (1 oz)	45	2	tr	8
Cheddar Fat Free	1 piece (1 oz)	45	2	tr	8
Fat Free Singles	1 slice (0.66 oz)	25	tr	0	5
Mozzarella Fat Free	1 piece (1 oz)	45	2	tr	8
Borden					
American Slices	1 oz	110	1	9	6
Swiss Slices	1 oz	100	1	8	7
Cheez Whiz					
Light	2 tbsp (1.2 oz)	80	6	3	6
Spread	2 tbsp (1.2 oz)	90	2	7	5
Spread Hot Salsa	2 tbsp (1.2 oz)	90	2	7	5
Squeezable	2 tbsp (1.2 oz)	100	4	8	2
Cracker Barrel					
Cheddar Extra Sharp	2 tbsp (1.1 oz)	100	3	8	5
Delico					
Alouette Cajun	2 tbsp (0.8 oz)	70	1	7	1
Alouette Garden Vegetable	2 tbsp (0.8 oz)	60	1	6	1
Dorman's					
Lo-Chol Cheddar	1 oz	100	1	7	7
Lo-Chol Muenster	1 oz	100	1	7	7
Formagg					
Formaggio D'Oro	1 oz	70	1	5	6
Handi-Snacks					
Cheez'n Breadsticks	1 pkg (1.1 oz)	130	11	7	4

FOOD	PORTION	CALS.	CARB.	FAT	PRO.
Handi-Snacks (CONT.)					
Cheez'n Pretzels	1 pkg (1 oz)	110	11	6	4
Cheez'n Crackers	1 pkg (1.1 oz)	130	10	8	4
Mozzarella String Cheese	1 stick (1 oz)	80	tr	6	7
Harvest Moon					
American	1 slice (0.7 oz)	70	0	6	4
Healthy Choice					
American Singles White	1 slice (0.7 oz)	30	2	0	5
American Singles Yellow	1 slice (0.7 oz)	30	2	0	5
Heluva Good Cheese					
American	1 slice (0.7 oz)	45	2	5	4
Cold Pack Cheddar Sharp With Horseradish	2 tbsp (1 oz)	90	3	7	5
Kraft					
American Grated	1 tbsp (0.2 oz)	25	1	2	1
Cheese With Jalapeno Peppers	1 oz	60	2	7	5
Deluxe American	1 slice (0.7 oz)	70	tr	6	4
Deluxe American White	1 slice (0.7 oz)	70	tr	6	4
Deluxe Swiss	1 slice (1 oz)	90	tr	7	7
Free Singles	1 slice (0.7 oz)	30	3	0	5
Free Singles Swiss	1 slice (0.7 oz)	30	3	0	5
Spread Pimento	2 tbsp (1.1 oz)	80	3	6	2
Lactaid					
American	3.5 oz	328	7	25	20
Land O'Lakes					
American Less Salt	1 oz	110	tr	9	6
American Light	1 oz	70	2	5	7
Jalapeno Light	1 oz	70	1	4	7
Laughing Cow					
Assorted Wedge	1 (1 oz)	70	1	6	4
Cheesebits	6 pieces (1 oz)	70	1	6	4
Original Wedge	1 (1 oz)	70	1	6	4
Light N'Lively					
Singles 50% Less Fat American	0.7 oz	50	2	3	5
Mohawk Valley					
Spread Limburger	2 tbsp (1.1 oz)	80	0	7	4
Old English					
American Sharp	1 oz	100	tr	9	6
Roka					
Spread Blue	2 tbsp (1.1 oz)	80	2	7	3

FOOD	PORTION	CALS.	CARB.	FAT	PRO.
Rondele					
Light Soft Spreadable Garlic & Herb	2 tbsp (0.9 oz)	60	2	4	4
Soft Spreadable Garlic & Herbs	2 tbsp (1 oz)	100	1	9	2
Smart Beat					
American	1 slice (0.6 oz)	35	2	2	4
Low Sodium	1 slice (0.6 oz)	35	2	2	4
Sharp	1 slice (0.6 oz)	35	2	2	4
Spreadery					
Vermont Sharp White Cheddar	2 tbsp (1.1 oz)	80	3	5	5
Velveeta					
Cheese	1 slice (0.7 oz)	60	2	5	4
Light	1 oz	60	3	3	6
Shredded	¼ cup (1.3 oz)	130	3	9	8
Weight Watchers					
American Slices Low Sodium White	2 slices (⅔ oz)	35	2	1	4
American Slices Low Sodium Yellow	2 slices (⅔ oz)	35	2	1	4
American Slices White	2 slices (⅔ oz)	35	1	1	4
American Slices Yellow	2 slices (⅔ oz)	35	1	1	4
Swiss Slices	2 slices (⅔ oz)	35	2	1	4
WisPride					
Hickory Smoked Cup	2 tbsp (1.1 oz)	100	4	7	4
Port Wine Ball	2 tbsp (1.1 oz)	100	4	8	4
Port Wine Cup	2 tbsp (1.1 oz)	100	4	7	4
Port Wine Light Cup	2 tbsp (1.1 oz)	80	5	3	5

CHEESE DISHES
HOME RECIPE

FOOD	PORTION	CALS.	CARB.	FAT	PRO.
welsh rarebit as prep w/ 1 white toast	1 slice	228	14	16	8
TAKE-OUT					
cheese omelette as prep w/ 2 eggs	1 (6.8 oz)	519	tr	44	31
fondue	½ cup (3.8 oz)	247	4	15	15
macaroni & cheese	6.3 oz	320	25	19	13

CHEESE SUBSTITUTES

FOOD	PORTION	CALS.	CARB.	FAT	PRO.
mozzarella	1 oz	70	7	3	3
Borden					
Taco-Mate	1 oz	100	2	7	6
Cheese Two	1 oz	90	2	7	5

FOOD	PORTION	CALS.	CARB.	FAT	PRO.
Formagg					
American White	1 slice (0.66 oz)	60	tr	4	4
American Yellow	1 slice (0.66 oz)	60	tr	4	4
Caesar's Italian Garden American	1 oz	60	1	3	7
Cheddar	1 slice (0.66 oz)	60	tr	4	4
Cheddar Shredded	1 oz	60	1	3	7
Classic American	1 oz	60	1	3	7
Macaroni And Cheese Sauce	⅔ cup (5 oz)	190	35	2	7
Mozzarella Shredded	1 oz	60	1	3	7
Old World Mozzarella	1 oz	60	1	3	7
Parmesan Grated	2 tsp (5 g)	15	tr	1	2
Swiss	1 oz	60	1	3	7
Swiss White	1 slice (0.66 oz)	60	tr	4	4
Vintage Provolone	1 oz	60	1	3	7
Zesty Jalapeno American	1 oz	60	1	3	7
Frigo					
Imitation Cheddar	1 oz	90	1	7	5
Imitation Mozzeralla	1 oz	90	1	7	6
Georgio's					
Imitation Cheddar Shredded	¼ cup (1 oz)	90	1	7	6
Imitation Mozzarella Shredded	¼ cup (1 oz)	90	1	7	6
Golden Image					
American	0.7 oz	70	1	5	5
Harvest Moon					
American Shredded	¼ cup (1.3 oz)	120	3	9	6
Cheddar Shredded	¼ cup (1.3 oz)	120	3	9	6
Mozzarella Shredded	¼ cup (1.3 oz)	110	1	8	8
Lunchwagon					
American	1 slice (0.7 oz)	70	1	5	4
Sargento					
Classic Supreme Cheddar Shredded	¼ cup (1 oz)	90	2	6	5
Classic Supreme Mozzarella Shredded	¼ cup (1 oz)	80	tr	6	6
Fancy Supreme Cheddar Shredded	¼ cup (1 oz)	90	2	6	5
White Wave					
Soy A Melt Cheddar	1 oz	80	1	5	8
Soy A Melt Fat Free Cheddar	1 oz	40	3	tr	7

FOOD	PORTION	CALS.	CARB.	FAT	PRO.
White Wave (CONT.)					
Soy A Melt Fat Free Mozzarella	1 oz	40	3	tr	7
Soy A Melt Garlic Herb	1 oz	80	1	5	8
Soy A Melt Jalapeno Jack	1 oz	80	1	5	8
Soy A Melt Monterey Jack	1 oz	80	1	5	8
Soy A Melt Mozzarella	1 oz	80	1	5	8
Soy A Melt Singles American	1 slice (¾ oz)	60	1	4	5
Soy A Melt Singles Mozzarella	1 slice (¾ oz)	60	1	4	5

CHERIMOYA
fresh	1	515	131	2	7

CHERRIES
CANNED
sour in heavy syrup	½ cup	232	60	tr	2
sour in light syrup	½ cup	189	49	tr	2
sour water packed	1 cup	87	22	tr	2
sweet in heavy syrup	½ cup	107	27	tr	1
sweet in light syrup	½ cup	85	22	tr	1
sweet juice pack	½ cup	68	17	tr	1
sweet water pack	½ cup	57	15	tr	1
Del Monte					
Dark Pitted In Heavy Syrup	½ cup (4.2 oz)	120	24	0	tr
Sweet Dark Whole Unpitted In Heavy Syrup	½ cup (4.2 oz)	120	24	0	tr
DRIED					
Chukar					
Bing	2 oz	160	35	1	2
Rainer	2 oz	160	35	1	2
Tart	2 oz	170	43	0	2
Tart 'n Sweet	2 oz	180	43	0	2
Sonoma					
Pitted	¼ cup (1.4 oz)	140	34	0	1
FRESH					
sour	1 cup	51	13	tr	1
sweet	10	49	11	1	1
Dole					
Cherries	1 cup	90	19	1	1

FOOD	PORTION	CALS.	CARB.	FAT	PRO.
FROZEN					
sour unsweetened	1 cup	72	17	1	1
sweet sweetened	1 cup	232	58	tr	3
Big Valley					
Dark Sweet	¾ cup (4.9 oz)	90	20	0	1
CHERRY JUICE					
After The Fall					
Black Cherry	1 can (12 oz)	170	42	0	0
Hi-C					
Box	8.45 fl oz	140	35	0	0
Drink	8 fl oz	130	33	0	0
Juicy Juice					
Drink	1 box (8.45 fl oz)	130	30	0	1
Drink	1 bottle (6 fl oz)	90	23	0	1
Kool-Aid					
Black Cherry	8 oz	98	25	0	0
Drink	8 oz	98	25	0	0
Koolers	1 (8.45 oz)	142	38	0	0
Sugar Free	8 oz	3	0	0	0
Smucker's					
Black Cherry	8 oz	130	31	0	0
Black Cherry Sparkler	10 oz	120	30	tr	tr
Tang					
Fruit Box	8.45 oz	121	32	0	0
Tree Of Life					
Concentrate	8 tsp (1.4 oz)	110	28	0	0
Wylers					
Drink Mix Unsweetened Cherry	8 oz	2	1	0	0
Drink Mix Wild Cherry	8 oz	81	21	0	0
CHESTNUTS					
chinese cooked	1 oz	44	10	tr	1
chinese dried	1 oz	103	23	tr	2
chinese raw	1 oz	64	14	tr	1
chinese roasted	1 oz	68	15	tr	1
cooked	1 oz	37	8	tr	1
dried peeled	1 oz	105	22	1	1
japanese cooked	1 oz	16	4	tr	tr
japanese dried	1 oz	102	23	tr	1
japanese raw	1 oz	44	10	tr	1
japanese roasted	1 oz	57	13	tr	1

FOOD	PORTION	CALS.	CARB.	FAT	PRO.
raw peeled	1 oz	56	13	tr	tr
roasted	1 cup	350	76	3	5
roasted	1 oz	70	15	1	1

CHEWING GUM

FOOD	PORTION	CALS.	CARB.	FAT	PRO.
bubble gum	1 block (8 g)	27	8	0	0
stick	1 (3 g)	10	3	0	0
Bazooka					
Fruit Chunk	1 piece (6 g)	25	5	0	0
Fruit Soft	1 piece (6 g)	25	5	0	0
Gum	1 piece (4 g)	15	4	0	0
Gum	1 piece (6 g)	25	5	0	0
Beech-Nut					
Peppermint	1 stick (3 g)	10	2	0	0
Spearmint	1 stick (3 g)	10	2	0	0
Big Red					
Stick	1	10	2	tr	tr
Brock					
Bubble Gum	1 piece (0.2 oz)	20	4	0	0
Bubble Yum					
Bananaberry Split	1 piece (0.3 oz)	25	6	0	0
Cotton Candy	1 piece (0.3 oz)	25	6	0	0
Grape	1 piece (0.3 oz)	25	6	0	0
Luscious Lime	1 piece (0.3 oz)	25	6	0	0
Peppermint Sugarless	1 piece (0.2 oz)	15	3	0	0
Regular	1 piece (0.3 oz)	25	6	0	0
Sour Apple	1 piece (0.3 oz)	25	6	0	0
Sour Cherry	1 piece (0.3 oz)	25	6	0	0
Sugarless	1 piece (0.2 oz)	15	3	0	0
Sugarless Grape	1 piece (0.2 oz)	15	3	0	0
Sugarless Strawberry	1 piece (0.2 oz)	15	3	0	0
Sugarless Variety	1 piece (0.2 oz)	15	3	0	0
Variety Pack	1 piece (0.3 oz)	25	6	0	0
Watermelon	1 piece (0.3 oz)	25	6	0	0
Wild Strawberry	1 piece (0.3 oz)	25	6	0	0
Bubblicious					
Gum	1 piece (7.9 g)	25	6	0	0
*Care*Free*					
Bubble Gum Sugarless	1 stick (3 g)	10	2	0	0
Sugarless Cinnamon	1 piece (3 g)	5	2	0	0
Sugarless Peppermint	1 piece (3 g)	5	2	0	0
Sugarless Spearmint	1 piece (3 g)	5	2	0	0
Wild Cherry Sugarless	1 stick (3 g)	10	2	0	0
Chiclets					
Original	1 piece (1.59 g)	6	2	0	0

FOOD	PORTION	CALS.	CARB.	FAT	PRO.
Chiclets (CONT.)					
Tiny Size	8 pieces (0.13 g)	tr	tr	0	0
Clorets	1 piece (1.59 g)	6	2	0	0
Dentyne					
Cinn-A-Burst	1 piece (3.2 g)	9	2	0	0
Gum	1 piece (1.88 g)	6	1	0	0
Sugar Free	1 piece (1.88 g)	5	1	0	0
Doublemint					
Chewing Gum	1 piece	10	2	tr	tr
Extra Sugar Free					
Cinnamon	1 piece	8	tr	tr	tr
Spearmint & Peppermint	1 stick	8	tr	tr	tr
Winter Fresh	1 piece	8	tr	tr	tr
Freedent					
Spearmint Peppermint & Cinnamon	1 stick	10	3	tr	tr
Freshen-Up					
Gum	1 piece (4.2 g)	13	3	0	0
Fruit Stripe					
Bubble Gum Jumbo Pack	1 stick (3 g)	10	2	0	0
Variety Pack Chewing & Bubble Gum	1 stick (3 g)	10	2	0	0
Hubba Bubba					
Bubble Gum Cola	1 piece	23	6	tr	tr
Bubble Gum Sugarfree Grape	1 piece	13	tr	tr	tr
Bubble Gum Sugarfree Original	1 piece	14	tr	tr	tr
Original	1 piece	23	6	tr	tr
Strawberry Grape Raspberry	1 piece	23	6	tr	tr
Juicy Fruit					
Stick	1	10	2	tr	tr
Rain-Blo					
Bubble Gum Balls	1 piece (2 g)	5	2	0	0
Stick*Free					
Sugarless Peppermint	1 stick (3 g)	10	2	0	0
Sugarless Spearmint	1 stick (3 g)	10	2	0	0
Swell					
Bubble Gum	1 piece (3 g)	10	2	0	0
Trident					
Gum	1 piece (1.88 g)	5	1	0	0

FOOD	PORTION	CALS.	CARB.	FAT	PRO.
Trident (cont.)					
Soft Bubble Gum	1 piece (3.3 g)	9	2	0	0
Wrigley's					
Spearmint	1 stick	10	2	tr	tr

CHICKEN

(*see also* CHICKEN DISHES, CHICKEN SUBSTITUTES, DINNER, HOT DOGS)

FOOD	PORTION	CALS.	CARB.	FAT	PRO.
CANNED					
chicken spread	1 tbsp	25	1	2	2
w/ broth	1 can (5 oz)	234	0	11	31
Hormel					
No Salt Chunk Breast	2 oz	60	0	2	12
FRESH					
broiler/fryer breast w/ skin batter dipped & fried	½ breast (4.9 oz)	364	13	18	35
broiler/fryer breast w/ skin roasted	½ breast (3.4 oz)	193	0	8	29
broiler/fryer breast w/ skin stewed	½ breast (3.9 oz)	202	0	8	30
broiler/fryer breast w/o skin roasted	½ breast (3 oz)	142	0	3	27
broiler/fryer drumstick w/ skin batter dipped & fried	1 (2.6 oz)	193	6	11	16
broiler/fryer drumstick w/ skin floured & fried	1 (1.7 oz)	120	1	7	13
broiler/fryer drumstick w/ skin roasted	1 (1.8 oz)	112	0	6	14
broiler/fryer drumstick w/ skin stewed	1 (2 oz)	116	0	6	14
broiler/fryer drumstick w/o skin fried	1 (1.5 oz)	82	0	3	12
broiler/fryer drumstick w/o skin roasted	1 (1.5 oz)	76	0	2	12
broiler/fryer drumstick w/o skin stewed	1 (1.6 oz)	78	0	3	13
broiler/fryer leg w/ skin batter dipped & fried	1 (5.5 oz)	431	14	26	34
broiler/fryer leg w/ skin floured & fried	1 (3.9 oz)	285	3	16	30
broiler/fryer leg w/ skin roasted	1 (4 oz)	265	0	15	30
broiler/fryer leg w/ skin stewed	1 (4.4 oz)	275	0	16	30

FOOD	PORTION	CALS.	CARB.	FAT	PRO.
broiler/fryer leg w/o skin fried	1 (3.3 oz)	195	1	9	27
broiler/fryer leg w/o skin roasted	1 (3.3 oz)	182	0	8	26
broiler/fryer leg w/o skin stewed	1 (3.5 oz)	187	0	8	26
broiler/fryer neck w/ skin stewed	1 (1.3 oz)	94	0	7	7
broiler/fryer skin roasted	from ½ chicken (2 oz)	254	0	23	11
broiler/fryer thigh w/ skin batter dipped & fried	1 (3 oz)	238	8	14	19
broiler/fryer thigh w/ skin floured & fried	1 (2.2 oz)	162	2	9	17
broiler/fryer thigh w/ skin roasted	1 (2.2 oz)	153	0	10	16
broiler/fryer thigh w/ skin stewed	1 (2.4 oz)	158	0	10	16
broiler/fryer thigh w/o skin fried	1 (1.8 oz)	113	1	5	15
broiler/fryer thigh w/o skin roasted	1 (1.8 oz)	109	0	6	13
broiler/fryer thigh w/o skin stewed	1 (1.9 oz)	107	0	5	14
broiler/fryer w/ skin floured & fried	½ chicken (11 oz)	844	10	47	90
broiler/fryer w/ skin fried	½ chicken (16.4 oz)	1347	44	81	81
broiler/fryer w/ skin roasted	½ chicken (10.5 oz)	715	0	41	82
broiler/fryer w/ skin stewed	½ chicken (11.7 oz)	730	0	42	82
broiler/fryer w/o skin roasted	1 cup (5 oz)	266	0	10	41
broiler/fryer w/o skin stewed	1 cup (5 oz)	248	0	9	38
broiler/fryer wing w/ skin batter dipped & fried	1 (1.7 oz)	159	5	11	10
broiler/fryer wing w/ skin floured & fried	1 (1.1 oz)	103	1	7	8
broiler/fryer wing w/ skin roasted	1 (1.2 oz)	99	0	7	9
broiler/fryer wing w/ skin stewed	1 (1.4 oz)	100	0	7	9
cornish hen w/o skin & bone roasted	½ hen (2 oz)	72	0	2	13

FOOD	PORTION	CALS.	CARB.	FAT	PRO.
cornish hen w/o skin & bone roasted	1 hen (3.8 oz)	144	0	4	25
cornish hen w/skin roasted	1 hen (8 oz)	595	0	42	51
cornish hen w/skin roasted	½ hen (4 oz)	296	0	21	25
Perdue					
Breast Skinless Boneless cooked	1 oz	30	0	tr	6
Breast Split Fresh Young w/ Skin cooked	1 oz	45	0	3	6
Breast Thin-Sliced Skinless & Boneless Oven Stuffer cooked	1 oz	31	0	tr	7
Wampler Longacre					
Ground raw	1 oz	50	0	4	4
FROZEN					
Tyson					
Boneless Breasts	3.5 oz	210	0	12	26
Boneless Skinless Breast	3.5 oz	130	0	2	27
Boneless Skinless Thighs	3.5 oz	200	0	10	26
Drums & Thighs	3.5 oz	270	0	17	28
Skinless Breast Tenders	3.5 oz	120	0	1	28
FROZEN PREPARED					
Banquet					
Country Fried	1 serv (3 oz)	270	13	18	14
Drum Snackers	2.25 oz	190	12	13	9
Fried Breast	1 piece (4.45 oz)	240	18	26	23
Fried Chicken Thigh & Drumsticks	1 serv (3 oz)	260	10	18	15
Hot & Spicy Nuggets	2.5 oz	230	11	17	9
Wings Hot & Spicy	4 pieces (5 oz)	230	5	16	15
Country Skillet					
Chicken Nuggets	10 (3.3 oz)	280	16	18	14
Chicken Patties	2.5 oz	190	12	12	9
Empire					
Nuggets	5 (3 oz)	180	12	9	13
Stix	4 (3.1 oz)	180	6	9	18
Sensible Chef					
Fried Breast	1 (3 oz)	200	8	10	21
Swanson					
Chicken Nuggets	3 oz	230	14	14	13
Fried Chicken Breast Portion	4½ oz	360	21	20	23

FOOD	PORTION	CALS.	CARB.	FAT	PRO.
Tyson					
BBQ Breast Fillets	3 oz	110	13	2	14
Chick'n Cheddar	2.6 oz	220	11	15	11
Cordon Blue Mini	1	90	5	4	8
Grilled Sandwich	3.5 oz	200	25	5	15
Hors D'Oeuvres Mesquite Chunks	3.5 oz	100	1	1	22
Hot BBQ Breast Tenders	2.75 oz	110	4	3	16
Mesquite Breast Fillets	2.75 oz	100	3	2	16
Microwave Chunks	3.5 oz	220	11	15	10
Microwave Chunks BBQ Sandwich	4 oz	230	27	6	16
Weaver					
Breast Fillets	4.5 oz	270	18	13	20
Breast Patties	3 oz	205	14	11	12
Chicken Nuggets	2.6 oz	190	10	12	10
Crispy Dutch Frye Assorted	3.6 oz	290	16	18	16
Crispy Dutch Frye Breasts	4.5 oz	350	17	22	22
Crispy Dutch Frye Drums & Thighs	3.5 oz	290	14	19	16
Crispy Dutch Frye Wings	4 oz	400	20	28	16
Crispy Light Skinless	2.9 oz	170	9	9	14
Croquettes	2 pieces	280	22	16	14
Croquettes With Gravy	2 pieces + ½ cup gravy	282	26	18	15
Hot Wings	2.7 oz	170	1	11	17
Mini Drums Crispy	3 oz	210	13	12	13
Mini Drums Herbs & Spice	3 oz	200	13	11	13
Rondelets Cheese	1 (2.6 oz)	190	12	11	11
Rondelets Italian	1 (2.6 oz)	190	11	11	11
Rondelets Original	1 (3 oz)	190	13	10	13
Weight Watchers					
Chicken Nuggets	5.9 oz	220	23	7	16
READY-TO-USE					
chicken roll light meat	2 oz	90	1	4	11
poultry salad sandwich spread	1 tbsp (13 g)	109	1	2	2
Carl Buddig					
Chicken	1 oz	50	1	3	5
Chicken By George					
Cajun	1 breast (4 oz)	120	2	4	20

FOOD	PORTION	CALS.	CARB.	FAT	PRO.
Chicken By George (CONT.)					
Caribbean Grill	1 breast (4 oz)	150	8	4	21
Garlic & Herb	1 breast (4 oz)	120	3	3	20
Lemon Oregano	1 breast (4 oz)	130	3	4	20
Mesquite Barbecue	1 breast (4 oz)	120	5	2	20
Mustard Dill	1 breast (4 oz)	140	2	5	20
Roasted	1 breast (4 oz)	110	1	3	20
Teriyaki	1 breast (4 oz)	130	6	3	20
Empire					
Barbacue Whole	5 oz	280	1	17	31
Battered & Breaded Cutlets	1 (3.3 oz)	200	11	9	18
Battered & Breaded Nuggets	5 (3 oz)	200	9	13	13
Battered & Breaded Fried Breasts	3 oz	170	3	8	21
Bologna	3 slices (1.8 oz)	200	2	7	7
Fried Drum & Thigh	3 oz	240	7	16	16
Falls					
BBQ	3 oz	150	—	8	18
Healthy Choice					
Deli-Thin Oven Roasted Breast	6 slices (2 oz)	45	0	0	11
Deli-Thin Smoked Breast	6 slices (2 oz)	60	1	2	11
Oven Roasted Breast	1 slice (1 oz)	25	0	0	6
Hebrew National					
Deli Thin Oven Roasted	1.8 oz	45	—	1	10
Hillshire					
Deli Select Oven Roasted Breast	1 slice	10	tr	tr	2
Deli Select Smoked Breast	1 slice	10	tr	tr	2
Flavor Pack 90-99% Fat Free Smoked Breast	1 slice (0.75 oz)	20	tr	tr	4
Lunch 'N Munch Smoked Chicken/ Monterey Jack	1 pkg (4.5 oz)	350	19	20	22
Lunch 'N Munch Smoked Chicken/ Monterey/ Snickers	1 pkg (4.25 oz)	400	31	23	19
Louis Rich					
Deli-Thin Oven Roasted Breast	4 slices (1.8 oz)	60	1	2	9

FOOD	PORTION	CALS.	CARB.	FAT	PRO.
Mr. Turkey					
Deli Cuts Hardwood Smoked	3 slices	30	2	tr	5
Oscar Mayer					
Deli-Thin Honey Glazed Breast	4 slices (1.8 oz)	60	2	1	10
Free Oven Roasted Breast	4 slices (1.8 oz)	45	1	0	9
Healthy Favorites Oven Roasted Breast	4 slices (1.8 oz)	40	1	0	9
Lunchables Chicken/ Monterey Jack	1 pkg (4.5 oz)	350	20	21	20
Lunchables Deluxe Chicken/Turkey	1 pkg (5.1 oz)	380	24	22	22
Lunchables Dessert Chocolate Pudding/ Chicken/ Jack	1 pkg (6.2 oz)	370	33	18	19
Perdue					
BBQ Drumsticks	1 oz	53	2	2	6
BBQ Thighs	1 oz	59	1	3	6
BBQ Wings	1 oz	62	1	4	6
Cornish Hen Roasted Dark Meat	1 oz	45	tr	3	5
Cornish Hen Roasted White Meat	1 oz	39	tr	1	6
Nuggets Cheese	1 (.67 oz)	54	3	4	3
Nuggets Fun Shaped	1 (.73 oz)	54	4	3	3
Roasted Breast	1 oz	45	1	2	7
Roasted Drumsticks	1 oz	40	0	1	7
Roasted Thighs	1 oz	46	tr	2	6
Wings Garlic & Herb	1 oz	61	tr	4	7
Tyson					
Bologna	1 slice	44	4	1	2
Wings Barbecue	6-7 (3.5 oz)	218	0	14	23
Wings Hot & Spicy	6-7 (3.5 oz)	218	0	14	23
Wings Roasted	6-7 (3.5 oz)	218	0	14	23
Wings Teriyaki	6-7 (3.5 oz)	218	0	14	23
Wampler Longacre					
Breast	1 oz	35	1	1	5
Roll Sliced	1 slice (0.8 oz)	50	1	4	4
Weaver					
Roasted Wings	1 oz	70	—	5	6
Weight Watchers					
Roasted Ham	2 slices (¾ oz)	25	tr	1	4

FOOD	PORTION	CALS.	CARB.	FAT	PRO.
TAKE-OUT					
boneless breaded & fried w/ barbecue sauce	6 pieces (4.6 oz)	330	25	18	17
boneless breaded & fried w/ honey	6 pieces (4 oz)	339	27	18	17
boneless breaded & fried w/ mustard sauce	6 pieces (4.6 oz)	323	21	17	17
boneless breaded & fried w/ sweet & sour sauce	6 pieces (4.6 oz)	346	29	18	17
breast & wing breaded & fried	2 pieces (5.7 oz)	494	20	30	36
drumstick breaded & fried	2 pieces (5.2 oz)	430	16	27	30
oven roasted breast of chicken	2 oz	60	0	1	11
thigh breaded & fried	2 pieces (5.2 oz)	430	16	27	30

CHICKEN DISHES
(see also CHICKEN SUBSTITUTES, DINNER)

FOOD	PORTION	CALS.	CARB.	FAT	PRO.
CANNED					
Dinty Moore					
American Classics Chicken & Noodles	1 bowl (10 oz)	260	26	8	21
American Classics Chicken With Mashed Potatoes	1 bowl (10 oz)	220	24	4	22
Chicken Stew	1 cup (7.5 oz)	180	18	8	10
Microwave Cup Chicken & Dumpling	1 cup (7.5 oz)	190	20	6	15
Stew	1 cup (8.5 oz)	220	16	11	12
Swanson					
Chicken & Dumplings	7½ oz	220	19	11	11
Chicken Ala King	5¼ oz	190	9	12	10
Top Shelf					
Chicken Acapulco Fiesta Chicken	1 bowl (10 oz)	420	45	16	26
Chicken Cacciatore	1 bowl (10 oz)	210	26	3	21
Glazed Breast Of Chicken	1 bowl (10 oz)	200	17	5	22
FROZEN					
Croissant Pocket					
Stuffed Sandwich Chicken Broccoli & Cheddar	1 piece (4.5 oz)	300	37	11	14
Hot Pocket					
Stuffed Sandwich Chicken & Cheddar With Broccoli	1 (4.5 oz)	300	37	12	12

FOOD	PORTION	CALS.	CARB.	FAT	PRO.
Jimmy Dean					
Grilled Breast Sandwich	1 (5.5 oz)	330	27	11	28
Lean Pockets					
Stuffed Sandwich Chicken Fijita	1 (4.5 oz)	260	36	8	12
Stuffed Sandwich Chicken Parmesan	1 (4.5 oz)	260	34	8	12
Stuffed Sandwich Glazed Chicken Supreme	1 (4.5 oz)	240	34	7	10
Luigino's					
Chicken A La King With Noodles	1 pkg (8 oz)	240	28	7	18
Noodles With Chicken Peas & Carrots	1 pkg (8 oz)	300	38	11	13
Noodles With Chicken Peas & Carrots	1 cup (6.3 oz)	260	33	10	11
Sweet & Sour Chicken With Rice	1 pkg (8 oz)	300	50	6	12
MicroMagic					
Chicken Sandwich	1 pkg (4.5 oz)	390	42	16	13
Ovenstuffs					
Chicken Turnover	1 (4.75 oz)	350	36	16	15
Tyson					
Microwave Breast Sandwich	4.25 oz	328	33	14	16
Weight Watchers					
Chicken & Broccoli Pita	1 (5.4 oz)	190	19	5	15
Grilled Chicken Sandwich	1 (4 oz)	210	22	6	18
White Castle					
Grilled Chicken Sandwich	2 (4 oz)	250	24	9	17
Grilled Chicken Sandwich w/ Sauce	2 (4.8 oz)	290	33	9	17
MIX					
Lipton					
Microeasy Barbeque Chicken	¼ pkg	108	24	1	2
Microeasy Country Chicken	¼ pkg	78	15	1	3
Skillet Chicken Helper					
Cheesy Broccoli as prep	⅕ pkg (7.5 oz)	270	34	6	19
Creamy Chicken as prep	⅕ pkg (8.25 oz)	290	29	10	21
Creamy Mushroom as prep	⅕ pkg (8 oz)	280	31	8	21

FOOD	PORTION	CALS.	CARB.	FAT	PRO.
Skillet Chicken Helper (CONT.)					
Fettucine Alfredo as prep	⅕ pkg (7.5 oz)	270	29	8	21
Stir-Fried Chicken as prep	⅕ pkg (7 oz)	330	36	11	4
READY-TO-USE					
Wampler Longacre					
Cacciatore	1 serv (4 oz)	118	5	3	14
Salad	1 oz	70	3	3	3
Salad Lite	1 oz	45	3	2	3
Smokey Barbecue	1 serv (4 oz)	175	11	7	17
Sweet N Sour	1 serv (4 oz)	106	16	tr	9
Szechwan With Peanuts	1 serv (4 oz)	112	6	4	13
SHELF-STABLE					
Lunch Bucket					
Dumplings'n Chicken	1 pkg (7.5 oz)	140	25	2	4
Light'n Healthy Chicken Fiesta	1 pkg (7.5 oz)	170	28	3	7
TAKE-OUT					
chicken cacciatore	¾ cup	394	9	24	33
chicken & dumplings	¾ cup	256	12	12	23
chicken & noodles	1 cup	365	26	18	22
chicken a la king	1 cup	470	12	34	27
chicken pie w/ top crust	1 slice (5.6 oz)	472	32	31	19
fillet sandwich plain	1	515	39	29	24
fillet sandwich w/ cheese lettuce mayonnaise & tomato	1	632	42	39	29

CHICKEN SUBSTITUTES

FOOD	PORTION	CALS.	CARB.	FAT	PRO.
Harvest Direct					
TVP Poultry Chunks	3.5 oz	280	32	1	52
TVP Poultry Ground	3.5 oz	280	32	1	52
Jaclyn's					
Salsa Chicken Style Dinner	11.5 oz	325	35	9	28
Sesame Chicken Style Dinner	11.5 oz	345	40	8	31
Knox Mountain Farm					
Chick'N Wheat Mix	1 serv (1/9 pkg)	110	3	1	13
LaLoma					
Chicken Supreme not prep	¼ cup (16 g)	50	4	0	9
Chik Nuggets	5 nuggets (85 g)	270	8	20	15
Fried Chicken	1 piece (57 g)	180	2	14	11

FOOD	PORTION	CALS.	CARB.	FAT	PRO.
LaLoma (CONT.)					
Fried Chicken w/ Gravy	2 piece (85 g)	140	4	10	9
White Wave					
Meatless Sandwich Slices	2 slices (1.6 oz)	80	8	0	12
Worthington					
Chick-ketts	½ cup (84 g)	160	6	7	19
ChickStiks	1 (47 g)	110	4	7	9
Chicken Sliced	2 slices (57 g)	130	3	9	9
CrispyChik	6 nuggets (85 g)	280	17	19	10
CrispyChik	1 patty (71 g)	220	13	15	8
Cutlets	1.5 slices (92 g)	100	4	2	16
Diced Chik	¼ cup (60 g)	90	2	8	4
FriChik	2 pieces (90 g)	180	13	13	4
Golden Croquettes	5 pieces (106 g)	280	20	14	19
Savory Slices	2 slices (60 g)	90	2	8	4
Vegetarian Chicken Pie	1 (227 g)	380	43	20	7
CHICKPEAS					
CANNED					
chickpeas	1 cup	285	54	3	12
Allen					
Garbanzo	½ cup (4.4 oz)	120	19	3	5
East Texas Fair					
Garbanzo	½ cup (4.4 oz)	120	19	3	5
Eden					
Organic	½ cup (4.1 oz)	110	17	2	6
Goya					
Spanish Style	7.5 oz	150	32	2	9
Green Giant					
Garbanzo	½ cup	90	18	2	6
Old El Paso					
Garbanzo	½ cup	190	16	tr	5
Progresso					
Chickpeas	½ cup	110	22	1	9
S&W					
Garbanzo Lite 50% Less Salt	½ cup	110	21	0	6
Garbanzo Premium Large	½ cup	110	20	1	6
Garbanzo Water Pack	½ cup	105	19	1	26
DRIED					
cooked	1 cup	269	45	4	15
Bean Cuisine					
Garbanzo	½ cup	115	—	1	8

FOOD	PORTION	CALS.	CARB.	FAT	PRO.
CHICORY					
greens raw chopped	½ cup	21	4	tr	2
root raw	1 (2.1 oz)	44	11	tr	1
roots raw cut up	½ cup (1.6 oz)	33	8	tr	1
witloof head raw	1 (1.9 oz)	9	2	tr	tr
witloof raw	½ cup (1.6 oz)	8	2	tr	tr
CHILI					
CANNED					
chili w/ beans	1 cup	286	30	14	15
Allen					
Mexican Chili Beans	½ cup (4.5 oz)	120	22	1	6
Armour					
Chili No Beans	1 cup (8.7 oz)	470	18	38	14
Chili With Beans	1 cup (8.9 oz)	440	34	28	14
Chili With Beans Hot	1 cup (8.9 oz)	440	34	28	14
Chili With Beans Western Style	1 cup (8.8 oz)	460	29	32	14
Brown Beauty					
Mexican Chili Beans	½ cup (4.5 oz)	120	22	1	6
Chi-Chi's					
San Antonio	1 cup (8.5 oz)	240	23	19	19
Del Monte					
Sauce	1 tbsp (0.6 oz)	20	0	0	1
Gebhardt					
Hot With Beans	1 cup	470	47	27	16
Plain	1 cup	530	20	43	21
With Beans	1 cup	495	47	28	20
Hain					
Spicy Tempeh	7½ oz	160	24	4	7
Spicy Vegetarian	7½ oz	160	29	1	7
Spicy Vegetarian Reduced Sodium	7½ oz	170	31	1	7
Spicy With Chicken	7½ oz	130	19	2	11
Health Valley					
Mild Vegetarian With Beans	5 oz	160	21	3	10
Mild Vegetarian With Beans No Salt Added	5 oz	160	21	3	10
Mild Vegetarian With Lentils	5 oz	140	15	4	8
Mild Vegetarian With Lentils No Salt Added	5 oz	140	15	4	8
Spicy Vegetarian With Beans	5 oz	160	21	4	10

FOOD	PORTION	CALS.	CARB.	FAT	PRO.
Hormel					
Chili Mac	1 can (7.5 oz)	200	17	9	11
Chili No Beans	1 cup (8.3 oz)	410	16	30	19
Chili With Beans	1 cup (8.7 oz)	340	30	17	18
Chunky Chili With Beans	1 cup (8.7 oz)	330	30	16	17
Hot Chili No Beans	1 cup (8.3 oz)	410	16	30	19
Hot Chili With Beans	1 cup (8.7 oz)	340	30	17	18
Hot With Beans	1 can (7.5 oz)	250	23	11	15
No Beans	1 can (7.5 oz)	390	13	30	18
Turkey Chili With Beans	1 cup (8.7 oz)	220	28	3	20
Turkey Chili No Beans	1 cup (8.3 oz)	190	17	3	23
With Beans	1 can (7.5 oz)	250	23	11	15
Hunt's					
Chili Beans	4 oz	100	18	tr	6
Just Rite					
Hot With Beans	4 oz	195	16	10	11
With Beans	4 oz	200	16	11	10
Without Beans	4 oz	180	9	11	13
Manwich					
Chili Fixin's as prep	8 oz	290	20	14	20
Micro Cup Meals					
Chili Mac	1 cup (7.5 oz)	200	17	9	11
Chili No Beans	1 cup (7.5 oz)	290	15	17	18
Chili With Beans	1 cup (7.5 oz)	250	23	11	15
Chili With Beans	1 cup (10.4 oz)	410	41	17	23
Hot Chili With Beans	1 cup (7.5 oz)	250	23	11	15
Natural Touch					
Vegetarian	⅔ cup (190 g)	230	19	12	12
Old El Paso					
Chili With Beans	1 cup	217	17	10	15
S&W					
Chili Beans	½ cup	130	23	1	7
Chili Makin's Original	½ cup	100	20	1	5
Van Camp's					
Chilee Beanee Weenee	1 can (8 oz)	240	27	12	14
Chili With Beans	1 cup (8.9 oz)	350	28	21	19
Wolf Brand					
Chili-Mac	7.5 oz	317	23	20	12
Extra Spicy With Beans	7.5 oz	324	21	21	14
Extra Spicy Without Beans	7.5 oz	363	15	25	19
Plain	7.5 oz	330	10	22	25
With Beans	7.5 oz	345	22	22	15
Without Beans	1 cup	387	16	27	21

FOOD	PORTION	CALS.	CARB.	FAT	PRO.
Worthington					
Chili	⅔ cup (141 g)	190	15	10	10
DRIED					
powder	1 tsp	8	1	tr	tr
Gebhardt					
Chili Powder	1 tsp	15	3	tr	tr
Chili Quik Seasoning	1 tsp	10	2	tr	tr
Hain					
Hot Chili	¼ pkg	30	5	1	1
Medium Chili	¼ pkg	30	5	1	1
Mild Chili	¼ pkg	30	5	1	1
Nile Spice					
Chili'n Beans Original	1 pkg	150	25	2	8
Chili'n Beans Spicy	1 pkg	150	25	2	8
Old El Paso					
Chili Seasoning Mix	⅕ pkg	21	4	1	1
Watkins					
Chili Seasoning	1¼ tsp (4 g)	15	2	0	0
Powder	¼ tsp (0.5 g)	0	0	0	0
FROZEN					
Lean Cuisine					
Three Bean	1 pkg (9 oz)	210	32	6	8
Lightlife					
Chili	4.3 oz	110	14	3	7
Luigino's					
Chili-Mac	1 pkg (8 oz)	230	29	7	14
Stouffer's					
With Beans	1 pkg (8.75 oz)	270	29	10	15
Swanson					
Homestyle Chili Con Carne	8¼ oz	270	26	10	20
Tabatchnick					
Vegetarian	7.5 oz	210	28	6	12
Tyson					
Chicken Chili	3.5 oz	105	11	3	8
SHELF-STABLE					
Lunch Bucket					
Chili With Beans	1 pkg (7.5 oz)	300	26	14	16
Wampler Longacre					
Turkey	1 serv (4 oz)	118	10	3	10
TAKE-OUT					
con carne w/ beans	8.9 oz	254	22	8	25

FOOD	PORTION	CALS.	CARB.	FAT	PRO.

CHINESE CABBAGE
(see CABBAGE)

CHINESE FOOD
(see ORIENTAL FOOD)

CHIPS
(see also POPCORN, PRETZELS, SNACKS)

FOOD	PORTION	CALS.	CARB.	FAT	PRO.
CORN					
barbecue	1 oz	148	16	9	2
barbecue	1 bag (7 oz)	1036	111	65	14
cones nacho	1 oz	152	17	9	2
cones plain	1 oz	145	18	8	2
onion	1 oz	142	19	6	2
plain	1 oz	153	16	10	2
plain	1 bag (7 oz)	1067	113	66	13
puffs cheese	1 oz	157	15	10	2
puffs cheese	1 bag (8 oz)	1256	122	78	17
twists cheese	1 oz	157	15	10	2
twists cheese	1 bag (8 oz)	1256	122	78	17
Energy Food Factory					
Corn Pops Fat Free	½ oz	50	11	0	1
Corn Pops Nacho	½ oz	50	12	1	1
Corn Pops Original	½ oz	50	11	1	1
Fritos					
Chili Cheese	34 pieces (1 oz)	160	15	10	2
Chips	34 pieces (1 oz)	150	16	10	2
Crisp 'N Thin	18 pieces (1 oz)	160	16	10	2
Dip Size	13 pieces (1 oz)	150	16	10	1
Non-Stop Nacho Cheese	34 pieces (1 oz)	150	16	9	2
Rowdy Rustlers Bar-B-Q	34 pieces (1 oz)	150	17	9	2
Wild 'N Mild	32 pieces (1 oz)	160	16	9	2
Health Valley					
Chips	1 oz	160	13	11	1
No Salt Added	1 oz	160	13	11	1
With Cheddar Cheese	1 oz	160	15	10	3
Lance					
BBQ	1 pkg (50 g)	260	25	16	3
Chips	1 pkg (50 g)	270	26	17	3
Planters					
Corn Chips	34 chips (1 oz)	170	17	10	2
King Size	17 chips (1 oz)	160	16	10	2
Snacks To Go	1 pkg (1.5 oz)	240	23	15	3
Snyder's					
BBQ	1 oz	160	14	11	2

FOOD	PORTION	CALS.	CARB.	FAT	PRO.
Snyder's (CONT.)					
Chips	1 oz	160	14	11	2
Weight Watchers					
Corn Snacker	½ oz	60	10	2	1
Corn Snackers Nacho Cheese	½ oz	60	10	2	1
Wise					
Corn	1 oz	160	15	10	2
Corn Crunchies	1 oz	160	15	10	2
Crispy Corn	1 oz	160	15	10	2
Crispy Corn Nacho Cheese	1 oz	160	16	10	2
MULTIGRAIN					
Sunchips					
Chips	12 pieces (1 oz)	150	18	8	2
French Onion	12 pieces (1 oz)	140	18	7	3
POTATO					
barbecue	1 bag (7 oz)	971	105	64	15
barbecue	1 oz	139	15	9	2
cheese	1 bag (6 oz)	842	98	46	14
cheese	1 oz	140	16	8	2
light	1 bag (6 oz)	801	114	35	12
light	1 oz	134	19	6	2
potato	1 oz	152	15	10	2
potato	1 pkg (8 oz)	1217	120	79	16
sour cream & onion	1 bag (7 oz)	1051	102	67	16
sour cream & onion	1 oz	150	15	10	2
sticks	½ cup (0.6 oz)	94	10	6	1
sticks	1 oz	148	15	10	2
sticks	1 pkg (1 oz)	148	15	10	2
sticks	½ cup	94	10	6	1
Barrel O' Fun					
Barbeque	1 oz	145	16	9	2
Chips	1 oz	150	15	9	2
Sour Cream & Onion	1 oz	150	15	9	2
Butterfield					
Sticks	⅔ cup (1 oz)	150	16	9	2
Sticks	1 pkg (1.7 oz)	250	26	15	3
Cape Cod					
Chips	19 chips (1 oz)	150	17	8	2
Cottage Fries					
No Salt Added	1 oz	160	14	11	2
Eagle					
BBQ Thins	1 oz	150	15	10	2

FOOD	PORTION	CALS.	CARB.	FAT	PRO.
Eagle (CONT.)					
Kettle Fry BBQ Crunchy	1 oz	150	16	8	2
Kettle Fry Cape Cod	1 oz	150	16	8	2
Kettle Fry Cape Cod No Salt	1 oz	150	16	8	2
Kettle Fry Cape Cod Waves	1 oz	150	16	8	2
Kettle Fry Cape Cod Waves No Salt	1 oz	150	16	8	2
Kettle Fry Dill & Sour Cream	1 oz	150	16	8	2
Kettle Fry Dill & Sour Cream No Salt	1 oz	150	16	8	2
Kettle Fry Extra Crunchy	1 oz	150	16	8	2
Kettle Fry Idaho Russet	1 oz	150	16	8	2
Kettle Fry Louisiana BBQ	1 oz	150	16	8	2
Ranch Ridged	1 oz	160	15	10	2
Ridged	1 oz	150	15	10	2
Sour Cream & Onion	1 oz	150	15	10	2
Thins	1 oz	150	15	10	2
Energy Food Factory					
Potato Pops Au Gratin	½ oz	60	12	2	1
Potato Pops Fat Free	½ oz	50	13	0	1
Potato Pops Herb & Garlic	½ oz	50	11	1	1
Potato Pops Mesquite	½ oz	50	12	1	1
Potato Pops Original	½ oz	50	11	1	1
Potato Pops Salt N' Vinegar	½ oz	50	11	1	1
Health Valley					
Country Ripple	1 oz	160	15	10	2
Country Ripple No Salt Added	1 oz	160	15	10	2
Dip Chips	1 oz	160	15	10	2
Dip Chips No Salt Added	1 oz	160	15	10	2
Natural	1 oz	160	15	10	2
Natural No Salt Added	1 oz	160	15	10	2
Kelly's					
Bar-B-Q	1 oz	150	15	9	2
Chips	1 oz	150	14	9	2
Crunchy	1 oz	150	17	9	2
Rippled	1 oz	150	14	9	2
Sour Cream n' Onion	1 oz	150	15	9	2
Unsalted	1 oz	150	14	10	2

FOOD	PORTION	CALS.	CARB.	FAT	PRO.
Lance					
BBQ	1 pkg (32 g)	190	18	12	3
Cajun Style	1 pkg (32 g)	160	16	11	2
Chips	1 pkg (32 g)	190	12	15	2
Hot Fries	1 pkg (28 g)	160	14	10	2
Ripple	1 pkg (32 g)	190	12	15	2
Sour Cream & Onion	1 pkg (32 g)	190	18	12	3
Lay's					
Bar-B-Q	17 pieces (1 oz)	150	15	9	1
Cheddar Cheese	17 pieces (1 oz)	150	14	10	2
Chips	17 pieces (1 oz)	150	15	10	1
Crunch Tators	16 pieces (1 oz)	150	17	8	2
Crunch Tators Amazin' Cajun	16 pieces (1 oz)	150	17	8	2
Crunch Tators Hoppin' Jalapeno	16 pieces (1 oz)	140	18	7	1
Crunch Tators Mighty Mesquite	16 pieces (1 oz)	150	17	8	2
Crunch Tators Supreme Sour Cream	16 pieces (1 oz)	150	16	8	2
Flamin' Hot	17 pieces (1 oz)	150	15	9	2
Kansas City Style Bar-B-Q	17 pieces (1 oz)	150	15	9	2
Salt & Vinegar	17 pieces (1 oz)	150	14	10	1
Sour Cream & Onion	17 pieces (1 oz)	160	15	10	2
Tangy Ranch	17 pieces (1 oz)	160	15	10	2
Unsalted	17 pieces (1 oz)	150	15	10	2
Louise's					
"1g" Mesquite BBQ	1 oz	110	24	1	2
"1g" Original	1 oz	110	24	1	2
70% Less Fat Mesquite BBQ	1 oz	110	21	3	2
70% Less Fat Original	1 oz	110	21	3	2
Fat-Free Maui Onion	1 oz	110	23	0	3
Fat-Free Mesquite BBQ	1 oz	110	23	0	3
Fat-Free No Salt	1 oz	110	24	0	3
Fat-Free Original	1 oz	110	23	0	3
Fat-Free Vinegar & Salt	1 oz	110	23	0	3
Mr. Phipps					
Tater Crisps Bar-B-Que	21 (1 oz)	130	21	4	2
Tater Crisps Original	23 (1 oz)	120	20	7	2
Tater Crisps Sour Cream 'n Onion	22 (1 oz)	130	21	4	1

FOOD	PORTION	CALS.	CARB.	FAT	PRO.
New York Deli					
Chips	1 oz	160	14	11	2
Old Dutch Foods					
Augratin	1 oz	150	15	8	2
BBQ	1 oz	140	16	8	2
Chips	1 oz	150	16	9	2
Dill Flavored	1 oz	150	16	8	2
Onion & Garlic	1 oz	150	15	9	2
Ripple	1 oz	150	16	9	2
Sour Cream & Onion	1 oz	150	15	10	2
Pringles					
BBQ	14 chips (1 oz)	150	15	6	2
Cheez-ums	14 chips (1 oz)	150	—	10	2
Original	14 chips (1 oz)	160	—	11	2
Ranch	14 chips (1 oz)	150	—	10	2
Ridges Cheddar & Sour Cream	12 chips (1 oz)	150	—	10	1
Ridges Mesquite BBQ	12 chips (1 oz)	150	—	10	1
Ridges Original	12 chips (1 oz)	150	—	10	1
Right BBQ	16 chips (1 oz)	140	18	7	2
Right Original	16 chips (1 oz)	140		7	1
Right Ranch	16 chips (1 oz)	140	18	7	2
Right Sour Cream 'N Onion	16 chips (1 oz)	140	18	7	2
Rippled Original	10 chips (1 oz)	160	15	11	2
Sour Cream N'Onion	14 chips (1 oz)	160	15	10	2
Ruffles					
Cheddar Cheese & Sour Cream	18 chips (1 oz)	160	15	10	2
Chips	18 chips (1 oz)	150	15	10	2
Light	18 chips (1 oz)	130	19	6	2
Light Sour Cream & Onion	18 chips (1 oz)	130	18	6	3
Mesquite Grille B-B-Q	18 chips (1 oz)	160	15	10	2
Monterey Jack Cheese Attack	18 chips (1 oz)	160	15	10	2
Ranch	18 chips (1 oz)	160	15	10	2
Sour Cream & Onion	18 chips (1 oz)	160	15	10	2
Snyder's					
BBQ	1 oz	150	13	10	2
Cheddar Bacon	1 oz	150	13	10	2
Chips	1 oz	150	13	10	2
Coney Island	1 oz	150	13	10	2
Grilled Steak & Onion	1 oz	150	13	10	2

FOOD	PORTION	CALS.	CARB.	FAT	PRO.
Snyder's (CONT.)					
Hot Buffalo Wings	1 oz	150	13	10	2
Kosher Dill	1 oz	150	13	10	2
No Salt	1 oz	150	13	10	2
Salt & Vinegar	1 oz	150	13	10	2
Sausage Pizza	1 oz	150	13	10	2
Sour Cream & Onion	1 oz	150	13	10	2
Sour Cream & Onion Unsalted	1 oz	150	13	10	2
State Line					
Chips	1 pkg (0.5 oz)	80	7	5	1
Suprimos					
Cheddar & Jack	1 oz	140	17	6	4
Cool Onion	1 oz	140	17	6	4
Weight Watchers					
Great Snackers Barbecue	½ oz	70	10	3	1
Great Snackers Cheddar Cheese	½ oz	70	10	3	1
Great Snackers Sour Cream & Onion	½ oz	70	10	3	1
Wise					
Natural	1 oz	160	14	11	2
Ridgies Barbecue	1 oz	150	14	10	2
TORTILLA					
nacho	1 oz	141	18	7	2
nacho	1 bag (8 oz)	1131	142	58	18
nacho light	1 bag (6 oz)	757	122	26	15
nacho light	1 oz	126	20	4	3
plain	1 bag (7.5 oz)	1067	134	56	15
plain	1 oz	142	18	7	2
ranch	1 oz	139	18	7	2
ranch	1 bag (7 oz)	969	128	47	15
taco	1 bag (8 oz)	1089	143	55	18
taco	1 oz	136	18	7	2
Barrel O' Fun					
Nacho	1 oz	140	19	6	2
Tostada Yellow	1 oz	140	19	6	2
White	1 oz	140	20	6	2
Doritos					
Lightly Salted	16 chips (1 oz)	150	18	7	2
Eagle					
Chips	1 oz	150	18	8	2
Nacho	1 oz	150	17	8	2

FOOD	PORTION	CALS.	CARB.	FAT	PRO.
Eagle (CONT.)					
Ranch	1 oz	150	17	8	2
Restaurant Style	1 oz	150	18	7	2
Strips	1 oz	150	18	8	2
Frito Lay					
Salsa 'N Cheese	16 (1 oz)	150	17	8	2
Guiltless Gourmet					
Baked	22-26 chips (1 oz)	110	21	1	3
Hain					
Sesame	1 oz	140	19	7	2
Sesame Cheese	1 oz	160	20	8	2
Sesame No Salt Added	1 oz	140	19	7	2
Taco Style	1 oz	160	15	11	2
La FAMOUS					
No Salt Added	1 oz	140	18	7	2
Tortilla	1 oz	140	18	7	2
Lance					
Nacho	1 pkg (32 g)	160	19	8	3
Louise's					
95% Fat-Free	1 oz	120	23	2	2
Mr. Phipps					
Nacho	28 (1 oz)	130	20	4	2
Original	28 (1 oz)	130	21	4	2
Old El Paso					
NACHIPS	9 chips (1 oz)	150	18	7	2
White Corn	12 chips (1 oz)	150	16	8	2
Santitas					
Cantina Style	1 oz	140	19	6	2
Cantina Style Fajita	1 oz	140	19	7	2
Chips	1 oz	140	19	7	2
Strips	1 oz	140	19	7	2
Snyder's					
Chips	1 oz	140	18	7	2
Enchilada	1 oz	140	18	7	2
Nacho Cheese	1 oz	140	18	7	2
No Salt	1 oz	140	18	7	2
Ranch	1 oz	140	18	7	2
Tostitos					
Baked	1 oz	110	24	1	2
Baked Cool Ranch	1 oz	130	21	3	2
Baked Unsalted	1 oz	110	24	1	2
Bite Size	16 pieces (1 oz)	150	18	8	2
Chips	11 pieces (1 oz)	140	18	8	2
Restaurant Style Lime 'N Chili	7 pieces (1 oz)	150	18	7	2

FOOD	PORTION	CALS.	CARB.	FAT	PRO.
Tostitos (CONT.)					
Restaurant Style White Corn	7 pieces (1 oz)	150	20	6	2
Tyson					
Nacho Cheese	1 oz	140	17	7	2
Ranch Flavor	1 oz	140	17	2	2
Traditional	1 oz	140	17	7	2
Unsalted	1 oz	140	17	7	2
Wise					
Bravos	1 oz	150	18	8	2
VEGETABLE					
taro	1 oz	141	19	7	1
taro	10 (0.8 oz)	115	16	6	1
Eden					
Vegetable Chips	50 (1 oz)	130	24	4	tr
Wasabi Chip Hot & Spicy	50 (1 oz)	130	24	4	tr
Hain					
Carrot Chips	1 oz	150	16	9	2
Carrot Chips Barbecue	1 oz	140	16	8	2
Carrot Chips No Salt Added	1 oz	150	16	7	2
Health Valley					
Carrot Lites	0.5 oz	75	9	4	1
Terra Chips					
Sweet Potato	1 oz	140	18	7	1
Sweet Potato Spiced	1 oz	140	16	7	1
Taro Spiced	1 oz	130	20	5	1
Vegetable	1 oz	140	18	7	1
Top Banana					
Plantain Chips	1 oz	150	17	8	1

CHITTERLINGS

FOOD	PORTION	CALS.	CARB.	FAT	PRO.
pork, simmered	3 oz	258	0	24	24

CHIVES

FOOD	PORTION	CALS.	CARB.	FAT	PRO.
freeze-dried	1 tbsp	1	tr	tr	tr
fresh chopped	1 tbsp	1	tr	tr	tr
fresh chopped	1 tsp	0	tr	tr	tr

CHOCOLATE

(*see also* CANDY, CAROB, COCOA, ICE CREAM TOPPINGS, MILK DRINKS)

FOOD	PORTION	CALS.	CARB.	FAT	PRO.
BAKING					
baking	1 oz	145	8	15	3
grated unsweetened	1 cup (4.6 oz)	690	37	73	14
liquid unsweetened	1 oz	134	10	14	3

FOOD	PORTION	CALS.	CARB.	FAT	PRO.
squares unsweetened	1 square (1 oz)	148	8	16	3
Baker's					
German Sweet	¼ cup	200	27	12	2
German Sweet	1 oz	143	17	10	1
Semi-Sweet	1 oz	135	17	9	2
Unsweetened	1 oz	141	9	15	3
Hershey					
Premium Semi-Sweet	1 oz	140	16	8	1
Premium Unsweetened	1 oz	190	7	16	4
Nestle					
Choco Bake	½ oz	80	5	8	1
Premier White	½ oz	80	8	5	1
Semi-Sweet	½ oz	70	9	4	<1
Unsweetened	½ oz	80	5	7	2
CHIPS					
milk chocolate	1 cup (6 oz)	862	100	52	12
semisweet	1 cup (6 oz)	804	106	50	7
semisweet	60 pieces (1 oz)	136	18	9	1
Baker's					
Big Milk Chocolate	¼ cup	239	30	14	3
Big Semi-Sweet	¼ cup	220	31	13	2
Chips	1 oz	143	18	8	2
Real Semi-Sweet	¼ cup	198	28	12	2
Semi-Sweet	¼ cup	197	30	9	2
Hershey					
Chunks Milk Chocolate	1 oz	160	16	9	2
Chunks Semi-Sweet	1 oz	140	15	8	1
Milk Chocolate	1 oz	150	27	12	2
Mint Chocolate	¼ cup	230	28	12	2
Semi-Sweet	¼ cup (1.5 oz)	220	26	12	2
Semi-Sweet Miniature	¼ cup (1.5 oz)	220	26	12	2
M&M's					
Baking Bits Milk Chocolate	0.5 oz	70	10	3	7
Baking Bits Semi-Sweet	0.5 oz	70	9	4	1
Nestle					
Morsels Milk Chocolate	1 tbsp	70	10	4	0
Morsels Mini Semi-Sweet	1 tbsp	70	9	4	0
Morsels Mint Chocolate	1 tbsp	70	9	4	0
Morsels Rainbow	1 tbsp	70	10	3	0
Semi-Sweet Morsels	1 tbsp	40	9	4	0

FOOD	PORTION	CALS.	CARB.	FAT	PRO.
MIX					
powder	2-3 heaping tsp	75	20	1	1
powder as prep w/ whole milk	9 oz	226	31	9	9
Hershey					
Chocolate Milk Mix	3 tbsp	90	22	4	1
SYRUP					
chocolate	1 cup	653	177	3	6
chocolate	2 tbsp	82	22	tr	1
chocolate as prep w/ whole milk	9 oz	232	34	9	9
chocolate fudge	1 tbsp (0.7 oz)	73	12	3	1
chocolate fudge	1 cup (11.9 oz)	1176	200	46	15
Crumpy					
Chocolate Hazelnut Spread	1 tbsp (0.5 oz)	80	8	5	tr
Estee					
Choco-Syp	2 tbsp (1.2 oz)	50	11	0	tr
Hershey					
Syrup	2 tbsp	80	17	1	1
Marzetti					
Syrup	2 tbsp	40	21	4	1
Quik					
Syrup Chocolate	1 ⅔ tbsp	100	22	1	1
Red Wing					
Syrup	2 tbsp (1.4 oz)	110	25	1	1

CHOCOLATE MILK

(*see* CHOCOLATE, COCOA, MILK DRINKS)

CHUTNEY

apple	1.2 oz	68	18	0	tr
apple cranberry	1 tbsp	16	4	0	tr
tomato	1.2 oz	54	14	0	tr
Sonoma					
Dried Tomato	1 tbsp (0.7 g)	35	9	0	0

CILANTRO

fresh	¼ cup	1	tr	tr	tr
Watkins					
Dried	¼ tsp (0.5 oz)	0	0	0	0

CINNAMON

ground	1 tsp	6	2	tr	tr
sticks	0.5 oz	39	8	tr	1

FOOD	PORTION	CALS.	CARB.	FAT	PRO.
Watkins					
Ground	¼ tsp (0.5 g)	0	0	0	0
CLAMS					
CANNED					
liquid only	1 cup	6	tr	tr	1
liquid only	3 oz	2	tr	tr	tr
meat only	1 cup	236	8	3	41
meat only	3 oz	126	4	2	22
American Original					
Quahogs	4 oz	66	2	tr	12
Doxsee					
Chopped	6.5 oz	90	6	tr	16
Clam Juice	3 fl oz	4	0	0	tr
Empress					
Whole Baby	4 oz	60	2	1	11
Gorton's					
Minced & Chopped	½ can	70	4	1	12
Progresso					
Clams	½ cup	70	2	tr	12
Red Clam Sauce	½ cup	70	7	3	5
White Clam Sauce	½ cup	110	1	8	9
S&W					
Fancy Chopped	2 oz	28	2	0	5
Fancy Minced	2 oz	28	2	0	5
Whole Baby Chowder	2 oz	33	1	0	6
Clams					
Snow's					
Minced	6.5 oz	90	6	tr	16
FRESH					
cooked	3 oz	126	4	2	22
cooked	20 sm	133	5	2	23
raw	20 sm (180 g)	133	5	2	23
raw	9 lg (180 g)	133	5	2	23
raw	3 oz	63	2	1	11
FROZEN					
Gorton's					
Microwave Chrunchy	3.5 oz	330	24	22	10
Clam Strips					
Mrs. Paul's					
Fried	2½ oz	200	21	9	10
Microwave Fried Clams	2.5 oz	260	23	15	8
HOME RECIPE					
breaded & fried	3 oz	171	9	9	12

FOOD	PORTION	CALS.	CARB.	FAT	PRO.
breaded & fried	20 sm	379	19	21	27
TAKE-OUT					
breaded & fried	¾ cup	451	39	26	13

COCOA
(*see also* CHOCOLATE)

FOOD	PORTION	CALS.	CARB.	FAT	PRO.
hot cocoa	1 cup	218	26	9	9
mix as prep w/ water	7 oz	103	23	1	3
mix w/ nutrasweet as prep w/ water	7 oz	48	9	tr	4
powder unsweetened	1 tbsp (5 g)	11	3	1	1
powder unsweetened	1 cup (3 oz)	197	47	12	17
Hershey					
Cocoa	⅓ cup (1 oz)	120	13	4	7
European Cocoa	1 oz	90	8	3	7
Nestle					
Cocoa	1 tbsp	15	3	1	1
Hot Cocoa Mix	1 oz	110	23	1	2
Hot Cocoa Mix With Marshmallows	1 oz	120	23	1	2
Hot Cocoa Mix With Marshmallows as prep w/ 2% milk	6 oz	220	32	5	8
Hot Cocoa Mix With Marshmallows as prep w/ skim milk	6 oz	190	32	1	8
Hot Cocoa Mix With Marshmallows as prep w/ whole milk	6 oz	240	32	8	8
Hot Cocoa Mix as prep w/ 2% milk	6 oz	210	32	5	8
Hot Cocoa Mix as prep w/ skim milk	6 oz	180	32	1	8
Hot Cocoa Mix as prep w/ whole milk	6 oz	230	32	8	8
Swiss Miss					
Cocoa Diet	6 oz	20	3	tr	2
Hot Cocoa Bavarian Chocolate	6 oz	110	20	3	1
Hot Cocoa Double Rich	6 oz	110	22	1	2
Hot Cocoa Milk Chocolate	6 oz	110	24	1	2
Hot Cocoa With Mini Marshmallows	6 oz	110	23	1	1

FOOD	PORTION	CALS.	CARB.	FAT	PRO.
Swiss Miss (CONT.)					
Lite as prep	6 oz	70	17	tr	1
Sugar Free With Sugar Free Marshmallows as prep	6 oz	50	9	tr	3
Sugar Free as prep	6 oz	60	10	tr	3
Ultra Slim-Fast					
Hot Cocoa as prep w/ water	8 oz	190	35	tr	14
Weight Watchers					
Cocoa	1 pkg	60	10	0	6
COCONUT					
coconut water	1 cup	46	9	tr	2
coconut water	1 tbsp	3	1	tr	tr
cream canned	1 tbsp	36	2	3	1
cream canned	1 cup	568	25	52	8
dried sweetened flaked	1 cup	351	35	24	2
dried sweetened flaked	7 oz pkg	944	95	64	7
dried sweetened flaked canned	1 cup	341	32	24	3
dried sweetened shredded	7 oz pkg	997	95	71	6
dried sweetened shredded	1 cup	466	44	33	2
dried toasted	1 oz	168	13	13	2
dried unsweetened	1 oz	187	7	18	2
fresh	1 piece (1½ oz)	159	7	15	2
fresh shredded	1 cup	283	12	27	3
milk canned	1 cup	445	6	48	5
milk canned	1 tbsp	30	tr	3	tr
milk frozen	1 tbsp	30	1	3	tr
milk frozen	1 cup	486	13	50	4
Baker's					
Angel Flake Toasted	⅓ cup	212	17	17	2
Premium Shred	⅓ cup	135	12	9	1
Coco Lopez					
Cream of Coconut	2 tbsp	120	20	5	0
COD					
CANNED					
atlantic	3 oz	89	0	1	19
atlantic	1 can (11 oz)	327	0	3	71
roe	3.5 oz	118	tr	3	22
DRIED					
atlantic	3 oz	246	0	2	53

FOOD	PORTION	CALS.	CARB.	FAT	PRO.
FRESH					
atlantic raw	3 oz	70	0	1	15
atlantic cooked	1 fillet (6.3 oz)	189	0	2	41
atlantic cooked	3 oz	89	0	1	19
pacific baked	3 oz	95	0	1	21
roe baked w/ butter & lemon juice	3.5 oz	126	2	3	22
roe raw	3½ oz	130	2	2	24
FROZEN					
Gorton's					
Fishmarket Fresh	5 oz	110	0	1	26
Mrs. Paul's					
Light Fillets	1 fillet	240	22	11	15
Van De Kamp's					
Light Fillets	1 piece	250	20	11	17
Natural Fillets	4 oz	90	0	1	20

COFFEE

(see also COFFEE BEVERAGES, COFFEE SUBSTITUTES)

FOOD	PORTION	CALS.	CARB.	FAT	PRO.
INSTANT					
cappuccino mix as prep	7 oz	62	11	2	tr
decaffeinated	1 rounded tsp (1.8 g)	4	1	0	tr
decaffeinated as prep	6 oz	4	1	0	tr
french mix as prep	7 oz	57	7	3	1
mocha mix as prep	7 oz	51	8	2	1
regular	1 rounded tsp	4	1	0	tr
regular as prep	6 oz	4	1	0	tr
regular w/ chicory	1 rounded tsp	6	1	0	tr
regular w/ chicory as prep	6 oz	6	1	0	tr
Kava					
Instant	1 tsp	2	1	0	0
REGULAR					
brewed	6 oz	4	1	0	tr
Folgers					
Colombian Supreme	1 tbsp	16	3	tr	tr
Custom Roast	1 tbsp	16	3	tr	tr
Decaffeinated	1 tbsp	17	3	tr	1
French Roast	1 tbsp	16	3	tr	tr
Gourmet Supreme	1 tbsp	16	3	tr	tr
Instant	1 tsp	8	1	tr	tr
Instant Decaffeinated	1 tsp	8	2	tr	tr
Singles	1 bag	21	4	tr	1
Singles Decaffeinated	1 bag	21	4	tr	1

FOOD	PORTION	CALS.	CARB.	FAT	PRO.
Folgers (CONT.)					
Special Roast	1 tbsp	16	3	tr	tr
Vacuum Pack	1 tbsp	16	3	tr	tr
Maryland Club					
Ground	1 tbsp	16	3	tr	tr
TAKE-OUT					
cafe au lait	1 cup (8 fl oz)	77	6	4	4
cafe brulot	1 cup (4.8 fl oz)	48	3	0	tr
capuccino	1 cup (8 fl oz)	77	6	4	4
coffee con leche	1 cup (8 fl oz)	77	6	4	4
espresso	1 cup (3 fl oz)	2	tr	0	tr
irish coffee	1 serving (9 fl oz)	107	3	3	1
mocha	1 mug (9.6 fl oz)	202	17	15	3

COFFEE BEVERAGES
(*see also* COFFEE SUBSTITUTES)

Chock o'ccino					
Cinnamon	8 oz	120	25	2	2
Coffee	8 oz	120	25	2	2
Mocha	8 oz	120	25	2	2

COFFEE SUBSTITUTES

powder	1 tsp	9	2	tr	tr
powder as prep	6 oz	9	2	tr	tr
powder as prep w/ milk	6 oz	121	10	6	6
Natural Touch					
Kaffree Roma	1 tsp	6	1	0	0
Postum					
Instant	6 oz	11	3	0	0
Instant Coffee Flavored	6 oz	11	3	0	0

COFFEE WHITENERS
(*see also* MILK SUBSTITUTES)
LIQUID

nondairy frzn	1 tbsp	20	2	2	tr
Coffee-Mate					
Liquid	1 tbsp (0.5 fl oz)	16	2	1	0
Hood					
Non Dairy	1 tbsp (0.5 fl oz)	20	2	2	0
International Delight					
Amaretto	1 tbsp (0.6 fl oz)	45	7	2	0
Cinnamon Hazelnut	1 tbsp (0.6 fl oz)	45	7	2	0
Irish Creme	1 tbsp (0.6 fl oz)	45	7	2	0
No Fat Amaretto	1 tbsp (0.5 fl oz)	30	7	0	0
No Fat French Vanilla Royale	1 tbsp (0.5 fl oz)	30	7	0	0

FOOD	PORTION	CALS.	CARB.	FAT	PRO.
International Delight (CONT.)					
No Fat Hawaiian Macadamia	1 tbsp (0.5 fl oz)	30	7	0	0
No Fat Irish Creme	1 tbsp (0.5 fl oz)	30	7	0	0
Suisse Chocolate Mocha	1 tbsp (0.6 fl oz)	45	7	2	0
Mocha Mix					
Fat-Free	1 tbsp (0.5 fl oz)	10	1	0	0
Lite	1 tbsp (0.5 fl oz)	10	tr	tr	0
Lite	4 fl oz	80	3	7	1
Original	1 tbsp (0.5 fl oz)	20	1	2	0
Signature Flavors French Vanilla	1 tbsp (0.5 fl oz)	35	8	0	0
Signature Flavors Irish Creme	1 tbsp (0.5 fl oz)	35	8	0	0
Signature Flavors Kahlua	1 tbsp (0.5 fl oz)	35	8	0	0
Signature Flavors Mauna Loa Macadamia Nut	1 tbsp (0.5 fl oz)	35	8	0	0
POWDER					
nondairy	1 tsp	11	1	tr	tr
Coffee-Mate					
Powder	1 tsp (2 g)	10	1	1	tr
Cremora					
Whitener	1 tsp	12	1	1	0
N-Rich Creamer					
Whitener	1 tsp	10	1	tr	tr
Weight Watchers					
Dairy Creamer Instant Nonfat Dry Milk	1 pkg	10	1	0	1

COLESLAW

(*see* CABBAGE, SALAD DRESSING)

COLLARDS

CANNED
Allen

Collards	½ cup (4.1 oz)	30	5	1	1

Sunshine

Collards	½ cup (4.1 oz)	30	5	1	1

FRESH

cooked	½ cup	17	4	tr	1
raw chopped	½ cup	6	1	tr	tr

FROZEN

chopped cooked	½ cup	31	6	tr	3

COOKIES

(*see also* BROWNIE, CAKE, DOUGHNUT, PIE)

READY-TO-EAT

animal crackers	1 box (2.4 oz)	299	51	9	4

FOOD	PORTION	CALS.	CARB.	FAT	PRO.
animal crackers	1 (2.5 g)	11	2	tr	tr
butter	1 (5 g)	23	3	1	tr
chocolate chip	1 (0.4 oz)	48	7	2	1
chocolate chip	1 box (1.9 oz)	233	36	12	3
chocolate chip low fat	1 (0.25 oz)	45	7	2	1
chocolate chip low sugar low sodium	1 (0.24 oz)	31	5	1	tr
chocolate chip soft-type	1 (0.5 oz)	69	9	4	1
chocolate w/ creme filling	1 (0.35 oz)	47	7	2	1
chocolate w/ creme filling chocolate coated	1 (0.60 oz)	82	11	5	1
chocolate w/ creme filling sugar free low sodium	1 (0.35 oz)	46	7	2	1
chocolate wafer	1 (0.2 oz)	26	4	1	tr
chocolate wafer cookie crumbs	½ cup (5.9 oz)	728	120	25	11
fig bars	1 (0.56 oz)	56	11	1	1
fortune	1 (0.28 oz)	30	7	tr	tr
fudge	1 (0.73 oz)	73	17	1	1
gingersnaps	1 (0.24 oz)	29	5	1	tr
graham	1 square (0.24 oz)	30	5	1	1
graham chocolate covered	1 (0.49 oz)	68	9	3	1
graham cracker crumbs	½ cup (4.4 oz)	540	97	13	9
graham honey	1 (0.24 oz)	30	5	1	1
ladyfingers	1 (0.38 oz)	40	7	1	1
marshmallow chocolate coated	1 (0.46 oz)	55	9	2	1
molasses	1 (0.5 oz)	65	11	2	1
oatmeal	1 (0.6 oz)	81	12	3	1
oatmeal soft-type	1 (0.5 oz)	61	10	2	1
oatmeal raisin	1 (0.6 oz)	81	12	3	1
oatmeal raisin low sugar no sodium	1 (0.24 oz)	31	5	1	tr
oatmeal raisin soft-type	1 (0.5 oz)	61	10	2	1
peanut butter sandwich	1 (0.5 oz)	67	9	3	1
peanut butter sandwich sugar free low sodium	1 (0.35 oz)	54	5	3	1
peanut butter soft-type	1 (0.5 oz)	69	9	4	1
raisin soft-type	1 (0.5 oz)	60	10	2	1
shortbread	1 (0.28 oz)	40	5	2	1
shortbread pecan	1 (0.49 oz)	79	8	5	1
sugar	1 (0.52 oz)	72	10	3	1
sugar low sugar sodium free	1 (0.24 oz)	30	5	1	1

FOOD	PORTION	CALS.	CARB.	FAT	PRO.
sugar wafers w/ creme filling	1 (0.12 oz)	18	3	1	tr
sugar wafers w/ creme filling sugar free sodium free	1 (0.14 oz)	20	3	1	tr
vanilla sandwich	1 (0.35 oz)	48	7	2	tr
vanilla wafers	1 (0.21 oz)	28	4	1	tr
Archway					
Almond Crescents	2 (0.8 oz)	100	17	4	1
Cookie Jar Hermits	1 (1 oz)	110	19	3	1
Frosty Lemon	1 (1 oz)	120	19	5	1
Fudge Nut Bar	1 (1 oz)	110	17	5	2
Iced Oatmeal	1 (1 oz)	120	19	5	2
Pfeffernusse	2 (1.3 oz)	140	32	1	1
Biscos					
Sugar Wafers	8 (1 oz)	140	21	6	tr
Chip-A-Roos					
Cookies	3 (1.3 oz)	190	23	10	2
Chips Ahoy!					
Real Chocolate Chip	3 (1.1 oz)	160	21	8	2
Reduced Fat	3 (1.1 oz)	150	23	6	2
Cookie Lover's					
Classic Shortbread	1 (0.8 oz)	110	12	7	1
Old-Time Raisin	1 (0.8 oz)	90	14	3	1
Drake's					
Chocolate Chip	2 (1 oz)	140	18	6	1
Coconut Macaroon	1 (1 oz)	135	17	7	1
Entenmann's					
Chocolate Chip	3 (0.9 oz)	140	19	7	1
Estee					
Coconut	4 (1 oz)	140	19	6	2
Creme Wafers Chocolate	7 (1.1 oz)	160	21	8	tr
Creme Wafers Lemon	5 (1.2 oz)	170	23	8	1
Creme Wafers Peanut Butter	5 (1.2 oz)	170	21	9	3
Creme Wafers Triple Decker Banana Split	3 (0.9 oz)	140	18	7	1
Creme Wafers Triple Decker Chocolate Caramel & Peanut Butter	3 (0.9 oz)	140	17	7	2
Creme Wafers Vanilla	7 (1.1 oz)	160	22	7	tr
Creme Wafers Vanilla & Strawberry	5 (1.2 oz)	170	23	8	1

FOOD	PORTION	CALS.	CARB.	FAT	PRO.
Estee (CONT.)					
Fig Bars Apple Low Fat	2 (1 oz)	100	22	1	1
Fig Bars Cranberry Low Fat	2 (1 oz)	100	22	1	1
Fig Bars Low Fat	2 (1 oz)	100	23	0	1
Fudge	4 (1 oz)	150	19	7	2
Lemon	4 (1 oz)	140	19	6	2
Oatmeal Raisin	4 (1 oz)	130	19	5	2
Sandwich Chocolate	3 (1.2 oz)	160	24	6	2
Sandwich Original	3 (1.2 oz)	160	24	6	2
Sandwich Peanut Butter	3 (1.2 oz)	160	22	7	4
Sandwich Vanilla	3 (1.2 oz)	160	25	5	2
Shortbread Reduced Fat	4 (1 oz)	130	22	4	2
Vanilla	4 (1 oz)	140	19	6	2
Famous Amos					
Chocolate Chip	3 (1 oz)	140	20	6	2
Freihofer's					
Chocolate Chip	2 (0.9 oz)	120	16	6	1
Frookie					
Animal Frackers	6	60	9	2	1
Apple Cinnamon Oat Bran	1	45	7	2	tr
General Mills					
Dunkaroos	1 pkg (1 oz)	130	19	5	1
FundaMiddles Vanilla Creme In Chocolate Graham Shells	1 pkg (0.8 oz)	110	18	4	1
Glenny's					
Noah'N Friends Animal Peanut Butter	0.5 oz	65	9	3	1
Noah'N Friends Animal Vanilla	0.5 oz	65	10	2	1
Noah'N Friends Animal Wheat-Free Oatmeal	0.5 oz	65	10	2	1
Nookie Bar	1 (1.15 oz)	138	18	3	2
Sesame Nookie	1 (0.5 oz)	60	6	4	1
Golden Fruit					
Apple	1 (0.7 oz)	80	15	2	1
Cranberry	1 (0.7 oz)	70	15	1	1
Cranberry Low Fat	1 (0.7 oz)	70	15	1	1
Raisin	1 (0.7 oz)	80	15	2	1
Grandma's					
Old Time Molasses	2 (2.75 oz)	320	58	9	4
Raisin Soft	2 (2.75 oz)	320	54	10	3

FOOD	PORTION	CALS.	CARB.	FAT	PRO.
Health Valley					
Amaranth Cookies	1	70	12	3	2
Fruit & Fitness	5	200	34	6	4
Honey Jumbos Fancy Oat Bran	2	130	20	4	4
The Great Tofu	2	90	14	3	2
The Great Wheat Free	2	80	14	3	2
Heyday					
Caramel & Peanut	1 (0.8 oz)	110	13	5	2
Fudge	1 (0.8 oz)	110	13	5	2
Honey Maid					
Cinnamon Grahams	10 (1.1 oz)	140	26	3	2
Honey Grahams	8 (1 oz)	120	22	3	2
Hydrox					
Original	3	150	21	7	2
Reduced Fat	3 (1.1 oz)	130	24	4	1
Keebler					
French Vanilla Creme	1	80	12	4	tr
Graham Kitchen Rich	2	60	9	2	1
Pitter Patter	1	90	12	4	2
Vanilla Wafers	4	80	10	4	tr
LU					
Chocolatiers	4 (1.1 oz)	170	20	8	2
Little Schoolboy Milk Chocolate	2 (0.9 oz)	130	15	7	2
Marie Lu	3 (1.2 oz)	170	25	6	2
Truffle Lu	4 (1.2 oz)	180	18	11	2
La Choy					
Fortune	1	15	4	tr	tr
Lance					
Coated Graham	1 pkg (50 g)	200	24	10	3
Peanut Butter Creme Filled Wafer	1 pkg (50 g)	240	34	10	4
Little Debbie					
Chocolate Chip Chewy	1 pkg (2 oz)	370	47	19	3
Figaroos	1 pkg (2 oz)	200	40	5	2
Peanut Butter	1 pkg (1.5 oz)	210	27	10	2
Peanut Butter & Jelly Sandwiches	1 pkg (1.1 oz)	130	22	5	2
Lorna Doone	4 (1 oz)	140	19	7	2
Mallomars					
Cookies	2 (0.9 oz)	120	17	5	1
Mallopuffs					
Cookies	1 (0.6 oz)	70	12	2	1

FOOD	PORTION	CALS.	CARB.	FAT	PRO.
Manischewitz					
Macaroons Chocolate	2 (0.9 oz)	90	15	4	2
Mother's					
Double Fudge	3	170	22	8	2
Striped Shortbread	3	170	22	8	2
Mystic Mint					
Cookies	1 (0.5 oz)	90	11	4	1
Nabisco					
Brown Edge Wafers	5 (1 oz)	140	21	6	1
Cameo	2 (1 oz)	130	21	5	1
Chocolate Grahams	3 (1.1 oz)	160	21	8	2
Grahams	8 (1 oz)	120	22	3	2
Nilla Wafers	8 (1.1 oz)	140	24	5	2
National					
Arrowroot	1 (5 g)	20	3	1	0
Newtons					
Apple Fat Free	2 (1 oz)	100	24	0	1
Cranberry Fat Free	2 (1 oz)	100	23	0	1
Fig	2 (1.1 oz)	110	20	3	1
Fig Fat Free	1 (1 oz)	100	22	0	1
Raspberry Fat Free	2 (1 oz)	100	23	0	1
Strawberry Fat Free	2 (1 oz)	100	23	0	1
Nutra/Balance					
Chocolate Chip	1 (2 oz)	260	34	14	3
Nutter Butter					
Peanut Butter Sandwich	2 (1 oz)	130	19	6	3
Oreo					
Cookies	3 (1.2 oz)	160	23	7	2
Reduced Fat	3 (1.2 oz)	140	24	5	2
Pepperidge Farm					
Bordeaux	2	70	11	3	1
Brussels	2	110	13	5	1
Brussels Mint	2	130	17	7	1
Butter Chessman	2	90	12	4	1
Capri	1	80	10	5	0
Geneva	2	130	14	6	1
Gingerman	2	70	10	3	1
Lemon Nut Crunch	2	110	13	7	1
Lido	1	90	10	5	1
Linzer	1	120	20	4	2
Milano	2	120	15	6	1
Pirouettes Chocolate Laced	2	70	8	4	1
Pirouettes Original	2	70	9	4	0

FOOD	PORTION	CALS.	CARB.	FAT	PRO.
Pepperidge Farm (CONT.)					
Sausalito Milk Chocolate Macadamia	1	120	14	7	1
Shortbread	2	150	17	8	1
Sugar	2	100	13	5	1
Zurich	1	60	10	2	1
Sargento					
MooTown Snackers Cookies & Creme Honey Graham Sticks & Vanilla Creme w/Sprinkle	1 pkg (1.1 oz)	140	19	7	2
MooTown Snackers Cookies & Creme Vanilla Sticks & Chocolate Fudge Creme	1 pkg (1.1 oz)	140	20	7	1
Snackwell's					
Fat Free Cinnamon Grahams	20 (1 oz)	110	26	0	2
Fat Free Devil's Food	1 (0.5 oz)	50	13	0	1
Fat Free Double Fudge	1 (0.5 oz)	50	12	0	1
Reduced Fat Chocolate Sandwich With Chocolate Creme	2 (0.9 oz)	100	20	3	1
Reduced Fat Chocolate Chip	13 (1 oz)	130	22	4	2
Reduced Fat Oatmeal Raisin	2 (1 oz)	110	20	3	2
Reduced Fat Vanilla Sandwich With Vanilla Creme	2 (0.9 oz)	110	21	3	1
Social Tea					
Cookies	6 (1 oz)	120	20	4	2
Stella D'Oro					
Anisette Toast	1	50	9	1	1
Apple Pastry Low Sodium	1	80	14	3	1
Egg Biscuits Low Sodium	3	120	20	3	4
Egg Jumbo	1	50	9	1	1
Fruit Delight Apple Cinnamon Fat Free	1	70	17	0	tr

FOOD	PORTION	CALS.	CARB.	FAT	PRO.
Stella D'Oro (CONT.)					
Kichel Low Sodium	21	150	13	9	4
Sunshine					
Classics Chocolate Chip With Pecans	1 (0.7 oz)	110	11	7	1
Grahams Cinnamon	2 (1.1 oz) (1.9 oz)	140	22	6	2
Grahams Fudge Dipped	4 (1.2 oz)	170	21	9	2
Grahams Honey	2 (1 oz)	120	20	4	2
Grahamy Bears	10 (1.1 oz)	140	22	5	2
Vanilla Wafers	7 (1.1 oz)	150	20	7	2
Vienna Fingers	2 (1 oz)	140	21	6	2
Tastykake					
Vanilla Sugar Wafer	1 (6 g)	36	4	2	0
Teddy Grahams					
Chocolate	24 (1 oz)	140	22	5	2
Cinnamon	24 (1 oz)	140	23	4	2
Honey	24 (1 oz)	140	22	4	2
Tree Of Life					
Fat Free Classic Carrot Cake	1 (0.8 oz)	60	14	0	1
Fat Free Devil's Food Chocolate	1 (0.8 oz)	70	15	0	2
Fruit Bars Apple Spice	2 (1.3 oz)	120	22	3	1
Fruit Bars Fat Free Fig	1 (0.8 oz)	70	16	0	1
Wheat-Free American Oatmeal	1 (0.8 oz)	90	11	5	1
Wheat-Free California Carob	1 (0.8 oz)	105	14	5	1
Vienna Fingers					
Low Fat	2 (1 oz)	130	23	4	1
Weight Watchers					
Apple Raisin Bar	1	100	18	3	1
Chocolate	3	80	13	3	1
Chocolate Chip	2	90	18	2	1
Chocolate Sandwich	2	90	15	3	1
Fruit Filled Bar Apple	1	80	21	tr	tr
Fruit Filled Bar Raspberry	1	80	22	tr	tr
Oatmeal Raisin	2	90	20	tr	1
Oatmeal Spice	3	80	13	2	1
Shortbread	3	80	13	2	1
TAKE-OUT					
biscotti with nuts chocolate dipped	1 (1.3 oz)	117	16	6	2

FOOD	PORTION	CALS.	CARB.	FAT	PRO.

CORN

(see also BRAN, CEREAL, CORNMEAL, FLOUR)

CANNED

FOOD	PORTION	CALS.	CARB.	FAT	PRO.
cream style	½ cup	93	23	1	2
w/ red & green peppers	½ cup	86	21	1	3
white	½ cup	66	15	1	2
yellow	½ cup	66	15	1	2
Del Monte					
Cream Style Golden	½ cup (4.4 oz)	90	20	1	2
Cream Style Golden 50% Less Salt	½ cup (4.4 oz)	90	20	1	2
Cream Style Golden No Salt Added	½ cup (4.4 oz)	90	20	1	2
Cream Style Supersweet Golden	½ cup (4.4 oz)	60	14	1	1
Cream Style White	½ cup (4.4 oz)	100	21	0	2
Whole Kernel Golden	½ cup (4.4 oz)	90	18	0	2
Whole Kernel Golden Supersweet 50% Less Salt	½ cup (4.4 oz)	60	11	1	2
Whole Kernel Golden Supersweet No Salt Added	½ cup (4.4 oz)	60	11	1	2
Whole Kernel Golden Supersweet No Sugar	½ cup (4.4 oz)	60	11	0	2
Whole Kernel Golden Supersweet Vacuum Packed	½ cup (3.7 oz)	70	13	1	2
Whole Kernel Golden Supersweet Vacuum Packed No Salt Added	½ cup (3.7 oz)	70	13	1	2
Whole Kernel White Sweet	½ cup (4.4 oz)	80	17	0	2
Green Giant					
50% Less Salt No Sugar Added	½ cup	50	11	1	2
Corn	½ cup	70	10	0	2
Cream Style	½ cup	100	24	tr	2
Deli Corn	½ cup	80	19	tr	2
Golden Kernel 50% Less Salt	½ cup	70	16	tr	2
Golden Vacuum Packed	½ cup	80	20	0	2
Mexi Corn	½ cup	80	19	tr	2

FOOD	PORTION	CALS.	CARB.	FAT	PRO.
Green Giant (CONT.)					
No Salt No Sugar	½ cup	80	18	tr	3
Sweet Select	½ cup	60	12	1	2
White Vacuum Packed	½ cup	80	20	0	2
Ka-Me					
Baby	½ cup (4.5 oz)	20	3	0	1
Stir Fry	½ cup (4.5 oz)	20	3	0	1
S&W					
Cream Style Premium Homestyle	½ cup	105	25	1	2
Cream Style Diet	½ cup	100	21	1	3
Sweet 'N Natural	½ cup	90	20	1	2
Whole Kernel Tender Young	½ cup	90	20	1	2
Whole Kernel Water Pack	½ cup	80	15	1	2
Seneca					
Cream Style	½ cup	80	18	0	2
Whole Kernel	½ cup	90	21	0	2
Whole Kernel Natural Pack	½ cup	80	18	1	3
FRESH					
on-the-cob w/ butter cooked	1 ear	155	32	3	4
white cooked	½ cup	89	21	1	3
white raw	½ cup	66	15	1	2
yellow cooked	1 ear (2.7 oz)	83	19	1	3
yellow cooked	½ cup	89	21	1	3
yellow raw	½ cup	66	15	1	2
yellow raw	1 ear (3 oz)	77	17	1	3
FROZEN					
cooked	½ cup	67	17	tr	2
on-the-cob cooked	1 ear (2.2 oz)	59	14	tr	2
Birds Eye					
Big Ears	1 ear	160	37	1	5
In Butter Sauce	½ cup	90	19	2	2
Little Ears	2 ears	130	30	1	4
On The Cob	1 ear	120	29	1	4
Polybag Cut	½ cup	80	19	1	3
Polybag Deluxe Tender Sweet	½ cup	80	20	1	3
Sweet	½ cup	80	20	1	3
Fresh Like					
Cob Corn	1 ear (5 in)	96	23	1	3

FOOD	PORTION	CALS.	CARB.	FAT	PRO.
Fresh Like (CONT.)					
Cob Corn	1 ear (3 in)	96	24	1	3
Cut	3.5 oz	85	21	1	3
Green Giant					
Cream Style	½ cup	110	25	1	3
Harvest Fresh Niblets	½ cup	80	17	1	2
Harvest Fresh White Shoepeg	½ cup	90	19	1	3
In Butter Sauce	½ cup	100	19	2	3
Nibblers Corn On The Cob	2 ears	120	27	1	4
Niblet Ears	1 ear	120	27	1	4
Niblets	½ cup	90	19	tr	2
One Serve Niblets In Butter Sauce	1 pkg	120	24	2	3
One Serve On The Cob	1 pkg	120	26	1	4
Super Sweet Nibblers Corn On The Cob	2 ears	90	19	2	3
Super Sweet Niblet Ears	1 ear	90	19	2	3
Super Sweet Niblet Select	½ cup	60	13	1	2
White In Butter Sauce	½ cup	100	20	2	2
White Select	½ cup	90	19	1	2
Mrs. Paul's					
Fritters	2	240	35	9	5
Ore Ida					
Cob Corn	1 ear (6.1 oz)	180	33	3	6
Cob Corn Mini-Gold	1 ear (3.1 oz)	90	16	1	3
Stouffer's					
Souffle	½ cup (2.4 oz)	170	21	7	5
Tree Of Life					
Corn	⅔ cup (3.2 oz)	80	19	1	3
SHELF-STABLE					
Pantry Express					
Golden Whole Kernel	½ cup	60	18	tr	2
TAKE-OUT					
fritters	1 (1 oz)	62	9	2	2
scalloped	½ cup	258	43	7	7

CORN CHIPS
(see CHIPS)

CORNISH HENS
(see CHICKEN)

CORNMEAL

| corn grits cooked | 1 cup | 146 | 31 | tr | 4 |

FOOD	PORTION	CALS.	CARB.	FAT	PRO.
corn grits uncooked	1 cup	579	124	2	14
degermed	1 cup	506	107	2	12
self-rising degermed	1 cup	489	103	2	12
whole grain	1 cup	442	94	4	10
Albers					
White	3 tbsp	110	34	0	2
Yellow	3 tbsp	110	34	0	2
Arrowhead					
Yellow	¼ cup (1.2 oz)	120	27	1	3
Aunt Jemima					
White	3 tbsp	102	22	1	2
Yellow	3 tbsp	102	22	1	2
Quaker					
White	3 tbsp	102	22	1	2
Yellow	3 tbsp	102	22	1	2
HOME RECIPE					
hush puppies	5 (2.7 oz)	256	35	12	5
hush puppies	1 (¾ oz)	74	10	3	3
MIX					
Arrowhead					
Corn Bread	¼ cup (1.2 oz)	120	24	1	5
Aunt Jemima					
Bolded White Mix	3 tbsp	99	21	1	2
Buttermilk Self Rising White Mix	3 tbsp	101	21	1	3
Self Rising White Mix	3 tbsp	98	21	1	2
Self Rising Yellow Mix	3 tbsp	100	21	1	2
Golden Dipt					
Corny Dog Batter Mix	1 oz	100	22	0	3
Hush Puppy Deluxe Mix	1¼ oz	120	26	0	3
Hush Puppy Jalapeno Mix	1¼ oz	120	27	0	3
Hush Puppy With Onion	1¼ oz	120	27	0	3
Hodgson Mill					
Yellow Self Rising	¼ oup (1 oz)	90	21	1	3
Yellow	¼ cup (1 oz)	100	22	1	3
Kentucky Kernel					
White Corn Meal Mix	¼ cup (1 oz)	100	22	1	3
Miracle Maize					
Complete as prep	1 piece (1.5 oz)	193	34	3	4
Country Style as prep	1 piece 2 in x 2 in (1.8 oz)	230	38	5	5
Sweet as prep	1 piece 2 in x 2 in (1.8 oz)	236	41	5	5

FOOD	PORTION	CALS.	CARB.	FAT	PRO.
Stone-Buhr					
Yellow Corn Meal	¼ cup (1 oz)	100	23	0	2
READY-TO-USE					
Aurora					
Polenta	½ cup (5 oz)	110	24	0	2
CORNSTARCH					
cornstarch	⅓ cup	164	39	tr	tr
COTTAGE CHEESE					
creamed	1 cup	217	6	9	26
creamed	4 oz	117	3	5	14
creamed w/ fruit	4 oz	140	15	4	11
dry curd	1 cup	123	3	1	25
dry curd	4 oz	96	2	tr	20
lowfat 1%	1 cup	164	6	2	28
lowfat 1%	4 oz	82	3	1	14
lowfat 2%	4 oz	101	4	2	16
lowfat 2%	1 cup	203	8	4	31
Axelrod					
Nonfat	½ cup (4.4 oz)	90	7	0	15
Borden					
4%	½ cup	120	4	5	14
Dry Curd 0.5%	½ cup	80	3	1	18
Unsalted 4%	½ cup	120	4	5	14
Breakstone					
2% Fat Large Curd	½ cup (4.2 oz)	90	4	3	14
2% Fat Small Curd	½ cup (4.2 oz)	90	4	3	15
4% Fat Large Curd	½ cup (4.2 oz)	120	4	5	14
4% Fat Small Curd	½ cup (4.2 oz)	120	4	5	14
Dry Curd ½% Fat	¼ cup (1.9 oz)	45	3	0	8
Cabot					
Cottage Cheese	4 oz	120	3	5	14
Light	4 oz	90	3	1	14
Friendship					
California Style	½ cup (4 oz)	115	4	5	15
Lowfat No Salt Added	½ cup (4 oz)	90	4	1	16
Lowfat Pineapple	½ cup (4 oz)	120	17	1	12
Lowfat 1%	½ cup (4 oz)	90	4	1	16
Nonfat	½ cup (4 oz)	80	5	0	15
Nonfat Plus Peach	½ cup (4 oz)	110	15	0	12
Pot Style	½ cup (4 oz)	90	3	3	15
With Pineapple	½ cup (4 oz)	140	15	4	16
Hood					
1% Fat	½ cup (4 oz)	90	6	2	13

FOOD	PORTION	CALS.	CARB.	FAT	PRO.
Hood (cont.)					
1% Fat Chive & Onion	½ cup (4 oz)	90	6	2	13
1% Fat No Salt Added	½ cup (4 oz)	90	6	2	13
1% Fat Pepper & Herb	½ cup (4 oz)	90	6	2	13
1% Fat Pineapple Cherry	½ cup (4 oz)	110	15	1	10
4% Fat	½ cup (4 oz)	120	5	4	13
4% Fat Chive	½ cup (4 oz)	130	5	4	13
4% Fat Pineapple	½ cup (4 oz)	130	15	4	10
Nonfat	½ cup (4 oz)	80	6	0	13
Nonfat Pineapple	½ cup (4 oz)	110	16	0	10
Knudsen					
1.5% Fat Peach	4 oz	110	12	2	11
1.5% Fat Pineapple	4 oz	110	11	2	11
1.5% Fat Strawberry	4 oz	110	12	2	11
1.5% Fat Tropical Fruit	4 oz	120	15	2	11
2% Fat Small Curd	½ cup (4.2 oz)	100	3	3	16
4% Fat Large Curd	½ cup (4.5 oz)	130	3	5	16
4% Fat Small Curd	½ cup (4.3 oz)	120	2	5	15
Free	½ cup (4.3 oz)	80	4	0	15
Lactaid					
1%	4 oz	72	3	1	12
Light N'Lively					
1% Fat	½ cup (4 oz)	80	4	2	14
1% Fat Garden Salad	½ cup (4.2 oz)	90	5	2	13
1% Fat Peach & Pineapple	½ cup (4.3 oz)	120	14	1	12
Free	½ cup (4.4 oz)	80	5	0	14
Lite Line					
Lowfat 1½%	½ cup	90	4	2	14
Sealtest					
2% Fat Small Curd	½ cup (4.2 oz)	90	4	3	14
4% Fat Large Curd	½ cup (4.2 oz)	120	4	5	14
4% Fat Small Curd	½ cup (4.2 oz)	120	4	5	14
Viva					
Nonfat	½ cup	70	5	0	13
Weight Watchers					
1%	½ cup	90	4	1	14
2%	½ cup	100	4	2	14
COTTONSEED					
kernels roasted	1 tbsp	51	2	4	3
COUSCOUS					
cooked	½ cup	101	21	tr	3
dry	½ cup	346	71	tr	12

FOOD	PORTION	CALS.	CARB.	FAT	PRO.
Casbah					
Almond Chicken Vegetarian	1 pkg (1.5 oz)	160	29	2	5
Asparagus Au Gratin Organic	1 pkg (1.5 oz)	150	28	2	14
Cheddar Broccoli	1 pkg (1.3 oz)	130	23	2	11
Hearty Harvest Zestful Organic as prep	1 pkg (10 fl oz)	180	36	1	6
Moroccan Stew	1 pkg (2 oz)	180	36	1	5
Pilaf as prep	1 cup	200	40	tr	8
Tomato Parmesan	1 pkg (1.8 oz)	170	34	2	7
Kitchen Del Sol					
Aegean Citrus as prep	½ cup (1.1 oz)	110	20	3	3
Moroccan Ginger as prep	½ cup (1.1 oz)	120	21	3	3
Spicy Vegetable as prep	½ cup (1.1 oz)	120	20	3	3
Tomato & Olive	½ cup (1 oz)	120	19	4	3
Tomato & Olive	½ cup (1.1 oz)	120	19	4	3
Near East					
As Prep	1¼ cup	260	46	6	8
CRAB					
CANNED					
blue	3 oz	84	0	1	17
blue	1 cup	133	0	2	28
S&W					
Dungeness Crab	3.25 oz	81	1	2	18
FRESH					
alaska king cooked	1 leg (4.7 oz)	129	0	2	26
alaska king cooked	3 oz	82	0	1	16
alaska king raw	1 leg (6 oz)	144	0	1	32
alaska king raw	3 oz	71	0	1	16
blue cooked	3 oz	87	0	2	17
blue cooked	1 cup	138	0	2	27
blue raw	3 oz	74	tr	1	15
blue raw	1 crab (.7 oz)	18	tr	tr	4
dungeness raw	3 oz	73	1	1	15
dungeness raw	1 crab (5.7 oz)	140	1	2	28
queen steamed	3 oz	98	0	1	20
FROZEN					
Mrs. Paul's					
Deviled Crab	1 cake	180	18	9	8
Deviled Crab Miniatures	3½ oz	240	25	12	9
READY-TO-USE					
crab cakes	1 cake (2.1 oz)	93	tr	5	12

FOOD	PORTION	CALS.	CARB.	FAT	PRO.
TAKE-OUT					
baked	1 (3.8 oz)	160	4	2	29
cake	1 (2 oz)	160	5	10	11
soft-shell fried	1 (4.4 oz)	334	31	18	11
CRACKER CRUMBS					
cracker meal	1 cup (4 oz)	440	93	2	11
Golden Dipt					
Cracker Meal	1 oz	100	22	0	3
Honey Maid					
Graham Cracker	0.5 oz	70	13	2	1
Keebler					
Cracker Meal	1 cup	100	23	3	3
Graham Crumbs	1 cup	520	90	14	8
Zesty Meal	1 cup	85	61	10	8
Kellogg's					
Corn Flake Crumbs	2 tbsp (0.4 oz)	40	9	0	1
Lance					
Cracker Meal	1 oz	100	21	1	3
Nabisco					
Nilla Cookie Crumbs	2 tbsp (0.5 oz)	70	13	3	1
Oreo					
Cookie Crumbs	2 tbsp (0.5 oz)	80	13	3	1
Premium					
Fat Free Cracker Crumbs	¼ cup (1 oz)	100	23	0	3
Ritz					
Cracker Crumbs	⅓ cup (1 oz)	140	17	7	2
Sunshine					
Graham	3 tbsp (0.6 oz)	80	13	2	2
CRACKERS					
(*see also* CRACKER CRUMBS)					
cheese	1 (1 in sq) (1 g)	5	1	tr	tr
cheese	14 (½ oz)	71	8	4	1
cheese low sodium	1 (1 in sq) (1 g)	5	1	tr	tr
cheese low sodium	14 (½ oz)	71	8	4	1
cheese w/ peanut butter filling	1 (0.24 oz)	34	4	2	1
crispbread	3	61	9	2	1
crispbread rye	1 (0.35 oz)	37	8	tr	1
crispbread rye	3	77	17	1	2
melba toast plain	1 (5 g)	19	4	tr	1
melba toast pumpernickel	1 (5 g)	19	4	tr	1
melba toast rye	1 (5 g)	19	4	tr	1
melba toast wheat	1 (5 g)	19	4	tr	1

FOOD	PORTION	CALS.	CARB.	FAT	PRO.
milk	1 (0.42 oz)	55	8	2	1
oyster cracker	1 (1 g)	4	1	tr	tr
peanut butter sandwich	1 (7 g)	34	4	2	1
rusk toast	1 (0.35 oz)	41	7	1	1
rye w/ cheese filling	1 (0.24 oz)	34	4	2	1
rye wafers plain	1 (0.9 oz)	84	20	tr	2
rye wafers seasoned	1 (0.8 oz)	84	16	2	2
saltines	1 (3 g)	13	2	tr	tr
saltines fat free low sodium	3 (0.5 oz)	59	12	tr	2
saltines fat free low sodium	6 (1 oz)	118	25	tr	3
saltines low salt	1 (3 g)	13	2	tr	tr
snack cracker	1 (3 g)	15	2	1	tr
snack cracker low salt	1 (3 g)	15	2	1	tr
snack cracker w/ cheese filling	1 (7 g)	33	4	2	1
soup cracker	1 (1 g)	4	1	tr	tr
water biscuits	3	92	16	3	2
wheat w/ cheese filling	1 (0.24 oz)	35	4	2	1
wheat w/ peanut butter filling	1 (0.24 oz)	35	4	2	1
wheat thins	1 (2 g)	9	1	tr	tr
wheat thins	7 (0.5 oz)	67	9	3	1
wheat thins low salt	7 (0.5 oz)	67	9	3	1
whole wheat	1 (4 g)	18	3	1	tr
whole wheat low salt	1 (4 g)	18	3	1	tr
zwieback	3½ oz	374	73	4	9
Adrienne's					
Gourmet Flatbread Caraway & Rye	2	20	4	tr	1
Gourmet Flatbread Classic Island	2	20	3	tr	1
Gourmet Flatbread Slightly Onion	2	20	3	tr	tr
Gourmet Flatbread Ten Grain	2	20	3	tr	1
American Heritage					
Sesame	9 (1.1 oz) (1.9 oz)	160	17	9	4
Wheat & Bran	9 (1 oz) (1.9 oz)	140	17	7	3
Better Cheddars					
Crackers	22 (1 oz)	70	17	8	4
Low Sodium	22 (1 oz)	150	18	7	3
Reduced Fat	24 (1 oz)	140	19	6	3
Burns & Ricker					
Bagel Crisps Garlic	5 (1 oz)	100	22	0	5

FOOD	PORTION	CALS.	CARB.	FAT	PRO.
Cheez-It					
Crackers	27 (1 oz)	160	16	8	4
Crackers	1 pkg (2 oz) (1.9 oz)	290	31	16	7
Crackers	1 pkg (1.5 oz) (1.9 oz)	220	23	12	6
Hot & Spicy	26 (1 oz) (1.9 oz)	160	17	8	3
Hot & Spicy	1 pkg (1.5 oz) (1.9 oz)	220	25	12	4
Low Sodium	27 (1 oz)	160	16	8	4
Party Mix	½ cup (1 oz)	140	19	5	4
Reduced Fat	30 (1 oz) (1.9 oz)	130	19	5	4
White Cheddar	26 (1 oz) (1.9 oz)	160	17	9	3
White Cheddar	1 pkg (1.5 oz) (1.9 oz)	220	24	12	4
Crown Pilot					
Crackers	1 (0.5 oz)	70	13	2	1
Devonsheer					
Melba Rounds Garlic	½ oz	56	9	1	2
Melba Rounds Honey Bran	½ oz	52	9	1	2
Melba Rounds Onion	½ oz	51	10	1	2
Melba Rounds Plain	½ oz	53	10	1	2
Melba Rounds Plain Unsalted	½ oz	52	10	1	2
Melba Rounds Rye	½ oz	53	10	1	2
Melba Rounds Sesame	½ oz	57	8	2	2
Eagle					
Bacon Cheese	1 oz	140	18	6	3
Cheese	1 oz	130	18	6	3
Peanut Butter & Cheese	1 oz	280	26	16	7
Eden					
Brown Rice	5 (1 oz)	120	22	2	3
Escort					
Crackers	3 (0.5 oz)	70	9	4	1
Estee					
Unsalted	1 (0.5 oz)	70	10	2	1
Frito Lay					
Cheese Filled	6 (1.5 oz)	210	24	10	4
Cracker Snacks Cheddar	13-16 (1 oz)	70	8	4	1
Cracker Snacks Zesty Italian	13-16 (1 oz)	70	9	3	1
Peanut Butter Filled	6 (1.5 oz)	210	24	10	6

FOOD	PORTION	CALS.	CARB.	FAT	PRO.
Goya					
Butter Crackers	1	40	6	1	0
Crackers	1	30	5	0	1
Hain					
Cheese	1 oz	130	17	6	3
Onion	1 oz	130	17	6	3
Onion No Salt Added	1 oz	130	17	6	3
Rich	1 oz	130	18	5	3
Rich No Salt Added	1 oz	130	18	5	3
Rye	1 oz	120	19	4	3
Rye No Salt Added	1 oz	120	19	4	3
Sesame	1 oz	140	16	7	3
Sesame No Salt Added	1 oz	140	16	7	3
Sour Cream & Chive	1 oz	130	15	6	3
Sour Cream & Chive No Salt Added	1 oz	130	15	6	3
Sourdough	½ oz	65	9	3	2
Sourdough Low Salt	1 oz	130	18	5	3
Vegetable	1 oz	130	10	5	3
Vegetable No Salt Added	1 oz	130	10	5	3
Harvest Crisps					
5 Grain	13 (1.1 oz)	130	23	4	3
Oat	13 (1.1 oz)	140	22	5	3
Health Valley					
Herb Stoned Wheat	13	55	9	2	1
Herb Stoned Wheat No Salt	13	55	9	2	1
Rice Bran	7	130	19	4	4
Sesame Stoned Wheat	13	55	9	2	1
Sesame Stoned Wheat No Salt Added	13	55	9	2	1
Seven Grain Vegetable Stoned Wheat	13	55	9	2	1
Seven Grain Vegetable Stoned Wheat No Salt Added	13	55	9	2	1
Stoned Wheat	13	55	9	2	1
Stoned Wheat No Salt Added	13	55	9	2	1
Hi Ho					
Butter Flavored	9 (1.1 oz)	160	19	9	2
Cracked Pepper	9 (1.1 oz)	160	18	9	2
Crackers	9	160	18	9	2
Low Salt	9 (1.1 oz)	160	18	9	2

FOOD	PORTION	CALS.	CARB.	FAT	PRO.
Hi Ho (CONT.)					
Multi Grain	9 (1.1 oz)	160	18	9	2
Reduced Fat	10 (1.1 oz)	140	21	5	2
Whole Wheat	9 (1.1 oz)	150	18	8	3
Ideal Crispbread					
Extra Thin	3	48	9	0	1
Fiber Thins	2	41	8	1	2
Oatbran Thins	2	50	8	0	2
J.J. Flats					
Breadflats Caraway	1	52	10	1	2
Breadflats Caraway And Salt	1	51	9	1	2
Breadflats Cinnamon	1	53	10	1	2
Breadflats Flavorall	1	52	10	1	2
Breadflats Garlic	1	52	10	1	2
Breadflats Oat Bran	1	49	8	1	2
Breadflats Onion	1	53	10	1	2
Breadflats Plain	1	53	10	1	1
Breadflats Poppy	1	53	9	1	2
Breadflats Sesame	1	55	9	2	2
Kavli					
Crackers	1 piece	40	10	tr	1
Keebler					
Club	2	30	4	2	tr
Melba Toast Garlic	2	25	4	tr	1
Melba Toast Long	2	30	7	tr	1
Melba Toast Onion	2	25	4	tr	1
Melba Toast Plain	2	25	4	tr	1
Melba Toast Sesame	2	25	4	tr	1
Oyster Crackers Large	26	80	13	2	2
Oyster Crackers Small	50	80	13	2	2
Snack Crackers Toasted Rye	2	30	4	2	tr
Snack Crackers Toasted Sesame	2	30	4	2	tr
Snack Crackers Toasted Wheat	2	30	4	2	tr
Toasted Snack Bacon	2	30	4	2	tr
Toasted Snack Onion	2	30	4	2	tr
Toasted Snack Pumpernickel	2	30	4	2	tr
Wholegrain Wheat	2	30	5	1	1
Krispy					
Cracked Pepper	5 (0.5 oz)	60	10	2	2

FOOD	PORTION	CALS.	CARB.	FAT	PRO.
Krispy (CONT.)					
Fat Free	5 (0.5 oz)	60	12	0	2
Mild Cheddar	5 (0.5 oz)	60	10	2	2
Original	5 (0.5 oz)	60	10	2	2
Soup & Oyster Crackers	17 (0.5 oz)	60	11	2	2
Unsalted Tops	5 (0.5 oz)	60	10	2	2
Whole Wheat	5 (0.5 oz)	60	10	2	2
Lance					
Bonnie	1 pkg (34 g)	160	24	7	2
Captain Wafers	2	30	5	1	1
Captain Wafers Very Low Sodium	2	30	5	1	1
Captain Wafers w/ Cream Cheese & Chives	1 pkg (37 g)	170	23	9	4
Cheese-On-Wheat	1 pkg (37 g)	180	22	9	4
Lanchee	1 pkg (35 g)	180	19	11	5
Melba Toast Oblong	2	30	7	0	1
Melba Toast Plain	2	20	4	0	1
Melba Toast Round Garlic	2	20	4	0	1
Melba Toast Round Onion	2	20	4	0	1
Melba Toast Sesame	2	25	4	0	1
Nekot	1 pkg (42 g)	210	24	10	6
Nip-Chee	1 pkg (37 g)	180	21	8	4
Oyster Crackers	1 pkg (14 g)	70	10	2	2
Peanut Butter Wheat	1 pkg (37 g)	190	18	11	6
Rye Twins	2	30	5	1	1
Rye-Chee	1 pkg (41 g)	190	22	9	4
Saltines	2	25	4	1	1
Saltines Slug Pack	4 crackers	50	8	1	1
Sesame Twins	2	40	6	1	1
Toastchee	1 pkg (39 g)	190	19	11	6
Toasty	1 pkg (35 g)	180	17	10	5
Wheat Twins	2	30	5	1	1
Wheatswafer	2	30	4	1	1
Lavash					
Bread Crisp Original	2 (0.5 oz)	60	11	1	2
Bread Crisp Sesame	2 (0.5 oz)	60	10	1	2
Little Debbie					
Cheese Crackers With Peanut Butter	1 pkg (1.4 oz)	210	23	10	5
Cheese Crackers With Peanut Butter	1 pkg (0.9 oz)	140	16	7	3

FOOD	PORTION	CALS.	CARB.	FAT	PRO.
Little Debbie (cont.)					
Toasty Crackers With Peanut Butter	1 pkg (0.9 oz)	140	16	7	3
Toasty Crackers With Peanut Butter	1 pkg (1.4 oz)	200	20	10	5
Wheat Crackers With Cheddar Cheese	1 pkg (0.9 oz)	140	16	7	3
Manischewitz					
Tam Tams	10	147	17	8	2
Tam Tams No Salt	10	138	18	7	2
Tams Garlic	10	153	19	8	2
Tams Onion	10	150	18	8	2
Tams Wheat	10	150	18	8	2
McCrackens					
Cracker Crisp Country Butter	1 oz	140	18	8	2
Cracker Crisp Sour Cream & Chives	1 oz	140	18	8	2
Cracker Crisp Tangy Cheddar	1 oz	140	18	8	2
Cracker Crisp Toasted Wheat	1 oz	140	18	8	2
NABS					
Cheese Peanut Butter Sandwich	6 (1.4 oz)	190	24	10	4
Peanut Butter Toast Sandwich	6 (1.4 oz)	190	24	10	4
Nabisco					
Bacon Flavored	15 (1.1 oz)	160	19	8	3
Chicken In A Biskit	14 (1 oz)	160	17	9	2
Garden Crisps	15 (1 oz)	130	22	4	2
Oat Thins	18 (1 oz)	140	20	1	3
Royal Lunch	1 (0.4 oz)	50	8	2	tr
Swiss	15 (1 oz)	140	18	7	2
Tid-Bit Cheese	32 (1 oz)	150	17	8	2
Vegetable Thins	14 (1.1 oz)	160	19	9	2
Wheat Thins Original	16 (1 oz)	140	19	6	2
Wheat Thins Reduced Fat	18 (1 oz)	120	21	4	2
Zings!	1 pkg (1.8 oz)	240	34	11	3
Nips					
Cheese	29 (1 oz)	150	18	6	3
Old London					
Melba Toast Pumpernickel	½ oz	54	10	1	2

118 • CRACKERS

FOOD	PORTION	CALS.	CARB.	FAT	PRO.
Old London (CONT.)					
Melba Toast Rye	½ oz	52	10	1	2
Melba Toast Sesame	½ oz	55	8	2	2
Melba Toast Sesame Unsalted	½ oz	55	8	2	2
Melba Toast Wheat	½ oz	51	10	1	2
Melba Toast White	½ oz	51	10	1	2
Melba Toast White Unsalted	½ oz	51	10	1	2
Melba Toast Whole Grain	½ oz	52	9	1	2
Melba Toast Whole Grain Unsalted	½ oz	53	10	1	2
Rounds Bacon	½ oz	53	9	1	2
Rounds Garlic	½ oz	56	9	1	2
Rounds Onion	½ oz	52	10	1	2
Rounds Rye	½ oz	52	10	1	2
Rounds Sesame	½ oz	56	8	2	2
Rounds White	½ oz	48	9	1	2
Rounds Whole Grain	½ oz	54	9	1	2
Oysterettes					
Crackers	19 (0.5 oz)	60	10	3	1
Pepperidge Farm					
Butter Thins	4	70	10	3	1
Cracked Wheat	3	100	14	4	2
Crispy Graham	4	70	13	2	1
English Water Biscuits	4	70	13	1	2
Flutters Garden Herb	¾ oz	100	14	4	2
Flutters Golden Sesame	¾ oz	110	13	5	2
Flutters Original Butter	¾ oz	100	15	4	2
Flutters Toasted Wheat	¾ oz	110	13	5	2
Garden Vegetable	5	60	10	2	1
Goldfish Cheddar Cheese	1 pkg (1½ oz)	190	28	6	6
Goldfish Cheddar Cheese	1 oz	120	19	4	4
Goldfish Cheese Thins	4	50	—	2	18
Goldfish Original	1 oz	130	18	5	3
Goldfish Parmesan Cheese	1 oz	120	19	4	4
Goldfish Pizza Flavored	1 oz	130	19	5	4
Goldfish Pretzel	1 oz	110	20	3	3
Hearty Wheat	4	100	13	5	2
Multi Grain	4	70	12	2	1
Sesame	4	80	12	4	2

FOOD	PORTION	CALS.	CARB.	FAT	PRO.
Pepperidge Farm (CONT.)					
Snack Mix Classic	1 oz	140	14	8	4
Snack Mix Lightly Smoked	1 oz	150	13	9	4
Snack Sticks Cheese	8	130	19	5	4
Snack Sticks Pretzel	8	120	23	3	3
Snack Sticks Pumpernickel	8	140	20	6	3
Snack Sticks Sesame	8	140	19	5	4
Spicy Lightly Smoked	1 oz	140	14	8	4
Toasted Rice	4	60	10	2	2
Toasted Wheat With Onion	4	80	12	3	2
Planters					
Cheese Peanut Butter Sandwiches	1 pkg (1.4 oz)	190	24	10	4
Toast Peanut Butter Sandwiches	1 pkg (1.4 oz)	190	24	10	4
Premium					
Saltine Fat Free	5 (0.5 oz)	50	11	0	1
Saltine Low Sodium	5 (0.5 oz)	60	10	1	1
Saltine Original	5 (0.5 oz)	60	10	2	1
Saltine Unsalted Tops	5 (0.5 oz)	60	10	2	1
Saltine Bits	34 (1 oz)	150	19	7	2
Soup & Oyster	23 (0.5 oz)	60	11	2	1
Ralston					
Oat Bran Krisp	2	60	6	3	1
Ritz					
Bits	48 (1 oz)	160	18	9	2
Bits Sandwiches With Peanut Butter	13 (1 oz)	150	17	8	4
Bits Sandwiches With Real Cheese	14 (1.1 oz)	160	17	10	3
Crackers	5 (0.5 oz)	80	10	4	1
Low Sodium	5 (0.5 oz)	80	10	4	1
Sandwiches With Real Cheese	1 pkg (1.4 oz)	210	21	12	4
Rykrisp					
Natural	2	40	7	0	1
Seasoned	2	45	8	1	1
Seasoned Twindividuals	2	45	8	1	1
Sesame	2	50	7	2	1
Sesmark					
Brown Rice	15 (1 oz)	120	25	2	2

FOOD	PORTION	CALS.	CARB.	FAT	PRO.
Sesmark (CONT.)					
Cheese Thins	15 (1 oz)	130	26	3	2
Rice Thins Original	15 (1 oz)	130	24	3	2
Rice Thins Teriyaki Flavored	13 (1 oz)	130	24	3	2
Savory Thins Original	15 (1 oz)	125	25	2	3
Sesame Thins Cheddar	9 (1 oz)	150	15	8	5
Sesame Thins Garlic	9 (1 oz)	150	16	8	4
Sesame Thins Original	9 (1 oz)	150	16	8	5
Sesame Thins Unsalted	11 (1 oz)	150	17	8	5
Snackwell's					
Cracked Pepper	7 (0.5 oz)	60	13	0	2
Fat Free Wheat	5 (0.5 oz)	60	12	0	2
Reduced Fat Cheese	38 (1 oz)	130	23	2	4
Reduced Fat Classic Golden	6 (0.5 oz)	60	11	1	1
Snorkles					
Cheddar	56 (1 oz)	140	19	5	4
Sociables					
Crackers	7 (0.5 oz)	80	9	4	1
Sunshine					
Saltines Cracked Pepper	5 (0.5 oz)	60	10	2	2
Town House					
Crackers	2	35	4	2	tr
Tree Of Life					
Bite Size Fat Free Corn & Salsa	12	60	12	0	1
Bite Size Fat Free Cracked Pepper	12	55	12	0	1
Bite Size Fat Free Garden Vegetable	12	55	12	0	2
Bite Size Fat Free Garlic & Herb	12	55	12	0	2
Bite Size Fat Free Soya Nut	12	60	12	0	2
Bite Size Fat Free Toasted Onion	12	60	12	0	2
Bite Size Fat Free Whole Wheat	12	60	12	0	2
Fat Free Oyster	40 (0.5 oz)	60	13	0	2
Saltine Cracked Pepper Fat Free	4 (0.5 oz)	60	13	0	2
Saltine Fat Free	4 (0.5 oz)	50	11	0	2
Triscuit					
Crackers	7 (1.1 oz)	140	21	5	3

FOOD	PORTION	CALS.	CARB.	FAT	PRO.
Triscuit (CONT.)					
Deli-Style Rye	7 (1.1 oz)	140	22	5	3
Garden Herb	6 (1 oz)	130	20	5	3
Low Sodium	7 (1.1 oz)	150	21	6	3
Reduced Fat	8 (1.1 oz)	130	24	3	3
Wheat 'n Bran	7 (1.1 oz)	140	22	5	3
Twigs					
Sesame & Cheese Sticks	15 (1 oz)	150	17	7	4
Uneeda Biscuit					
Unsalted Tops	2 (0.5 oz)	60	11	2	1
Venus					
Armenian Thin Bread	2 (0.9 oz)	100	19	1	3
Bran Wafers Salt Free	5 (0.5 oz)	60	11	1	1
Corn Crackers Salt Free	5 (0.5 oz)	60	10	1	2
Cracked Wheat Wafers Salt Free	5 (0.5 oz)	60	11	1	1
Cracker Bread	5 (0.5 oz)	60	11	1	2
Hors D'oeuvre	3 (0.5 oz)	60	11	2	1
Oat Bran Wafers	5 (0.5 oz)	60	11	1	2
Oat Bran Wafers Salt Free	5 (0.5 oz)	60	11	1	2
Old Brussels Cheddar Waferettes	5 (0.5 oz)	80	7	5	1
Old Brussels Jalapeno Waferettes	5 (0.5 oz)	80	7	5	1
Rye Wafers Low Salt	5 (0.5 oz)	60	11	1	2
Stoned Wheat Wafers Bite Size	7 (0.5 oz)	60	11	1	1
Water Crackers Fat Free	5 (0.5 oz)	55	11	0	2
Wheat Wafers Low Salt	5 (0.5 oz)	60	10	2	2
Waldorf					
Sodium Free	2	30	5	1	tr
Wasa Crispbread					
Breakfast	1	50	9	1	2
Extra Crisp	1	25	5	0	1
Falu Rye	1	30	6	0	1
Fiber Plus	1	35	5	1	1
Golden Rye	1	30	7	0	1
Hearty Rye	1	50	10	0	2
Light Rye	1	25	5	0	1
Royal	½	26	6	0	1
Savory Sesame	1	30	4	1	1
Sesame Rye	1	30	4	1	1
Sesame Wheat	1	60	9	2	2

FOOD	PORTION	CALS.	CARB.	FAT	PRO.
Wasa Crispbread (CONT.)					
Toasted Wheat	1	50	9	1	2
Waverly					
Crackers	5 (0.5 oz)	70	10	4	1
Weight Watchers					
Crispbread Garlic	2	30	7	0	tr
Wheat Thins					
Low Salt	16 (1 oz)	140	20	6	2
Multi-Grain	17 (1 oz)	130	21	4	2
Wheatworth					
Stone Ground	5 (0.5 oz)	80	10	4	2
Zesta					
Saltine	2	25	4	1	tr
Saltine Unsalted Top	2	25	4	1	tr
Zwieback					
Crackers	1 (8 g)	35	5	1	1

CRANBERRIES
CANNED

FOOD	PORTION	CALS.	CARB.	FAT	PRO.
cranberry sauce sweetened	½ cup	209	54	tr	tr
Ocean Spray					
CranFruit Cranberry Raspberry Sauce	2 oz	100	23	0	0
CranFruit Cranberry Strawberry Sauce	2 oz	100	23	0	0
CranFruit Cranberry Orange Sauce	2 oz	100	23	0	0
Cranberry Sauce Jellied	2 oz	90	22	0	0
Whole Berry Sauce	2 oz	90	23	0	0
S&W					
Cranberry Sauce Jellied Old Fashioned	½ cup	90	22	0	0
Cranberry Sauce Whole Berry Old Fashioned	½ cup	90	22	0	0
FRESH					
chopped	1 cup	54	14	tr	tr
Ocean Spray					
Fresh	½ cup	25	6	0	0

CRANBERRY BEANS
CANNED

FOOD	PORTION	CALS.	CARB.	FAT	PRO.
cranberry beans	1 cup	216	39	1	14
DRIED					
cooked	1 cup	240	43	1	17

FOOD	PORTION	CALS.	CARB.	FAT	PRO.
Bean Cuisine					
Dried	½ cup	115	—	1	8
CRANBERRY JUICE					
cocktail	1 cup	147	38	tr	tr
cranberry juice cocktail	6 oz	108	27	tr	0
cranberry juice cocktail low calorie	6 oz	33	9	0	0
cranberry juice cocktail frzn	12 oz can	821	210	0	tr
cranberry juice cocktail frzn as prep	6 oz	102	26	0	0
After The Fall					
Cape Cod Cranberry	1 bottle (10 oz)	130	30	0	0
Cranberry Ginger Ale	1 can (12 oz)	140	35	0	1
Apple & Eve					
Juice	6 fl oz	100	25	0	0
Ocean Spray					
Cocktail	8 fl oz	140	34	0	0
Cocktail Reduced Calorie	8 fl oz	50	13	0	0
Lightstyle Low Calorie Cranberry Juice Cocktail	8 fl oz	40	10	0	0
Seneca					
Cocktail frzn as prep	8 fl oz	140	36	0	0
Smucker's					
Juice Sparkler	10 oz	140	34	tr	1
Snapple					
Cranberry Royal	10 fl oz	150	37	0	0
Tree Of Life					
Concentrate	8 tsp (1.4 oz)	110	28	0	0
Tropicana					
Twister Ruby Red	1 bottle (10 fl oz)	150	37	0	0
Twister Ruby Red	8 fl oz	120	30	0	0
Veryfine					
Drink	8 oz	160	40	0	0
CRAYFISH					
(see also LOBSTER)					
cooked	3 oz	97	0	1	20
raw	3 oz	76	0	1	16
raw	8	24	0	tr	5
CREAM					
(see also SOUR CREAM, SOUR CREAM SUBSTITUTES, WHIPPED TOPPINGS)					
LIQUID					
half & half	1 tbsp	20	1	2	tr

FOOD	PORTION	CALS.	CARB.	FAT	PRO.
half & half	1 cup	315	10	28	7
heavy whipping	1 tbsp	52	tr	6	tr
light coffee	1 cup	496	9	46	6
light coffee	1 tbsp	29	1	3	tr
light whipping	1 tbsp	44	tr	5	tr
Farmland					
Half & Half	2 tbsp	40	2	3	1
Light Cream	2 tbsp	30	1	3	1
Hood					
Half & Half	2 tbsp (1 oz)	40	1	4	1
Heavy	1 tbsp (0.5 oz)	50	0	5	0
Light	1 tbsp (0.5 oz)	30	tr	3	1
Whipping Cream	1 tbsp (0.5 oz)	45	tr	5	0
Parmalat					
Half & Half	2 tbsp (1 oz)	40	2	3	1
WHIPPED					
heavy whipping	1 cup	411	7	44	5
light whipping	1 cup	345	7	37	5

CREAM CHEESE

FOOD	PORTION	CALS.	CARB.	FAT	PRO.
cream cheese	1 oz	99	1	10	2
cream cheese	1 pkg (3 oz)	297	2	30	6
Alpine Lace					
Fat Free Garden Vegetable	2 tbsp (1 oz)	30	1	tr	5
Fat Free Garlic & Herbs	2 tbsp (1 oz)	30	1	tr	5
Breakstone					
Temp-Tee Whipped	3 tbsp (1.2 oz)	110	1	10	3
Fleur De Lait					
Bermuda Onion & Chives	2 tbsp (0.9 oz)	90	2	8	1
Cinnamon Raisin	2 tbsp (0.9 oz)	90	6	8	1
Date Nut Rum	2 tbsp (0.9 oz)	90	4	8	2
Fresh Cut Garden Vegetable	2 tbsp (0.9 oz)	80	1	8	2
Garden Vegetable	2 tbsp (0.9 oz)	80	1	8	2
Garlic & Spice	2 tbsp (0.9 oz)	90	1	9	2
Herb & Spice	2 tbsp (0.9 oz)	90	2	9	2
Irish Creme	2 tbsp (0.9 oz)	100	2	9	2
Lemon	2 tbsp (0.9 oz)	90	5	7	1
Lox	2 tbsp (0.9 oz)	90	1	8	2
Mandarin Orange	2 tbsp (0.9 oz)	90	3	7	1
Peach	2 tbsp (0.9 oz)	90	3	7	1
Pineapple	2 tbsp (0.9 oz)	90	3	8	1

FOOD	PORTION	CALS.	CARB.	FAT	PRO.
Fleur De Lait (CONT.)					
Plain	2 tbsp (1 oz)	100	1	10	2
Strawberry	2 tbsp (0.9 oz)	90	3	8	1
Toasted Onion	2 tbsp (0.9 oz)	90	2	9	2
Wildberry	2 tbsp (0.9 oz)	90	4	7	1
Fresh Cut					
Bac'n & Horseradish	2 tbsp (0.9 oz)	90	1	9	2
Bermuda Onion & Chives	2 tbsp (0.9 oz)	90	2	8	1
Date Nut & Rum	2 tbsp (0.9 oz)	90	4	8	2
Garlic & Spice	2 tbsp (0.9 oz)	90	1	9	2
Herb & Spice	2 tbsp (0.9 oz)	90	2	9	2
Lox	2 tbsp (0.9 oz)	90	1	8	2
Peaches & Cream	2 tbsp (0.9 oz)	90	3	7	1
Strawberry	2 tbsp (0.9 oz)	90	3	8	1
Friendship					
NY Style Reduced Fat	2 tbsp (1 oz)	50	0	3	5
Healthy Choice					
Herbs & Garlic	2 tbsp (1 oz)	25	2	0	4
Plain	2 tbsp (1 oz)	25	2	0	4
Strawberry	2 tbsp (1 oz)	30	5	0	4
Heluva Good Cheese					
Cream Cheese	1 tbsp (1 oz)	100	1	10	2
Philadelphia					
Free	1 oz	25	2	0	4
Free Soft	2 tbsp (1.2 oz)	30	2	0	5
Light Soft	2 tbsp (1.1 oz)	70	2	5	3
Regular	1 oz	100	tr	10	2
Soft	2 tbsp (1 oz)	100	1	10	2
Soft Herb & Garlic	2 tbsp (1.1 oz)	110	2	10	1
Soft Olive & Pimento	2 tbsp (1.1 oz)	100	2	9	2
Soft Pineapple	2 tbsp (1.1 oz)	100	4	9	2
Soft Smoked Salmon	2 tbsp (1.1 oz)	100	1	9	2
Soft Strawberries	2 tbsp (1.1 oz)	100	5	9	1
Soft With Chives & Onions	2 tbsp (1.1 oz)	110	2	10	2
Whipped	3 tbsp (1.1 oz)	110	1	11	2
Whipped Smoked Salmon	3 tbsp (1.1 oz)	100	2	9	2
With Chives	1 oz	90	tr	9	2
With Pimentos	1 oz	90	tr	9	2
Ultra Delight					
Cheddar Cream Cheese	2 tbsp (0.9 oz)	60	2	4	3
Chive	2 tbsp (0.9 oz)	60	2	4	3

FOOD	PORTION	CALS.	CARB.	FAT	PRO.
Ultra Delight (CONT.)					
Garlic	2 tbsp (0.9 oz)	60	2	4	3
Mixed Berry	2 tbsp (0.9 oz)	70	5	4	2
Nacho	2 tbsp (0.9 oz)	60	2	4	3
Salsa	2 tbsp (0.9 oz)	60	2	4	2
Shrimp	2 tbsp (0.9 oz)	60	2	4	3
Strawberry	2 tbsp (0.9 oz)	60	4	4	2
Vegetable	2 tbsp (0.9 oz)	50	2	4	2
Weight Watchers					
Reduced Fat	2 tbsp	35	1	2	3

CREAM CHEESE SUBSTITUTES
Tofutti

Better Than Cream Cheese French Onion	1 oz	80	1	8	1
Better Than Cream Cheese Herb & Chive	1 oz	80	1	8	1
Better Than Cream Cheese Plain	1 oz	80	1	8	1

CREAM OF TARTAR
cream of tartar	1 tsp	8	2	0	0

CRESS
(see also WATERCRESS)

garden cooked	½ cup	16	3	tr	1
garden raw	½ cup	8	1	tr	tr

CROAKER
atlantic breaded & fried	3 oz	188	6	11	15
atlantic raw	3 oz	89	0	3	15

CROISSANT
apple	1 (2 oz)	145	21	5	4
cheese	1 (2 oz)	236	27	12	5
plain	1 (2 oz)	232	26	12	5
plain	1 mini (1 oz)	115	13	6	2
Pepperidge Farm					
Croissant Sandwich Quartet	1	170	22	7	4
Petite All Butter	1	120	13	6	3
Rudy's Farm					
Ham & Swiss Sandwich	1 (3.4 oz)	310	27	18	12
Sara Lee					
All Butter	1	170	19	9	4
All Butter Petite Size	1	120	13	6	3

FOOD	PORTION	CALS.	CARB.	FAT	PRO.
TAKE-OUT					
w/ egg & cheese	1	369	24	25	13
w/ egg cheese & bacon	1	413	24	28	16
w/ egg cheese & ham	1	475	24	34	19
w/ egg cheese & sausage	1	524	25	38	20
CROUTONS					
plain	1 cup (1 oz)	122	22	2	4
seasoned	1 cup (1.4 oz)	186	25	7	4
Arnold					
Crispy Cheddar Romano	½ oz	64	8	3	2
Crispy Cheese Garlic	½ oz	60	9	2	2
Crispy Fine Herbs	½ oz	50	10	1	2
Crispy Italian	½ oz	60	8	3	2
Crispy Onion & Garlic	½ oz	60	9	2	2
Crispy Seasoned	½ oz	60	8	3	2
Brownberry					
Ceasar Salad	½ oz	62	8	3	2
Cheddar Cheese	½ oz	63	8	3	2
Onion & Garlic	½ oz	60	9	2	2
Seasoned	½ oz	59	8	2	2
Toasted	½ oz	56	10	1	2
Pepperidge Farm					
Cheddar & Romano Cheese	½ oz	60	10	2	2
Cheese & Garlic	½ oz	70	9	3	2
Onion & Garlic	½ oz	70	9	3	2
Seasoned	½ oz	70	9	3	2
Sour Cream & Chive	½ oz	70	9	3	2
CUCUMBER					
FRESH					
raw	1 (11 oz)	38	8	tr	2
raw sliced	½ cup (1.8 oz)	7	1	tr	tr
JARRED					
Rosoff's					
Salad	3 slices (1 oz)	12	3	0	0
Schorr's					
Cucumber Garden Salad	3 slices (1 oz)	12	3	0	0
TAKE-OUT					
cucumber salad	3.5 oz	50	11	tr	1
CURRANT JUICE					
black currant nectar	3½ oz	55	13	0	tr
red currant nectar	3½ oz	54	13	tr	tr

FOOD	PORTION	CALS.	CARB.	FAT	PRO.
CURRANTS					
black fresh	½ cup	36	9	tr	1
zante dried	½ cup	204	53	tr	3
CUSK					
fillet baked	3 oz	106	0	1	23
CUSTARD					
HOME RECIPE					
baked	½ cup (5 oz)	148	15	7	7
baked	1 recipe 4 serv (19.8 oz)	549	60	26	29
flan	½ cup (5.4 oz)	220	35	6	7
flan	1 recipe 10 serv (53.7 oz)	2206	349	63	70
MIX					
as prep w/ 2% milk	½ cup (4.7 oz)	148	24	4	7
as prep w/ 2% milk	1 recipe 4 serv (18.7 oz)	595	95	15	22
as prep w/ whole milk	1 recipe 4 serv (18.7 oz)	652	94	22	22
as prep w/ whole milk	½ cup (4.7 oz)	163	23	5	6
flan as prep w/ 2% milk	1 recipe 4 serv (18.7 oz)	542	102	9	16
flan as prep w/ 2% milk	½ cup (4.7 oz)	135	26	2	4
flan as prep w/ whole milk	1 recipe 4 serv (18.7 oz)	600	102	16	16
flan as prep w/ whole milk	½ cup (4.7 oz)	150	25	4	4
Jell-O					
Flan	½ cup	151	26	4	4
Golden Egg Americana as prep	½ cup	160	23	6	5
Royal					
Custard	mix for 1 serving	60	16	0	0
Flan Caramel Custard	mix for 1 serving	60	15	0	0
TAKE-OUT					
baked	½ cup (5 oz)	148	15	7	7
zabaione	½ cup (57.2 g)	135	13	5	3
CUTTLEFISH					
steamed	3 oz	134	1	1	28
DANDELION GREENS					
fresh cooked	½ cup	17	3	tr	1
raw chopped	½ cup	13	3	tr	1

FOOD	PORTION	CALS.	CARB.	FAT	PRO.
DANISH PASTRY					
FROZEN					
Morton					
Honey Buns	1 (2.28 oz)	250	35	10	3
Honey Buns Mini	1 (1.23 oz)	160	19	8	2
Pepperidge Farm					
Apple	1	220	35	8	2
Cheese	1	240	25	14	3
Cinnamon Raisin	1	250	35	11	3
Raspberry	1	220	31	9	3
Sara Lee					
Apple	1	120	15	6	2
Apple Free & Light	1 slice (2 oz)	130	30	0	2
Apple Danish Twist	1 slice (1.9 oz)	190	22	10	3
Cheese	1	130	13	8	2
Cheese Danish Twist	1 slice (1.9 oz)	200	21	12	3
Cinnamon Raisin	1	150	17	8	2
Raspberry Danish Twist	1 slice (1.9 oz)	200	25	9	3
READY-TO-EAT					
plain ring	1 (12 oz)	1305	152	71	21
Hostess					
Apple	1 (3.8 oz)	400	47	22	4
Apple Fruit Roll	1 (2 oz)	180	33	4	4
Coffee Cake Raspberry	1 (1.2 oz)	110	21	3	2
REFRIGERATED					
Pillsbury					
Caramel Danish w/ Nuts	1	160	19	8	2
Cinnamon Raisin Danish w/ Icing	1	150	20	7	2
Orange Danish w/ Icing	1	150	19	7	2
TAKE-OUT					
almond	1 (4¼ in) (2.3 oz)	280	30	16	5
apple	1 (4¼ in) (2.5 oz)	264	34	13	4
cheese	1 (3 oz)	353	29	25	6
cheese	1 (4¼ in) (2.5 oz)	266	26	16	6
cinnamon	1 (3 oz)	349	47	17	5
cinnamon	1 (4¼ in) (2.3 oz)	262	29	15	5
cinnamon nut	1 (4¼ in) (2.3 oz)	280	30	16	5
fruit	1 (3.3 oz)	335	45	16	5
lemon	1 (4¼ in) (2.5 oz)	264	34	13	4
raisin	1 (4¼ in) (2.5 oz)	264	34	13	4
raisin nut	1 (4¼ in) (2.3 oz)	280	30	16	5
raspberry	1 (4¼ in) (2.5 oz)	264	34	13	4
strawberry	1 (4¼ in) (2.5 oz)	264	34	13	4

FOOD	PORTION	CALS.	CARB.	FAT	PRO.
DATES					
DRIED					
chopped	1 cup	489	131	1	4
whole	10	228	61	tr	2
Bordo					
Diced	2 oz	203	48	1	1
Dole					
Chopped	½ cup	230	56	0	0
Pitted	½ cup	280	62	0	8
Dromedary					
Chopped	¼ cup	130	31	0	1
Pitted	5	100	23	0	1
Sonoma					
Dried	5-6 (1.4 oz)	110	30	0	1

DEER

(*see* VENISON)

DELI MEATS/COLD CUTS

(*see also* CHICKEN, HAM, MEAT SUBSTITUTES, TURKEY)

FOOD	PORTION	CALS.	CARB.	FAT	PRO.
barbecue loaf pork & beef	1 oz	49	2	3	4
beerwurst beef	1 slice (2¾ in x ¹⁄₁₆ in)	20	tr	2	1
beerwurst beef	1 slice (4 in x ⅛ in)	75	tr	7	3
beerwurst pork	1 slice (2¾ in x ¹⁄₁₆ in)	14	tr	1	1
beerwurst pork	1 slice (4 in x ⅛ in)	55	tr	4	4
berliner pork & beef	1 oz	65	1	4	4
blood sausage	1 oz	95	tr	9	4
bologna beef	1 oz	88	tr	8	4
bologna beef & pork	1 oz	89	1	8	3
bologna pork	1 oz	70	tr	6	4
braunschweiger pork	1 oz	102	1	9	4
braunschweiger pork	1 slice (2½ in x ¼ in)	65	1	6	2
corned beef loaf	1 oz	43	0	2	7
dutch brand loaf pork & beef	1 oz	68	2	5	4
headcheese pork	1 oz	60	tr	5	5
honey loaf pork & beef	1 oz	36	2	1	4
honey roll sausage beef	1 oz	42	1	2	4
lebanon bologna beef	1 oz	60	1	4	6
liver cheese pork	1 oz	86	1	7	4
liverwurst pork	1 oz	92	1	8	4
luncheon meat beef	1 oz	87	1	7	4
luncheon meat pork & beef	1 oz	100	1	9	4

FOOD	PORTION	CALS.	CARB.	FAT	PRO.
luncheon meat pork canned	1 oz	95	1	9	4
luncheon sausage pork & beef	1 oz	74	tr	6	4
luxury loaf pork	1 oz	40	1	1	5
mortadella beef & pork	1 oz	88	1	7	5
mother's loaf pork	1 oz	80	2	6	3
new england sausage pork & beef	1 oz	46	1	2	5
olive loaf pork	1 oz	67	3	5	3
peppered loaf pork & beef	1 oz	42	1	2	5
pepperoni pork & beef	1 slice (0.2 oz)	27	tr	2	1
pepperoni pork & beef	1 (9 oz)	1248	7	110	53
pickle & pimiento loaf pork	1 oz	74	2	6	3
picnic loaf pork & beef	1 oz	66	1	5	4
salami cooked beef & pork	1 oz	71	1	6	4
salami hard pork	1 pkg (4 oz)	460	2	38	26
salami hard pork	1 slice (⅓ oz)	41	3	4	2
salami hard pork & beef	1 slice (⅛ oz)	42	tr	3	2
salami hard pork & beef	1 pkg (4 oz)	472	3	39	26
sandwich spread pork & beef	1 tbsp	35	2	3	1
sandwich spread pork & beef	1 oz	67	3	5	2
summer sausage thuringer cervelat	1 oz	98	1	8	5
Carl Buddig					
Beef	1 oz	40	1	2	5
Corned Beef	1 oz	40	1	2	5
Pastrami	1 oz	40	1	2	5
DiLusso					
Genoa	1 oz	100	0	8	6
Hansel n'Gretel					
Healthy Deli Bologna Beef & Pork	1 oz	41	1	2	4
Healthy Deli Cooked Corn Beef	1 oz	35	1	1	6
Healthy Deli Italian Roast Beef	1 oz	31	tr	1	6
Healthy Deli Pastrami Round	1 oz	34	1	1	5
Healthy Deli Regular Roast Beef	1 oz	30	tr	tr	6

FOOD	PORTION	CALS.	CARB.	FAT	PRO.
Hansel n'Gretel (CONT.)					
Healthy Deli St Paddy's Corned Beef	1 oz	24	1	tr	4
Healthy Choice					
Bologna	1 slice (1 oz)	30	1	1	4
Bologna Beef	1 slice (1 oz)	35	3	1	4
Deli-Thin Bologna	4 slices (1.8 oz)	60	3	2	8
Well-Pack Bologna	1 slice (1 oz)	30	1	1	4
Hebrew National					
Bologna Beef	2 oz	180	—	16	7
Bologna Beef Reduced Fat	2 oz	130	—	12	6
Bologna Lean Chub	2 oz	90	—	6	8
Bologna Midget	2 oz	180	—	16	7
Deli Pastrami	2 oz	80	—	3	12
Deli Express Corned Beef	2 oz	80	—	3	15
Deli Express Tongue Sliced	2 oz	120	—	9	10
Salami Beef	2 oz	170	—	14	8
Salami Beef Reduced Fat	2 oz	110	—	8	8
Salami Sean Chub	2 oz	90	—	6	9
Salami Midget	2 oz	170	—	14	8
Hillshire					
Bologna Large	1 oz	90	tr	8	3
Bologna Ring	1 oz	90	tr	8	3
Braunschweiger	1 oz	95	2	8	4
Deli Select Corned Beef	1 slice	10	tr	tr	2
Deli Select Light Bologna	1 slice	12	tr	1	1
Deli Select Oven Roasted Cured Beef	1 slice	10	tr	tr	2
Deli Select Pastrami	1 slice	10	tr	tr	2
Deli Select Roast Beef	1 slice	10	tr	tr	2
Deli Select Smoked Beef	1 slice	10	tr	tr	2
Flavor Pack 90-99% Fat Free Light Bologna	1 slice (0.73 oz)	30	1	2	3
Flavor Pack 90-99% Fat Free Pastrami	1 slice (0.6 oz)	18	tr	tr	4
Lunch 'N Munch Bologna/ American/ Snickers	1 pkg (4.25 oz)	490	31	34	15
Lunch 'N Munch Bologna/ American/ Snickers/Hi-C	1 pkg (4.25 oz + 6 fl oz)	590	55	34	15

FOOD	PORTION	CALS.	CARB.	FAT	PRO.
Hillshire (CONT.)					
Lunch 'N Munch Bologna/American	1 pkg (4.5 oz)	480	20	37	17
Lunch 'N Munch Cotto Salami/ Monterey Jack	1 pkg (4.5 oz)	440	21	32	18
Lunch 'N Munch Pepperoni/ American	1 pkg (4.5 oz)	570	20	46	22
Pepperoni	1 oz	110	0	10	5
Salami Hard	1 oz	100	0	9	5
Salami Hard	1 oz	90	1	7	5
Summer Sausage	2 oz	180	1	16	9
Summer Sausage Beef	2 oz	190	1	17	9
Summer Sausage Light	2 oz	150	1	12	10
Summer Sausage w/ Cheddar Cheese	2 oz	200	1	18	9
Homeland					
Hard Salami	1 oz	110	0	10	5
Hormel					
Liverwurst Spread	4 tbsp (2 oz)	130	2	10	8
Pepperoni Chunk	1 oz	140	0	13	5
Pepperoni Sliced	15 slices (1 oz)	140	0	13	5
Pepperoni Twin	1 oz	140	0	13	5
Pillow Pack Genoa Salami	4 slices (1.1 oz)	120	0	10	7
Pillow Pack Pepperoni	16 slices (1 oz)	140	0	13	5
Pillow Pack Pepperoni	1 oz	140	0	13	5
Jones					
Liver Sausage	1 slice	80	tr	7	3
Liver Sausage Chub	1 slice	80	tr	7	5
Oscar Mayer					
Bologna Beef	1 slice (1 oz)	90	1	8	3
Bologna Garlic	1 slice (1.4 oz)	110	1	12	5
Bologna Light	1 slice (1 oz)	60	2	4	3
Bologna Light Beef	1 slice (1 oz)	60	2	4	3
Bologna Pork & Chicken & Beef	1 slice (1 oz)	90	0	8	3
Bologna Wisconsin Made Ring	2 oz	140	1	16	7
Braunschweiger	1 slice (1 oz)	100	1	9	4
Braunschweiger	2 oz	190	2	17	8
Braunschweiger German Brand	2 oz	200	1	18	8
Cotto Salami	2 slices (1.6 oz)	100	1	8	6

FOOD	PORTION	CALS.	CARB.	FAT	PRO.
Oscar Mayer (CONT.)					
Cotto Salami Beef	2 slices (1.6 oz)	90	0	7	6
Free Bologna	2 slices (1.6 oz)	35	2	0	6
Genoa Salami	3 slices (1 oz)	100	0	9	5
Hard Salami	3 slices (1 oz)	100	0	9	6
Head Cheese	1 slice (1 oz)	50	0	4	5
Healthy Favorites Bologna	2 slices (1.6 oz)	45	2	1	7
Honey Loaf	1 slice (1 oz)	35	1	1	5
Liver Cheese	1 slice (1.3 oz)	120	1	10	6
Lunchables Bologna/ American	1 pkg (4.5 oz)	450	19	34	18
Lunchables Deluxe Turkey/Ham	1 pkg (5.1 oz)	360	23	19	23
Lunchables Dessert Jello/Honey Turkey/ Cheddar	1 pkg (5.7 oz)	320	27	16	17
Lunchables Fun Pack Bologna/Wild Cherry	1 pkg (11.2 oz)	530	58	29	13
Lunchables Fun Pack Ham/Fruit Punch	1 pkg (11.2 oz)	450	53	20	15
Lunchables Ham/Swiss	1 pkg (4.5 oz)	320	19	17	22
Lunchables Pepperoni/ American	1 pkg (4.5 oz)	480	19	36	20
Lunchables Salami/ American	1 pkg (4.5 oz)	430	18	32	18
Luncheon Loaf Spiced	1 slice (1 oz)	70	2	5	4
New England Brand Sausage	2 slices (1.6 oz)	60	1	3	8
Old Fashioned Loaf	1 slice (1 oz)	60	2	5	4
Olive Loaf	1 slice (1 oz)	70	2	5	3
Peppered Loaf	1 slice (1 oz)	39	1	2	5
Pickle And Pimiento Loaf	1 slice (1 oz)	70	2	6	3
Salami For Beer	1 slice (1.6 oz)	110	1	9	6
Salami Machaich Brand Beef	2 slices (1.6 oz)	120	1	10	6
Sandwich Spread	2 oz	140	9	10	4
Summer Sausage	2 slices (1.6 oz)	140	0	13	7
Summer Sausage Beef	2 slices (1.6 oz)	140	1	12	7
Russer					
Bologna	2 oz	180	3	15	6
Bologna Jalapeno Pepper	2 oz	170	3	14	6
Bologna Wunderbar German Brand	2 oz	190	5	16	6

FOOD	PORTION	CALS.	CARB.	FAT	PRO.
Russer (CONT.)					
Bologna Beef	2 oz	180	3	15	6
Bologna Garlic	2 oz	180	3	16	6
Bologna Italian Brand Sweet Red Pepper	2 oz	180	3	15	6
Braunschweiger	2 oz	170	3	14	8
Cooked Salami	2 oz	120	3	8	8
Dutch Brand	2 oz	130	6	8	7
Hot Cooked Salami	2 oz	110	3	7	8
Italian Brand Loaf	2 oz	130	5	8	7
Jalapeno Loaf With Monterey Jack Cheese	2 oz	160	4	13	6
Kielbasa Loaf	2 oz	120	5	8	7
Light Bologna	2 oz	120	3	8	8
Light Bologna Beef	2 oz	120	3	8	8
Light Braunschweiger	2 oz	120	3	8	8
Light Old Fashioned Loaf	2 oz	90	4	4	8
Light P&P Loaf	2 oz	100	4	6	8
Light Salami Cooked	2 oz	90	4	5	8
Olive Loaf	2 oz	160	4	13	6
P&P Loaf	2 oz	160	4	13	6
Pepper Loaf	2 oz	90	6	3	8
Polish Loaf	2 oz	140	7	10	7
Sara Lee					
Pastrami Beef	2 oz	100	1	6	10
Peppered Beef	2 oz	70	1	2	12
Shofar					
Salami Beef	2 oz	160	0	15	7
Spam					
Less Salt	2 oz	170	0	16	7
Lite	2 oz	110	0	8	9
Original	2 oz	170	0	16	7
Underwood					
Liverwurst	2.08 oz	180	4	15	8
Weight Watchers					
Bologna	2 slices (¾ oz)	35	1	2	3
TAKE-OUT					
corned beef	2 oz	70	0	2	12
corned beef brisket	2 oz	90	0	5	11
submarine w/ salami ham, cheese lettuce tomato onion & oil	1	456	51	19	22

DIETING AIDS
(*see* NUTRITIONAL SUPPLEMENTS)

FOOD	PORTION	CALS.	CARB.	FAT	PRO.

DINNER

(see also BEEF DISHES, PASTA DINNERS, POT PIES, ORIENTAL FOOD, SPANISH FOODS, VEAL DISHES)

FROZEN

Armour

FOOD	PORTION	CALS.	CARB.	FAT	PRO.
Classics Chicken Parmigiana	1 meal (10.75 oz)	360	25	18	24
Classics Chicken & Noodles	1 meal (11 oz)	280	30	9	19
Classics Chicken Mesquite	1 meal (9.5 oz)	280	39	13	21
Classics Chicken w/ Wine & Mushroom	1 meal (10 oz)	260	20	11	20
Classics Glazed Chicken	1 meal (10.75 oz)	280	20	14	19
Classics Meatloaf	1 meal (11.25 oz)	300	33	10	19
Classics Salisbury Steak	1 meal (11.25 oz)	330	20	18	23
Classics Swedish Meatballs	1 meal (10 oz)	300	20	17	18
Classics Turkey and Dressing	1 meal (11.25 oz)	270	34	7	17
Classics Veal Parmigiana	1 meal (11.25 oz)	400	35	22	16
Classics Lite Beef Pepper	1 meal (11 oz)	210	29	4	16
Classics Lite Chicken Burgundy	1 meal (10 oz)	210	20	5	20
Classics Lite Salisbury Steak	1 meal (11.5 oz)	260	26	7	22
Classics Lite Shrimp Creole	1 meal (10 oz)	220	49	1	6
Classics Lite Sweet & Sour Chicken	1 meal (11 oz)	220	38	1	16

Banquet

FOOD	PORTION	CALS.	CARB.	FAT	PRO.
BBQ Style Chicken	1 meal (9 oz)	320	36	12	18
Beef	1 meal (9 oz)	240	19	7	26
Chicken Parmigiana	1 pkg (9.5 oz)	290	27	15	14
Chicken & Dumplings	1 meal (10 oz)	260	35	8	13
Chicken Fried Steak	1 pkg (10 oz)	400	39	20	15
Chicken Nuggets	1 pkg (6.75 oz)	410	38	21	18
Extra Helping All White Chicken	1 meal (18 oz)	820	72	41	40
Extra Helping Chicken Parmigiana	1 meal (19 oz)	650	64	33	24
Extra Helping Chicken Fried Steak	1 meal (18.5 oz)	800	73	44	29

FOOD	PORTION	CALS.	CARB.	FAT	PRO.
Banquet (CONT.)					
Extra Helping Fried Chicken	1 meal (18 oz)	790	72	39	37
Extra Helping Meatloaf	1 meal (19 oz)	650	49	38	29
Extra Helping Mexican Style	1 meal (22 oz)	820	100	34	28
Extra Helping Salisbury Steak	1 meal (19 oz)	740	52	46	31
Extra Helping Southern Fried Chicken	1 meal (17.5 oz)	750	67	37	38
Extra Helping Turkey Dinner	1 meal (18.8 oz)	560	63	20	32
Family Entree Beef Stew	1 serv (8.13 oz)	160	17	4	14
Family Entree Chicken Parmigiana	1 serv (4.67 oz)	240	18	13	11
Family Entree Chicken & Dumplings	1 serv (7.47 oz)	290	30	14	12
Family Entree Gravy & Sliced Turkey	1 serv (4.8 oz)	100	5	5	8
Family Entree Gravy w/ Charbroiled Beef	1 serv (4.67 oz)	180	7	13	8
Family Entree Onion Gravy w/ Beef	1 serv (4.67 oz)	180	7	14	8
Family Entree Salisbury Steak	1 serv (4.67 oz)	200	7	14	12
Family Entree Veal Parmigiana	1 serv (4.67 oz)	230	19	14	9
Family Entrees Dumplings & Chicken	7 oz	280	28	14	12
Family Entrees Gravy & Sliced Beef	1 serv (5.6 oz)	100	7	3	13
Family Entrees Gravy & Sliced Turkey	6 oz	120	6	6	9
Fried Chicken	1 meal (9 oz)	470	35	27	21
Gravy w/ Beef Patty	1 pkg (9.5 oz)	300	21	20	11
Hot Sandwich Toppers Chicken Ala King	1 pkg (4.5 oz)	100	7	4	9
Hot Sandwich Toppers Creamed Chipped Beef	1 pkg (4 oz)	100	8	3	9
Hot Sandwich Toppers Gravy & Sliced Beef	1 pkg (4 oz)	70	5	2	8
Hot Sandwich Toppers Gravy & Sliced Turkey	1 pkg (5 oz)	90	7	4	8

FOOD	PORTION	CALS.	CARB.	FAT	PRO.
Banquet (CONT.)					
Hot Sandwich Toppers Salisbury Steak	1 pkg (5 oz)	220	8	16	9
Hot Sandwich Toppers Sloppy Joe	1 meal (4 oz)	140	12	7	7
Meatloaf	1 meal (9.5 oz)	280	23	17	12
Mexican Style Combo Meal	1 pkg (11 oz)	380	55	11	15
Mexican Style Meal	1 pkg (11 oz)	340	56	13	14
Oriental Style Chicken	1 pkg (9 oz)	260	34	9	12
Salisbury Steak	1 meal (9.5 oz)	310	28	16	14
Southern Fried Chicken Meal	1 pkg (8.75 oz)	260	44	30	22
Turkey	1 meal (9.25 oz)	270	31	10	15
Veal Parmagiana	1 pkg (9 oz)	530	35	14	13
Western Style Meal	1 meal (9.5 oz)	210	28	20	14
White Meat Chicken Meal	1 pkg (8.75 oz)	470	33	28	22
Birds Eye					
Easy Recipe Beef Burgundy not prep	½ pkg	120	17	5	4
Easy Recipe Beef Fajitas not prep	½ pkg	80	14	3	3
Budget Gourmet					
Beef Cantonese	1 meal (9.1 oz)	270	31	9	15
Beef Stroganoff	1 meal (8.75 oz)	260	27	10	19
Chicken And Egg Noodles	1 meal (10 oz)	440	28	26	24
Chicken Au Gratin	1 meal (9.1 oz)	230	23	8	18
Chicken Breast Parmigiana	1 pkg (11 oz)	270	30	9	22
Chicken Marsala	1 meal (9 oz)	260	31	8	17
Chicken With Fettucini	1 meal (10 oz)	400	29	21	24
Chinese Style Vegetables & Chicken	1 meal (10 oz)	280	47	7	11
French Recipe Chicken	1 meal (10 oz)	220	21	9	17
Glazed Turkey	1 meal (9 oz)	260	38	5	16
Ham & Asparagus Au Gratin	1 meal (8.7 oz)	300	26	14	17
Herbed Chicken Breast With Fettucini	1 pkg (11 oz)	240	30	6	21
Italian Style Vegetables & Chicken	1 meal (10.25 oz)	310	50	8	14
Mandarin Chicken	1 meal (10 oz)	240	38	5	15

FOOD	PORTION	CALS.	CARB.	FAT	PRO.
Budget Gourmet (CONT.)					
Mesquite Chicken Breast	1 pkg (11 oz)	250	33	6	23
Orange Glazed Chicken	1 meal (9 oz)	270	46	3	17
Oriental Beef	1 meal (10 oz)	290	36	8	18
Oriental Chicken With Vegetables	1 meal (9 oz)	280	44	6	19
Pepper Steak With Rice	1 meal (10 oz)	300	40	8	18
Pot Roast Beef	1 meal (10.5 oz)	230	19	7	25
Roast Chicken With Homestyle Gravy	1 meal (11 oz)	280	36	8	20
Roast Sirloin Supreme	1 meal (9 oz)	320	28	15	19
Sirloin Salisbury Steak	1 meal (9 oz)	220	24	8	16
Sirloin Salisbury Steak	1 meal (11 oz)	280	30	9	21
Sirloin Cheddar Melt	1 meal (9.4 oz)	380	29	21	18
Sirloin Of Beef In Herb Sauce	1 meal (9.5 oz)	250	21	9	20
Sirloin Of Beef In Wine Sauce	1 pkg (11 oz)	280	36	8	21
Sirloin Tips And Country Vegetables	1 meal (10 oz)	290	19	17	17
Special Recipe Sirloin Of Beef	1 meal (11 oz)	250	29	9	18
Stuffed Turkey Breast	1 pkg (11 oz)	250	31	6	21
Swedish Meatballs With Noodles	1 meal (10 oz)	590	37	38	24
Sweet And Sour Chicken	1 meal (10 oz)	340	55	5	17
Teriyaki Beef	1 pkg (10.75 oz)	260	37	7	19
Teriyaki Chicken Breast	1 meal (11 oz)	300	41	8	18
Healthy Choice					
Beef & Peppers Cantonese	1 meal (11.5 oz)	270	40	5	16
Beef Pepper Steak Oriental	1 meal (9.5 oz)	250	34	4	19
Beef Tips Francais	1 meal (9.5 oz)	280	40	5	20
Beef Tips With Sauce	1 meal (11 oz)	290	40	6	19
Chicken & Vegetables Marsala	1 meal (11.5 oz)	220	32	1	22
Chicken Bangkok	1 meal (9.5 oz)	270	35	4	25
Chicken Cantonese	1 meal (11.25)	210	31	1	19
Chicken Dijon	1 meal (11 oz)	280	41	4	21
Chicken Imperial	1 meal (9 oz)	230	31	4	17
Chicken Parmigiana	1 meal (11.5 oz)	300	47	2	23
Chicken Picante	1 meal (11.25 oz)	220	30	2	19
Chicken Teriyaki	1 meal (12.25 oz)	270	42	2	21

FOOD	PORTION	CALS.	CARB.	FAT	PRO.
Healthy Choice (CONT.)					
Classics Beef Broccoli Beijing	1 meal (12 oz)	330	55	3	20
Classics Cacciatore Chicken	1 meal (12.5 oz)	260	36	3	22
Classics Chicken Fransesca	1 meal (12.5 oz)	360	51	5	27
Classics Country Inn Roast Turkey	1 meal (10 oz)	250	29	4	26
Classics Ginger Chicken Hunan	1 meal (12.6 oz)	350	59	3	24
Classics Mesquite Beef Barbecue	1 meal (11 oz)	310	45	4	23
Classics Salisbury Steak	1 meal (11 oz)	260	32	6	18
Classics Sesame Chicken Shanghai	1 meal (12 oz)	310	42	5	24
Classics Shrimp & Vegetables Maria	1 meal (12.5 oz)	260	46	2	15
Country Glazed Chicken	1 meal (8.5 oz)	200	30	2	17
Country Herb Chicken	1 meal (11.5 oz)	270	40	4	20
Country Roast Turkey With Mushroom	1 meal (8.5 oz)	220	28	4	19
Country Turkey & Pasta	1 meal (12.6 oz)	300	42	4	22
Homestyle Turkey With Vegetables	1 meal (9.5 oz)	260	34	2	26
Honey Mustard Chicken	1 meal (9.5 oz)	260	40	2	21
Lemon Pepper Fish	1 meal (10.7 oz)	290	47	5	14
Mandarin Chicken	1 meal (10 oz)	280	44	3	20
Mesquite Chicken Barbecue	1 meal (10.5 oz)	320	55	2	19
Shrimp Marinara	1 meal (10.5 oz)	220	44	1	10
Smoky Chicken Barbecue	1 meal (12.75 oz)	380	57	5	25
Southwestern Glazed Chicken	1 meal (12.5 oz)	300	48	3	20
Sweet & Sour Chicken	1 meal (11.5 oz)	310	42	5	23
Traditional Breast Of Turkey	1 meal (10.5 oz)	280	40	3	22
Traditional Meat Loaf	1 meal (12 oz)	320	46	8	16
Traditional Beef Tips	1 meal (11.25 oz)	260	32	5	20
Traditional Salisbury Steak	1 meal (11.5 oz)	320	48	6	18
Yankee Pot Roast	1 meal (11 oz)	280	38	5	19

FOOD	PORTION	CALS.	CARB.	FAT	PRO.
Kid Cuisine					
Chicken Sandwich	1 pkg (9.43 oz)	480	71	15	17
Chicken Nuggets	1 pkg (9.1 oz)	440	54	16	18
Fish Sticks	1 pkg (8.25 oz)	370	55	12	11
Fried Chicken	1 pkg (10.1 oz)	440	49	19	18
Hot Dogs w/ Buns	6.7 oz	450	57	19	13
Macaroni & Beef	1 pkg (9.6 oz)	370	58	9	12
Le Menu					
Beef Sirloin Tips	11½ oz	400	29	18	30
Beef Stroganoff	10 oz	430	28	24	26
Chicken Parmigiana	11¾ oz	410	31	20	26
Chicken A La King	10¼ oz	330	29	13	23
Chicken Cordon Bleu	11 oz	460	47	20	23
Chicken In Wine Sauce	10 oz	280	27	7	26
Chopped Sirloin Beef	12¼ oz	430	28	24	25
Entree LightStyle Chicken A La King	8¼ oz	240	29	5	19
Entree LightStyle Chicken Dijon	8 oz	240	21	7	22
Entree LightStyle Empress Chicken	8¼ oz	210	26	5	16
Entree LightStyle Glazed Turkey	8¼ oz	260	34	6	18
Entree LightStyle Herb Roast Chicken	7¾ oz	260	29	6	22
Entree LightStyle Swedish Meatballs	8 oz	260	30	8	18
Entree LightStyle Traditional Turkey	8 oz	200	19	5	19
Ham Steak	10 oz	300	31	11	19
LightStyle Glazed Chicken Breast	10 oz	230	25	3	25
LightStyle Herb Roasted Chicken	10 oz	240	18	7	27
LightStyle Salisbury Steak	10 oz	280	31	9	18
LightStyle Sliced Turkey	10 oz	210	21	5	21
LightStyle Sweet & Sour Chicken	10 oz	250	29	7	18
LightStyle Turkey Divan	10 oz	260	23	7	25
LightStyle Veal Marsala	10 oz	230	28	3	22
Pepper Steak	11½ oz	370	36	13	26
Salisbury Steak	10½ oz	370	28	20	20
Sliced Breast Of Turkey w/ Mushroom Gravy	10½ oz	300	38	7	22

FOOD	PORTION	CALS.	CARB.	FAT	PRO.
Le Menu (CONT.)					
Sweet & Sour Chicken	11¼ oz	400	41	18	19
Veal Parmigiana	11½ oz	390	36	17	24
Yankee Pot Roast	10 oz	330	27	13	26
Lean Cuisine					
Baked Chicken	1 meal (8 oz)	240	31	5	18
Beef Pot Roast	1 meal (9 oz)	210	21	7	16
Chicken & Vegetables	1 meal (10.5 oz)	240	30	5	19
Chicken A L'Orange	1 meal (8 oz)	260	40	3	19
Chicken In Honey Barbecue Sauce	1 pkg (8.75 oz)	250	35	5	18
Chicken In Peanut Sauce	1 pkg (9 oz)	280	33	6	23
Chicken Italiano	1 pkg (9 oz)	270	31	6	22
Chicken Marsala	1 meal (8.1 oz)	180	13	4	22
Chicken Oriental	1 pkg (9 oz)	260	30	6	21
Chicken Parmesan	1 meal (10.9 oz)	220	22	5	22
Chicken Pie	1 meal (9.5 oz)	320	39	10	18
Fiesta Chicken	1 pkg (8.5 oz)	240	31	5	18
Fish Divan	1 pkg (10.4 oz)	210	15	6	25
Glazed Chicken	1 meal (8.5 oz)	240	24	6	22
Homestyle Turkey	1 pkg (9.4 oz)	230	26	5	18
Honey Mustard Chicken	1 pkg (7.5 oz)	250	32	5	20
Meatloaf	1 pkg (9.4 oz)	270	24	10	21
Oriental Beef	1 meal (9 oz)	250	30	8	14
Roasted Turkey Breast	1 pkg (9.75 oz)	290	48	40	16
Salisbury Steak With Macaroni & Cheese	1 meal (9.5 oz)	200	22	10	27
Stuffed Cabbage	1 meal (9.5 oz)	220	27	7	11
Swedish Meatballs	1 pkg (9.1 oz)	290	32	8	22
Sweet & Sour Chicken	1 pkg (10.4 oz)	260	43	3	17
Turkey Pie	1 pkg (9.5 oz)	300	34	9	20
Life Choice					
Garden Potato Casserole	1 meal (13.4 oz)	160	37	1	8
Morton					
Breaded Chicken Pattie	1 meal (6.75 oz)	280	24	15	11
Chicken Nugget	1 meal (7 oz)	320	30	17	13
Fried Chicken	1 meal (9 oz)	420	30	25	20
Meatloaf	1 meal (9 oz)	250	24	13	9
Mexican	1 meal (10 oz)	260	40	7	8
Salisbury Steak	1 meal (9 oz)	210	23	9	9
Turkey	1 meal (9 oz)	230	27	8	14
Veal Parmagiana	1 meal (8.75 oz)	280	30	13	8
Western	1 meal (9 oz)	290	26	16	11
Patio					
Chili	1 cup (8 oz)	260	13	13	23

FOOD	PORTION	CALS.	CARB.	FAT	PRO.
Patio (CONT.)					
Ranchera	1 pkg (13 oz)	410	14	15	13
Stouffer's					
Chicken A La King	1 pkg (9.5 oz)	320	43	10	15
Chicken Divan	1 pkg (8 oz)	210	10	10	21
Creamed Chicken	1 pkg (6.5 oz)	280	8	20	17
Creamed Chipped Beef	½ cup (4.5 oz)	150	6	11	10
Creamed Chipped Beef Over Country Biscuit	1 pkg (9 oz)	460	40	28	18
Escalloped Chicken & Noodles	1 pkg (10 oz)	440	28	29	16
Green Pepper Steak	1 pkg (10.5 oz)	330	45	9	17
Ham & Asparagus Bake	1 pkg (9.5 oz)	520	32	36	16
Homestyle Baked Chicken	1 pkg (8.9 oz)	270	19	12	22
Homestyle Beef Pot Roast	1 pkg (8.9 oz)	270	25	10	19
Homestyle Breaded Chicken Tenders	1 pkg (6.6 oz)	380	33	18	21
Homestyle Chicken & Noodles	1 pkg (10 oz)	310	23	14	22
Homestyle Chicken Monterey	1 pkg (9.4 oz)	410	35	20	23
Homestyle Chicken Parmigiana	1 pkg (10.9 oz)	320	30	10	27
Homestyle Fish Filet With Macaroni & Cheese	1 pkg (9 oz)	430	37	21	24
Homestyle Fried Chicken	1 pkg (7.1 oz)	330	29	16	18
Homestyle Meatloaf	1 pkg (9.9 oz)	380	24	24	20
Homestyle Roast Turkey	1 pkg (7.9 oz)	280	25	11	19
Homestyle Salisbury Steak	1 pkg (9.6 oz)	370	26	19	24
Homestyle Sliced Beef & Potatoes	1 pkg (8.1 oz)	270	25	10	19
Homestyle Veal Parmigiana	1 pkg (11.9 oz)	420	43	19	20
Lunch Express Chicken With Garden Vegetables	1 pkg (9.9 oz)	340	45	11	15
Lunch Express Mandarin Chicken	1 pkg (9.75 oz)	270	41	6	12
Lunch Express Mexican Style Rice With Chicken	1 pkg (9 oz)	270	39	8	10

FOOD	PORTION	CALS.	CARB.	FAT	PRO.
Stouffer's (CONT.)					
Lunch Express Oriental Beef	1 pkg (6.2 oz)	260	34	8	12
Lunch Express Stir-Fry Rice & Chicken	1 pkg (9 oz)	280	39	9	11
Stuffed Pepper	1 pkg (10 oz)	200	24	8	9
Swedish Meatballs	1 pkg (9.25 oz)	440	36	23	23
Swanson					
Beans & Franks	10½ oz	440	53	19	14
Beef	11¼ oz	310	38	6	26
Beef In Barbecue Sauce	11 oz	460	51	17	30
Chopped Sirloin Beef	10¾ oz	340	28	16	20
Fish 'n' Chips	10 oz	500	60	21	20
Fried Chicken Dark Meat	9¾ oz	560	55	28	22
Fried Chicken White Meat	10¼ oz	550	60	25	22
Homestyle Chicken Cacciatore	10.95 oz	260	33	8	15
Homestyle Chicken Nibbles	4¼ oz	340	29	20	10
Homestyle Fish & Fries	6½ oz	340	37	16	11
Homestyle Fried Chicken	7 oz	390	33	21	18
Homestyle Salisbury Steak	10 oz	320	22	16	21
Homestyle Scalloped Potatoes & Ham	9 oz	300	26	13	19
Homestyle Seafood Creole With Rice	9 oz	240	40	6	7
Homestyle Sirloin Tips In Burgundy Sauce	7 oz	160	16	5	12
Homestyle Turkey With Dressing & Potatoes	9 oz	290	30	11	18
Homestyle Veal Parmigiana	10 oz	330	33	13	19
Hungry-Man Turkey	17 oz	550	61	18	36
Hungry-Man Boneless Chicken	17¾ oz	700	65	28	48
Hungry-Man Chopped Beef Steak	16¾ oz	640	41	37	35
Hungry-Man Fried Chicken Dark Meat	14¼ oz	860	77	45	36
Hungry-Man Fried Chicken White Meat	14¼ oz	870	80	46	35
Hungry-Man Salisbury Steak	16½ oz	680	37	41	41

FOOD	PORTION	CALS.	CARB.	FAT	PRO.
Swanson (CONT.)					
Hungry-Man Sliced Beef	15¼ oz	450	49	12	37
Hungry-Man Veal Parmigiana	18¼ oz	590	57	26	32
Loin Of Pork	10¾ oz	280	27	12	20
Macaroni & Beef	12 oz	370	48	15	12
Meatloaf	10¾ oz	360	41	15	15
Noodles & Chicken	10½ oz	280	45	8	7
Salisbury Steak	10¾ oz	400	43	17	18
Swiss Steak	10 oz	350	37	11	26
Swedish Meatballs	8½ oz	360	26	20	19
Turkey	11½ oz	350	42	11	21
Veal Parmigiana	12¼ oz	430	42	20	20
Western Style	11½ oz	430	43	19	22
Tyson					
Beef Champignon	1 pkg (10.5 oz)	370	31	15	27
Chicken Picante	1 pkg (9 oz)	250	26	4	28
Chicken Supreme	1 pkg (9 oz)	230	23	6	21
Francais	1 pkg (9.5 oz)	280	20	14	19
Glazed Chicken With Sauce	1 pkg (9.25 oz)	240	29	4	22
Grilled Chicken	1 pkg (7.75 oz)	220	22	3	26
Grilled Italian Chicken	1 pkg (9 oz)	210	19	3	28
Healthy Portions BBQ Chicken	1 pkg (12.5 oz)	400	56	8	27
Healthy Portions Chicken Marinara	1 pkg (13.75 oz)	340	37	7	31
Healthy Portions Herb Chicken	1 pkg (13.75 oz)	340	43	4	32
Healthy Portions Honey Mustard Chicken	1 pkg (13.75 oz)	390	52	6	31
Healthy Portions Italian Style Chicken	1 pkg (13.75 oz)	310	38	4	30
Healthy Portions Mesquite Chicken	1 pkg (13.25 oz)	330	38	5	34
Healthy Portions Salsa Chicken	1 pkg (13.75 oz)	370	52	6	27
Healthy Portions Sesame Chicken	1 pkg (13.5 oz)	400	59	6	27
Honey Roasted Chicken	1 pkg (9 oz)	220	23	4	26
Kiev	1 pkg (9.25 oz)	450	39	25	18
Marsala	1 pkg (9 oz)	200	19	4	22
Mesquite	1 pkg (9 oz)	320	39	8	23
Picatta	1 pkg (9 oz)	200	18	4	24

FOOD	PORTION	CALS.	CARB.	FAT	PRO.
Tyson (CONT.)					
Roasted Chicken	1 pkg (9 oz)	200	21	2	21
Sweet & Sour	1 pkg (11 oz)	420	50	15	22
Turkey With Gravy	1 pkg (9.5 oz)	320	34	12	19
Ultra Slim-Fast					
Beef Pepper Steak	12 oz	270	36	4	22
Chicken Fettucini	12 oz	380	38	12	31
Chicken & Vegetable	12 oz	290	45	3	24
Country Style Vegetable & Beef Tips	12 oz	230	26	5	21
Mesquite Chicken	12 oz	360	61	1	29
Roasted Chicken In Mushroom Sauce	12 oz	280	30	6	25
Shrimp Creole	12 oz	240	45	4	12
Shrimp Marinara	12 oz	290	53	3	17
Sweet & Sour Chicken	12 oz	330	57	2	20
Turkey Medallions In Herb Sauce	12 oz	280	33	6	23
Weight Watchers					
Barbecue Glazed Chicken	7 oz	200	22	6	19
Beef Sirloin Tips	7.5 oz	210	20	6	20
Beef Stroganoff	8.5 oz	280	29	9	21
Chicken Ala King	9 oz	230	30	4	18
Chicken Cordon Bleu	7.7 oz	170	15	5	19
Chicken Kiev	7 oz	190	22	5	14
Homestyle Chicken & Noodles	9 oz	240	25	7	19
Imperial Chicken	8.5 oz	210	26	4	18
London Broil	7.5 oz	110	4	3	17
Oven Baked Fish	7 oz	150	6	4	20
Southern Baked Chicken	6.3 oz	170	10	7	17
Stuffed Turkey Breast	8.5 oz	270	31	8	18
Veal Patty Parmigiana	8.2 oz	150	5	4	22
SHELF-STABLE					
My Own Meal					
Beef Stew	1 pkg (10 oz)	260	22	11	19
Chicken Mediterranean	1 pkg (10 oz)	270	28	9	19
Chicken Noodles	1 pkg (10 oz)	270	29	8	20
Chicken & Black Beans	1 pkg (10 oz)	240	30	5	20
Old World Stew	1 pkg (10 oz)	310	31	12	20

DIP
Breakstone

Sour Cream Bacon & Onion	2 tbsp (1.1 oz)	60	2	5	1

FOOD	PORTION	CALS.	CARB.	FAT	PRO.
Breakstone (CONT.)					
Sour Cream Chesapeake Clam	2 tbsp (1.1 oz)	50	2	4	1
Sour Cream French Onion	2 tbsp (1.1 oz)	50	2	4	1
Sour Cream Jalapeno Cheddar	2 tbsp (1.1 oz)	60	2	4	1
Sour Cream Toasted Onion	2 tbsp (1.1 oz)	50	2	4	1
Chi-Chi's					
Fiesta Bean	2 tbsp (0.9 oz)	35	4	2	1
Fiesta Cheese	2 tbsp (0.9 oz)	40	3	3	1
Eagle					
Bean	1 oz	35	4	2	2
Frito Lay					
Cheddar Cheese	1 oz	45	3	3	1
French Onion	1 oz	50	3	4	1
Jalapeno Bean	1 oz	30	4	1	1
Picante Sauce	1 oz	10	3	0	0
Guiltless Gourmet					
Black Bean Mild	1 oz	25	5	0	2
Black Bean Spicy	1 oz	25	5	0	2
Pinto Bean	1 oz	25	5	0	2
Hain					
Hot Bean	4 tbsp	70	10	1	4
Mexican Bean	4 tbsp	60	9	1	4
Onion Bean	4 tbsp	70	10	1	4
Taco Dip & Sauce	4 tbsp	25	1	1	5
Heluva Good Cheese					
Bacon Horseradish	2 tbsp (1.1 oz)	60	2	5	1
Clam	2 tbsp (1.1 oz)	50	2	5	1
French Onion	2 tbsp (1.1 oz)	50	2	5	1
Homestyle Onion	2 tbsp (1.1 oz)	60	3	5	1
Light French Onion	2 tbsp (1.1 oz)	35	3	2	1
Light Jalapeno Cheddar	2 tbsp (1.1 oz)	40	3	2	2
Ranch	2 tbsp (1.1 oz)	60	2	5	1
Knudsen					
Nacho Cheese	2 tbsp (1.1 oz)	60	3	4	2
Sour Cream Bacon & Onion	2 tbsp (1.1 oz)	60	2	5	1
Sour Cream French Onion	2 tbsp (1.1 oz)	50	2	4	1
Kraft					
Avocado	2 tbsp (1.1 oz)	60	4	4	1

FOOD	PORTION	CALS.	CARB.	FAT	PRO.
Kraft (CONT.)					
Bacon & Horseradish	2 tbsp (1.1 oz)	60	3	5	1
Clam	2 tbsp (1.1 oz)	60	3	4	1
French Onion	2 tbsp (1.1 oz)	60	4	4	1
Green Onion	2 tbsp (1.1 oz)	60	4	4	1
Jalapeno	2 tbsp (1.1 oz)	60	3	4	1
Jalapeno Cheese	2 tbsp (1.1 oz)	60	1	5	2
Premium Bacon & Horseradish	2 tbsp (1.1 oz)	50	2	5	1
Premium Bacon & Onion	2 tbsp (1.1 oz)	60	2	5	1
Premium Blue Cheese	2 tbsp (1.1 oz)	45	2	4	1
Premium Clam	2 tbsp (1.1 oz)	45	2	4	1
Premium Creamy Cucumber	2 tbsp (1.1 oz)	50	2	4	tr
Premium Creamy Onion	2 tbsp (1.1 oz)	45	2	4	tr
Premium French Onion	2 tbsp (1.1 oz)	50	2	4	tr
Premium Nacho Cheese	2 tbsp (1.1 oz)	60	2	5	2
Ranch	2 tbsp (1.1 oz)	60	3	4	1
Louise's					
Fat Free Honey Mustard	1 oz	40	9	0	1
Fat Free Sour Cream & Onion	1 oz	25	4	0	1
Fat Free White Cheese Peppercorn	1 oz	25	4	0	1
Marzetti					
Blue Cheese Veggie	2 tbsp	200	1	21	1
Lemon Dill Veggie	2 tbsp	140	2	14	1
Light Ranch Veggie	2 tbsp	60	5	7	0
Ranch Veggie	2 tbsp	140	1	14	1
Sour Cream & Onion	2 tbsp	130	2	14	1
Southwestern Veggie	2 tbsp	130	1	14	1
Spinach Veggie	2 tbsp	130	1	13	1
Old El Paso					
Chunky Salsa Medium	2 tbsp	10	1	0	1
Chunky Salsa Mild	2 tbsp	10	1	0	1
Jalapeno Bean Mild	1 tbsp	14	2	0	1
Sealtest					
French Onion	2 tbsp (1.1 oz)	50	2	4	1
Snyder's					
Mustard Pretzel	2 tbsp (1.2 oz)	90	13	4	1
Wise					
Jalapeno Bean	2 tbsp	25	5	0	1
Taco	2 tbsp	12	3	0	0

FOOD	PORTION	CALS.	CARB.	FAT	PRO.
DOCK					
fresh cooked	3½ oz	20	3	1	2
raw chopped	½ cup	15	2	tr	1
DOGFISH					
raw	3½ oz	193	0	15	13
DOLPHINFISH					
fresh baked	3 oz	93	0	1	20
fresh fillet baked	5.6 oz	174	0	1	38
DOUGHNUTS					
cake type unsugared	1 (1.6 oz)	198	23	11	2
chocolate glazed	1 (1.5 oz)	175	24	8	2
chocolate sugared	1 (1.5 oz)	175	24	8	2
chocolate coated	1 (1.5 oz)	204	21	13	2
creme filled	1 (3 oz)	307	26	21	6
french cruller glazed	1 (1.4 oz)	169	24	8	1
frosted	1 (1.5 oz)	204	21	13	2
honey bun	1 (2.1 oz)	242	27	14	4
jelly	1 (3 oz)	289	33	16	5
old fashioned	1 (1.6 oz)	198	23	11	2
sugared	1 (1.6 oz)	192	23	10	2
wheat glazed	1 (1.6 oz)	162	19	9	3
wheat sugared	1 (1.6 oz)	162	19	9	3
yeast glazed	1 (2.1 oz)	242	27	14	4
Drake's					
Old Fashion Donuts	1 (1.7 oz)	182	25	8	3
Powdered Sugar Donut Delites	7 (2.5 oz)	300	38	15	3
Dutch Mill					
Cider	1 (2.1 oz)	240	35	10	3
Cinnamon	1 (1.8 oz)	210	26	11	3
Donut Holes Double-Dipped Chocolate	3 (1.4 oz)	220	19	16	2
Donut Holes Shootin' Stars	3 (1.4 oz)	190	23	10	2
Double-Dipped Chocolate	1 (2.1 oz)	280	31	17	3
Glazed	1 (2.1 oz)	250	34	12	3
Glazed Chocolate	1 (2.4 oz)	270	40	11	3
Plain	1 (1.8 oz)	210	25	12	3
Sugared	1 (1.8 oz)	220	27	11	3
Entenmann's					
Crumb Topped	1 (2.1 oz)	260	34	12	3

FOOD	PORTION	CALS.	CARB.	FAT	PRO.
Entenmann's (CONT.)					
Devil's Food Crumb	1 (2.1 oz)	250	34	12	3
Rich Frosted	1 (2 oz)	280	27	18	3
Freihofer's					
Assorted	1 (2 oz)	270	26	17	2
Hostess					
Assorted Regular	1 (1.6 oz)	200	23	11	3
Cinnamon Family Pack	1 (1 oz)	110	15	5	2
Cinnamon Swirl	1 (1.6 oz)	180	28	7	3
Crumb Regular	1 (1 oz)	130	14	8	1
Frosted Regular	1 (1.4 oz)	180	20	11	2
Gem Donettes Cinnamon	6 (3 oz)	320	53	11	5
Gem Donettes Frosted	6 (3 oz)	390	42	23	5
Gem Donettes Frosted Strawberry Filled	3 (3 oz)	240	29	13	3
Gem Donettes Powdered	6 (3 oz)	350	47	16	4
Gem Donettes Powdered Strawberry Filled	3 (3 oz)	210	31	9	3
Glazed Party	1 (2.3 oz)	260	39	10	4
Jumbo Frosted	1 (2 oz)	260	28	16	3
Jumbo Plain	1 (1.1 oz)	140	16	7	2
Jumbo Powdered	1 (1.3 oz)	160	19	9	2
Mini Chocolate	5 (2 oz)	220	33	9	4
O's Raspberry Filled Powdered	1 (2.2 oz)	230	35	10	3
Old Fashioned Glazed	1 (2.1 oz)	250	33	12	3
Old Fashioned Glazed Honey Wheat	1 (2.1 oz)	250	33	12	3
Old Fashioned Plain	1 (1.5 oz)	170	21	9	3
Plain Regular	1 (1 oz)	120	13	6	2
Powdered Family Pack	1 (1 oz)	110	15	6	1
Little Debbie					
Donut Sticks	1 pkg (1.6 oz)	210	25	13	2
Donut Sticks	1 pkg (3 oz)	390	45	23	4
Donut Sticks	1 pkg (2.5 oz)	320	37	19	3
Donut Sticks	1 pkg (2 oz)	250	30	15	2
Tastykake					
Cinnamon	1 (47 g)	180	26	8	3
Frosted Rich	1 (57 g)	260	28	16	4
Frosted Rich Mini	1 (14 g)	44	8	3	1
Honey Wheat	1 (57 g)	210	32	8	3
Honey Wheat Mini	1 (12 g)	40	7	1	1
Orange Glazed	1 (57 g)	210	32	9	3
Plain	1 (47 g)	190	22	10	3

FOOD	PORTION	CALS.	CARB.	FAT	PRO.
Tastykake (CONT.)					
Powdered Sugar	1 (46 g)	180	24	9	3
Powdered Sugar Mini	1 (12 g)	40	7	1	1

DRESSING
(*see* STUFFING/DRESSING)

DRINK MIXERS
(*see also* SODA, MINERAL/BOTTLED WATER)

whiskey sour mix	2 oz	55	14	0	0
whiskey sour mix as prep	3.6 oz	169	16	0	tr
Bacardi					
Margarita Mix w/ rum	8 fl oz	160	24	0	0
Margarita Mix w/o liquor	8 fl oz	100	25	0	0
Pina Colada	8 fl oz	140	34	0	0
Rum Runner	8 fl oz	140	35	0	0
Strawberry Daiquiri w/o liquor	8 fl oz	140	35	0	0
Canada Dry					
Collins Mixer	8 fl oz	120	25	0	0
Sour Mixer	8 fl oz	90	22	0	0
Libby					
Bloody Mary Mix	6 oz	40	8	0	2
McIlhenny					
Tabasco Bloody Mary Mix	8 fl oz	56	11	tr	2
Schweppes					
Collins Mixer	8 fl oz	100	24	0	0
Tabasco					
Bloody Mary Mix Extra Spicy	8 fl oz	58	11	tr	3

DRUM

freshwater fillet baked	5.4 oz	236	0	10	35
freshwater baked	3 oz	130	0	5	19

DUCK
FRESH

w/ skin roasted	½ duck (13.4 oz)	1287	0	108	73
w/ skin roasted	6 oz	583	0	49	33
w/o skin roasted	3.5 oz	201	0	11	23
w/o skin roasted	½ duck (7.8 oz)	445	0	25	52
wild breast w/o skin raw	½ breast (2.9 oz)	102	0	4	16
wild w/ skin raw	½ duck (9.5 oz)	571	0	41	47

FOOD	PORTION	CALS.	CARB.	FAT	PRO.
DUMPLING					
FROZEN					
Pepperidge Farm					
Apple Dumpling	1 (3 oz)	260	33	13	2
DURIAN					
fresh	3½ oz	141	29	2	3
EEL					
fresh cooked	1 fillet (5.6 oz)	375	0	24	38
fresh cooked	3 oz	200	0	13	20
raw	3 oz	156	0	10	16
smoked	3.5 oz	330	0	28	19
EGG					
(*see also* EGG DISHES, EGG SUBSTITUTES)					
CHICKEN					
fried w/ margarine	1	91	1	7	6
frozen	1 cup	363	3	24	30
frozen	1	75	1	5	6
hard cooked	1	77	1	5	6
hard cooked chopped	1 cup	210	2	14	17
poached	1	74	1	5	6
raw	1	75	1	5	6
scrambled plain	2	200	2	15	13
scrambled w/ whole milk & margarine	1 cup	365	5	27	24
scrambled w/ whole milk & margarine	1	101	1	7	7
white only	1 cup	121	2	0	26
white only	1	17	tr	0	4
OTHER POULTRY					
duck raw	1	130	1	10	9
goose raw	1	267	2	19	20
quail raw	1	14	tr	1	1
turkey raw	1	135	1	9	9
EGG DISHES					
FROZEN					
Downyflake					
Scrambled Eggs With Ham & Hash Browns	1 pkg (6.25 oz)	360	17	26	13
Scrambled Eggs With Ham & Pecan Twirl	1 pkg (6.25 oz)	470	40	28	15
Scrambled Eggs With Hash Browns & Sausage	1 pkg (6.25 oz)	420	17	34	12

FOOD	PORTION	CALS.	CARB.	FAT	PRO.
Downyflake (CONT.)					
Scrambled Eggs With Sausage & Pecan Twirl	1 pkg (6.25 oz)	510	39	33	16
Great Starts					
Egg Sausage & Cheese	5½ oz	460	35	28	18
Omelets With Cheese & Ham	7 oz	390	15	29	19
Reduced Cholesterol Eggs With Mini Oatbran Muffins	4¾ oz	250	27	12	10
Scrambled Eggs With Cheese & Cinnamon Pancakes	3.4 oz	290	14	23	7
Scrambled Eggs & Bacon With Home Fries	5.6 oz	340	16	26	11
Scrambled Eggs & Home Fries	4.6 oz	260	14	19	7
Scrambled Eggs & Sausage With Hash Browns	6½ oz	430	19	34	13
Quaker					
Scrambled Eggs Cheddar Cheese & Fried Potatoes	1 pkg (5.9 oz)	250	22	13	11
Scrambled Eggs & Sausage With Hash Browns	1 pkg (5.7 oz)	290	14	20	12
Scrambled Eggs & Sausage With Pancakes	1 pkg (5.2 oz)	270	21	14	13
Weight Watchers					
Garden Vegetable Omelet Sandwich	1 (3.6 oz)	210	28	6	9
Ham & Cheese Handy Omelet	4 oz	180	18	5	14
TAKE-OUT					
deviled	2 halves	145	1	13	6
salad	½ cup	307	2	28	13
sandwich w/ cheese	1	340	26	19	16
sandwich w/ cheese & ham	1	348	31	16	19
scotch egg	1 (4.2 oz)	301	16	21	14

FOOD	PORTION	CALS.	CARB.	FAT	PRO.
EGG SUBSTITUTES					
frozen	¼ cup	96	2	7	7
frozen	1 cup	384	8	27	27
liquid	1½ oz	40	tr	2	6
liquid	1 cup	211	2	8	30
powder	0.35 oz	44	2	1	5
powder	0.7 oz	88	4	3	11
Egg Beaters					
Eggs Substitute	¼ cup	25	1	0	5
Omelette Cheese	½ cup	110	2	5	14
Omelette Vegetable	½ cup	50	5	0	7
Egg Watchers					
Egg Substitute	2 oz	50	2	2	7
Healthy Choice					
Cholesterol Free	¼ cup (2 oz)	25	tr	0	6
LaLoma					
Scramblers Links Muffins	1 pkg (4 oz)	220	22	10	11
Morningstar Farms					
Better'n Eggs	¼ cup (57 g)	30	1	0	6
Scramblers	¼ cup (57 g)	60	3	3	6
Scramblers Links Hash Browns	1 pkg (5 oz)	240	20	13	11
Scramblers Sandwich w/ Cheese	1 (3.5 oz)	220	29	7	11
Scramblers Sandwich w/ Pattie	1 (4.5 oz)	300	29	12	18
Scramblers Sandwich w/ Pattie Cheese	1 (5 oz)	350	33	15	20
Scramblers Cheese Home Fries	1 pkg (5 oz)	210	20	9	11
Second Nature					
No Cholesterol	2 fl oz	60	3	2	6
No Fat	2 fl oz	40	3	0	6
No Fat With Garden Vegetables	2.5 fl oz	40	4	0	6
Simply Eggs					
Egg Substitue	1.75 fl oz	35	1	1	5
EGGNOG					
eggnog	1 cup	342	34	19	10
eggnog	1 qt	1368	138	76	39
eggnog flavor mix as prep w/ milk	9 oz	260	39	8	8

FOOD	PORTION	CALS.	CARB.	FAT	PRO.
Borden					
Eggnog	4 fl oz	160	16	9	3
Light	½ cup	130	23	2	5
Hood					
Fat Free	4 fl oz	100	21	0	4
Golden	4 fl oz	180	22	8	4
Light	4 fl oz	120	23	2	4
Select	4 fl oz	210	22	12	4

EGGPLANT
CANNED
Progresso

Caponata	2 tbsp (1 oz)	30	2	2	0
FRESH					
cubed cooked	½ cup	13	3	tr	tr
raw cut up	½ cup (1.4 oz)	11	2	tr	tr
slices, cooked	4 (7 oz)	38	0	0	2
whole peeled raw	1 (1 lb)	117	28	1	5
FROZEN					
Mrs. Paul's					
Parmigiana	5 oz	240	18	16	6
TAKE-OUT					
baba ghannouj	¼ cup	55	5	4	2

ELDERBERRIES

fresh	1 cup	105	27	1	1

ELDERBERRY JUICE

elderberry	3½ oz	38	8	0	2

ELK

roasted	3 oz	124	0	2	26

ENDIVE

fresh	3½ oz	9	tr	tr	2
raw chopped	½ cup	4	1	tr	tr

ENGLISH MUFFIN
FROZEN
Great Starts

Egg Beefsteak & Cheese	5.9 oz	360	27	20	17
Egg Canadian Bacon & Cheese	4.1 oz	290	25	15	15
Weight Watchers					
Sandwich With Egg Ham & Cheese	1 (4 oz)	230	25	8	13

FOOD	PORTION	CALS.	CARB.	FAT	PRO.
HOME RECIPE					
cinnamon raisin	1	186	38	3	5
english muffin	1	158	30	2	4
honey bran	1	153	30	3	4
whole wheat	1	167	34	tr	6
READY-TO-EAT					
apple cinnamon	1	138	28	2	4
granola	1	155	31	1	6
mixed grain	1	155	31	1	6
plain	1	134	26	1	4
plain toasted	1	133	26	1	4
raisin cinnamon	1	138	28	2	4
sourdough	1	134	26	1	4
wheat	1	127	26	1	5
whole wheat	1	134	27	1	6
Arnold					
Extra Crisp	1	130	26	1	4
Sourdough	1	130	25	1	4
Matthew's					
9 Grain & Nut	1	140	26	4	10
Cinnamon Raisin	1	160	33	2	6
Golden White	1	140	23	4	5
Whole Wheat	1	150	31	2	7
Pepperidge Farm					
Cinnamon Apple	1	140	27	1	4
Cinnamon Chip	1	160	28	3	4
Cinnamon Raisin	1	150	29	2	4
Plain	1	140	27	1	5
Sourdough	1	135	27	1	4
Roman Meal					
English Muffin	1 (2.2 oz)	135	25	1	6
Tastykake					
Cinnamon Raisin	1 (64 g)	150	31	1	4
English Muffin	1 (57 g)	130	26	1	5
Sourdough	1 (57 g)	130	25	1	5
Thomas'					
Honey Wheat	1	128	24	1	5
Oat Bran	1	116	26	1	4
Raisin Cinnamon	1	151	31	1	4
Regular	1	130	25	1	4
Sandwich Size	1 (92 g)	210	42	2	7
Sour Dough	1	131	25	1	4
Wonder					
English Muffin	1 (2 oz)	120	25	1	5

FOOD	PORTION	CALS.	CARB.	FAT	PRO.
Wonder (CONT.)					
Raisin Rounds	1 (2.1 oz)	150	30	2	5
Sourdough	1 (2 oz)	120	25	1	5
REFRIGERATED					
Roman Meal					
English Muffin	½ muffin (1.1 oz)	66	14	tr	2
Honey Nut Oat Bran	½ muffin (1.1 oz)	81	16	1	2
TAKE-OUT					
w/ butter	1	189	30	6	5
w/ cheese & sausage	1	394	29	24	15
w/ egg cheese & bacon	1	487	31	31	22
w/ egg cheese & canadian bacon	1	383	31	20	20

FALAFEL

MIX
Casbah

as prep	5	130	20	3	6
Near East					
as prep	2½ patties	230	18	15	10
TAKE-OUT					
falafel	3 (1.8 oz)	170	16	9	7
falafel	1 (1.2 oz)	57	5	3	2

FAT

(*see also* BUTTER, BUTTER BLENDS, BUTTER SUBSTITUTES, MARGARINE, OIL)

beef cooked	1 oz	193	0	20	3
beef suet	1 oz	242	0	27	tr
beef tallow	1 tbsp (13 g)	115	0	13	0
chicken	1 cup	1846	0	205	0
chicken	1 tbsp	115	0	13	0
cocoa butter	1 tbsp	120	0	14	0
duck	1 tbsp	115	0	13	0
goose	1 tbsp	115	0	13	0
goose	3.5 oz	900	0	100	0
lamb new zealand raw	1 oz	182	0	19	2
lard	1 tbsp (13 g)	115	0	13	0
lard	1 cup (205 g)	1849	0	205	0
nutmeg butter	1 tbsp	120	0	14	0
pork, cooked	1 oz	200	0	21	2
salt pork	1 oz	212	0	23	23
shortening	1 tbsp	113	0	13	0
shortening	1 cup	1812	0	205	0
turkey	1 tbsp	115	0	13	0

FOOD	PORTION	CALS.	CARB.	FAT	PRO.
ucuhuba butter	1 tbsp	120	0	14	0
Crisco					
Butter Flavor	1 tbsp	110	0	12	0
Shortening	1 tbsp	110	0	12	0
Shortening	1 tbsp (0.4 oz)	110	0	12	0
Sticks	1 tbsp (0.4 oz)	110	0	12	0
Sticks Butter Flavor	1 tbsp (0.4 oz)	110	0	12	0
Empire					
Chicken Fat Rendered	1 tbsp (0.5 oz)	120	tr	13	0
Wesson					
Shortening	1 tbsp	100	0	12	0

FAVA BEANS
CANNED
Progresso

Fava Beans	½ cup	90	15	tr	7

FEIJOA

fresh	1 (1.75 oz)	25	5	tr	1
puree	1 cup	119	26	2	3

FENNEL

fresh bulb	1 (8.2 oz)	72	17	tr	3
fresh sliced	1 cup	27	6	tr	1
leaves	3.5 oz	24	3	tr	2
seed	1 tsp	7	1	tr	tr

FIBER
Delta

Natural Fiber	½ cup (1 oz)	20	2	tr	3

FIGS
CANNED

in heavy syrup	3	75	19	tr	tr
in light syrup	3	58	15	tr	tr
water pack	3	42	11	tr	tr
S&W					
Kadota Figs Whole Fancy	½ cup	100	28	0	0
DRIED					
California	½ cup (3.5 oz)	200	58	1	4
cooked	½ cup	140	16	1	2
whole	10	477	122	2	6
Sonoma					
White Misson	3-4 (1.4 oz)	110	26	0	1
FRESH					
fig	1 med	50	10	tr	tr

FOOD	PORTION	CALS.	CARB.	FAT	PRO.
FISH					
(see also FISH SUBSTITUTES, INDIVIDUAL NAMES, SUSHI)					
CANNED					
Holmes					
Finest Kippered Snacks drained	1 can (3.2 oz)	135	0	8	17
Port Clyde					
Fish Steaks In Louisiana Hot Sauce	1 can (3.75 oz)	150	2	9	17
Fish Steaks In Mustard Sauce	1 can (3.75 oz)	140	1	7	18
Fish Steaks In Soybean Oil With Hot Chilies drained	1 can (3.3 oz)	155	0	8	20
Fish Steaks In Soybean Oil drained	1 can (3.3 oz)	220	0	17	19
Progresso					
Mixed Seafood Sauce	½ cup	110	12	6	5
Seafood	½ cup	190	5	15	7
FROZEN					
breaded fillet	1 (2 oz)	155	14	7	9
sticks	1 stick (1 oz)	76	7	3	4
Cajun Cookin'					
Seafood Gumbo	17 oz	330	51	7	16
Gorton's					
Crispy Batter Dipped Fillets	2	290	18	19	11
Crispy Batter Sticks	4	260	16	18	9
Crunch Fillets	2	230	16	13	13
Crunchy Sticks	4	210	15	13	7
Light Recipe Lightly Breaded Fish Fillets	1 fillet	180	16	8	11
Light Recipe Tempura Fillets	1 fillet	200	8	14	10
Micorwave Fillets	2	340	17	26	10
Microwave Crispy Batter Large Cut Fillets	1	320	20	21	12
Microwave Entree Fillets In Herb Butter	1 pkg	190	3	8	26
Microwave Larger Cut Fillets	1	320	20	22	11
Microwave Larger Cut Ranch Fillet	1	330	24	21	12

FOOD	PORTION	CALS.	CARB.	FAT	PRO.
Gorton's (CONT.)					
Microwave Sticks	6	340	24	22	11
Potato Crisp Fillets	2	300	18	20	12
Potato Crisp Sticks	4	260	21	16	8
Value Pack Portions	1 portion	180	13	11	7
Value Pack Sticks	4	190	17	9	9
Kineret					
Fish Sticks	5 pieces (4 oz)	280	27	14	12
Mrs. Paul's					
Buttered Fillet Microwave	1 fillet	80	10	4	10
Entree Light Seafood Dijon	8¾ oz	200	17	5	21
Entree Light Seafood Florentine	8 oz	220	10	8	25
Entrees Light Seafood Mornay	9 oz	230	12	10	24
Fillet Sandwich Microwave	1	280	27	15	10
Fillets Microwave	1 fillet	280	16	19	12
Fish Cakes	2	190	24	7	9
Fish Fillets Batter Dipped	2 fillets	330	28	17	16
Fish Fillets Crispy Crunchy	2 fillets	220	23	9	13
Fish Fillets Crunchy Batter	2 fillets	280	26	14	12
Fish Sticks 40 Crunchy	4 (2.75 oz)	200	18	10	10
Fish Sticks Crispy Crunchy	4 sticks	190	18	8	9
Fish Sticks Microwave	5	290	18	20	10
In Butter Sauce Light Fillets	1 fillet	140	1	6	20
Portions Battered Fish	2 portions	300	21	19	11
Portions Crispy Crunchy Breaded Fish	2 portions	230	14	15	10
Seafood Platter Combination	9 oz	600	55	33	19
Sticks Battered Fish	4 sticks	210	15	12	7
Sticks Crispy Crunchy Breaded Fish	4 sticks	140	14	6	7
Van De Kamp's					
Crispy Microwave Fillets	1 piece	140	9	9	6
Crispy Microwave Fish Sticks	3 pieces	130	11	7	7

FOOD	PORTION	CALS.	CARB.	FAT	PRO.
Van De Kamp's (CONT.)					
Crispy Microwave Large Fillets	1 piece	290	21	17	12
Fish Fillets Battered	1	170	13	10	7
Fish Fillets Breaded	2	280	18	18	11
Fish Sticks Battered	4	160	12	9	8
Fish Sticks Breaded	4	200	15	12	9
Fish Sticks Breaded Value Pack	4	170	13	10	8
MIX					
Golden Dipt					
Beer Batter Fry	1 oz	100	22	0	2
Cajun Style Fish Fry	⅔ oz	60	14	0	2
Fish & Chips Batter Mix	1¼ oz	120	27	0	2
Fish Fry	⅔ oz	60	14	0	2
Seafood Frying Mix	⅔ oz	60	14	0	1
Tempura Batter Mix	1 oz	100	22	0	3
TAKE-OUT					
fish cake	1 (4.7 oz)	166	6	7	18
kedgeree	5.6 oz	242	15	11	21
sandwich w/ tartar sauce	1	431	41	55	17
sandwich w/ tartar sauce & cheese	1	524	48	29	21
stew	1 cup (7.9 oz)	157	10	4	19
taramasalata	3.5 oz	446	4	46	3
FISH PASTE					
fish paste	2 tsp	15	tr	1	1
FISH SUBSTITUTES					
LaLoma					
Ocean Platter mix not prep	¼ cup (16 g)	50	5	0	8
Worthington					
Fillets	2 (85 g)	180	9	9	15
Tuno	2 oz (57 g)	100	3	7	5
FLAXSEED					
Arrowhead					
Flaxseed	3 tbsp (1 oz)	140	11	10	5
Stone-Buhr					
Flaxseed	1 tsp (1 oz)	150	11	10	5
FLOUNDER					
FRESH					
cooked	1 fillet (4.5 oz)	148	0	2	31
cooked	3 oz	99	0	1	21

FOOD	PORTION	CALS.	CARB.	FAT	PRO.
FROZEN					
Gorton's					
Fishmarket Fresh	5 oz	110	1	1	23
Microwave Entree Stuffed	1 pkg	350	21	18	25
Mrs. Paul's					
Crunchy Batter Fillets	2 fillets	220	23	9	12
Light Fillets	1 fillet	240	20	10	16
Van De Kamp's					
Light Fillets	1 piece	260	21	12	18
Natural Fillets	4 oz	100	0	2	22
TAKE-OUT					
battered & fried	3.2 oz	211	15	11	13
breaded & fried	3.2 oz	211	15	11	13
FLOUR					
corn masa	1 cup	416	87	4	11
corn whole grain	1 cup	422	90	5	8
cottonseed lowfat	1 oz	94	10	tr	14
peanut defatted	1 cup	196	21	tr	31
peanut defatted	1 oz	92	10	tr	15
peanut lowfat	1 cup	257	19	13	20
potato	1 cup (6.3 oz)	628	143	1	14
rice brown	1 cup	574	121	4	11
rice white	1 cup	578	127	2	9
rye dark	1 cup	415	88	3	18
rye light	1 cup	374	82	1	9
rye medium	1 cup	361	79	2	10
sesame lowfat	1 oz	95	10	tr	14
triticale whole grain	1 cup	440	95	2	17
white all-purpose	1 cup	455	95	1	13
white bread	1 cup	495	99	2	16
white cake	1 cup	395	85	tr	9
white self-rising	1 cup	442	93	1	12
whole wheat	1 cup	407	87	2	16
Arrowhead					
Kamut	¼ cup (1.2 oz)	110	25	1	4
Pastry	⅓ cup (1.1 oz)	100	22	1	4
Rye Whole Grain	¼ cup (1.6 oz)	160	34	1	6
Spelt	¼ cup (1.2 oz)	100	24	1	4
Teff	¼ cup (1.4 oz)	140	29	1	5
Unbleached White	⅓ cup (1.6 oz)	160	33	1	5
Whole Grain Wheat	¼ cup (1.6 oz)	160	34	1	6
Whole Wheat	¼ cup (1.2 oz)	130	25	1	5

FOOD	PORTION	CALS.	CARB.	FAT	PRO.
Aunt Jemima					
Self-Rising	3 tbsp	90	20	0	3
Ballard					
All Purpose	1 cup	400	87	1	11
Self-Rising	1 cup	380	84	1	9
Ceresota					
All Purpose	1 cup	390	83	1	12
Whole Wheat	1 cup	400	80	2	15
Gold Medal					
All Purpose	1 cup	400	87	1	11
Oat Blend	1 cup	390	81	3	14
Self-Rising	1 cup	380	83	1	10
Unbleached	1 cup	400	87	1	11
Whole Wheat	1 cup	350	78	2	16
Whole Wheat Blend	1 cup	380	84	2	14
Heckers					
All Purpose	1 cup	390	83	1	12
Whole Wheat	1 cup	400	80	2	15
Hodgson Mill					
50/50 Flour	¼ cup (1 oz)	100	21	1	4
Best For Bread	¼ cup (1 oz)	100	22	0	4
Buckwheat	⅓ cup (1.6 oz)	160	33	1	7
Oat Bran Blend	¼ cup (1 oz)	110	24	1	3
Oat Bran Flour	¼ cup (1 oz)	110	23	2	3
Rye	¼ cup (1 oz)	90	22	1	3
Seasoned Flour	¼ cup (1 oz)	90	20	0	3
White	¼ cup (1 oz)	100	23	0	3
Whole Wheat	¼ cup (1 oz)	100	22	1	3
King Arthur					
All Purpose Unbleached	¼ cup (1 oz)	100	22	0	3
Pillsbury					
All Purpose Best	1 cup	400	87	1	11
Bohemian Style Rye and Wheat Best	1 cup	400	86	1	11
Bread Best	1 cup	400	83	2	14
Rye Medium Best	1 cup	400	83	2	12
Self-Rising Best	1 cup	380	84	1	9
Shake & Blend Best	2 tbsp	50	11	0	1
Unbleached Best	1 cup	400	86	1	12
Whole Wheat Best	1 cup	400	80	2	15
Robin Hood					
All Purpose	1 cup	400	85	1	13
Rye Stone Ground	1 cup	360	86	2	13
Self-Rising	1 cup	380	83	1	10
Unbleached	1 cup	400	85	1	13

FOOD	PORTION	CALS.	CARB.	FAT	PRO.
Stone Ground Mills					
White Unbleached Organic	¼ cup (1.4 oz)	130	25	0	5
Whole Wheat 100% Stone Ground	3 tbsp (1 oz)	90	20	1	4

FRANKFURTER
(see HOT DOG)

FRENCH BEANS

dried cooked	1 cup	228	43	1	12

FRENCH FRIES
(see POTATOES)

FRENCH TOAST
FROZEN

french toast	1 slice (2 oz)	126	19	4	4
Aunt Jemima					
Cinnamon Swirl	2 pieces (4.1 oz)	240	37	6	9
Slices	2 pieces (4.1 oz)	240	38	6	9
Downyflake	2	270	34	12	6
Extra Thick	1	150	11	9	5
Texas Style & Sausage	1 pkg (4.25 oz)	400	37	24	10
Great Starts					
Cinnamon Swirl With Sausage	5½ oz	390	37	21	12
French Toast With Sausage	5½ oz	380	35	21	12
Mini French Toast With Sausage	2½ oz	190	22	9	6
Oatmeal French Toast With Lite Links	4.65 oz	310	35	13	13
Healthy Starts					
French Toast With LeanLinks	6.5 oz	400	51	13	20
Quaker					
French Toast Sticks & Syrup	1 pkg (5.2 oz)	400	48	20	7
French Toast Wedges & Sausage	1 pkg (5.3 oz)	360	40	17	13
Weight Watchers					
French Toast With Cinnamon	2 slices (3 oz)	160	24	5	8
French Toast With Links	4.5 oz	270	24	11	15
HOME RECIPE					
as prep w/ 2% milk	1 slice	149	16	7	7

FOOD	PORTION	CALS.	CARB.	FAT	PRO.
as prep w/ whole milk	1 slice	151	16	7	7
TAKE-OUT					
w/ butter	2 slices	356	36	19	10

FROG'S LEGS

frog leg as prep w/ seasoned flour & fried	1 (0.8)	70	15	5	4

FROSTING
(*see* CAKE)

FRUCTOSE
Estee

Fructose	1 tsp (4 g)	15	4	0	0
Packet	1 pkg (3 g)	10	3	0	0

FRUIT DRINKS
(*see also* LEMONADE)
FROZEN

citrus juice drink as prep	1 cup	114	28	0	1
citrus juice drink not prep	1 can (12 fl oz)	684	171	tr	5
fruit punch as prep w/water	1 cup	113	29	tr	tr
fruit punch not prep	1 can (12 fl oz)	678	173	tr	1
limeade	1 can (6 oz)	408	108	tr	tr
limeade as prep w/ water	1 cup	102	27	tr	tr
Bright & Early					
Fruit Punch	8 fl oz	130	31	0	0
Dole					
100% Juice Blend Country Raspberry as prep	8 fl oz	140	34	0	1
100% Juice Blend Orchard Peach as prep	8 fl oz	140	34	0	1
Mountain Cherry 100% Juice Blend as prep	8 fl oz	120	30	0	0
Pineapple Grapefruit as prep	8 fl oz	130	29	0	1
Pineapple Passion Banana as prep	8 fl oz	120	30	0	1
Pineapple Orange Banana as prep	8 fl oz	130	31	0	1
Pineapple Orange Banana as prep	8 fl oz	130	32	0	1
Pineapple Orange Guava as prep	8 fl oz	120	30	0	1

FOOD	PORTION	CALS.	CARB.	FAT	PRO.
Dole (CONT.)					
Pineapple Orange as prep	8 fl oz	120	29	0	1
Tropical Fruit as prep	8 fl oz	140	34	0	1
Five Alive					
Berry Citrus	8 fl oz	120	30	0	0
Citrus	8 fl oz	120	30	0	0
Tropical Citrus	8 fl oz	120	29	0	0
Minute Maid					
Berry Punch	8 fl oz	130	31	0	0
Citrus Punch	8 fl oz	120	31	0	0
Fruit Punch	8 fl oz	120	31	0	0
Limeade	8 fl oz	100	26	0	0
Pineapple Orange	8 fl oz	120	31	0	0
Tropical Punch	8 fl oz	120	31	0	0
Seneca					
Cranberry-Apple Juice Cocktail frzn as prep	8 fl oz	140	33	0	0
Raspberry-Cranberry Juice Cocktail frzn as prep	8 fl oz	140	36	0	0
Tree Top					
Apple Citrus as prep	6 oz	90	22	0	1
Apple Cranberry as prep	6 oz	100	25	0	0
Apple Grape as prep	6 oz	100	25	0	0
Apple Pear as prep	6 oz	90	22	0	0
Apple Raspberry as prep	6 oz	80	21	0	0
MIX					
fruit punch as prep w/water	9 oz	97	25	0	tr
Crystal Light					
Berry Blend Sugar Free	8 oz	3	0	0	0
Fruit Punch Sugar Free	8 oz	3	0	0	0
Lemon-Lime	8 oz	4	0	0	0
Tropic Quencher	8 oz	5	0	0	0
Kool-Aid					
Lemon-Lime	8 oz	98	25	0	0
Purplesaurus Rex	8 oz	98	25	0	0
Rainbow Punch	8 oz	98	25	0	0
Sharkleberry Fin	8 oz	98	25	0	0
Sugar Free Berry Blue	8 oz	3	0	0	0
Sugar Free Berry Punch	8 oz	3	0	0	0
Sugar Free Purplesaurus Rex	8 oz	3	0	0	0
Sugar Free Rainbow Punch	8 oz	4	0	0	0

FOOD	PORTION	CALS.	CARB.	FAT	PRO.
Kool-Aid (CONT.)					
Sugar Free Sharkleberry Fin	8 oz	3	0	0	0
Sugar Free Tropical Punch	8 oz	3	0	0	0
Sugar Sweetened Mountain Berry Punch	8 oz	98	25	0	0
Sugar Sweetened Purplesaurus Rex	8 oz	84	21	0	0
Sugar Sweetened Rainbow Punch	8 oz	84	21	0	0
Sugar Sweetened Sharkleberry Fin	8 oz	84	21	0	0
Sugar Sweetened Sunshine Punch	8 oz	83	21	0	0
Sugar Sweetened Surfin' Berry Punch	8 oz	79	20	0	0
Sugar Sweetened Tropical Punch	8 oz	84	21	0	0
Tropical Punch	8 oz	98	25	0	0
Unsweetened Berry Blue	8 oz	98	25	0	0
Wylers					
Drink Mix Unsweetened Bunch O' Berries	8 oz	2	1	0	0
Drink Mix Unsweetened Pink	8 fl oz	3	1	0	0
Drink Mix Unsweetened Tropical Punch	8 oz	2	1	0	0
READY-TO-DRINK					
cranberry apple drink	6 fl oz	123	32	0	tr
cranberry apricot drink	6 fl oz	118	30	0	0
fruit punch	6 fl oz	87	22	tr	tr
orange grapefruit juice	8 fl oz	107	25	tr	1
orange & apricot	8 fl oz	128	32	tr	1
pineapple & grapefruit	8 fl oz	117	29	tr	1
pineapple & orange drink	8 fl oz	125	29	0	3
After The Fall					
Amaretto Almond	1 can (12 oz)	170	42	0	tr
American Pie Cherry	1 can (12 oz)	190	35	0	tr
Apple Apricot	1 cup (8 oz)	100	26	0	1
Apple Raspberry	1 bottle (10 oz)	110	29	0	0
Apple Strawberry	1 bottle (10 oz)	120	30	0	1
Banana Casablanca	1 bottle (10 oz)	120	24	0	1
Berrymeister	1 can (12 oz)	160	40	0	1

FOOD	PORTION	CALS.	CARB.	FAT	PRO.
After The Fall (CONT.)					
Cranberry Meets Raspberry	1 bottle (10 oz)	120	29	0	0
Georgia Peach Blend	1 bottle (10 oz)	130	33	0	1
Mango Montage	1 bottle (10 oz)	140	33	0	1
Maui Grove	1 bottle (10 oz)	120	29	0	1
Nantucket Ginger Ale	1 can (12 oz)	140	35	0	1
Orange Icicle Cream	1 can (12 oz)	170	42	0	tr
Oregon Berry	1 bottle (10 oz)	130	31	0	0
Passion Of The Islands	1 bottle (10 oz)	125	32	0	1
Peach Vanilla	1 can (12 oz)	170	42	0	tr
Strawberry Vanilla	1 can (12 oz)	160	42	0	tr
Twist O' Strawberry	1 can (12 oz)	190	37	0	tr
Vanilla Bean Cream	1 can (12 oz)	170	42	0	tr
Apple & Eve					
Apple Cranberry	6 fl oz	80	19	0	0
Apple Grape	6 fl oz	120	29	0	1
Cranberry Grape	6 fl oz	100	23	0	1
Fruit Punch	6 fl oz	78	18	0	0
Raspberry Cranberry	6 fl oz	90	21	0	0
BAMA					
Fruit Punch	8.45 fl oz	130	32	0	0
Boku					
White Grape Raspberry	16 fl oz	120	29	0	0
Crystal Geyser					
Juice Squeeze Citrus Grape	1 bottle (12 fl oz)	145	35	0	1
Juice Squeeze Orange & Passion Fruit	1 bottle (12 fl oz)	130	31	0	0
Juice Squeeze Passion Fruit & Mango	1 bottle (12 fl oz)	125	31	0	0
Juice Squeeze Wild Berry	1 bottle (12 fl oz)	130	31	0	1
Dole					
Pineapple Passion Banana	6 fl oz	100	21	0	tr
Pineapple Orange	6 fl oz	90	22	0	0
Pineapple Orange Banana	6 fl oz	100	23	0	0
Pineapple Orange Guava	6 fl oz	100	21	0	tr
Five Alive					
Citrus	1 bottle (16 fl oz)	120	31	0	0
Citrus	6 fl oz	90	22	0	0
Citrus	1 can (11.5 fl oz)	170	43	0	0

FOOD	PORTION	CALS.	CARB.	FAT	PRO.
Five Alive (CONT.)					
Citrus Chilled	8 fl oz	120	30	0	0
Hi-C					
Boppin Berry Box	8.45 fl oz	140	33	0	0
Boppin' Berry	8 fl oz	130	32	0	0
Double Fruit Box	8.45 fl oz	130	32	0	0
Double Fruit Cooler	8 fl oz	130	31	0	0
Ecto Cooler	8 fl oz	130	32	0	0
Ecto Cooler	1 can (11.5 fl oz)	180	45	0	0
Ecto Cooler Box	8.45 fl oz	130	32	0	0
Fruit Punch	8 fl oz	130	32	0	0
Fruit Punch	1 can (11.5 fl oz)	190	46	0	0
Fruit Punch Box	8.45 fl oz	140	32	0	0
Fruity Bubble Gum	8 fl oz	120	30	0	0
Fruity Bubble Gum Box	8.45 fl oz	130	32	0	0
Hula Punch	8 fl oz	120	29	0	0
Hula Punch	1 can (11.5 fl oz)	170	42	0	0
Hula Punch Box	8.45 fl oz	120	30	0	0
Jammin' Apple Box	8.45 fl oz	130	33	0	0
Stompin' Banana Berry	8 fl oz	130	31	0	0
Stompin' Banana Berry Box	8.45 fl oz	130	32	0	0
Wild Berry	8 fl oz	120	30	0	0
Wild Berry Box	8.45 fl oz	130	32	0	0
Hood					
Natural Blenders Apple Wild Blueberry Strawberry	1 cup (8 oz)	120	30	0	0
Natural Blenders Apple Cranberry Raspberry	1 cup (8 oz)	130	32	0	0
Natural Blenders Apple Grape Cherry	1 cup (8 oz)	130	32	0	0
Natural Blenders Apple Peach Pear	1 cup (8 oz)	120	30	0	0
Natural Blenders Pineapple Orange Kiwi	1 cup (8 oz)	120	30	0	0
Juicy Juice					
Apple Grape	1 box (8.45 fl oz)	120	29	0	1
Berry	1 box (8.45 fl oz)	130	30	0	1
Berry	1 bottle (6 fl oz)	90	22	0	1
Punch	1 box (8.45 fl oz)	140	33	0	1
Punch	1 bottle (6 fl oz)	100	23	0	1
Tropical	1 bottle (6 fl oz)	110	26	0	1
Tropical	1 box (8.45 fl oz)	150	36	0	1

FOOD	PORTION	CALS.	CARB.	FAT	PRO.
Kern's					
Apple Strawberry Nectar	6 fl oz	110	26	0	0
Apricot Pineapple Nectar	6 fl oz	110	27	0	0
Banana Pineapple Nectar	6 fl oz	110	27	0	1
Coconut Pineapple Nectar	6 fl oz	140	26	0	1
Orange Banana Nectar	6 fl oz	110	25	0	1
Strawberry Banana Nectar	6 fl oz	110	28	0	0
Tropical Nectar	6 fl oz	110	27	0	0
Kool-Aid					
Koolers Mountainberry Punch	1 pkg (8.45 fl oz)	142	37	0	0
Koolers Rainbow Punch	1 pkg (8.45 fl oz)	135	36	0	0
Koolers Sharkleberry Fin	1 pkg (8.45 fl oz)	140	37	0	0
Koolers Tropical Punch	1 pkg (8.45 fl oz)	132	35	0	0
Libby					
Strawberry Banana Nectar	1 can (11.5 fl oz)	220	51	0	tr
Lifesavers					
Fruit Punch	8 fl oz	140	34	0	0
Lime Punch	8 fl oz	140	34	0	0
Mauna La'i					
Island Guava Hawaiian Guava Fruit Juice Drink	8 fl oz	130	32	0	0
Mango & Hawaiian Guava Fruit Juice Drink	8 fl oz	130	33	0	0
Paradise Guava Hawaiian Guava & Passion Fruit Juice Drink	8 fl oz	130	32	0	0
Minute Maid					
Berry Punch Box	8.45 fl oz	130	31	0	0
Berry Punch Chilled	8 fl oz	130	31	0	0
Citrus Punch Chilled	8 fl oz	130	31	0	0
Fruit Punch Box	8.45 fl oz	120	31	0	0
Fruit Punch Chilled	8 fl oz	120	31	0	0
Juices To Go Citrus Punch	1 can (11.5 fl oz)	180	45	0	0
Juices To Go Citrus Punch	1 bottle (10 fl oz)	160	39	0	0
Juices To Go Concord Punch	1 can (11.5 fl oz)	180	46	0	0

FOOD	PORTION	CALS.	CARB.	FAT	PRO.
Minute Maid (CONT.)					
Juices To Go Concord Punch	1 bottle (10 fl oz)	160	40	0	0
Juices To Go Concord Punch	1 bottle (16 fl oz)	130	32	0	0
Juices To Go Fruit Punch	1 bottle (10 fl oz)	160	39	0	0
Juices To Go Fruit Punch	1 can (11.5 fl oz)	180	44	0	0
Juices To Go Fruit Punch	1 bottle (16 fl oz)	120	31	0	0
Juices To Go Orange Blend	1 can (11.5 fl oz)	170	43	0	0
Juices To Go Orange Blend	1 bottle (10 fl oz)	150	37	0	0
Naturals Apple Cranberry	8 fl oz	170	42	0	0
Naturals Concord Medley	8 fl oz	130	32	0	0
Naturals Fruit Medley	8 fl oz	120	31	0	0
Naturals Orange Grape Medley	8 fl oz	120	30	0	0
Naturals Tropical Medley	8 fl oz	120	31	0	0
Tropical Punch Box	8.45 fl oz	130	32	0	0
Tropical Punch Chilled	8 fl oz	120	31	0	0
Mott's					
Apple Cranberry Blend	10 fl oz	180	44	0	0
Apple Cranberry From Concentrate as prep	8 fl oz	120	30	0	0
Apple Grape From Concentrate as prep	8 fl oz	120	30	0	0
Apple Raspberry Blend	10 fl oz	140	33	0	0
Apple Raspberry From Concentrate	8.45 fl oz	120	30	0	0
Fruit Basket Apple Raspberry Juice Cocktail as prep	8 fl oz	130	30	0	0
Fruit Basket Tropical Blend Juice Cocktail as prep	8 fl oz	120	30	0	0
Fruit Punch From Concentrate	8.45 fl oz	120	29	0	0
Fruit Punch From Concentrate	10 fl oz	170	42	0	0
Grape Apple	10 fl oz	170	41	0	0
Pineapple Orange	10 fl oz	170	42	0	0

FOOD	PORTION	CALS.	CARB.	FAT	PRO.
Ocean Spray					
Cran.Blueberry	8 fl oz	160	41	0	0
Cran.Cherry	6 fl oz	160	39	0	0
Cran.Grape	8 fl oz	170	41	0	0
Cran.Raspberry	8 fl oz	140	36	0	0
Cran.Raspberry Reduced Calorie	8 fl oz	50	13	0	0
Cran.Strawberry	8 fl oz	140	36	0	0
Cranapple	8 fl oz	160	41	0	0
Cranapple Reduced Calorie	8 fl oz	50	13	0	0
Cranicot	8 fl oz	160	40	0	0
Crantastic	8 fl oz	150	37	0	0
Fruit Punch	8 fl oz	130	32	0	0
Lightstyle Low Calorie Cran.Grape	8 fl oz	40	9	0	0
Lightstyle Low Calorie Cran.Raspberry	8 fl oz	40	10	0	0
Refreshers Juice Drink Citrus Cranberry	8 fl oz	140	35	0	0
Refreshers Juice Drink Citrus Peach	8 fl oz	120	30	0	0
Refreshers Juice Drink Orange Cranberry	8 fl oz	130	33	0	0
Ruby Red & Tangerine Grapefruit Juice Cocktail	8 fl oz	130	32	0	0
Odwalla					
Boyzenberry Mango	8 fl oz	140	34	0	1
C Monster	16 fl oz	300	72	0	4
Fruitshake Blackberry	8 fl oz	160	39	0	1
Guanaba Dabba Doo!	8 fl oz	130	29	0	2
Lotta Colada	8 fl oz	160	33	3	2
Mango Tango	8 fl oz	150	37	3	1
Mo Beta	16 fl oz	280	69	1	3
Raspberry Smoothie	8 fl oz	140	35	0	2
Strawberry Banana Smoothie	8 fl oz	100	26	0	1
Strawberry Go Man Go	8 fl oz	100	26	1	1
Super Protein	16 fl oz	400	40	6	10
Pek					
Mango Guava Ecstasy	1 bottle (20 fl oz)	110	27	0	0
Passionate Peach Grapefruit	8 fl oz	110	27	0	0

FOOD	PORTION	CALS.	CARB.	FAT	PRO.
S&W					
Apricot Pineapple Nectar	6 fl oz	120	29	0	1
Apricot Pineapple Nectar Diet	6 fl oz	80	20	0	0
Smucker's					
Apple Cranberry	8 oz	120	32	0	0
Orange Banana	8 oz	120	30	0	0
Snapple					
Diet Kiwi Strawberry	8 fl oz	13	3	0	0
Fruit Punch	8 fl oz	120	29	0	0
Kiwi Strawberry Cocktail	8 fl oz	130	33	0	0
Melonberry Cocktail	8 fl oz	120	29	0	0
Vitamin Supreme	10 fl oz	150	38	0	0
Squeezit					
Berry B. Wild	1 (6.75 fl oz)	90	22	0	0
Chucklin' Cherry	1 (6.75 fl oz)	90	23	0	0
Grumpy Grape	1 (6.75 fl oz)	90	23	0	0
Mean Green Puncher	1 (6.75 fl oz)	90	23	0	0
Silly Billy Strawberry	1 (6.75 fl oz)	90	23	0	0
Smarty Arty Orange	1 (6.75 fl oz)	90	23	0	0
Tang					
Mixed Fruit	8.45 fl oz	137	36	0	0
Tree Top					
Apple Citrus	6 fl oz	90	22	0	1
Apple Cranberry	6 fl oz	100	25	0	0
Apple Grape	6 fl oz	100	25	0	0
Apple Pear	6 fl oz	90	22	0	0
Apple Raspberry	6 fl oz	80	21	0	0
Tropicana					
Berry Punch	8 fl oz	120	29	0	0
Citrus Punch	1 bottle (10 fl oz)	180	45	0	0
Citrus Punch	8 fl oz	140	36	0	0
Cranberry Punch	1 can (11.5 fl oz)	200	49	0	0
Cranberry Punch	1 bottle (10 fl oz)	170	43	0	0
Cranberry Punch	8 fl oz	140	34	0	0
Fruit Punch	1 bottle (10 fl oz)	150	39	0	0
Fruit Punch	1 can (11.5 fl oz)	170	42	0	0
Fruit Punch	8 fl oz	130	31	0	0
Fruit Punch	1 container (10 fl oz)	160	39	0	0
Orange Pineapple	8 fl oz	110	27	0	tr
Orange Pineapple	1 bottle (10 fl oz)	130	32	0	tr
Pineapple Punch	8 fl oz	120	31	0	0

FOOD	PORTION	CALS.	CARB.	FAT	PRO.
Tropicana (CONT.)					
Pineapple Punch	1 bottle (10 fl oz)	160	39	0	0
Season's Best Cranberry Medley	8 fl oz	120	29	0	tr
Tropics Apple Cranberry Kiwi	8 fl oz	120	30	0	tr
Tropics Orange Kiwi Passion	8 fl oz	100	26	0	tr
Tropics Orange Peach Mango	8 fl oz	110	28	0	tr
Tropics Orange Pineapple	8 fl oz	110	27	0	tr
Tropics Orange Strawberry Banana	8 fl oz	110	27	0	tr
Tropics Pineapple Passion	8 fl oz	120	30	0	tr
Twister Apple Raspberry Blackberry	8 fl oz	120	31	0	0
Twister Apple Raspberry Blackberry	1 bottle (10 fl oz)	150	38	0	0
Twister Apple Raspberry Blackberry	1 can (11.5 fl oz)	180	44	0	0
Twister Cranberry Raspberry Strawberry	8 fl oz	120	31	0	0
Twister Cranberry Raspberry Strawberry	1 bottle (10 fl oz)	160	39	0	tr
Twister Light Cranberry Raspberry Strawberry	8 fl oz	45	11	0	tr
Twister Light Cranberry Raspberry Strawberry	1 container (10 fl oz)	50	13	0	tr
Twister Light Orange Cranberry	8 fl oz	30	7	0	0
Twister Light Orange Cranberry	1 container (10 fl oz)	35	9	0	0
Twister Light Orange Raspberry	8 fl oz	35	9	0	0
Twister Light Orange Strawberry Banana	8 fl oz	35	9	0	0
Twister Light Orange Strawberry Banana	1 container (10 fl oz)	45	11	0	tr

FOOD	PORTION	CALS.	CARB.	FAT	PRO.
Tropicana (CONT.)					
Twister Orange Cranberry	1 container (10 fl oz)	140	35	0	tr
Twister Orange Cranberry	1 bottle (10 fl oz)	140	36	0	tr
Twister Orange Cranberry	8 fl oz	120	29	0	tr
Twister Orange Peach	1 can (11.5 fl oz)	160	41	0	tr
Twister Orange Peach	1 bottle (10 fl oz)	140	36	0	tr
Twister Orange Peach	8 fl oz	120	29	0	tr
Twister Orange Raspberry	1 bottle (10 fl oz)	140	36	0	tr
Twister Orange Raspberry	8 fl oz	120	29	0	0
Twister Orange Strawberry Banana	1 container (10 fl oz)	140	35	0	tr
Twister Strawberry Banana	1 bottle (10 fl oz)	140	35	0	tr
Twister Strawberry Banana	8 fl oz	120	29	0	tr
Twister Strawberry Banana	1 can (11.5 fl oz)	160	41	0	tr
Twister Strawberry Guava	1 bottle (10 fl oz)	140	35	0	tr
Twister Strawberry Guava	8 fl oz	110	28	0	tr
Veryfine					
Apple Cherryberry	8 fl oz	130	33	0	0
Apple Cranberry	8 fl oz	130	33	0	0
Apple Raspberry	8 fl oz	110	27	0	0
Fruit Punch	8 fl oz	130	33	0	0
Guava Strawberry	8 fl oz	120	30	0	0
Lemon & Lime	8 fl oz	120	30	0	0
Papaya Punch	8 fl oz	120	30	0	0
Passionfruit Orange	8 fl oz	110	26	0	0
Pineapple Orange	8 fl oz	130	32	0	0
White House					
Apple Cherry	6 fl oz	90	22	0	0

FRUIT MIXED
(see also individual names)
CANNED

FOOD	PORTION	CALS.	CARB.	FAT	PRO.
fruit cocktail in heavy syrup	½ cup	93	24	tr	1

FOOD	PORTION	CALS.	CARB.	FAT	PRO.
fruit cocktail juice pack	½ cup	56	15	tr	1
fruit cocktail water pack	½ cup	40	10	tr	1
fruit salad in heavy syrup	½ cup	94	24	tr	tr
fruit salad in light syrup	½ cup	73	19	tr	tr
fruit salad juice pack	½ cup	62	16	tr	1
fruit salad water pack	½ cup	37	10	tr	tr
mixed fruit in heavy syrup	½ cup	92	24	tr	tr
tropical fruit salad in heavy syrup	½ cup	110	29	tr	1
Del Monte					
Fruit Cocktail Fruit Naturals	½ cup (4.4 oz)	60	15	0	0
Fruit Cocktail In Heavy Syrup	½ cup (4.5 oz)	100	24	0	0
Fruit Cocktail Lite	½ cup (4.4 oz)	60	15	0	0
Lite Mixed Fruits Chunky	½ cup (4.4 oz)	60	15	0	0
Mixed Fruits Chunky Fruit Naturals	½ cup (4.4 oz)	60	15	0	0
Mixed Fruits Chunky In Heavy Syrup	½ cup (4.5 oz)	100	24	0	0
Snack Cups Mixed Fruit Fruit Naturals	1 serv (4.5 oz)	60	16	0	0
Snack Cups Mixed Fruit Fruit Naturals EZ-Open Lid	1 serv (4.5 oz)	60	15	0	0
Snack Cups Mixed Fruit In Heavy Syrup	1 serv (4.5 oz)	100	24	0	0
Snack Cups Mixed Fruit In Heavy Syrup EZ-Open Lid	1 serv (4.2 oz)	90	23	0	0
Snack Cups Mixed Fruit Lite	1 serv (4.5 oz)	60	16	0	0
Snack Cups Mixed Fruit Lite EZ-Open Lid	1 serv (4.5 oz)	60	15	0	0
Dole					
Tropical Fruit Salad	½ cup	70	17	0	0
Hunt's					
Fruit Cocktail	4 oz	90	23	tr	tr
Libby					
Chunky Mixed Lite	½ cup (4.3 oz)	60	14	0	0
Fruit Cocktail Lite	½ cup (4.3 oz)	60	15	0	0
S&W					
Chunky Mixed Diet	½ cup	40	10	0	0
Chunky Mixed Natural Style	½ cup	90	21	0	1

FOOD	PORTION	CALS.	CARB.	FAT	PRO.
S&W (CONT.)					
Chunky Mixed Unsweetened	½ cup	40	10	0	0
Fruit Cocktail Diet	½ cup	40	10	0	0
Fruit Cocktail Heavy Syrup	½ cup	90	24	0	0
Fruit Cocktail Natural Lite	½ cup	60	15	0	0
Fruit Cocktail Natural Style	½ cup	90	21	0	1
Fruit Cocktail Unsweetened	½ cup	40	10	0	0
DRIED					
mixed	11 oz pkg	712	188	1	7
Del Monte					
Mixed	⅓ cup (1.4 oz)	110	30	0	0
Planters					
Fruit'n Nut Mix	1 oz	140	13	9	4
Sonoma					
Diced	⅓ cup (1.4 oz)	120	31	0	1
Mixed Fruit	5-8 pieces (1.4 oz)	120	30	0	1
Trail Mix	¼ cup (1.4 oz)	160	24	7	3
FROZEN					
mixed fruit sweetened	1 cup	245	61	tr	4
Big Valley					
Burst O' Berries	⅔ cup (4.9 oz)	70	16	0	1
California Tropics	⅔ cup (4.9 oz)	60	15	0	1
Cup A Fruit	1 pkg (4 oz)	50	7	0	tr
Mixed	4.9 oz	60	14	0	1
Birds Eye					
Mixed Fruit	½ cup	120	31	0	1
Dole					
Applesauce Strawberry	1 pkg (4 oz)	60	15	0	tr
FRUIT SNACKS					
fruit leather	1 bar (0.8 oz)	81	18	1	tr
fruit leather pieces	1 pkg (0.9 oz)	92	21	2	tr
fruit leather pieces	1 oz	97	22	2	tr
fruit leather rolls	1 lg (0.7 oz)	73	18	1	tr
fruit leather rolls	1 sm (0.5 oz)	49	12	tr	tr
Betty Crocker					
String Thing Berry 'N Blue	1 pkg (0.7 oz)	80	17	1	0
String Thing Cherry	1 pkg (0.7 oz)	80	17	1	0

FOOD	PORTION	CALS.	CARB.	FAT	PRO.
Betty Crocker (CONT.)					
String Thing Strawberry	1 pkg (0.7 oz)	80	17	1	0
Brock					
Beauty & The Beast	1 pkg (0.9 oz)	90	21	0	1
Cinderella	1 pkg (0.9 oz)	90	21	0	1
Dinosaurs	1 pkg (0.9 oz)	90	21	0	1
Ninja Trolls	1 pkg (0.9 oz)	90	21	0	1
Sharks	1 pkg (0.9 oz)	90	21	0	1
Del Monte					
Sierra Trail Mix	¼ cup (1.2 oz)	150	20	8	4
Sierra Trail Mix	1 pkg (1 oz)	120	16	6	3
Sierra Trail Mix	1 pkg (0.9 oz)	110	15	6	3
Fruit By The Foot					
Cherry	1	80	18	2	tr
Grape	1	80	18	2	tr
Strawberry	1	80	18	2	tr
Fruit Roll-Ups					
Cherry	1 (½ oz)	50	12	tr	tr
Crazy Colors	1 (½ oz)	50	12	tr	tr
Fruit Punch	1 (½ oz)	50	12	tr	tr
Grape	1 (½ oz)	50	12	tr	tr
Raspberry	1 (½ oz)	50	12	tr	tr
Strawberry	1 (½ oz)	50	12	tr	tr
General Mills					
Garfield And Friends 1-2 Punch	1 pkg	100	22	1	tr
Garfield And Friends Cat Cooler	1 pkg	100	22	1	tr
Garfield And Friends Fat Cat Funnies	1 (½ oz)	50	12	tr	tr
Garfield And Friends Fruit Party	1 (½ oz)	50	12	tr	tr
Garfield And Friends Very Strawberry	1 pkg	100	22	1	tr
Shark Bites & Berry Bears Assorted Fruit	1 pkg	100	22	tr	tr
Shark Bites & Berry Bears Fruit Punch	1 pkg	100	22	tr	tr
Surf's Up! Sun Splash	1 pkg	100	22	1	tr
Surf's Up! Tutti Frutti	1 pkg	100	22	1	tr
Thunder Jets Assorted Fruit Squadron	1 pkg	100	24	1	tr
Thunder Jets Mach 1 Fruit Mix	1 pkg	100	24	1	tr

FOOD	PORTION	CALS.	CARB.	FAT	PRO.
Health Valley					
Bakes Apple	1 bar	100	16	3	2
Bakes Date	1 bar	100	16	3	3
Bakes Raisin	1 bar	100	16	3	2
Fat Free Fruit Bars 100% Organic Apple	1 bar	140	33	tr	3
Fat Free Fruit Bars 100% Organic Date	1 bar	140	33	tr	3
Fat Free Fruit Bars 100% Organic Raisin	1 bar	140	33	tr	3
Fat Free Fruit Bars 100%Fruit Organic Apricot	1 bar	140	33	tr	3
Fruit & Fitness Bars	2 bars	200	35	5	4
Oat Bran Bakes Apricot	1 bar	100	16	3	2
Oat Bran Bakes Fig & Nut	1 bar	110	16	3	2
Oat Bran Jumbo Fruit Bar Almond & Date	1 bar	170	28	5	4
Oat Bran Jumbo Fruit Bars Raisin & Cinnamon	1 bar	160	32	2	3
Rice Bran Jumbo Fruit Bars Almond & Date	1 bar	160	27	5	3
Lipton					
Hanna Barbera Flintstones	1 pkg (1 oz)	100	22	0	2
Hanna Barbera Jetsons	1 pkg (1 oz)	100	22	0	2
Hanna Barbera Yo Yogi!	1 pkg (1 oz)	100	22	0	2
Tiny Toons Bunch Of Berries	1 pkg (0.9 oz)	100	22	1	0
Tiny Toons Fruit Assortment	1 pkg (0.9 oz)	100	22	1	0
Tiny Toons Paaaarrrty Punch	1 pkg (0.9 oz)	100	22	1	0
Sovex					
Fruit Bites Jungle Pals	1 pkg (0.9 oz)	90	21	1	0
Stretch Island					
Fruit Leather Berry Blackberry	2 pieces (1 oz)	90	24	0	0
Fruit Leather Chunky Cherry	2 pieces (1 oz)	90	24	0	0
Fruit Leather Great Grape	2 pieces (1 oz)	90	24	0	0

FOOD	PORTION	CALS.	CARB.	FAT	PRO.
Stretch Island (CONT.)					
Fruit Leather Organic Apple	2 pieces (1 oz)	90	24	0	0
Fruit Leather Organic Grape	2 pieces (1 oz)	90	24	0	0
Fruit Leather Organic Raspberry	2 pieces (1 oz)	90	25	0	0
Fruit Leather Rare Raspberry	2 pieces (1 oz)	90	24	0	0
Fruit Leather Snappy Apple	2 pieces (1 oz)	90	25	0	0
Fruit Leather Tangy Apricot	2 pieces (1 oz)	90	23	0	1
Fruit Leather Truly Tropical	2 pieces (1 oz)	90	22	0	tr
Sunbelt					
Fruit Booster Strawberry	1 (1.3 oz)	130	27	2	1
Fruit Boosters Apple	1 (1.3 oz)	130	27	2	1
Fruit Boosters Blueberry	1 (1.3 oz)	130	27	2	1
Fruit Jammers	1 (1 oz)	100	23	1	0
Sunkist					
Fruit Flippits Cherry	0.8 oz	107	18	4	1
Fruit Flippits Strawberry	0.8 oz	107	18	4	1
Fruit Roll Apricot	1	76	18	1	tr
Fruit Roll Cherry	1	75	18	tr	tr
Fruit Roll Grape	1	76	19	tr	tr
Fruit Roll Raspberry	1	75	18	tr	tr
Fruit Roll Strawberry	1	74	18	tr	tr
Fun Fruit Animals	0.9 oz	100	22	1	tr
Fun Fruit Dinosaurs Strawberry	0.9 oz	100	22	1	tr
Fun Fruit Galactic Gems	0.9 oz	100	22	1	1
Fun Fruit Mario Nintendo	0.9 oz	100	22	tr	1
Fun Fruit Meteorites	0.9 oz	100	22	1	tr
Fun Fruit Spooky Fruit	1 pkg	100	22	1	tr
Fun Fruit Strawberry	0.9 oz	100	22	1	tr
Fun Fruit Wacky Players	0.9 oz	100	22	1	tr
Weight Watchers					
Apple	½ oz	50	13	tr	tr
Apple Chips	¾ oz	70	19	0	0
Cinnamon	½ oz	50	13	tr	tr
Peach	½ oz	50	13	tr	tr

FOOD	PORTION	CALS.	CARB.	FAT	PRO.
Weight Watchers (CONT.)					
Strawberry	½ oz	50	13	tr	tr
GARBANZO					
(*see* CHICKPEAS)					
GARLIC					
clove	1	4	1	tr	tr
powder	1 tsp	9	2	tr	tr
Watkins					
Garlic & Chive Seasoning	1 tbsp (7 g)	25	2	2	1
Garlic Lover's Herb Blend	¼ tsp (0.5 oz)	0	0	0	0
Liquid Spice	1 tbsp (0.5 oz)	120	0	14	0
GEFILTE FISH					
READY-TO-USE					
sweet	1 piece (1.5 oz)	35	3	1	4
Manischewitz					
Gefilte Fish	1 piece	107	4	4	14
Gefiltefish & Pike	1 piece	99	5	4	13
Gefiltefish & Pike Sweet	1 piece	129	9	4	15
Homestyle	1 piece	111	6	4	14
Sweet	1 piece	132	9	4	15
GELATIN					
DRINKS					
Knox					
Orange Flavored Drinking Gelatin w/ Nutrasweet	1 pkg	39	4	tr	6
MIX					
low calorie	½ cup	8	0	0	2
mix artificially sweetened as prep	1 pkg 4 serv (16.5 oz)	33	3	0	5
mix artificially sweetened as prep	½ cup (4.1 oz)	8	1	0	1
mix as prep	½ cup (4.7 oz)	80	19	0	2
mix as prep	1 pkg 4 serv (19 oz)	319	76	0	7
mix not prep	1 pkg (3 oz)	324	77	0	7
mix w/ fruit as prep	½ cup (3.7 oz)	73	18	tr	1
mix w/ fruit as prep	1 pkg 8 serv (19 oz)	588	144	2	10
powder unsweetened	1 oz	94	0	0	24
powder unsweetened	1 pkg (7 g)	23	0	0	6

FOOD	PORTION	CALS.	CARB.	FAT	PRO.
D-Zerta					
Cherry	½ cup	8	0	0	2
Lemon	½ cup	8	0	0	2
Lime	½ cup	9	0	0	2
Orange	½ cup	8	0	0	2
Raspberry	½ cup	8	0	0	2
Strawberry	½ cup	8	0	0	2
Emes					
Kosher-Jel	½ cup (4 fl oz)	60	15	0	tr
Kosher-Jel Plain	1 tbsp (7 g)	21	5	0	tr
Jell-O					
Apricot	½ cup	82	19	tr	2
Black Cherry	½ cup	82	19	tr	2
Black Raspberry	½ cup	82	19	tr	2
Blackberry	½ cup	82	19	tr	2
Cherry Sugar Free	½ cup	9	0	0	1
Concord Grape	½ cup	82	19	tr	2
Hawaiian Pineapple Sugar Free	½ cup	8	0	tr	1
Lemon	½ cup	82	19	tr	2
Lemon Sugar Free	½ cup	8	0	0	1
Lime	½ cup	82	19	tr	2
Lime Sugar Free	½ cup	9	0	0	1
Mixed Fruit	½ cup	82	19	tr	2
Mixed Fruit Sugar Free	½ cup	8	0	0	1
Orange	½ cup	82	19	tr	2
Orange Sugar Free	½ cup	8	0	0	1
Peach Sugar Free	½ cup	8	0	tr	1
Raspberry Sugar Free	½ cup	8	0	0	1
Strawberry Banana Sugar Free	½ cup	9	0	0	1
Strawberry Sugar Free	½ cup	9	0	0	1
Triple Berry Sugar Free	½ cup	8	0	tr	1
Wild Strawberry	½ cup	81	19	tr	2
Kojel					
Diet	1 serv	10	4	tr	1
Royal					
Apple	½ cup	80	19	0	2
Blackberry	½ cup	80	19	0	2
Cherry	½ cup	80	19	0	2
Cherry Sugar Free	½ cup	8	1	0	1
Concord Grape	½ cup	80	19	0	2
Fruit Punch	½ cup	80	19	0	2
Lemon	½ cup	80	19	0	2

FOOD	PORTION	CALS.	CARB.	FAT	PRO.
Royal (CONT.)					
Lemon-Lime	½ cup	80	19	0	2
Lime	½ cup	80	19	0	2
Lime Sugar Free	½ cup	8	1	0	1
Mixed Berry	½ cup	80	19	0	2
Orange	½ cup	80	19	0	2
Orange Sugar Free	½ cup	10	1	0	1
Peach	½ cup	80	19	0	2
Pineapple	½ cup	80	19	0	2
Raspberry	½ cup	80	19	0	2
Raspberry Sugar Free	½ cup	8	1	0	1
Strawberry	½ cup	80	19	0	2
Strawberry Banana Sugar Free	½ cup	8	1	0	1
Strawberry Orange	½ cup	80	19	0	2
Strawberry Sugar Free	½ cup	8	1	0	1
Tropical Fruit	½ cup	80	19	0	2
READY-TO-USE					
Del Monte					
Gel Snack Cups Blue Berry	1 serv (3.5 oz)	70	19	0	0
Gel Snack Cups Cherry	1 serv (3.5 oz)	70	19	0	0
Gel Snack Cups Orange	1 serv (3.5 oz)	70	19	0	0
Gel Snack Cups Strawberry	1 serv (3.5 oz)	70	19	0	0
GIBLETS					
capon simmered	1 cup (5 oz)	238	0	8	38
chicken floured & fried	1 cup (5 oz)	402	6	19	47
chicken simmered	1 cup (5 oz)	228	1	7	37
turkey simmered	1 cup (5 oz)	243	3	7	39
GINGER					
root fresh sliced	¼ cup	17	4	tr	tr
Ka-Me					
Crystallized Slices	5 pieces (1 oz)	100	25	0	0
GINKGO NUTS					
canned	1 oz	32	6	tr	1
dried	1 oz	99	21	tr	3
GIZZARDS					
chicken simmered	1 cup (5 oz)	222	2	5	5
turkey simmered	1 cup (5 oz)	236	1	6	43
GOAT					
roasted	3 oz	122	0	3	23

FOOD	PORTION	CALS.	CARB.	FAT	PRO.
GOOSE					
w/ skin roasted	6.6 oz	574	0	41	47
w/ skin roasted	½ goose (1.7 lbs)	2362	0	170	195
w/o skin roasted	5 oz	340	0	18	41
w/o skin roasted	½ goose (1.3 lbs)	1406	0	75	171
GOOSEBERRIES					
fresh	1 cup	67	15	1	1
CANNED					
in light syrup	½ cup	93	24	tr	1
GRANOLA					
BARS					
almond	1 (0.8 oz)	117	15	6	2
almond	1 (1 oz)	140	18	7	2
chewy chocolate coated chocolate chip	1 (1 oz)	132	18	7	2
chewy chocolate coated chocolate chip	1 (1.25 oz)	165	23	9	2
chewy chocolate coated peanut butter	1 (1 oz)	144	15	9	3
chewy chocolate coated peanut butter	1 (1.3 oz)	187	20	11	4
chewy raisin	1 (1 oz)	127	19	5	2
chewy raisin	1 (1.5 oz)	191	28	8	3
chocolate chip	1 (1 oz)	124	20	5	2
chocolate chip	1 (0.8 oz)	103	17	4	2
chocolate chip chewy	1 (1.5 oz)	178	29	7	3
chocolate chip chewy	1 (1 oz)	119	10	5	2
chocolate chip, graham & marshmallow chewy	1 (1 oz)	121	20	4	2
nut & raisin chewy	1 (1 oz)	129	18	6	2
peanut	1 (1 oz)	136	18	6	3
peanut	1 (0.8 oz)	113	15	5	3
peanut butter	1 (0.8 oz)	114	15	6	2
peanut butter	1 (1 oz)	137	18	7	3
peanut butter chewy	1 (1 oz)	121	18	5	3
peanut butter & chocolate chip chewy	1 (1 oz)	122	18	6	3
plain	1 (1 oz)	134	18	7	3
plain	1 (0.9 oz)	115	19	4	3
plain chewy	1 (1 oz)	126	19	5	2
Carnation					
Chocolate Chunk	1 (1.26 oz)	140	23	5	2
Honey & Oats	1 (1.26 oz)	130	23	4	2

FOOD	PORTION	CALS.	CARB.	FAT	PRO.
Fi-Bar					
Coconut	1	120	20	4	2
Peanut Butter	1	130	20	4	3
General Mills					
Nature Valley Cinnnamon	1	120	17	5	2
Nature Valley Oat Bran Honey Graham	1	110	16	4	2
Nature Valley Oats N'Honey	1	120	17	5	2
Nature Valley Peanut Butter	1	120	15	6	2
Nature Valley Rice Bran Cinnamon Graham	1	90	13	4	1
Grist Mill					
Chew Chocolate Chip	1 (1 oz)	130	21	4	2
Chewy Apple Cinnamon	1 (1 oz)	120	21	4	2
Chewy Chunky Nut & Raisin	1 (1 oz)	130	18	6	3
Chewy Peanut Butter	1 (1 oz)	130	20	5	3
Chewy Peanut Butter Chocolate	1 (1 oz)	130	20	4	3
Chocolate Snack Chocolate Chip	1 (1.2 oz)	180	21	10	3
Chocolate Snack Nutty Fudge	1 (1.3 oz)	190	19	11	3
Crunchy Cinnamon	1 (0.8 oz)	110	16	5	3
Crunchy Oasts 'N Honey	1 (0.8 oz)	110	15	5	3
Hershey					
Chocolate Covered Chocolate Chip	1 (1.2 oz)	170	22	8	2
Chocolate Covered Cookies & Creme	1 (1.2 oz)	170	22	8	2
Chocolate Covered Cocoa Creme	1 (1.2 oz)	180	22	9	2
Chocolate Covered Peanut Butter	1 (1.2 oz)	180	19	10	4
Kellogg's					
Low Fat Crunchy Almond & Brown Sugar	1 (0.7 oz)	80	16	2	2
Low Fat Crunchy Apple Spice	1 (0.7 oz)	80	16	2	2
Low Fat Crunchy Cinnamon Raisin	1 (0.7 oz)	80	16	2	2

FOOD	PORTION	CALS.	CARB.	FAT	PRO.
Kudos					
Chocolate Chunk	1 (0.7 oz)	90	13	3	1
Chocolate Coated Chocolate Chip	1 (1 oz)	120	18	5	2
Chocolate Coated Milk & Cookies	1 (1 oz)	130	18	5	2
Chocolate Coated Nutty Fudge	1 (1 oz)	130	18	5	2
Chocolate Coated Peanut Butter	1 (1 oz)	130	18	5	2
Low Fat Blueberry	1 (0.7 oz)	90	15	2	1
Low Fat Strawberry	1 (0.7 oz)	80	15	2	1
New Country					
Chocolate Covered Cookies & Creme	1	200	23	11	2
Quaker					
Chewy Chocolate Chip	1	128	19	5	2
Chewy Chunky Nut & Raisin	1	131	17	6	3
Chewy Cinnamon Raisin	1	128	19	5	2
Chewy Honey & Oats	1	125	19	4	2
Chewy Peanut Butter	1	128	18	5	3
Chewy Peanut Butter Chocolate Chip	1	131	17	6	3
Dipps Caramel Nut	1	148	21	6	2
Dipps Chocolate Chip	1	139	19	6	2
Dipps Chocolate Fudge	1	160	20	8	2
Dipps Peanut Butter	1	170	9	9	4
Dipps Peanut Butter Chocolate Chip	1	174	10	10	4
Sunbelt					
Chewy Chocolate Chip	1 (1.8 oz)	220	32	10	3
Chewy Chocolate Chip	1 (1.25 oz)	160	23	7	2
Chewy Oats & Honey	1 (1.7 oz)	210	32	9	3
Chewy Oats & Honey	1 (1 oz)	130	19	5	2
Chewy With Almonds	1 (1.5 oz)	190	25	10	3
Chewy With Almonds	1 (1 oz)	130	17	7	2

FOOD	PORTION	CALS.	CARB.	FAT	PRO.
Sunbelt (CONT.)					
Chewy With Raisins	1 (1.2 oz)	150	25	6	2
Fudge Dipped Chewy Chocolate Chip	1 (1.5 oz)	190	28	8	3
Fudge Dipped Chewy Macaroo	1 bar (2 oz)	280	32	17	3
Fudge Dipped Chewy Macaroo	1 (1.4 oz)	200	22	13	2
Fudge Dipped Chewy With Peanuts	1 bar (1.5 oz)	210	24	12	3
CEREAL					
granola	¼ cup	138	16	8	4
Erewhon					
Date Nut	1 oz	130	17	6	3
Honey Almond	1 oz	130	17	6	3
Maple	1 oz	130	17	5	3
Spiced Apple	1 oz	130	17	6	3
Sunflower Crunch	1 oz	130	18	4	3
With Bran	1 oz	130	17	6	3
General Mills					
Nature Valley Cinnamon & Raisin	⅓ cup (1 oz)	120	20	4	2
Nature Valley Fruit & Nut	⅓ cup (1 oz)	130	19	5	2
Nature Valley Toasted Oat	⅓ cup (1 oz)	130	20	5	2
Good Shepherd					
Crunchy	1 oz	130	19	5	3
Honey Almond	1 oz	120	20	4	3
Organic 5 Grain Muesli	1 oz	160	27	3	4
Organic Brown Rice	1 oz	130	16	4	3
Organic Wheat Free	1 oz	90	39	3	3
Organic Wheat Free Apple Cinnamon	1 oz	125	20	4	3
Organic Wheat Free Blueberry Amaranth	1 oz	110	22	1	3
Organic Wheat Free Strawberry Amaranth	1 oz	110	22	1	3
Grist Mill					
Low-Fat With Raisins	⅔ cup (1.9 oz)	220	42	3	5
Kellogg's					
Low Fat	½ cup (1.9 oz)	210	43	3	5
Low Fat With Raisins	⅔ cup (1.9 oz)	210	43	3	5

FOOD	PORTION	CALS.	CARB.	FAT	PRO.
Post					
Post Hearty	¼ cup (1 oz)	128	21	4	2
Stone-Buhr					
Hot Apple	⅓ cup (1.6 oz)	153	31	1	5
Sun Country					
100% Natural With Almonds	¼ cup	130	19	5	3
100% Natural With Raisins & Dates	¼ cup	123	20	5	3
With Raisins	¼ cup	125	19	5	3
Sunbelt					
Banana Nut	1.9 oz	250	37	9	5
Fruit & Nut	1.9 oz	230	38	7	6
Low Fat	1.9 oz	200	42	3	5
Uncle Roy's					
Cashew Raisin	½ cup (1.6 oz)	180	32	6	8
Fat Free Apple Cinnamon	½ cup (1.6 oz)	175	38	1	8
Fat Free Wild Cherry	½ cup (1.6 oz)	175	38	1	6
Fruit & Nut	½ cup (1.6 oz)	175	30	5	6
Low Fat Berries Jubilee	½ cup (1.6 oz)	175	34	3	6
Low Fat Crispy	½ cup (1.4 oz)	160	31	3	4
Low Fat Luscious Raspberry	½ cup (1.6 oz)	175	34	3	6
Low Fat True Blueberry	½ cup (1.6 oz)	175	34	3	6
Maple Date Nut	½ cup (1.6 oz)	180	29	6	6
Nut Butter & Almonds	½ cup (1.6 oz)	195	29	8	6
Organic Golden Honey	½ cup (1.6 oz)	190	30	6	5
Organic Maple Nut'N Rice	½ cup (1.4 oz)	170	27	6	4
Organic Maple Raisin	½ cup (1.6 oz)	190	30	6	5

GRAPE JUICE

FOOD	PORTION	CALS.	CARB.	FAT	PRO.
bottled	1 cup	155	38	tr	1
frzn sweetened as prep	1 cup	128	32	tr	tr
frzn sweetened not prep	6 oz	386	96	1	1
grape drink	6 oz	84	22	0	0
BAMA					
Juice	8.45 fl oz	120	29	0	0
Bright & Early					
Frozen	8 fl oz	140	34	0	0
Hi-C					
Box	8.45 fl oz	130	33	0	0
Drink	1 can (11.5 fl oz)	180	46	0	0
Drink	8 fl oz	130	32	0	0

FOOD	PORTION	CALS.	CARB.	FAT	PRO.
Juicy Juice					
Drink	1 bottle (6 fl oz)	90	22	0	1
Drink	1 box	130	31	0	1
Kool-Aid					
Drink	8 oz	98	25	0	0
Sugar Free	8 oz	3	0	0	0
Sugar Sweetened	8 oz	80	21	0	0
Lifesavers					
Grape Punch	8 fl oz	150	36	0	0
Minute Maid					
Chilled	8 fl oz	130	33	0	0
Grape Punch frzn	8 fl oz	130	32	0	0
Punch Chilled	8 fl oz	130	32	0	0
Mott's					
Drink	10 fl oz	170	42	0	0
Fruit Basket Cocktail as prep	8 fl oz	130	32	0	1
S&W					
Concord Unsweetened	6 oz	100	25	0	1
Seneca					
Blush Grape Juice frzn as prep	8 fl oz	170	39	0	0
Fortified With Vitamin C frzn as prep	8 fl oz	170	39	0	0
Sweetened frzn as prep	8 fl oz	140	39	0	0
White Grape Juice frzn as prep	8 fl oz	140	33	0	0
Sippin' Pak					
100% Pure	8.45 fl	130	32	0	1
Snapple					
Grapeade	8 fl oz	120	30	0	0
Tang					
Fruit Box	8.45 oz	131	34	0	0
Tree Top					
Juice	6 oz	120	30	0	1
Sparkling Juice	6 oz	120	29	0	0
Tropicana					
Season's Best	8 fl oz	160	39	0	tr
Veryfine					
100%	8 oz	153	37	0	0
Grape Drink	8 oz	130	34	0	0
Wylers					
Drink Mix Unsweetened	8 oz	2	1	0	0

FOOD	PORTION	CALS.	CARB.	FAT	PRO.
GRAPE LEAVES					
Cedar's					
Grape Leaves Stuffed With Rice	6 pieces (4.9 oz)	180	22	8	4
GRAPEFRUIT					
CANNED					
juice pack	½ cup	46	11	tr	1
unsweetened	1 cup	93	22	tr	1
water pack	½ cup	44	11	tr	1
S&W					
Sections Unsweetened	½ cup	40	9	0	0
Sections In Light Syrup	½ cup	80	14	0	tr
Sections Natural Style	½ cup	40	9	0	0
FRESH					
pink	½	37	9	tr	1
pink sections	1 cup	69	18	tr	1
red	½	37	9	tr	1
red sections	1 cup	69	18	tr	1
white	½	39	10	tr	1
white sections	1 cup	76	19	tr	2
Dole					
Grapefruit	½	50	14	0	1
Ocean Spray					
Pink	½ med	50	13	0	1
White	½ med	45	12	0	1
GRAPEFRUIT JUICE					
fresh	1 cup	96	23	tr	1
frzn as prep	1 cup	102	24	tr	1
frzn not prep	6 oz	302	72	1	4
sweetened	1 cup	116	28	tr	1
After The Fall					
Pink	1 bottle (10 oz)	100	23	0	1
Crystal Geyser					
Juice Squeeze	1 bottle (12 fl oz)	150	36	0	1
Del Monte					
Juice	8 fl oz	100	24	0	2
Hood					
Select	1 cup (8 oz)	100	23	0	0
Minute Maid					
Frozen	8 fl oz	100	23	0	0
Juices To Go	1 can (11.5 fl oz)	140	33	0	0
Juices To Go	1 bottle (16 fl oz)	100	23	0	0
Juices To Go	1 bottle (10 fl oz)	120	29	0	0

FOOD	PORTION	CALS.	CARB.	FAT	PRO.
Minute Maid (cont.)					
Juices To Go Pink Cocktail	1 bottle (16 fl oz)	110	27	0	0
Juices To Go Pink Cocktail	1 bottle (10 fl oz)	140	34	0	0
Juices to Go Pink Cocktail	8 fl oz	160	39	0	0
Mott's					
From Concentrate as prep	8 fl oz	120	27	0	2
Ocean Spray					
100% Juice	8 oz	100	24	0	1
Lightstyle Low Calorie Pink Cocktail	8 fl oz	40	9	0	0
Pink Juice Cocktail	8 oz	110	28	0	tr
Ruby Red Drink	8 oz	130	33	0	0
Odwalla					
Juice	8 fl oz	90	20	0	2
S&W					
Unsweetened	6 oz	80	18	0	1
Snapple					
Juice	10 fl oz	110	25	0	0
Pink Grapefruit Cocktail	8 fl oz	120	31	0	0
Tree Of Life					
Juice	8 fl oz	100	26	0	1
Tree Top					
Juice	6 oz	80	19	0	1
Tropicana					
Juice	1 container (6 fl oz)	80	19	0	tr
Juice	8 fl oz	90	23	0	tr
Ruby Red	8 fl oz	100	25	0	tr
Ruby Red	1 container (10 fl oz)	120	30	0	tr
Season's Best	1 bottle (7 fl oz)	80	19	0	tr
Season's Best	1 bottle (10 fl oz)	110	27	0	tr
Season's Best	1 can (11.5 fl oz)	120	31	0	tr
Season's Best	8 fl oz	90	22	0	tr
Twister Light Pink	8 fl oz	40	10	0	tr
Twister Light Pink	1 container (10 fl oz)	50	12	0	tr
Twister Pink	1 can (11.5 fl oz)	160	40	0	tr
Twister Pink	8 fl oz	110	28	0	tr
Twister Pink	1 container (10 fl oz)	140	35	0	tr

FOOD	PORTION	CALS.	CARB.	FAT	PRO.
Veryfine					
100%	8 oz	101	23	0	0
Pink	8 oz	120	29	0	0

GRAPES
CANNED

thompson seedless in heavy syrup	½ cup	94	25	tr	1
thompson seedless water pack	½ cup	48	13	tr	1
S&W					
Thompson Seedless Premium	½ cup	100	25	0	0

FRESH

grapes	10	36	9	tr	tr
Dole					
Grapes	1½ cup	85	24	0	1

GRAVY
(see also SAUCE)
CANNED

au jus	1 cup	38	6	tr	3
beef	1 cup	124	11	6	9
beef	1 can (10 oz)	155	14	7	11
chicken	1 cup	189	13	14	5
mushroom	1 cup	120	13	6	3
turkey	1 cup	122	12	5	6
Franco-American					
Au Jus	2 oz	10	2	0	0
Beef	2 oz	25	4	1	0
Chicken	2 oz	45	3	4	0
Chicken Giblet	2 oz	30	3	2	1
Cream	2 oz	35	4	2	0
Mushroom	2 oz	25	3	1	0
Pork	2 oz	40	3	3	0
Turkey	2 oz	30	3	2	0
Gravymaster					
Seasoning	¼ tsp	3	1	0	tr
Rudy's Farm					
Sausage Gravy	¼ cup (2 oz)	50	7	1	3

DRY

au jus as prep w/ water	1 cup	32	4	1	1
brown as prep w/ water	1 cup	75	13	2	2
chicken as prep	1 cup	83	14	2	3

FOOD	PORTION	CALS.	CARB.	FAT	PRO.
mushroom as prep	1 cup	70	14	1	2
onion as prep w/ water	1 cup	77	16	1	2
pork as prep	1 cup	76	13	2	2
turkey as prep	1 cup	87	15	2	3
Bournvita					
Extract	2 heaping tsp	34	7	1	1
Bovril					
Extract	1 heaping tsp	9	tr	0	2
Cajun King					
Oil-Less Roux And Gravy Mix	3.5 oz	394	78	4	12
Hain					
Brown	¼ pkg	16	3	0	1
LaLoma					
Brown Gravy Quik as prep	2 tsp	45	2	4	tr
Chicken Gravy Quik as prep	2 tsp	45	2	4	tr
Country Quik Gravy as prep	2 tsp	10	2	tr	tr
Mushroom Quik Gravy as prep	2 tsp	10	2	tr	tr
Onion Quik Gravy as prep	2 tsp	10	2	tr	tr
Marmite					
Extract	1 heaping tsp	9	tr	0	2
Pillsbury					
Brown	¼ cup	15	3	0	tr
Chicken	¼ cup	25	4	1	tr
Home Style	¼ cup	15	3	0	tr

GREAT NORTHERN BEANS

FOOD	PORTION	CALS.	CARB.	FAT	PRO.
CANNED					
great northern	1 cup	300	55	1	19
Allen					
Great Northern	½ cup (4.5 oz)	100	19	1	6
Green Giant					
Great Northern	½ cup	80	18	1	6
Trappey					
With Sausage	½ cup (4.5 oz)	100	18	1	6
DRIED					
cooked	1 cup	210	37	1	15

FOOD	PORTION	CALS.	CARB.	FAT	PRO.
Bean Cuisine					
Dried	½ cup	115	—	1	8
GREEN BEANS					
CANNED					
Allen					
Cut	½ cup (4.2 oz)	30	6	1	0
Cut No Added Salt	½ cup (4.2 oz)	15	3	0	0
French Style	½ cup (4.2 oz)	25	4	0	tr
Italian	½ cup (4.2 oz)	35	7	1	1
Shell Outs	½ cup (4.5 oz)	30	6	0	2
Alma					
Cut	½ cup (4.2 oz)	30	6	1	0
Crest Top					
Cut	½ cup (4.2 oz)	30	6	1	0
Del Monte					
Cut	½ cup (4.3 oz)	20	4	0	1
Cut 50% Less Salt	½ cup (4.3 oz)	20	4	0	1
Cut Italian	½ cup (4.3 oz)	30	6	0	1
Cut No Salt Added	½ cup (4.3 oz)	20	4	0	1
French Style	½ cup (4.3 oz)	20	4	0	1
French Style 50% Less Salt	½ cup (4.3 oz)	20	4	0	1
French Style No Salt Added	½ cup (4.3 oz)	20	4	0	1
French Style Seasoned	½ cup (4.3 oz)	20	4	0	1
Whole	½ cup (4.3 oz)	20	4	0	1
GaBelle					
Cut	½ cup (4.2 oz)	30	6	1	0
Green Giant					
Almondine	½ cup	45	5	3	2
Cut	½ cup	16	4	0	1
French	½ cup	16	4	0	1
Kitchen Sliced	½ cup	16	4	0	1
S&W					
Cut Water Pack	½ cup	20	4	0	1
Cut Premium Blue Lake	½ cup	20	4	0	1
Dilled	½ cup	60	15	0	1
French Style Premium Blue Lake	½ cup	20	4	0	1
Green Beans & Wax Beans	½ cup	20	5	0	1
Whole Fancy Stringless	½ cup	20	4	0	1
Whole Vertical Pack	½ cup	20	4	0	1

FOOD	PORTION	CALS.	CARB.	FAT	PRO.
Seneca					
Cut	½ cup	20	6	0	1
Cuts Natural Pack	½ cup	25	6	0	1
French	½ cup	20	6	0	1
French Natural Pack	½ cup	25	6	0	1
Whole	½ cup	20	6	0	1
Sunshine					
Cut	½ cup (4.2 oz)	30	6	1	0
Italian	½ cup (4.2 oz)	35	7	1	1
FROZEN					
Birds Eye					
Cut	½ cup	25	6	0	1
Farm Fresh Whole	¾ cup	30	7	0	2
French Cut	½ cup	25	6	0	1
In Sauce French Green Beans With Toasted Almonds	½ cup	50	8	2	3
Italian	½ cup	30	7	0	2
Polybag Cut	½ cup	25	6	0	1
Polybag Deluxe Whole	½ cup	20	4	0	1
Polybag French Cut	½ cup	25	6	0	1
Whole Deluxe	½ cup	45	5	0	1
Fresh Like					
Cut	3.5 oz	29	7	tr	1
French	3.5 oz	29	7	tr	1
Italian	3.5 oz	35	8	tr	2
Whole	3.5 oz	29	6	tr	1
Green Giant					
Cut	½ cup	16	4	0	1
Cut In Butter Sauce	½ cup	30	4	1	1
Green Beans	½ cup	14	4	0	1
One Serve In Butter Sauce	1 pkg	60	8	2	2
Stouffer's					
Green Bean Mushroom Casserole	½ cup (1.9 oz)	130	13	8	3
Tree Of Life					
Green Beans	⅔ cup (2.8 oz)	25	4	0	1
SHELF-STABLE					
Pantry Express					
Cut	½ cup	12	3	0	tr

GREENS

CANNED

Allen

Mixed	½ cup (4.2 oz)	30	8	1	1

FOOD	PORTION	CALS.	CARB.	FAT	PRO.
Sunshine					
Mixed	½ cup (4.2 oz)	30	8	1	1
GROUPER					
cooked	3 oz	100	0	1	21
cooked	1 fillet (7.1 oz)	238	0	3	50
raw	3 oz	78	0	1	16
GUANABANA JUICE					
Libby					
Nectar	1 can (11.5 fl oz)	210	50	0	0
GUAVA					
fresh	1	45	11	1	1
guava sauce	½ cup	43	11	tr	tr
GUAVA JUICE					
Kern's					
Nectar	6 fl oz	110	28	0	0
Libby					
Nectar	6 oz	110	26	0	0
Nectar	1 can (11.5 fl oz)	220	54	0	0
Snapple					
Guava Mania	8 fl oz	110	29	0	0
GUINEA HEN					
w/ skin raw	½ hen (12.1 oz)	545	0	22	81
w/o skin raw	½ hen (9.3 oz)	292	0	7	55
HADDOCK					
FRESH					
cooked	1 fillet (5.3 oz)	168	0	1	36
cooked	3 oz	95	0	1	21
raw	3 oz	74	0	1	16
roe raw	3½ oz	130	2	2	24
FROZEN					
Gorton's					
Fishmarket Fresh	5 oz	110	0	1	25
Microwave Entree	1 pkg	360	19	21	23
Haddock In Lemon Butter					
Mrs. Paul's					
Crunchy Batter Fillets	2 fillets	190	22	5	14
Light Fillets	1 fillet	220	15	9	17
Van De Kamp's					
Battered	2 pieces	250	19	15	12
Breaded Fillets	2 pieces	270	19	16	12

FOOD	PORTION	CALS.	CARB.	FAT	PRO.
Van De Kamp's (CONT.)					
Light Fillets	1 piece	240	21	11	15
Natural Fillets	4 oz	90	0	1	21
SMOKED					
smoked	1 oz	33	0	tr	7
smoked	3 oz	99	0	1	21
HAKE					
raw	3½ oz	84	0	1	17
HALIBUT					
FRESH					
atlantic & pacific cooked	3 oz	119	0	2	23
atlantic & pacific cooked	½ fillet (5.6 oz)	223	0	5	42
atlantic & pacific raw	3 oz	93	0	2	18
greenland baked	3 oz	203	0	15	16
greenland baked	5.6 oz	380	0	28	29
FROZEN					
Van De Kamp's					
Battered	2 pieces	150	16	6	8
HALVA					
(*see* SESAME)					
HAM					
(*see also* HAM DISHES, PORK, TURKEY)					
canned 13% fat	3 oz	192	tr	13	17
canned extra lean 4% fat	3 oz	116	tr	4	18
center slice lean & fat	4 oz	229	tr	15	23
chopped	1 oz	65	0	5	5
chopped canned	1 oz	68	tr	5	5
ham & cheese loaf	1 oz	73	1	6	9
ham & cheese spread	1 tbsp	37	tr	3	2
ham & cheese spread	1 oz	69	1	5	5
ham salad spread	1 tbsp	32	2	2	1
ham salad spread	1 oz	61	3	4	2
minced	1 oz	75	1	6	5
sliced extra lean 5% fat	1 oz	37	tr	1	5
sliced regular 11% fat	1 oz	52	1	3	5
steak boneless extra lean	1 oz	35	1	1	6
Alpine Lace					
Boneless Cooked	2 oz	60	1	2	9
Armour					
Chopped Ham canned	2 oz	120	2	9	8
Deviled Ham canned	1 pkg (3 oz)	200	0	16	14
Lower Salt 93% Fat Free	1 oz	35	—	1	5

FOOD	PORTION	CALS.	CARB.	FAT	PRO.
Black Label					
Chopped	2 oz	140	3	11	7
Carl Buddig					
Ham	1 oz	50	1	3	5
Honey Ham	1 oz	50	1	3	5
Hansel n'Gretel					
Baked Virginia	1 oz	34	2	1	5
Black Forest	1 oz	32	tr	1	6
Cappy	1 oz	31	1	1	5
Cooked Fresh	1 oz	33	tr	1	6
Deluxe	1 oz	31	1	1	5
Honey Valley	1 oz	31	1	1	5
Jalapeno	1 oz	25	1	1	4
Lessalt	1 oz	30	1	1	5
Lessalt Virginia	1 oz	32	1	1	5
Light AM	1 oz	27	1	1	4
Travane	1 oz	31	tr	1	5
Healthy Choice					
Baked Cooked	3 slices (2.2 oz)	70	1	2	12
Cooked	3 slices (2.2 oz)	70	1	2	12
Deli-Thin Baked Cooked With Natural Juices	6 slices (2 oz)	60	2	2	10
Deli-Thin Cooked	6 slices (2 oz)	60	1	2	10
Deli-Thin Honey With Natural Juices	6 slices (2 oz)	60	2	2	10
Deli-Thin Smoked With Natural Juices	6 slices (2 oz)	60	1	2	10
Fresh-Trak Cooked	1 slice (1 oz)	30	1	1	5
Fresh-Trak Honey	1 slice (1 oz)	30	1	1	5
Honey Boneless	3 oz	100	5	3	15
Smoked	3 slices (2.2 oz)	70	1	2	13
Variety Pack Regular	3 slices (2.2 oz)	70	1	2	12
Hillshire					
Brown Sugar	1 oz	40	2	2	4
Cooked Ham	1 oz	30	tr	1	5
Deli Select Baked Ham	1 slice	10	tr	tr	2
Deli Select Brown Sugar Baked	1 slice	10	tr	tr	2
Deli Select Cajun Ham	1 slice	10	tr	tr	2
Deli Select Honey Ham	1 slice	10	tr	tr	2
Deli Select Lower Salt	1 slice	10	tr	tr	2
Deli Select Smoked Ham	1 slice	10	tr	tr	2
Flavor Pack 90-99% Fat Free Brown Sugar Baked	1 slice (0.6 oz)	20	1	tr	3

FOOD	PORTION	CALS.	CARB.	FAT	PRO.
Hillshire (CONT.)					
Flavor Pack 90-99% Fat Free Honey Ham	1 slice (0.6 oz)	20	1	tr	3
Flavor Pack 90-99% Fat Free Smoked	1 slice (0.6 oz)	20	tr	tr	3
Genuine Baked	1 oz	35	1	1	5
Honey Ham	1 oz	40	2	2	4
Lower Salt	1 oz	30	1	1	5
Lunch 'N Munch Cooked Ham/Swiss	1 pkg (4.5 oz)	360	19	22	20
Lunch 'N Munch Cooked Ham/Swiss Oreo	1 pkg (4.125 oz)	370	30	21	16
Lunch 'N Munch Cooked Ham/Swiss Snickers/ Hi-C	1 pkg (4.25 oz + 6 fl oz)	470	54	21	16
Lunch 'N Munch Honey Ham/ Cheddar/ Snickers/Hi-C	1 pkg (4.25 oz + 6 fl oz)	500	56	23	17
Hormel					
Black Label Canned (refrigerated)	3 oz	100	0	5	14
Black Label Canned (shelf stable)	3 oz	110	0	5	14
Canned Chunk	2 oz	90	0	6	9
Cure 81 Half Ham	3 oz	100	0	5	16
Curemaster	3 oz	80	0	3	14
Deli Cooked	1 oz	29	1	1	4
Deviled Ham	4 tbsp (2 oz)	150	1	12	9
Ham & Cheese Patties	1 patty (2 oz)	190	0	17	7
Light & Lean	3 oz	90	2	3	14
Light & Lean 97	3 oz	90	2	3	14
Light & Lean 97 Cuts	16 pieces (1 oz)	35	0	1	5
Light & Lean 97 Sliced	1 slice (1 oz)	25	0	1	4
Patties	1 patty (2 oz)	180	1	17	7
Primissimo Proscuitti	1 oz	70	0	5	7
Spread	4 tbsp (2 oz)	100	1	11	8
Supreme Cut Canned	1 oz	31	tr	1	5
Jones					
Family Ham	1 slice	40	tr	2	6
Ham Slices	1 slice	30	tr	1	5
Krakus					
Ham	1 oz	25	1	1	5
Louis Rich					
Carving Board Baked With Natural Juices	2 slices (1.6 oz)	45	1	1	8

FOOD	PORTION	CALS.	CARB.	FAT	PRO.
Louis Rich (CONT.)					
Carving Board Carved Thin Honey With Natural Juices	6 slices (2.1 oz)	70	2	2	11
Carving Board Honey With Natural Juices	2 slices (1.6 oz)	50	1	2	8
Carving Board Smoked Cooked With Natural Juices	1 slice (1.6 oz)	50	0	2	8
Dinned Slices Baked	1 slice (3.3 oz)	80	1	2	16
Mr. Turkey					
Deli Cuts Honey Cured	3 slices	35	1	1	5
Oscar Mayer					
Baked	3 slices (2.2 oz)	60	2	1	11
Boiled	3 slices (2.2 oz)	60	0	3	10
Chopped	1 slice (1 oz)	50	1	4	4
Deli-Thin Boiled	4 slices (1.8 oz)	50	0	2	9
Deli-Thin Honey Ham	4 slices (1.8 oz)	60	2	2	9
Deli-Thin Smoked	4 slices (1.8 oz)	50	0	2	9
Dinner Slice	3 oz	90	0	3	14
Dinner Steaks	1 (2 oz)	60	0	2	10
Ham & Cheese Loaf	1 slice (1 oz)	70	1	5	4
Healthy Favorites Baked	4 slices (1.8 oz)	50	1	1	9
Healthy Favorites Honey Ham	4 slices (1.8 oz)	50	2	2	9
Healthy Favorites Smoked Cooked	4 slices (1.8 oz)	50	0	2	9
Honey Ham	3 slices (2.2 oz)	70	2	3	10
Lower Sodium	3 slices (2.2 oz)	70	2	3	10
Lunchables Cookies/ Ham/ Swiss	1 pkg (4.2 oz)	360	29	19	18
Lunchables Dessert Chocolate Pudding/ Ham/ American	1 pkg (6.2 oz)	390	34	20	18
Lunchables Ham/ Cheddar	1 pkg (4.5 oz)	340	19	20	21
Lunchables Ham/Garden Vegetable Cheese	1 pkg (4.5 oz)	380	36	21	13
Lunchables Honey Ham/ Herb & Chive Cheese	1 pkg (4.5 oz)	390	37	21	13
Smoked Cooked	3 slices (2.2 oz)	60	0	3	10
Russer					
Baked	2 oz	70	4	3	9
Canadian Brand Maple	2 oz	70	4	2	9

FOOD	PORTION	CALS.	CARB.	FAT	PRO.
Russer (CONT.)					
Chopped	2 oz	130	5	9	7
Cooked Ham	2 oz	60	2	2	9
Ham & Cheese Loaf	2 oz	120	5	8	8
Honey & Maple Cured	2 oz	70	3	2	9
Honey Cured	2 oz	60	2	3	9
Hot	2 oz	70	3	2	9
Light Cooked	2 oz	60	2	2	9
Light Smoked	2 oz	60	2	2	9
Smoked Virginia	2 oz	70	3	3	9
Spiced	2 oz	160	5	12	7
Sara Lee					
Bavarian Brand Baked	2 oz	80	1	4	9
Bavarian Brand Baked Honey	2 oz	80	2	4	9
Golden Cure Smoked	2 oz	80	1	4	9
Honey Ham	2 oz	60	2	2	10
Honey Roasted	2 oz	90	3	5	9
Underwood					
Deviled	2.08 oz	220	tr	19	8
Deviled Light	2.08 oz	120	1	8	11
Deviled Smoked	2.08 oz	190	tr	18	9
Weight Watchers					
Deli Thin Oven Roasted	5 slices (⅓ oz)	12	tr	tr	2
Deli Thin Oven Roasted Honey Ham	5 slices (⅓ oz)	12	tr	tr	2
Deli Thin Premium Smoked	5 slices (⅓ oz)	12	tr	tr	2
Oven Roasted Honey Ham	2 slices (¾ oz)	25	tr	1	4
Oven Roasted Smoked	2 slices (¾ oz)	25	tr	1	4
Premium Cooked	2 slices (¾ oz)	25	tr	1	4

HAM DISHES
FROZEN
Croissant Pocket

Stuffed Sandwich Ham & Cheddar	1 piece (4.5 oz)	360	39	17	13
Hot Pocket					
Stuffed Sandwich Ham & Cheese	1 (4.5 oz)	340	37	15	14
Ovenstuffs					
Ham/Turkey Deli Melt	1 (4.75 oz)	360	35	15	20

FOOD	PORTION	CALS.	CARB.	FAT	PRO.
Weight Watchers					
Handy Pocket Cheese Sauce & Ham	1 (4 oz)	200	24	6	14
TAKE-OUT					
croquettes	1 (3.1 oz)	217	11	14	12
salad	½ cup	287	5	23	16
sandwich w/ cheese	1	353	33	15	21
HAMBURGER					
(see also BEEF)					
FROZEN					
Jimmy Dean					
Burger	1 (2 oz)	220	0	21	7
Flamed Broiled Cheeseburger	1 (6.3 oz)	540	34	34	28
Mini Cheeseburger	2 (3 oz)	270	23	14	14
Kid Cuisine					
Beef Patty Sandwich w/ Cheese	1 (8.5 oz)	410	58	15	12
MicroMagic					
Cheeseburger	1 pkg (4.75 oz)	450	29	25	17
Hamburger	1 pkg (4 oz)	350	26	18	13
Rudy's Farm					
Mild Burger	1 (3 oz)	360	0	35	11
White Castle					
Cheeseburger	2 (3.6 oz)	310	23	17	15
Hamburger	2 (3.2 oz)	270	23	14	12
TAKE-OUT					
double patty w/ bun	1 reg	544	43	28	30
double patty w/ catsup mayonnaise onion pickle tomato & bun	1 reg	649	53	35	30
double patty w/ catsup cheese mayonnaise mustard pickle tomato & bun	1 lg	706	40	44	38
double patty w/ catsup mustard mayonnaise onion pickle tomato & bun	1 lg	540	40	27	34
double patty w/ catsup mustard onion pickle & bun	1 reg	576	39	32	32
double patty w/ cheese & bun	1 reg	457	22	28	28

FOOD	PORTION	CALS.	CARB.	FAT	PRO.
double patty w/ cheese & double bun	1 reg	461	44	22	22
double patty w/ cheese catsup mayonnaise onion pickle tomato & bun	1 reg	416	35	21	21
single patty w/ bacon catsup cheese mustard onion pickle & bun	1 lg	609	37	37	32
single patty w/ bun	1 reg	275	31	12	12
single patty w/ bun	1 lg	400	25	23	23
single patty w/ catsup cheese ham mayonnaise pickle tomato & bun	1 lg	745	38	48	40
single patty w/ catsup mustard mayonnaise onion pickle tomato & bun	1 reg	279	27	13	13
single patty w/ cheese & bun	1 lg	608	47	33	30
single patty w/ cheese & bun	1 reg	320	32	15	15
triple patty w/ catsup mustard pickle & bun	1 lg	693	29	41	50
triple patty w/ cheese & bun	1 lg	769	27	51	56
HAZELNUTS					
dried blanched	1 oz	191	5	19	4
dried unblanched	1 oz	179	4	18	4
dry roasted unblanched	1 oz	188	5	19	3
oil roasted unblanched	1 oz	187	5	18	4
Crumpy					
Chocolate Hazelnut Spread	1 tbsp (0.5 oz)	80	8	5	tr
HEART					
beef simmered	3 oz	148	tr	5	24
chicken simmered	1 cup (5 oz)	268	tr	11	11
lamb braised	3 oz	158	2	7	21
turkey simmered	1 cup (5 oz)	257	3	9	39
veal braised	3 oz	158	tr	6	25
HEARTS OF PALM					
canned	1 (1.2 oz)	9	2	tr	1
canned	1 cup (5.1 oz)	41	7	1	4

FOOD	PORTION	CALS.	CARB.	FAT	PRO.
HERBAL TEA					
(see TEA/HERBAL TEA)					
HERRING					
CANNED					
roe	3.5 oz	118	tr	3	22
FRESH					
atlantic cooked	3 oz	172	0	10	20
atlantic cooked	1 fillet (5 oz)	290	0	17	33
atlantic raw	3 oz	134	0	8	15
pacific baked	3 oz	213	0	15	18
pacific fillet baked	5.1 oz	360	0	26	30
roe raw	3½ oz	130	2	2	24
READY-TO-USE					
atlantic kippered	1 fillet (1.4 oz)	87	0	5	10
atlantic pickled	½ oz	39	1	3	2
HICKORY NUTS					
dried	1 oz	187	5	18	4
HOMINY					
CANNED					
canned	½ cup	57	11	tr	1
Allen					
Golden	½ cup (4.5 oz)	120	27	1	2
Mexican	½ cup (4.5 oz)	120	25	1	2
White	½ cup (4.5 oz)	100	22	1	2
Uncle William					
Golden	½ cup (4.5 oz)	120	27	1	2
Mexican	½ cup (4.5 oz)	120	25	1	2
White	½ cup (4.5 oz)	100	22	1	2
Van Camp's					
Golden	½ cup (4.3 oz)	80	17	1	1
White	½ cup (4.3 oz)	80	15	1	1
HONEY					
honey	1 cup (11.9 oz)	1031	279	0	1
honey	1 tbsp (0.7 oz)	64	17	0	tr
Burleson's					
Clover	1 tbsp	60	16	0	tr
Creamed	1 tbsp	60	16	0	tr
Natural	1 tbsp	60	16	0	tr
Pure	1 tbsp	60	16	0	tr
Raw	1 tbsp	60	16	0	tr
Rocky Mountain Clover	1 tbsp	60	16	0	tr

FOOD	PORTION	CALS.	CARB.	FAT	PRO.
Golden Blossom					
Honey	1 tsp	20	5	0	0
Smucker's					
Single Serving	½ oz	45	11	0	0
Tree Of Life					
Alfalfa	1 tbsp (0.7 oz)	60	17	0	0
Avocado	1 tbsp (0.7 oz)	60	17	0	0
Buckwheat	1 tbsp (0.7 oz)	60	17	0	0
Clover	1 tbsp (0.7 oz)	60	17	0	0
Honeybear Wildflower	1 tbsp (0.7 oz)	60	17	0	0
Orange	1 tbsp (0.7 oz)	60	17	0	0
Tupelo	1 tbsp (0.7 oz)	60	17	0	0
Wildflower	1 tbsp (0.7 oz)	60	17	0	0

HONEYDEW
FRESH

FOOD	PORTION	CALS.	CARB.	FAT	PRO.
cubed	1 cup	60	16	tr	1
wedge	1/10	46	12	tr	1
Dole					
Honeydew	1/10	50	12	0	1
FROZEN					
Big Valley					
Balls	¾ cup (4.9 oz)	45	11	0	1

HORSERADISH

FOOD	PORTION	CALS.	CARB.	FAT	PRO.
Gold's					
Hot	1 tsp	4	tr	tr	tr
Red	1 tsp	4	tr	0	tr
White	1 tsp	4	tr	tr	tr
Hebrew National					
White	1 tbsp	7	1	0	0
Heluva Good Cheese					
Horseradish	1 tsp (5 g)	0	0	0	0
Ka-Me					
Wasabi Powder	¼ tsp (1 g)	0	1	0	0
Kraft					
Cream Style	1 tsp (0.2 oz)	0	0	0	0
Horseradish Mustard	1 tsp (0.2 oz)	0	0	0	0
Prepared	1 tsp (0.2 oz)	0	0	0	0
Rosoff's					
Red	1 tbsp (0.5 oz)	8	2	0	0
White	1 tbsp (0.5 oz)	7	1	0	0
Sauceworks					
Horseradish	1 tsp (0.2 oz)	20	tr	2	0

FOOD	PORTION	CALS.	CARB.	FAT	PRO.
Schorr's					
Red	1 tbsp (0.5 oz)	8	2	0	0
White	1 tbsp (0.5 oz)	7	1	0	0

HOT CAKES
(*see* PANCAKES)

HOT DOG
(*see also* MEAT SUBSTITUTES, SAUSAGE, SAUSAGE SUBSTITUTES)

FOOD	PORTION	CALS.	CARB.	FAT	PRO.
CHICKEN					
chicken	1 (1.5 oz)	116	3	9	6
Empire					
Hot Dog	1 (2 oz)	100	1	7	8
Health Valley					
Weiners	1	96	1	8	5
Tyson					
Cheese	1	145	1	11	7
Wampler Longacre					
Chicken	1 (2 oz)	130	0	11	8
Chicken	1 (1.6 oz)	110	0	9	6
MEAT					
beef	1 (2 oz)	180	1	16	7
beef	1 (1.5)	142	1	13	5
beef & pork	1 (2 oz)	183	1	17	6
beef & pork	1 (1.5 oz)	144	1	13	5
pork cheesefurter smokie	1 (1.5 oz)	141	1	12	6
Armour					
Star Jumbo Beef	1	190	—	18	6
Healthy Choice					
Beef	1 (1.8 oz)	60	5	2	7
Bunsize	1 (2 oz)	70	5	2	8
Franks	1 (1.6 oz)	50	4	2	6
Jumbo	1 (2 oz)	70	5	2	8
Hebrew National					
Beef	1 (1.7 oz)	150	—	14	6
Cocktail Beef	6 (1.8 oz)	160	—	15	6
Dinner Beef	1 (4 oz)	350	—	34	14
Reduced Fat Beef	1 (1.7 oz)	120	—	10	5
Hillshire					
Franks Bun Size Beef	2 oz	180	2	16	7
Light & Mild Franks Jumbo	1 link	110	2	8	7
Light & Mild Weiners	1 link	90	2	7	6
Lit'l Franks Beef	2 oz	180	1	16	7

FOOD	PORTION	CALS.	CARB.	FAT	PRO.
Hillshire (CONT.)					
Lit'l Wieners	2 oz	180	2	16	8
Weiners Bun Size	2 oz	180	2	16	7
Weiners Natural Casing	2 oz	180	2	17	6
Hormel					
Big 8	1 (2 oz)	170	1	15	6
Light & Lean 97	1 (1.6 oz)	45	4	1	5
Light & Lean 97 Beef	1 (1.6 oz)	45	4	1	5
Jimmy Dean					
Mini	1 (2 oz)	110	6	6	6
Nathan's					
Natural Casing Franks	1	158	1	14	7
Skinless Franks	1	176	1	16	7
Oscar Mayer					
Beef	1 (1.6 oz)	150	1	13	5
Big & Juicy Deli Style Beef	1 (2.7 oz)	250	1	23	9
Big & Juicy Hot 'N Spicy	1 (2.7 oz)	220	1	20	10
Big & Juicy Original	1 (2.7 oz)	240	0	23	9
Big & Juicy Original Beef	1 (2.7 oz)	230	1	21	10
Big & Juicy Quarter Pound Beef	1 (4 oz)	350	2	32	15
Big & Juicy Smokie Links	1 (2.7 oz)	200	1	18	10
Bun-Length Beef	1 (2 oz)	180	1	17	6
Cheese	1 (1.6 oz)	150	1	14	5
Free	1 (1.8 oz)	40	2	0	7
Healthy Favorites Turkey & Beef	1 (2 oz)	60	2	2	9
Light Beef	1 (2 oz)	110	2	8	6
Weiners Bun-Length Pork & Turkey	1 (2 oz)	180	1	17	6
Weiners Little	6 (2 oz)	170	1	16	6
Weiners Pork & Turkey	1 (1.6 oz)	150	1	13	5
Weiners Light Pork Turkey Beef	1 (2 oz)	110	2	8	7
Russer					
Lil'Salt Deli Franks	1 (2.67 oz)	160	3	11	11
Shofar					
Kosher Beef	1 (1.8 oz)	150	0	14	6
Kosher Beef Reduced Fat Reduced Sodium	1 (1.8 oz)	120	0	10	7
Wrangler					
Beef	1 (2 oz)	170	1	15	7

FOOD	PORTION	CALS.	CARB.	FAT	PRO.
Wrangler (CONT.)					
Cheese	1 (2 oz)	170	1	15	7
Smoked	1 (2 oz)	170	1	15	7
TAKE-OUT					
corndog	1	460	56	19	17
w/ bun chili	1	297	31	13	14
w/ bun plain	1	242	18	15	10
TURKEY					
turkey	1 (1.5 oz)	102	1	8	6
Empire					
Hot Dog	1 (2 oz)	90	1	6	9
Health Valley					
Weiners	1	96	1	8	5
Louis Rich					
Bun Length	1 (2 oz)	110	2	8	7
Turkey	1 (1.6 oz)	90	1	7	6
Turkey	1 (1.5 oz)	80	1	6	6
Turkey Cheese	1 (1.6 oz)	90	2	7	6
Mr. Turkey					
Bun Size	1	130	2	11	6
Cheese	1	140	2	12	7
Hot Dog	1	110	2	9	5
Wampler Longacre					
Turkey	1 (2 oz)	130	0	11	8
Turkey	1 (1.6 oz)	110	0	9	6
HUMMUS					
hummus	⅓ cup	140	17	7	4
hummus	1 cup	420	50	21	12
Casbah					
Mix as prep	¼ cup	120	15	5	5
Cedar's					
No Salt Added Hommus Tahini	2 tbsp (1 oz)	50	5	2	3
HYACINTH BEANS					
DRIED					
cooked	1 cup	228	40	1	16

ICE CREAM AND FROZEN DESSERTS

(*see also* ICES AND ICE POPS, PUDDING POPS, SHERBET, YOGURT FROZEN)

FOOD	PORTION	CALS.	CARB.	FAT	PRO.
chocolate	½ cup (4 fl oz)	143	19	7	3
dixie cup chocolate	1 (3.5 fl oz)	125	16	6	2
dixie cup strawberry	1 (3.5 fl oz)	112	16	5	2
dixie cup vanilla	1 (3.5 fl oz)	116	14	6	2

FOOD	PORTION	CALS.	CARB.	FAT	PRO.
french vanilla soft serve	½ gal	3014	306	180	56
french vanilla soft serve	½ cup (4 fl oz)	185	19	11	4
strawberry	½ cup (4 fl oz)	127	18	6	2
vanilla	½ cup (4 fl oz)	132	16	7	2
vanilla light	½ cup	92	15	3	3
vanilla rich	½ cup	178	17	12	3
vanilla soft serve	½ cup	111	19	2	4
vanilla 10% fat	½ gal	2153	254	115	38
vanilla 16% fat	½ gal	2805	256	190	33
vanilla light	½ gal	1469	232	45	41
vanilla light	1 cup	184	29	6	5
vanilla light soft serve	½ gal	1787	307	37	64
vanilla light soft serve	1 cup	223	38	5	8
3 Musketeers					
Single Chocolate	1 (2 fl oz)	160	16	10	2
Single Vanilla	1 (2 fl oz)	160	16	10	2
Snack Chocolate	1 (0.72 fl oz)	60	6	4	1
Snack Vanilla	1 (0.72 fl oz)	60	6	4	1
Avari					
Creme Glace All Flavors	1 oz	10	3	0	tr
Ben & Jerry's					
Banana Walnut	½ cup (3.9 oz)	290	26	21	5
Butter Pecan	½ cup (3.9 oz)	310	20	26	4
Cherry Garcia	½ cup (3.7 oz)	240	25	16	4
Cherry Vanilla	½ cup (3.9 oz)	240	26	15	3
Chocolate Chip Cookie Dough	½ cup (3.7 oz)	270	30	17	4
Chocolate Fudge Brownie	½ cup (3.7 oz)	250	31	14	4
Chunky Monkey	½ cup (3.7 oz)	280	29	19	4
Coconut Almond	½ cup (3.7 oz)	260	19	20	5
Coconut Almond Fudge Chip	½ cup (3.8 oz)	320	24	25	6
Coffee Almond Fudge	½ cup (3.7 oz)	290	24	20	6
Coffee Toffee Crunch	½ cup (3.7 oz)	280	28	19	4
English Toffee Crunch	½ cup (4 oz)	310	30	21	4
Mint Chocolate Cookie	½ cup (3.8 oz)	260	27	17	4
New York Super Fudge Chunk	½ cup (3.7 oz)	290	28	20	5
No Fat Strawberry	½ cup (3.3 oz)	140	31	0	3
No Fat Vanilla Fudge Swirl	½ cup (3.1 oz)	150	32	0	3
Peanut Butter Cup	½ cup (4.1 oz)	370	30	26	8
Pop Chocolate Chip Cookie Dough	1 (4.1 oz)	450	48	28	6

FOOD	PORTION	CALS.	CARB.	FAT	PRO.
Ben & Jerry's (CONT.)					
Pop English Toffee Crunch	1 (3.7 oz)	340	35	23	4
Pop Vanilla	1 (3.9 oz)	360	30	28	5
Rain Forest Crunch	½ cup (3.7 oz)	300	24	23	5
Smooth Aztec Harvest Coffee	½ cup (3.8 oz)	230	22	16	4
Smooth Deep Dark Chocolate	½ cup (3.9 oz)	260	32	15	4
Smooth Double Chocolate Fudge	½ cup (4.1 oz)	280	35	16	5
Smooth Mocho Fudge	½ cup (4 oz)	270	30	18	5
Smooth Vanilla	½ cup (3.8 oz)	230	21	17	4
Smooth Vanilla Bean	½ cup (3.8 oz)	230	21	17	4
Smooth Vanilla Caramel Fudge	½ cup (4.1 oz)	280	33	17	4
Smooth White Russian	½ cup (3.8 oz)	240	23	16	4
Vanilla	½ cup (3.7 oz)	230	21	17	4
Wavy Gravy	½ cup (4.1 oz)	330	29	24	6
Bon Bons					
Vanilla With Milk Chocolate Coating	5 pieces	200	17	14	2
Vanilla With Milk Chocolate Coating	8 pieces	330	27	23	3
Borden					
Buttered Pecan	½ cup	180	16	12	3
Chocolate Swirl	½ cup	130	18	6	2
Dutch Chocolate Olde Fashioned Recipe	½ cup	130	16	6	2
Fat Free Black Cherry	½ cup	90	21	tr	2
Fat Free Chocolate	½ cup	100	21	tr	3
Fat Free Peach	½ cup	90	21	tr	2
Fat Free Strawberry	½ cup	90	21	tr	2
Fat Free Vanilla	½ cup	90	20	tr	3
Ice Milk Chocolate	½ cup	100	18	2	3
Ice Milk Strawberry	½ cup	90	17	2	2
Ice Milk Vanilla	½ cup	90	17	2	2
Strawberries 'N Cream Olde Fashioned Recipe	½ cup	130	19	5	2
Strawberry	½ cup	130	18	6	2
Sundae Cone	1	210	23	12	3
Vanilla Olde Fashioned Recipe	½ cup	130	15	7	2

FOOD	PORTION	CALS.	CARB.	FAT	PRO.
Bounty					
Cherry/Dark	1 (0.84 fl oz)	70	8	5	1
Coconut/Dark	1 (0.84 fl oz)	70	7	5	1
Coconut/Milk	1 (0.84 fl oz)	70	7	5	1
Bresler's					
All Flavors Ice Cream	3.5 oz	230	23	12	3
All Flavors Royale Cremes	4 oz	260	24	16	4
All Flavors Royale Lites	4 oz	217	49	0	5
Breyers					
Bar Vanilla	1 (2.7 oz)	250	21	17	4
Bar Vanilla Caramel w/ Chocolate Brittle Coating	1 (2.7 oz)	260	26	15	4
Bar Vanilla With Chocolate Coating	1 (2.6 oz)	230	20	15	4
Butter Almond	½ cup	170	15	11	4
Butter Pecan	½ cup (2.6 oz)	180	15	12	4
Cherry Vanilla	½ cup	150	17	7	3
Chocolate	½ cup (2.6 oz)	160	19	8	3
Chocolate Chocolate Chip	½ cup (2.5 oz)	180	21	10	3
Chocolate Peanut Butter Twirl	½ cup (2.6 oz)	220	20	13	5
Chocolate Chip	½ cup (2.5 oz)	170	18	10	3
Chocolate Chip Cookie Dough	½ cup (2.5 oz)	190	20	10	3
Coffee	½ cup (2.6 oz)	150	15	8	3
Cookies n'Cream	½ cup (2.6 oz)	170	19	9	3
Deluxe Rocky Road	½ cup (2.5 oz)	190	24	9	3
French Vanilla	(2.5 oz)	170	15	10	4
Light Brownie Marble Fudge	½ cup (2.6 oz)	150	23	5	4
Light Chocolate	½ cup (2.4 oz)	130	19	4	4
Light Chocolate Fudge Twirl	½ cup (2.6 oz)	140	22	4	4
Light Heavenly Hash	½ cup. (2.4 oz)	150	22	5	4
Light Rocky Road Deluxe	½ cup (2.4 oz)	150	22	5	4
Light Strawberry	½ cup (2.4 oz)	120	18	4	3
Light Toffee Fudge Parfait	½ cup (2.6 oz)	150	23	5	4
Light Vanilla	½ cup (2.4 oz)	130	18	5	4
Light Vanilla Chocolate Strawberry	½ cup (2.4 oz)	120	18	4	4

FOOD	PORTION	CALS.	CARB.	FAT	PRO.
Breyers (CONT.)					
Mint Chocolate Chip	½ cup (2.6 oz)	170	18	10	3
Mocha Almond Fudge	½ cup (2.7 oz)	190	20	10	4
Peach	½ cup (2.6 oz)	130	18	6	2
Reduced Fat Chocolate Chocolate Chip	½ cup (2.4 oz)	150	21	5	3
Reduced Fat Heavenly Hash	½ cup (2.4 oz)	150	22	5	4
Reduced Fat Mocha Almond Fudge	½ cup (2.5 oz)	160	20	6	4
Reduced Fat Praline Almond Crunch	½ cup (2.4 oz)	140	20	5	4
Reduced Fat Swiss Almond Fudge Twirl	½ cup (2.5 oz)	160	22	6	4
Sandwich Vanilla	1 (2.8 oz)	250	32	11	5
Strawberry	½ cup (2.6 oz)	130	15	6	3
Toffee Bar Crunch	½ cup (2.5 oz)	180	18	11	3
Vanilla	½ cup (2.6 oz)	150	15	8	3
Vanilla Caramel Praline	½ cup (2.6 oz)	190	23	10	3
Vanilla Chocolate	½ cup (2.5 oz)	160	17	8	3
Vanilla Chocolate Strawberry	½ cup (2.5 oz)	150	16	8	3
Vanilla Peanut Butter Fudge Sundae	½ cup (2.5 oz)	170	18	9	4
Vanilla Fudge Twirl	½ cup (2.6 oz)	160	19	8	4
Butterfinger					
Bar	1 (2.5 oz)	170	14	12	2
Nuggets	8	340	29	24	3
Carnation					
Sundae Cup Strawberry	1 (3.3 oz)	200	29	8	2
Cool 'N Creamy					
Amarello With Chocolate Swirl	1 bar	62	10	2	2
Chocolate Vanilla	1 bar	54	7	2	2
Double Chocolate Fudge	1 bar	55	7	2	2
Orange Vanilla	1 bar	31	5	1	1
Cool Creations					
Cookies & Cream Sandwich	1 (3.5 oz)	240	34	11	2
Mini Sandwich	1 (2.3 oz)	110	16	5	1
Cyrk					
Chocolate	3 oz	209	18	16	3
Maple Walnut	3 oz	299	25	22	4
Mint Chocolate Chip	3 oz	258	22	18	3

FOOD	PORTION	CALS.	CARB.	FAT	PRO.
Cyrk (CONT.)					
Strawberry	3 oz	208	17	15	2
Vanilla	3 oz	209	16	16	2
DoveBar					
Almond	1 (3.67 fl oz)	335	30	22	5
Bite Size Almond Praline	1 (0.75 fl oz)	80	8	5	1
Bite Size Cherry Royale	1 (0.75 fl oz)	70	8	5	1
Bite Size Classic Vanilla	1 (0.75 fl oz)	70	7	5	1
Bite Size French Vanilla	1 (0.75 fl oz)	70	7	5	1
Bite Size Mint Supreme	1 (0.75 fl oz)	80	8	5	1
Caramel Pecan	1 (3.67 fl oz)	350	35	35	4
Chocolate Milk Chocolate	1 (3.8 fl oz)	340	35	21	4
Coffee Cashew	1 (3.67 fl oz)	335	31	22	4
Crunchy Cookie	1 (3.8 fl oz)	340	35	21	4
Peanut	1 (3.8 fl oz)	380	35	25	7
Single Vanilla/Dark	1 (2 fl oz)	200	24	12	2
Vanilla Dark Chocolate	1 (3.8 fl oz)	340	34	22	4
Vanilla Milk Chocolate	1 (3.8 fl oz)	340	34	21	4
Drumstick					
Cone Chocolate	1 (4.6 oz)	340	37	19	6
Cone Chocolate Dipped	1 (4.6 oz)	340	41	17	5
Cone Vanilla	1 (4.6 oz)	350	36	20	6
Cone Vanilla Caramel	1 (4.6 oz)	360	39	20	6
Cone Vanilla Fudge	1 (4.6 oz)	370	40	21	6
Eagle Brand					
Vanilla	½ cup	150	16	9	3
Edy's					
American Dream Chocolate	3 oz	90	20	1	2
American Dream Chocolate Chip	3 oz	100	22	1	2
American Dream Cookies'N'Cream	3 oz	100	22	1	2
American Dream Mocha Almond Fudge	3 oz	110	24	1	3
American Dream Rocky Road	3 oz	110	24	1	3
American Dream Strawberry	3 oz	70	16	tr	2
American Dream Toasted Almond	3 oz	110	24	1	3
American Dream Vanilla	3 oz	80	18	tr	2
American Dream Vanilla Chocolate Strawberry	3 oz	80	18	1	2

FOOD	PORTION	CALS.	CARB.	FAT	PRO.
Edy's (CONT.)					
Light Almond Praline	4 oz	140	18	5	5
Light Banana-Politan	4 oz	110	15	4	3
Light Butter Pecan	4 oz	140	18	5	5
Light Cafe Au Lait	4 oz	110	13	4	3
Light Candy Bar	4 oz	140	20	5	4
Light Chocolate Chip	4 oz	120	16	4	4
Light Chocolate Fudge Mousse	4 oz	130	18	5	4
Light Cookies'N'Cream	4 oz	120	18	5	3
Light Dreamy Caramel Cream	4 oz	140	16	4	4
Light Malt Ball 'N' Fudge	4 oz	140	20	5	4
Light Marble Fudge	4 oz	120	15	4	5
Light Mocha Almond Fudge	4 oz	140	19	5	6
Light Peanut Butter & Chocolate	4 oz	130	19	5	6
Light Raspberry Truffle	4 oz	110	19	5	4
Light Rocky Road	4 oz	130	17	5	4
Light Strawberry	4 oz	110	15	4	3
Light Vanilla	4 oz	100	13	4	3
Vanilla Chocolate Strawberry	4 oz	110	14	4	4
Fi-Bar					
Banana Cream	1 bar	93	21	tr	2
Cocoa-Fudge 'N Cream	1 bar	93	21	tr	2
Raspberries 'N Cream	1 bar	93	21	tr	2
Wildberry Cream	1 bar	93	21	tr	2
Flintstones					
Cool Cream	1 (2.75 oz)	90	18	2	1
Push-Up	1 (2.75 oz)	100	20	2	1
Friendly's					
Black Raspberry	½ cup	150	17	7	2
Chocolate Almond Chip	½ cup	170	18	10	3
Forbidden Chocolate	½ cup	150	14	9	3
Fudge Nut Brownie	½ cup	200	23	11	3
Heath English Toffee	½ cup (2.7 oz)	190	24	10	3
Purely Pistachio	½ cup	160	16	10	3
Vanilla	½ cup	150	16	8	2
Vanilla Chocolate Strawberry	½ cup	150	16	8	2
Vienna Mocha Chunk	½ cup	180	19	11	3

FOOD	PORTION	CALS.	CARB.	FAT	PRO.
Frusen Gladje					
Butter Pecan	½ cup	280	16	21	5
Chocolate	½ cup	240	17	17	5
Chocolate Chocolate Chip	½ cup	270	21	18	5
Strawberry	½ cup	230	20	15	4
Swiss Chocolate Candy Almond	½ cup	270	18	19	6
Vanilla	½ cup	230	16	17	5
Vanilla Swiss Almond	½ cup	270	18	19	6
Good Humor					
Banana Bob	1 (3 fl oz)	155	22	7	2
Bar Classic Almond	1 (3.1 fl oz)	210	21	12	2
Bar Classic Toasted Almond	1 (3.1 fl oz)	170	22	9	2
Bar Classic Vanilla	1 (3.1 fl oz)	190	22	10	2
Bar Sidewalk Sundae	1	280	21	20	4
Bubble O'Bill	1 (3.6 fl oz)	170	20	10	2
Bubble Play	1	110	25	1	0
Chip Burrrger	1 (4.7 oz)	320	44	15	4
Chip Sandwich	1 (4.7 oz)	320	44	15	4
Choco Taco	1 (4.4 oz)	320	38	17	3
Chocolate Eclair Classic	1 (3.1 fl oz)	170	21	9	2
Classic Candy Center Crunch Vanilla	1	280	21	21	2
Colonel Crunch Chocolate	1 (3.1 oz)	160	21	7	2
Colonel Crunch Strawberry	1 (3.1 oz)	170	22	8	1
Combo Cup	1 (6.2 fl oz)	200	25	10	3
Cone Olde Nut Sundae	1 (3.9 oz)	230	32	9	4
Cone Sidewalk Sundae	1 (4.2 oz)	270	31	14	4
Creamee Burrrger	1 (4.7 oz)	310	40	17	0
Crunch Classic Candy Center	1 (3.1 fl oz)	260	21	19	2
Dinosaur Bar	1	110	25	2	0
Far Frog	1 (3.6 fl oz)	150	19	8	1
Fun Box Ice Cream Sandwich	1 (3.1 fl oz)	160	27	5	3
King Cone	1 (5.7 fl oz)	300	38	14	5
King Cone Classic Vanilla	1 (4.8 oz)	300	48	10	4
King Cone Strawberry	1 (5.7 oz)	250	38	10	3
Light Chocolate Chocolate Chip	½ cup (2.4 oz)	130	20	4	3

FOOD	PORTION	CALS.	CARB.	FAT	PRO.
Good Humor (CONT.)					
Light Chocolate Chip	½ cup (2.4 oz)	130	20	4	3
Light Coffee	½ cup (2.4 oz)	110	18	3	3
Light Cookies N'Cream	½ cup (2.4 oz)	130	21	3	3
Light Heavenly Hash	½ cup (2.4 oz)	140	23	4	3
Light Praline Almond Crunch	½ cup (2.4 oz)	130	20	3	3
Light Toffee Bar Crunch	½ cup (2.4 oz)	130	20	4	3
Light Vanilla	½ cup (2.4 oz)	110	19	3	3
Light Vanilla Chocolate Strawberry	½ cup (2.4 oz)	110	19	3	3
Light Vanilla Fudge	½ cup (2.6 oz)	120	21	3	3
Magnum Almond	1 (4.2 fl oz)	270	35	12	5
Magnum Chocolate	1 (4.2 fl oz)	260	38	12	1
Number One Bar	1 (4.1 fl oz)	190	22	11	2
Popsicle Ice Cream Sandwich	1 (3.6 fl oz)	190	28	8	3
Popsicle Ice Cream Bar	1 (3.1 fl oz)	160	15	11	2
Sandwich Classic Chip Cookie	1 (4.1 fl oz)	300	43	13	3
Sandwich Giant Neapolitan	1 (5.2 fl oz)	260	39	10	3
Sandwich Giant Vanilla	1 (5.2 fl oz)	240	35	10	4
Sandwich Ice Cream	1	190	28	8	4
Sandwich Sidewalk Sundae	1 (3.1 oz)	160	27	5	3
Sandwich Sprinkle	1 (3.1 fl oz)	180	28	6	2
Strawberry Shortcake Bar Classic	1 (3.1 fl oz)	160	20	8	1
Sundae Twist Cup	1	160	33	3	2
Toffee Taco	1 (4.4 fl oz)	300	35	16	3
Viennetta Chocolate	1 (4.2 fl oz)	160	19	9	2
Viennetta Vanilla	1 (4.2 fl oz)	160	15	10	2
WWF Bar	1 (3.7 fl oz)	200	24	10	2
X-Men Bar	1 (3 fl oz)	150	23	6	2
Haagen-Dazs					
Baileys Original Irish Cream	½ cup (3.6 oz)	280	23	18	4
Brownies A La Mode	½ cup (3.7 oz)	280	25	18	5
Butter Pecan	½ cup (3.7 oz)	320	20	24	5
Cappuccino Commotion	½ cup (3.6 oz)	310	25	21	5
Caramel Cone Explosion	½ cup (3.6 oz)	310	27	20	5
Chocolate	½ cup (3.7 oz)	270	22	18	5
Chocolate Chocolate Chip	½ cup (3.7 oz)	300	26	20	5

FOOD	PORTION	CALS.	CARB.	FAT	PRO.
Haagen-Dazs (CONT.)					
Coffee	½ cup (3.7 oz)	270	21	18	5
Cookie Dough Dynamo	½ cup (3.6 oz)	300	29	19	4
Cookies & Cream	½ cup (3.6 oz)	270	23	17	5
DiSaronno Amaretto	½ cup (3.6 oz)	260	26	15	4
Macadamia Brittle	½ cup (3.7 oz)	300	25	20	4
Multi Pack Bars Caramel Cone Explosion	1 (3.1 oz)	330	30	22	4
Multi Pack Bars Chocolate & Dark Chocolate	1 (3.2 oz)	320	27	22	4
Multi Pack Bars Coffee & Almond Crunch	1 (3 oz)	290	22	21	4
Multi Pack Bars Iced Cappuccino Explosion	1 (2.9 oz)	290	21	21	4
Multi Pack Bars Triple Brownie Overload	1 (3 oz)	320	23	23	4
Multi Pack Bars Vanilla & Almonds	1 (3 oz)	300	21	22	5
Multi Pack Bars Vanilla & Dark Chocolate	1 (3.2 oz)	320	27	22	5
Multi Pack Bars Vanilla & Milk Chocolate	1 (3 oz)	280	20	20	4
Peanut Butter Burst	½ cup (3.6 oz)	330	26	22	6
Rum Raisin	½ cup (3.7 oz)	270	22	17	4
Single Pack Bars Caramel Cone Explosion	1 (3.3 oz)	350	32	23	4
Single Pack Bars Chocolate & Dark Chocolate	1 (3.9 oz)	400	33	27	5
Single Pack Bars Coffee & Almond Crunch	1 (3.7 oz)	360	27	26	5
Single Pack Bars Cookie Dough Dynamo	1 (3.5 oz)	380	34	25	4
Single Pack Bars Iced Cappuccino	1 (3.4 oz)	330	24	24	5
Single Pack Bars Triple Brownie Overload	1 (3.5 oz)	380	28	27	5
Single Pack Bars Vanilla & Almonds	1 (3.7 oz)	370	26	27	6

FOOD	PORTION	CALS.	CARB.	FAT	PRO.
Haagen-Dazs (CONT.)					
Single Pack Bars Vanilla & Dark Chocolate	1 (3.9 oz)	400	33	27	5
Single Pack Bars Vanilla & Milk Chocolate	1 (3.5 oz)	330	24	25	5
Strawberry	½ cup (3.7 oz)	250	23	16	4
Strawberry Cheesecake Craze	½ cup (3.7 oz)	290	28	18	4
Triple Brownie Overload	½ cup (3.5 oz)	300	26	20	5
Vanilla	½ cup (3.7 oz)	270	21	18	5
Vanilla Fudge	½ cup (3.7 oz)	280	25	18	5
Vanilla Swiss Almond	½ cup (3.7 oz)	310	23	21	6
Healthy Choice					
Black Forest	½ cup (2.5 oz)	120	23	2	3
Bordeaux Cherry Chocolate Chip	½ cup (2.5 oz)	110	19	2	3
Butter Pecan Crunch	½ cup (2.5 oz)	120	22	2	3
Cappuccino Chocolate Chunk	½ cup (2.5 oz)	120	32	2	3
Cookies 'N Cream	½ cup (2.5 oz)	120	21	2	3
Double Fudge Swirl	½ cup (2.5 oz)	120	21	2	3
Fudge Brownie	½ cup (2.5 oz)	120	22	2	3
Malt Caramel Cone	½ cup (2.5 oz)	120	22	2	3
Mint Chocolate Chip	½ cup (2.5 oz)	120	21	2	3
Peanut Butter Cookie Dough 'N Fudge	½ cup (2.5 oz)	120	22	2	3
Praline & Caramel	½ cup (2.5 oz)	130	25	2	3
Rocky Road	½ cup (2.5 oz)	140	28	2	3
Vanilla	½ cup	100	18	2	3
Heath					
Bar	1 (2.5 oz)	160	13	12	1
Nuggets	8	180	18	11	2
Hood					
Bar Orange Cream	1 bar (1.8 oz)	90	18	2	1
Bar Vanilla	1 bar (1.6 oz)	160	11	12	1
Caramel Butterscotch Blast	½ cup (2.3 oz)	160	20	8	2
Chocolate	½ cup (2.3 oz)	140	17	7	2
Chocolate Chip	½ cup (2.3 oz)	160	18	9	2
Chocolate Eclair	1 bar (1.6 oz)	150	14	10	1
Christmas Tree	½ cup (2.3 oz)	140	18	7	2
Coffee	½ cup (2.3 oz)	140	16	7	2

FOOD	PORTION	CALS.	CARB.	FAT	PRO.
Hood (CONT.)					
Cookie Dough Delight	½ cup (2.3 oz)	160	21	8	2
Cookies N Cream	½ cup (2.3 oz)	160	19	8	2
Cooler Cups	1 (2.1 oz)	80	18	1	tr
Crispy Bar	1 (1.9 oz)	180	15	13	2
Egg Nog	½ cup (2.3 oz)	130	17	6	2
Fabulous Fudge & Peanut Butter Swirled Fudge Bars	1 bar (2.1 oz)	110	17	4	1
Fabulous Fudgies Assorted Bars	1 bar (2.1 oz)	100	19	3	1
Fat Free Chocolate Passion	½ cup (2.5 oz)	100	23	0	3
Fat Free Classic Harlequin	½ cup (2.5 oz)	100	23	0	2
Fat Free Double Brownie Sundae	½ cup (2.5 oz)	120	27	0	2
Fat Free Heavenly Hash	½ cup (2.5 oz)	120	27	0	2
Fat Free Mississippi Mud Pie	½ cup (2.5 oz)	130	29	0	3
Fat Free Praline Pecan Delight	½ cup (2.5 oz)	120	27	0	2
Fat Free Raspberry Blush	½ cup (2.5 oz)	120	26	0	2
Fat Free Super Strawberry Swirl	½ cup (2.5 oz)	100	23	0	2
Fat Free Vanilla Fudge Twist	½ cup (2.5 oz)	120	26	0	2
Fat Free Very Vanilla	½ cup (2.5 oz)	100	23	0	2
Fudge Bars	1 bar (2.7 oz)	100	21	1	2
Grasshopper Pie	½ cup (2.3 oz)	160	22	7	2
Heavenly Hash	½ cup (2.3 oz)	140	21	6	2
Hendrie's Cherry Chocolate Dips	1 bar (1.3 oz)	120	11	9	1
Hoodsie Cup Vanilla & Chocolate	1 (1.7 oz)	100	12	5	2
Light Almond Praline Delight	½ cup (2.4 oz)	110	23	5	3
Light Brownie Nut Sundae	½ cup (2.4 oz)	140	22	5	3
Light Caribbean Coffee Royale	½ cup (2.4 oz)	110	18	4	2
Light Chocolate Chocolate Chip Cookie Dough	½ cup (2.4 oz)	140	21	5	3

FOOD	PORTION	CALS.	CARB.	FAT	PRO.
Hood (CONT.)					
Light Chocolate Almond Chip Sundae	½ cup (2.4 oz)	140	22	5	3
Light Cookies N Cream	½ cup (2.4 oz)	130	21	4	2
Light Heath Toffee Chunk Swirl	½ cup (2.4 oz)	140	23	5	2
Light Heavenly Hash	½ cup (2.4 oz)	130	22	4	2
Light Maple Sugar Shack	⅓ cup (2.4 oz)	130	23	4	2
Light Massachusetts Mud Pie	½ cup (2.4 oz)	140	20	5	3
Light Raspberry Swirl	½ cup (2.4 oz)	120	22	3	2
Light Strawberry Supreme	½ cup (2.4 oz)	110	19	3	2
Light Triple Nut Cluster Sundae	½ cup (2.4 oz)	140	22	5	3
Light Vanilla	½ cup (2.4 oz)	110	18	4	2
Light Vanilla Chocolate Strawberry	½ cup (2.4 oz)	110	18	4	2
Low Fat No Sugar Added Caramel Swirl	½ cup (2.4 oz)	120	18	3	3
Low Fat No Sugar Added Chocolate Supreme	½ cup (2.4 oz)	120	19	3	4
Low Fat No Sugar Added Mocha Fudge	½ cup (2.4 oz)	110	18	3	3
Low Fat No Sugar Added Raspberry Swirl	½ cup (2.4 oz)	110	17	3	3
Low Fat No Sugar Added Vanilla	½ cup (2.4 oz)	100	14	3	3
Maple Walnut	½ cup (2.3 oz)	160	16	9	3
Rockets	1 (2 oz)	120	18	5	1
Sandwich Light	1 (2.2 oz)	160	29	4	3
Sandwich Vanilla	1 (2.2 oz)	180	27	7	3
Sports Bar	1 (2.9 oz)	250	23	17	3
Spumoni	½ cup (2.3 oz)	140	17	9	2
Strawberry	½ cup (2.3 oz)	130	16	7	2
Super Sortment Chocolate & Banana Fudge Bar	1 bar (2.1 oz)	100	18	3	1
Super Sortment Root Beer Float & Orange Cream Bar	1 bar (1.5 oz)	70	12	3	1
Vanilla	½ cup (2.3 oz)	140	16	7	2
Vanilla Chocolate Patchwork	½ cup (2.3 oz)	140	17	7	2

FOOD	PORTION	CALS.	CARB.	FAT	PRO.
Hood (CONT.)					
Vanilla Chocolate Strawberry	½ cup (2.3 oz)	140	16	7	2
Vanilla Fudge	½ cup (2.3 oz)	140	20	6	2
Klondike					
Almond Bar	1 (5.2 fl oz)	310	26	21	3
Caramel Crunch	1 (5.2 fl oz)	300	31	18	3
Chocolate Chocolate Bar	1 (5.2 fl oz)	280	22	20	3
Coffee Bar	1 (5.2 fl oz)	290	25	20	3
Dark Chocolate Bar	1 (5.2 fl oz)	290	24	20	3
Gold Bar	1 (5.2 fl oz)	340	30	23	5
Krispy Bar	1 (5.2 fl oz)	300	28	20	3
Krunch	1 (3.1 fl oz)	200	17	13	3
Lite Bar	1 (2.3 fl oz)	110	14	6	3
Lite Bar Caramel	1 (2.4 fl oz)	120	18	6	3
Movie Bites Chocolate	8 pieces (4.6 fl oz)	340	22	26	3
Movie Bites Vanilla	8 pieces (4.6 fl oz)	320	27	22	3
Original Bar	1 (5.2 fl oz)	290	24	20	3
Sandwich Chocolate	1 (5.2 fl oz)	270	41	10	4
Sandwich Lite	1 (2.9 fl oz)	100	18	2	3
Sandwich Vanilla	1 (5.2 fl oz)	250	37	9	4
Mars					
Almond Bar	1 (1.85 fl oz)	210	20	14	4
Meadow Gold					
Sundae Cone	1	210	23	12	3
Milky Way					
Single Chocolate/Milk	1 (2 fl oz)	210	24	11	3
Snack Chocolate/Milk	1 (0.72 fl oz)	70	9	4	1
Snack Vanilla/Dark	1 (0.72 fl oz)	70	9	4	1
Mocha Mix					
Berry Berry Berry	½ cup	140	20	6	tr
Dutch Chocolate	½ cup (2.3 oz)	140	16	8	1
Mocha Almond Fudge	½ cup (2.3 oz)	150	19	8	1
Neapolitan	½ cup (2.3 oz)	140	18	7	1
Strawberry Swirl	½ cup (2.3 oz)	140	20	6	tr
Vanilla	½ cup (2.3 oz)	140	18	7	1
Nestle Crunch					
Chocolate	1 bar (3 oz)	200	18	14	2
Cones	1 (4.6 oz)	300	36	16	4
Crunch King	1 (4 oz)	270	21	19	3
Nuggets	8 pieces	140	12	9	2
Reduced Fat	1 (2.5 oz)	130	14	7	3
Vanilla	1 bar (3 oz)	200	17	14	2

FOOD	PORTION	CALS.	CARB.	FAT	PRO.
Rice Dream					
Bar Chocolate	1	270	33	16	1
Bar Chocolate Nutty	1	330	29	23	5
Bar Strawberry	1	260	31	15	1
Bar Vanilla	1	275	33	16	1
Bar Vanilla Nutty	1	330	29	23	5
Cappuccino	½ cup	130	17	5	1
Carob	½ cup	130	20	5	1
Carob Almond	½ cup	140	20	6	1
Carob Chip	½ cup	140	20	6	1
Carob Chip Mint	½ cup	140	20	6	1
Cocoa Marble Fudge	½ cup	140	19	6	1
Dream Pie Chocolate	1	380	47	19	3
Dream Pie Mint	1	380	47	19	3
Dream Pie Mocha	1	380	47	19	3
Dream Pie Vanilla	1	380	47	19	3
Lemon	½ cup	130	17	5	1
Peanut Butter Fudge	½ cup	160	19	7	4
Strawberry	½ cup	130	17	5	1
Vanilla	½ cup	130	17	5	1
Vanilla Fudge	½ cup	140	21	6	1
Vanilla Swiss Almond	½ cup	140	20	6	1
Wildberry	½ cup	130	17	5	1
Sealtest					
American Glory	½ cup (2.4 oz)	130	17	6	2
Butter Pecan	½ cup (2.4 oz)	160	16	9	3
Candy Cane Crunch	½ cup (2.4 oz)	150	21	6	2
Chocolate	½ cup (2.4 oz)	140	19	7	3
Chocolate Butter Pecan	½ cup (2.4 oz)	150	17	8	3
Chocolate Chip	½ cup (2.4 oz)	150	18	8	3
Coconut Chocolate	½ cup (2.4 oz)	160	18	8	3
Coffee	½ cup (2.4 oz)	140	16	7	2
Cupid's Scoops	½ cup (2.5 oz)	140	20	6	2
Dessert Bar Free Chocolate Fudge	1	90	19	0	3
Dessert Bar Free Vanilla Strawberry Swirl	1	80	17	0	2
Dessert Bar Free Vanilla Fudge	1	80	18	0	3
Free Black Cherry	½ cup	100	25	0	2
Free Chocolate	½ cup	100	23	0	3
Free Peach	½ cup	100	23	0	2
Free Strawberry	½ cup	100	23	0	2
Free Vanilla	½ cup	100	24	0	3

FOOD	PORTION	CALS.	CARB.	FAT	PRO.
Sealtest (CONT.)					
Free Vanilla Strawberry Royale	½ cup	100	25	0	3
Free Vanilla Fudge Royale	½ cup	100	24	0	3
French Vanilla	½ cup (2.4 oz)	140	16	8	3
Fudge Royale	½ cup (2.5 oz)	150	19	7	3
Heavenly Hash	½ cup (2.4 oz)	150	20	7	3
Maple Walnut	½ cup (2.4 oz)	160	16	9	3
Strawberry	½ cup (2.4 oz)	130	19	6	2
Triple Chocolate Passion	½ cup (2.5 oz)	160	21	7	3
Vanilla	½ cup (2.4 oz)	140	16	7	2
Vanilla Chocolate Strawberry	½ cup (2.4 oz)	140	18	6	2
Vanilla With Orange Sherbet	½ cup (2.7 oz)	130	22	4	2
Simple Pleasures					
Chocolate	4 oz	140	25	tr	9
Chocolate Caramel Sundae Light	4 oz	90	20	tr	5
Chocolate Light	4 oz	80	16	tr	5
Chocolate Chip	4 oz	150	25	3	6
Coffee	4 oz	120	22	tr	8
Cookies n' Cream	4 oz	150	25	2	6
Mint Chocolate Chip	4 oz	150	26	2	6
Peach	4 oz	120	21	tr	7
Pecan Praline	4 oz	140	25	2	6
Rum Raisin	4 oz	130	35	tr	7
Strawberry	4 oz	120	22	tr	8
Toffee Crunch	4 oz	130	22	tr	9
Vanilla	4 oz	120	22	tr	6
Vanilla Light	4 oz	80	16	tr	5
Vanilla Fudge Swirl Light	4 oz	90	20	tr	5
Snickers					
Single	1 (2 fl oz)	220	22	13	4
Snack	1 (1 fl oz)	110	11	7	2
Tofu Ice Creme					
Carob	4 fl oz	190	28	8	2
Vanilla	4 fl oz	190	28	8	2
Tofutti					
Frutti Vanilla Apple Orchard	4 fl oz	100	20	0	2
Turkey Hill					
Black Cherry	½ cup (2.3 oz)	140	18	7	2

FOOD	PORTION	CALS.	CARB.	FAT	PRO.
Turkey Hill (CONT.)					
Butter Pecan	½ cup (2.3 oz)	170	16	11	2
Choco Mint Chip	½ cup (2.3 oz)	160	17	10	2
Cookies 'N Cream	½ cup (2.3 oz)	160	19	9	2
Lite Butter Pecan	½ cup (2.3 oz)	130	17	6	3
Lite Choco Mint Chip	½ cup (2.3 oz)	140	19	5	3
Lite Cookies 'N Cream	½ cup (2.3 oz)	130	21	5	3
Lite Vanilla & Chocolate	½ cup (2.3 oz)	110	18	3	3
Lite Vanilla Bean	½ cup (2.3 oz)	110	18	3	3
Neapolitan	½ cup (2.3 oz)	150	18	8	2
Rocky Road	½ cup (2.3 oz)	170	23	8	3
Tin Roof Sundae	½ cup (2.3 oz)	160	19	9	2
Vanilla	½ cup (2.3 oz)	140	16	8	2
Vanilla & Chocolate	½ cup (2.3 oz)	150	17	8	2
Vanilla Bean	½ cup (2.3 oz)	140	16	8	2
Ultra Slim-Fast					
Bar Fudge	1	90	17	tr	2
Bar Vanilla Cookie Crunch	1	90	14	4	3
Chocolate	4 oz	100	19	tr	5
Chocolate Fudge	4 oz	120	24	tr	5
Peach	4 oz	100	22	tr	4
Pralines & Caramel	4 oz	120	25	tr	4
Sandwich Vanilla	1	140	28	2	4
Sandwich Vanilla Chocolate	1	140	28	2	4
Sandwich Vanilla Oatmeal	1	150	26	3	4
Vanilla	4 oz	90	19	tr	5
Vanilla Fudge Cookie	4 oz	110	24	tr	5
Weight Watchers					
Bar Chocolate Dip	1 (2 oz)	110	10	7	2
Bar Double Fudge	1 (1.75 oz)	60	12	1	3
Bar English Toffee Crunch	1 (2 oz)	120	11	11	2
Bar Fat Free Vanilla Sandwich	1 (2.5 oz)	130	30	0	3
Bar Sugar Free Chocolate Mousse	1 (1.75 oz)	35	9	tr	2
Bar Sugar Free Chocolate Treat	1 (2.75 oz)	90	18	0	5
Bar Sugar Free Fat Free Orange Vanilla Treat	1 (1.75 oz)	30	9	0	2

FOOD	PORTION	CALS.	CARB.	FAT	PRO.
Weight Watchers (CONT.)					
Fat Free Frozen Dessert Chocolate	½ cup	80	19	0	3
Fat Free Frozen Dessert Chocolate Swirl	½ cup	90	22	0	3
Fat Free Frozen Dessert Neapolitan	½ cup	80	19	0	3
Fat Free Frozen Dessert Vanilla	½ cup	80	20	0	3
Ice Milk Chocolate Chip	½ cup	120	18	4	4
Ice Milk Pecan Pralines 'n Cream	½ cup	130	20	4	4
ONE-ders Brownies'n Creme	4 oz	130	20	4	4
ONE-ders Chocolate Chip	4 oz	120	18	4	4
ONE-ders Heavenly Hash	4 oz	130	22	3	4
ONE-ders Pralines'n Creme	4 oz	130	19	4	4
ONE-ders Strawberry	4 oz	110	17	3	3
TAKE-OUT					
cone vanilla light soft serve	1 (4.6 oz)	164	24	6	4
gelato chocolate hazelnut	½ cup (5.3 oz)	370	26	29	9
gelato vanilla	½ cup (3 oz)	211	18	15	3
sundae caramel	1 (5.4 oz)	303	49	9	7
sundae hot fudge	1 (5.4 oz)	284	48	9	6
sundae strawberry	1 (5.4 oz)	269	45	8	6

ICE CREAM CONES AND CUPS

FOOD	PORTION	CALS.	CARB.	FAT	PRO.
sugar cone	1	40	8	tr	1
wafer cone	1	17	3	tr	tr
Comet					
Cups	1 (5 g)	20	1	0	0
Sugar Cones	1 (12 g)	50	11	0	tr
Waffle Cone	1 (17 g)	70	14	1	1
Dutch Mill					
Chocolate Covered Wafer Cups	1 (0.5 oz)	80	8	5	1
Keebler					
Sugar Cones	1	45	11	tr	1
Vanilla Cups	1	15	4	tr	tr
Oreo					
Chocolate Cones	1 (13 g)	50	10	1	1

FOOD	PORTION	CALS.	CARB.	FAT	PRO.
Teddy Grahams					
Cinnamon Cones	1 (0.5 oz)	60	13	1	1
ICE CREAM TOPPINGS					
(*see also* SYRUP)					
butterscotch	2 tbsp (1.4 oz)	103	27	tr	1
caramel	2 tbsp (1.4 oz)	103	27	tr	1
marshmallow cream	1 jar (7 oz)	615	157	tr	3
marshmallow cream	1 oz	88	23	tr	1
pineapple	1 cup (11.5 oz)	861	226	—	1
pineapple	2 tbsp (1.5 oz)	106	28	0	tr
strawberry	2 tbsp (1.5 oz)	107	28	tr	tr
strawberry	1 cup (11.5 oz)	863	225	1	1
walnuts in syrup	2 tbsp (1.4 oz)	167	22	9	2
Hershey					
Chocolate Fudge	2 tbsp	100	14	4	1
Chocolate Shoppe Candy Bar Sprinkles York	2 tbsp (1.1 oz)	170	22	8	2
Kraft					
Butterscotch	2 tbsp (1.4 oz)	130	28	2	tr
Caramel	2 tbsp (1.4 oz)	120	28	0	2
Chocolate	2 tbsp (1.4 oz)	110	26	0	2
Hot Fudge	2 tbsp (1.4 oz)	140	24	4	1
Pineapple	2 tbsp (1.4 oz)	110	28	0	0
Strawberry	2 tbsp (1.4 oz)	110	29	0	0
Marzetti					
Caramel Apple	2 tbsp	60	23	7	1
Caramel Apple Reduced Fat	2 tbsp	30	26	3	1
Peanut Butter Caramel	2 tbsp	60	21	6	3
Planters					
Nut	2 tbsp (0.5 oz)	100	3	9	3
Smucker's					
Butterscotch	2 tbsp	140	33	1	0
Butterscotch Special Recipe	2 tbsp	160	33	3	1
Caramel	2 tbsp	140	33	1	1
Chocolate	2 tbsp	130	27	0	1
Chocolate Fudge	2 tbsp	130	31	1	1
Dark Chocolate Special Recipe	2 tbsp	130	31	1	1
Hot Caramel	2 tbsp	150	28	4	1
Hot Fudge	2 tbsp	110	18	4	1
Hot Fudge Special Recipe	2 tbsp	150	23	5	2

FOOD	PORTION	CALS.	CARB.	FAT	PRO.
Smucker's (CONT.)					
Hot Fudge Light	2 tbsp	70	19	tr	2
Hot Toffee Fudge	2 tbsp	110	18	4	1
Magic Shell Chocolate	2 tbsp	190	16	15	1
Magic Shell Chocolate Fudge	2 tbsp	190	16	15	1
Magic Shell Chocolate Nut	2 tbsp	200	25	16	2
Marshmallow	2 tbsp	120	29	0	0
Peanut Butter Caramel	2 tbsp	150	29	2	3
Pecans in Syrup	2 tbsp	130	28	1	2
Pineapple	2 tbsp	130	32	0	0
Strawberry	2 tbsp	120	30	0	0
Swiss Milk Chocolate Fudge	2 tbsp	140	31	1	3
Walnuts in Syrup	2 tbsp	130	27	1	2

ICED TEA

(*see also* TEA/HERBAL TEA)

MIX

FOOD	PORTION	CALS.	CARB.	FAT	PRO.
instant artifically sweetened lemon flavored as prep w/ water	8 oz	5	1	0	tr
instant sweetened lemon flavor as prep w/ water	9 oz	87	22	tr	tr
instant unsweetened lemon flavor as prep w/ water	8 oz	4	0	0	tr
4C					
Instant	8 oz	90	22	0	0
Bigelow					
Nice Over Ice	5 fl oz	1	tr	tr	tr
Celestial Seasonings					
Iced Delight	8 fl oz	4	1	tr	tr
Crystal Light					
Decaffeinated Sugar Free	8 oz	2	0	0	0
Sugar Free	8 oz	3	0	0	0
Lipton					
Instant	6 oz	0	0	0	0
Instant Decaffeinated	6 oz	0	0	0	0
Instant Lemon	8 oz	3	1	0	tr
Instant Raspberry	8 oz	3	1	0	0
Lemon	6 oz	55	14	0	0
Lemon w/ Vitamin C	6 oz	58	15	0	0

FOOD	PORTION	CALS.	CARB.	FAT	PRO.
Lipton (CONT.)					
Sugar Free	8 oz	1	tr	0	0
Sugar Free Peach	8 oz	5	1	0	0
Sugar Free Raspberry	8 oz	5	1	0	0
With Nutrasweet	8 oz	3	1	0	0
With Nutrasweet Decaffeinated	8 oz	3	1	0	0
Nestea					
100% Instant Tea as prep	8 oz	2	0	0	0
Ice Teasers Citrus	8 oz	6	1	0	0
Ice Teasers Lemon	8 oz	6	1	0	0
Ice Teasers Orange	8 oz	6	1	0	0
Ice Teasers Tropical	8 oz	6	1	0	0
Ice Teasers Wild Cherry	8 oz	6	1	0	0
Lemon	8 oz	6	1	0	0
Peach	8 fl oz	88	22	tr	tr
Raspberry	8 fl oz	88	22	tr	tr
Sugarfree	8 oz	4	1	0	0
With Sugar & Lemon	1 bottle (16 fl oz)	176	44	0	0
With Sugar & Lemon	1 can (11.5 fl oz)	127	32	0	0
With Sugar & Lemon as prep	8 oz	70	19	0	0
READY-TO-DRINK					
Arizona					
Raspberry	8 fl oz	95	25	0	0
Royal Mistic					
Diet	12 fl oz	8	2	0	0
Lemon	12 fl oz	144	36	0	0
Orange	12 fl oz	144	36	0	0
Wild Berry	12 fl oz	144	36	0	0
Schweppes					
Ice Tea	8 fl oz	90	22	0	0
Snapple					
Cranberry	8 fl oz	110	27	0	0
Diet	8 fl oz	0	1	0	0
Diet Peach	8 fl oz	0	1	0	0
Diet Raspberry	8 fl oz	0	1	0	0
Lemon	8 fl oz	110	27	0	0
Mango	8 fl oz	110	27	0	0
Mint	8 fl oz	120	29	0	0
Old Fashioned	8 fl oz	80	20	0	0
Orange	8 fl oz	110	27	0	0
Peach	8 fl oz	110	27	0	0

FOOD	PORTION	CALS.	CARB.	FAT	PRO.
Snapple (CONT.)					
Raspberry	8 fl oz	120	29	0	0
Strawberry	8 fl oz	100	26	0	0
Tropicana					
Diet Lemon Fruit	8 fl oz	15	4	0	0
Lemon Fruit	8 fl oz	100	25	0	0
Peach Fruit	8 fl oz	120	28	0	0
Peach Fruit	1 can (11.5 fl oz)	160	41	0	0
Peach Fruit	1 bottle (10 fl oz)	140	35	0	0
Raspberry Fruit	1 can (11.5 fl oz)	160	41	0	0
Raspberry Fruit	8 fl oz	120	28	0	0
Raspberry Fruit	1 bottle (10 fl oz)	140	34	0	0
Tangerine Fruit	1 bottle (10 fl oz)	140	34	0	0
Tangerine Fruit	1 can (11.5 fl oz)	170	42	0	0
Tangerine Fruit	8 fl oz	110	27	0	0
Twister Apple Berry	8 fl oz	100	28	0	0
Twister Lemon Citrus	8 fl oz	110	28	0	0
Turkey Hill					
Diet Decaffeinated	1 cup (8 oz)	0	0	0	0
Raspberry Cooler	1 cup (8 oz)	110	28	0	0
Regular	1 cup (8 oz)	90	22	0	0
Veryfine					
With Lemon	8 oz	80	16	0	0

ICES AND ICE POPS

(see also ICE CREAM AND FROZEN DESSERTS, PUDDING POPS, SHERBET, SORBET, YOGURT FROZEN)

FOOD	PORTION	CALS.	CARB.	FAT	PRO.
fruit & juice bar	1 (3 fl oz)	75	19	tr	1
gelatin pop	1 (1.5 oz)	31	7	0	1
ice coconut pineapple	½ cup (4 fl oz)	109	23	3	0
ice fruit w/ Equal	1 bar (1.7 oz)	12	3	0	tr
ice lime	½ cup (4 fl oz)	75	31	0	tr
ice pop	1 (2 fl oz)	42	11	0	0
Ben & Jerry's					
Cherry Pop	1	330	28	24	4
Bresler's					
All Flavors Ice	3.5 oz	120	30	0	0
Cool Creations					
10 Pack	1 pop (2 oz)	60	14	0	0
Lion King Cone	1 (4 oz)	280	36	14	3
Mickey Mouse Bar	1 (2.5 oz)	110	12	7	1
Mickey Mouse Bar	1 (4 oz)	170	17	11	2
Surprise Pops	1 (2 oz)	60	14	0	0
Crystal Light					
Berry Blend	1 bar	13	2	0	0

FOOD	PORTION	CALS.	CARB.	FAT	PRO.
Crystal Light (CONT.)					
Cherry	1 bar	13	2	0	0
Fruit Punch	1 bar	14	2	0	0
Orange	1 bar	13	2	0	0
Pina Colada	1 bar	14	2	0	0
Pineapple	1 bar	14	2	0	0
Pink Lemonade	1 bar	14	2	0	0
Raspberry	1 bar	13	2	0	0
Strawberry	1 bar	13	2	0	0
Strawberry Daiquiri	1 bar	14	2	0	0
Cyrk					
Ice Chocolate	4 oz	85	21	1	3
Ice Vanilla	4 oz	75	17	tr	1
Sorbet Apricot	4 oz	104	27	tr	1
Sorbet Blueberry	4 oz	77	20	tr	tr
Sorbet Cherry	4 oz	98	25	tr	tr
Sorbet Lemon	4 oz	66	18	0	tr
Sorbet Mango	4 oz	83	22	tr	tr
Sorbet Pina Colada	4 oz	107	23	3	tr
Sorbet Plum	4 oz	90	23	tr	tr
Sorbet Raspberry	4 oz	88	23	tr	tr
Sorbet Strawberry	4 oz	79	21	tr	tr
Sorbet Sugar Free Apricot	4 oz	36	9	tr	1
Sorbet Sugar Free Mango	4 oz	48	13	tr	tr
Sorbet Sugar Free Pina Colada	4 oz	66	11	3	tr
Sorbet Sugar Free Raspberry	4 oz	35	9	tr	tr
Sorbet White Peach	4 oz	96	26	tr	tr
Dole					
Fruit 'n Juice Coconut	1 bar (4 oz)	210	33	7	3
Fruit 'n Juice Lemonade	1 bar (4 oz)	120	28	0	1r
Fruit 'n Juice Lime	1 bar (4 oz)	110	28	0	0
Fruit 'n Juice Peach Passion	1 bar (2.5 oz)	70	17	0	0
Fruit 'n Juice Pineapple Coconut	1 bar (4 oz)	140	27	4	1
Fruit 'n Juice Pineapple Orange Banana	1 bar (2.5 oz)	70	16	0	0
Fruit 'n Juice Pineapple Orange Banana	1 bar (4 oz)	110	26	0	0
Fruit 'n Juice Raspberry	1 bar (2.5 oz)	70	16	0	0

FOOD	PORTION	CALS.	CARB.	FAT	PRO.
Dole (CONT.)					
Fruit 'n Juice Strawberry	1 bar (4 oz)	110	26	0	0r
Fruit 'n Juice Strawberry	1 bar (2.5 oz)	70	17	0	0
Fruit Juice Grape	1 bar (1.75 oz)	45	11	0	0
Fruit Juice No Sugar Added Grape	1 bar (1.75 oz)	25	6	0	0
Fruit Juice No Sugar Added Strawberry	1 bar (1.75 oz)	25	6	0	0
Fruit Juice Raspberry	1 bar (1.75 oz)	45	11	0	0
Fruit Juice Strawberry	1 bar (1.75 oz)	45	11	0	0
Fi-Bar					
Juice Bar Lemoney-Lime	1 bar	63	15	tr	tr
Juice Bar Strawberry Nectar	1 bar	63	15	tr	tr
Juice Bar Tropical Delight	1 bar	63	15	tr	tr
Flintstones					
Rock Pops	1 (3.5 oz)	80	20	0	0
Frozfruit					
Strawberry	1 (4 oz)	80	20	0	0
Good Humor					
Big Stick Cherry Pineapple	1 (3.6 fl oz)	50	12	0	0
Big Stick Popsicle	1 (3.6 fl oz)	50	12	0	0
Calippo Cherry	1 (3.8 fl oz)	100	23	0	0
Calippo Grape Lemon	1 (3.9 fl oz)	90	22	0	0
Calippo Orange	1 (3.9 fl oz)	90	23	0	0
Citrus Bites	1 (1.8 fl oz)	35	9	0	0
Creamsicle Orange	1 (1.8 fl oz)	70	13	2	1
Creamsicle Orange	1 (2.8 fl oz)	110	20	3	1
Creamsicle Orange Raspberry	1 (2.6 fl oz)	100	19	3	1
Creamsicle Sugar Free	1 (1.8 fl oz)	25	5	0	0
Flintstones Push-Up Yabba Dabba Doo Orange	1 (2.75 fl oz)	90	20	1	1
Fudgsicle Pop	1 (1.8 fl oz)	60	12	1	2
Fudgsicle Sugar Free	1 (1.8 fl oz)	40	8	1	1
Fudgsicle Bar	1 (2.8 fl oz)	90	17	1	3
Fun Box Fudge Bar	1 (2.3 fl oz)	80	16	1	1
Fun Box Pops	1 (2 fl oz)	35	10	0	0
Fun Box Twin Box Cherry	1 (2.6 fl oz)	50	14	0	0
Fun Box Twin Pop Banana	1 (2.6 fl oz)	50	14	0	0

FOOD	PORTION	CALS.	CARB.	FAT	PRO.
Good Humor (CONT.)					
Fun Box Twin Pop Blue Raspberry	1 (2.6 fl oz)	50	14	0	0
Fun Box Twin Pop Cherry Lemon	1 (2.6 fl oz)	50	14	0	0
Fun Box Twin Pop Orange Cherry Grape	1 (2.6 oz)	50	14	0	0
Fun Box Twin Pop Root Beer	1 (2.6 fl oz)	50	14	0	0
Garfield Bar	1 (3.9 fl oz)	90	22	0	0
Great White	1 (3.1 fl oz)	70	18	1	0
Hyperstripe	1 (2.8 fl oz)	80	21	0	0
Ice Stripe Cherry Orange	1 (1.5 fl oz)	35	9	0	0
Ice Stripe Grape Lemon	1 (1.5 fl oz)	35	9	0	0
Jumbo Jet Star	1 (4.7 fl oz)	80	20	0	0
Laser Blazer	1 (2.6 oz)	70	16	0	0
Popsicle All Natural	1 (1.8 fl oz)	45	10	0	0
Popsicle Orange Cherry Grape	1 (1.8 fl oz)	45	11	0	0
Popsicle Rainbow Pops	1 (1.8 fl oz)	45	11	0	0
Popsicle Rootbeer Banana Lime	1 (1.8 fl oz)	45	11	0	0
Popsicle Strawberry Raspberry Wildberry	1 (1.8 fl oz)	45	11	0	0
Popsicle Supersicle Traffic Signal	1	80	20	0	0
Popsicle Twin Pop Cherry	1 (2.6 fl oz)	70	16	0	0
Popsicle Twin Pop Orange Cherry Grape Lime	1 (2.6 fl oz)	70	16	0	0
Snow Cone	1	60	14	0	0
Snowfruit Coconut Bar	1 (3.75 fl oz)	150	27	4	2
Snowfruit Orange Bar	1	140	34	0	tr
Snowfruit Strawberry Bar	1	120	31	0	0
Snowfruit Tropical Fruit Bar	1	110	28	0	0
Sugar Free Pop Orange Cherry Grape	1 (1.8 fl oz)	15	3	0	0
Super Mario Bar	1	120	27	1	0
Supersicle Cherry Banana	1 (4.7 fl oz)	80	20	0	0
Supersicle Cherry Cola	1 (4.7 fl oz)	80	20	0	0

FOOD	PORTION	CALS.	CARB.	FAT	PRO.
Good Humor (CONT.)					
Supersicle Double Fudge	1 (4.7 fl oz)	150	29	2	5
Supersicle Firecracker	1 (4.7 fl oz)	90	20	0	0
Supersicle Firecracker Jr.	1	72	10	0	0
Supersicle Sour Tower	1	80	20	0	0
Swirl Bubble Gum	1 (2.7 fl oz)	55	13	0	0
Swirl Cherry Banana	1 (2.7 fl oz)	55	13	0	0
Torpedo Cherry	1 (1.8 fl oz)	35	10	0	0
Twister Blue Raspberry Cherry Cherry Cola Cherry	1 (1.8 fl oz)	45	10	0	0
Twister Cherry Lemon Orange Lemon	1 (1.8 fl oz)	45	10	0	0
Vampire's Deadly Secret	1 (2.8 fl oz)	100	24	0	0
Watermelon Bar	1 (3.6 fl oz)	80	20	0	0
Haagen-Dazs					
Sorbet Chocolate	½ cup (4 oz)	130	30	0	2
Sorbet Mango	½ cup (4 oz)	120	30	0	0
Sorbet Raspberry	½ cup (4 oz)	120	29	0	0
Sorbet Strawberry	½ cup (4 oz)	130	33	0	0
Sorbet Zesty Lemon	½ cup (4 oz)	130	32	0	0
Sorbet & Cream Blueberry	4 oz	190	25	8	3
Sorbet & Cream Keylime	4 oz	190	29	7	2
Sorbet & Cream Orange	½ cup (3.7 oz)	200	27	9	2
Sorbet & Cream Orange	4 oz	190	27	8	3
Sorbet & Cream Raspberry	½ cup (3.7 oz)	190	23	9	3
Sorbet Bar Chocolate	1 (2.7 oz)	80	20	0	1
Sorbet Bar Wild Berry	1 (2.7 oz)	90	22	0	0
Hood					
Hendrie's Sizzle'N Sour Stix	1 bar (2 oz)	80	15	tr	0
Hoodsie Pop	1 (3.3 oz)	60	16	0	0
Natural Blenders Pineappple	1 bar (1 oz)	60	16	0	0
Natural Blenders Raspberry	1 bar (1 oz)	60	16	0	0
Natural Blenders Strawberry	1 bar (1 oz)	60	16	0	0
Pop Banana	1 (3.3 oz)	60	16	0	0
Pop Blue Raspberry	1 (3.3 oz)	60	16	0	0
Pop Cherry	1 (3.3 oz)	60	16	0	0

FOOD	PORTION	CALS.	CARB.	FAT	PRO.
Hood (CONT.)					
Pop Grape	1 (3.3 oz)	60	16	0	0
Pop Orange	1 (3.3 oz)	60	16	0	0
Pop Root Beer	1 (3.3 oz)	60	16	0	0
Super Sortment Juice Bars	1 bar (1.9 oz)	40	10	0	0
Jell-O					
Lemon Lime	1 bar	33	8	tr	1
Mixed Berry	1 bar	31	7	tr	1
Orange	1 bar	31	7	tr	1
Orange Pineapple	1 bar	31	7	tr	1
Raspberry	1 bar	29	7	tr	1
Raspberry Peach	1 bar	29	7	tr	1
Side By Side Apple Cherry	1 bar	36	8	tr	1
Side By Side Grape Lemon	1 bar	36	8	tr	1
Strawberry	1 bar	31	7	tr	1
Strawberry Banana	1 bar	31	7	tr	1
Kool-Aid					
Berry Punch	1 bar	31	7	tr	1
Cherry	1 bar	42	11	0	0
Grape	1 bar	42	11	0	0
Mountain Berry Punch	1 bar	42	11	0	0
Lifesavers					
Ice Pops	1 (1.75 oz)	35	9	0	0
Sunkist					
Orange Juice Bar	1 (3.4 fl oz)	80	19	1	0
Wildberry	1 (3.4 fl oz)	120	27	1	0
Tofutti					
Frutti Apricot Mango	4 fl oz	100	20	0	2
Frutti Three Berry	4 fl oz	100	20	0	2

ICING
(see CAKE)

INSTANT BREAKFAST
(see BREAKFAST DRINKS)

JACKFRUIT
fresh	3½ oz	70	4	tr	1

JALAPENO
(see PEPPERS)

JAM/JELLY/PRESERVES
all flavors jam	1 pkg (0.5 oz)	34	9	0	tr

FOOD	PORTION	CALS.	CARB.	FAT	PRO.
all flavors jam	1 tbsp (0.7 oz)	48	13	0	tr
all flavors jelly	1 tbsp (0.7 oz)	52	14	0	tr
all flavors jelly	1 pkg (0.5 oz)	38	10	0	tr
all flavors preserve	1 tbsp (0.7 oz)	48	13	0	tr
all flavors preserve	1 pkg (0.5 oz)	34	9	0	tr
apple butter	1 cup (9.9 oz)	519	135	1	tr
apple butter	1 tbsp (0.6 oz)	33	9	0	0
apple jelly	3½ oz	259	65	0	0
apple jelly	1 tbsp (0.7 oz)	52	14	0	tr
apple jelly	1 pkg (0.5 oz)	38	10	0	tr
apricot jam	3½ oz	250	62	0	tr
blackberry jam	3½ oz	237	59	0	1
cherry jam	3½ oz	250	62	0	tr
loganberry jam	0.5 oz	23	6	tr	tr
orange jam	3½ oz	243	60	0	tr
orange marmalade	1 tbsp (0.7 oz)	49	13	0	tr
orange marmalade	1 pkg (0.5 oz)	34	9	0	tr
plum jam	3½ oz	241	60	0	tr
quince jam	3½ oz	236	59	0	tr
raspberry jam	3½ oz	248	61	0	1
raspberry jelly	3½ oz	259	65	0	0
red currant jam	3½ oz	237	59	0	1
red currant jelly	3½ oz	265	66	0	0
rose hip jam	3½ oz	250	62	0	tr
strawberry jam	1 tbsp (0.7 oz)	48	13	0	tr
strawberry jam	1 pkg (0.5 oz)	34	9	0	tr
strawberry preserve	1 pkg (0.5 oz)	34	9	0	tr
strawberry preserve	1 tbsp (0.7 oz)	48	13	0	tr
BAMA					
Apple Butter	2 tsp	25	6	0	0
Apple Jelly	2 tsp	30	8	0	0
Grape Jelly	2 tsp	30	8	0	0
Peach Preserves	2 tsp	30	8	0	0
Red Plum Jam	2 tsp	30	8	0	0
Strawberry Preserves	2 tsp	30	8	0	0
Eden					
Apple Butter	1 tbsp (0.5 fl oz)	25	3	0	0
Estee					
Apple Reduced Calorie	1 pkg (0.5 oz)	10	2	0	0
Apple Slice	1 tbsp (0.5 oz)	10	2	0	0
Apricot	1 tbsp (0.5 oz)	5	1	0	0
Blackberry	1 tbsp (0.5 oz)	5	1	0	0
Cherry	1 tbsp (0.5 oz)	5	1	0	0
Grape	1 tbsp (0.5 oz)	10	2	0	0

FOOD	PORTION	CALS.	CARB.	FAT	PRO.
Estee (CONT.)					
Orange	1 tbsp (0.5 oz)	10	2	0	0
Peach	1 tbsp (0.5 oz)	5	1	0	0
Red Raspberry	1 tbsp (0.5 oz)	5	1	0	0
Strawberry	1 tbsp (0.5 oz)	10	2	0	0
Strawberry	1 tbsp (0.5 oz)	10	2	0	0
Harvest Moon					
Apricot Fruit Spread	1 tbsp (0.6 oz)	35	9	0	0
Blueberry Fruit Spread	1 tbsp (0.6 oz)	35	9	0	0
Cherry Fruit Spread	1 tbsp (0.6 oz)	35	9	0	0
Grape Fruit Spread	1 tbsp (0.6 oz)	35	9	0	0
Peach Fruit Spread	1 tbsp (0.6 oz)	35	9	0	0
Raspberry Fruit Spread	1 tbsp (0.6 oz)	35	9	0	0
Strawberry Fruit Spread	1 tbsp (0.6 oz)	35	9	0	0
Kraft					
Apple Jelly	1 tbsp (0.7 oz)	60	14	0	0
Apple Strawberry Jelly	1 tbsp (0.7 oz)	50	13	0	0
Apricot Preserves	1 tbsp (0.7 oz)	50	13	0	0
Blackberry Jelly	1 tbsp (0.7 oz)	50	13	0	0
Blackberry Preserves	1 tbsp (0.7 oz)	50	13	0	0
Grape Jam	1 tbsp (0.7 oz)	60	14	0	0
Grape Jelly	1 tbsp (0.7 oz)	50	14	0	0
Grape Reduced Calorie	1 tbsp (0.6 oz)	20	5	0	0
Guava Jelly	1 tbsp (0.7 oz)	50	13	0	0
Orange Marmalade	1 tbsp (0.7 oz)	50	14	0	0
Peach Preserves	1 tbsp (0.7 oz)	50	14	0	0
Pineapple Preserves	1 tbsp (0.7 oz)	50	14	0	0
Red Currant Jelly	1 tbsp (0.7 oz)	50	13	0	0
Red Plum Jam	1 tbsp (0.7 oz)	60	13	0	0
Red Raspberry Preserves	1 tbsp (0.7 oz)	50	13	0	0
Strawberry Jam	1 tbsp (0.7 oz)	50	13	0	0
Strawberry Jelly	1 tbsp (0.7 oz)	60	14	0	0
Strawberry Preserves	1 tbsp (0.7 oz)	50	13	0	0
Strawberry Reduced Calorie	1 tbsp	20	5	0	0
Red Wing					
Apple Jelly	1 tbsp (0.7 oz)	50	13	0	0
Apple Blackberry Jelly	1 tbsp (0.7 oz)	50	13	0	0
Apple Cherry Jelly	1 tbsp (0.7 oz)	50	13	0	0
Apple Currant Jelly	1 tbsp (0.7 oz)	50	13	0	0
Apple Grape Jelly	1 tbsp (0.7 oz)	50	13	0	0
Apple Raspberry Jelly	1 tbsp (0.7 oz)	50	13	0	0
Apple Strawberry Jelly	1 tbsp (0.7 oz)	50	13	0	0

FOOD	PORTION	CALS.	CARB.	FAT	PRO.
Red Wing (CONT.)					
Black Raspberry Jelly	1 tbsp (0.7 oz)	50	13	0	0
Blackberry Jelly	1 tbsp (0.7 oz)	50	13	0	0
Cherry Jelly	1 tbsp (0.7 oz)	50	13	0	0
Concord Grape Jelly	1 tbsp (0.7 oz)	50	13	0	0
Crabapple Jelly	1 tbsp (0.7 oz)	50	13	0	0
Cranberry Jelly	1 tbsp (0.7 oz)	50	13	0	0
Cranberry Grape Jelly	1 tbsp (0.7 oz)	50	13	0	0
Currant Jelly	1 tbsp (0.7 oz)	50	13	0	0
Damson Plum Jelly	1 tbsp (0.7 oz)	50	13	0	0
Elderberry Jelly	1 tbsp (0.7 oz)	50	13	0	0
Grape Jelly	1 tbsp (0.7 oz)	50	13	0	0
Mint Jelly	1 tbsp (0.7 oz)	50	13	0	0
Mint Apple Jelly	1 tbsp (0.7 oz)	50	13	0	0
Mixed Fruit Jelly	1 tbsp (0.7 oz)	50	13	0	0
Red Plum Jelly	1 tbsp (0.7 oz)	50	13	0	0
Red Raspberry Jelly	1 tbsp (0.7 oz)	50	13	0	0
Strawberry Jelly	1 tbsp (0.7 oz)	50	13	0	0
Strawberry Apple Jelly	1 tbsp (0.7 oz)	50	13	0	0
S&W					
Apricot Pineapple Reduced Calorie Preserves	1 tsp	4	1	0	0
Blueberry Reduced Calorie Jam	1 tsp	4	1	0	0
Concord Grape Reduced Calorie Jelly	1 tsp	4	1	0	0
Orange Marmalade Reduced Calorie	1 tsp	4	1	0	0
Red Raspberry Reduced Calorie Jam	1 tsp	4	1	0	0
Red Tart Cherry Reduced Calorie Preserves	1 tsp	4	1	0	0
Strawberry Reduced Calorie Jam	1 tsp	4	1	0	0
Smucker's					
All Flavors Jam	1 tsp	18	4	0	0
All Flavors Jelly	1 tsp	18	4	0	0
All Flavors Low Sugar Spread	1 tsp	8	2	0	0
All Flavors Preserves	1 tsp	18	4	0	0
All Flavors Simply Fruit	1 tsp	16	4	0	0
All Flavors Single Serving Jelly	½ oz	38	9	0	0

FOOD	PORTION	CALS.	CARB.	FAT	PRO.
Smucker's (CONT.)					
All Flavors Single Serving Preserves	½ oz	38	9	0	0
All Flavors Slenderella	1 tsp	7	2	0	0
Apple Butter Autumn Harvest	1 tsp	12	3	0	0
Apple Butter Simply Fruit	1 tsp	12	3	0	0
Apple Butter Natural	1 tsp	12	3	0	0
Apple Cider Butter	1 tsp	12	3	0	0
Blackberry Single Serving Imitation Jelly	1 pkg (0.4 oz)	4	1	0	0
Cherry Single Serving Imitation Jelly	1 pkg (0.4 oz)	4	1	0	0
Grape Single Serving Imitation Jelly	1 pkg (0.4 oz)	4	1	0	0
Orange Marmalade	1 tsp	18	4	0	0
Peach Butter	1 tsp	15	4	0	0
Pumpkin Butter Autumn Harvest	1 tsp	12	3	0	0
Tree Of Life					
Apricot Fruit Spread	1 tbsp (0.6 oz)	45	12	0	0
Blueberry Fruit Spread	1 tbsp (0.6 oz)	35	9	0	0
Cherry Fruit Spread	1 tbsp (0.6 oz)	40	10	0	0
Grape Fruit Spread	1 tbsp (0.6 oz)	35	8	0	0
Peach Fruit Spread	1 tbsp (0.6 oz)	45	12	0	0
Raspberry Fruit Spread	1 tbsp (0.6 oz)	30	7	0	0
Strawberry Fruit Spread	1 tbsp (0.6 oz)	35	9	0	0
Weight Watchers					
Grape Spread	1 tsp	8	2	0	0
Raspberry Spread	1 tsp	8	2	0	0
Strawberry Spread	1 tsp	8	2	0	0
Whistling Wings					
Blueberry Jam	1 oz	50	12	tr	tr
Raspberry Jam	1 oz	60	14	tr	tr
White House					
Apple Butter	1 oz	50	12	0	0

JAPANESE FOOD
(*see* ORIENTAL FOOD)

JAVA PLUM

FOOD	PORTION	CALS.	CARB.	FAT	PRO.
fresh	1 cup	82	21	tr	1
fresh	3	5	1	tr	tr

FOOD	PORTION	CALS.	CARB.	FAT	PRO.

JELLY
(see JAM/JELLY/PRESERVE)

JERUSALEM ARTICHOKE
(see ARTICHOKE)

KALE
FRESH

FOOD	PORTION	CALS.	CARB.	FAT	PRO.
chopped cooked	½ cup	21	4	tr	1
raw chopped	½ cup	21	3	tr	1
scotch chopped cooked	½ cup	18	4	tr	1
Dole					
Chopped	½ cup	17	3	1	1
FROZEN					
chopped cooked	½ cup	20	4	tr	2

KEFIR

FOOD	PORTION	CALS.	CARB.	FAT	PRO.
kefir	3½ oz	66	5	4	3

KETCHUP

FOOD	PORTION	CALS.	CARB.	FAT	PRO.
ketchup	1 tbsp	16	4	tr	tr
ketchup	1 pkg (0.2 oz)	6	2	tr	tr
low sodium	1 tbsp	16	4	tr	tr
Del Monte					
Ketchup	1 tbsp (0.5 oz)	15	4	0	0
Estee					
Imitation Sodium Free	1 pkg (0.5 oz)	15	3	0	0
Hain					
Natural	1 tbsp	16	4	0	0
Natural No Salt Added	1 tbsp	16	4	0	0
Healthy Choice					
Ketchup	1 tbsp (0.5 oz)	10	2	0	0
Heinz					
Hot	1 tbsp	16	4	0	0
Lite	1 tbsp	14	3	0	0
	1 tbsp	8	2	0	0
Hunt's					
Ketchup	1 tbsp (0.6 oz)	15	4	0	0
No Salt Added	1 tbsp	20	5	tr	tr
McIlhenny					
Ketchup	1 tbsp (0.6 oz)	23	5	tr	tr
Spicy	1 tbsp (0.6 oz)	23	5	tr	tr
Muir Glen					
Organic	1 tbsp (0.6 oz)	15	3	0	0
Red Wing					
Extra Fancy	1 tbsp (0.6 oz)	20	5	0	0

FOOD	PORTION	CALS.	CARB.	FAT	PRO.
Smucker's					
Ketchup	1 tsp	8	2	0	0
Tree Of Life					
Ketchup	1 tbsp (0.5 oz)	10	3	0	0
Salsa Ketchup	1 tbsp (0.5 oz)	10	3	0	0
Weight Watchers					
Ketchup	2 tsp	8	2	0	0
KIDNEY					
beef simmered	3 oz	122	0	3	22
lamb braised	3 oz	117	1	3	20
veal braised	3 oz	139	0	5	22
KIDNEY BEANS					
CANNED					
kidney beans	1 cup	208	38	1	13
red	1 cup	216	40	1	13
B&M					
Red Baked Beans	8 oz	250	42	7	15
Eden					
Organic	½ cup (4.4 oz)	100	18	0	8
Friends					
Red Beans	8 oz	340	57	4	17
Goya					
Spanish Style	7.5 oz	140	29	1	13
Green Giant					
Dark Red	½ cup	90	20	0	7
Light Red	½ cup	90	20	0	7
Hunt's					
Red	4 oz	100	20	tr	6
Progresso					
Red	½ cup	100	21	tr	9
S&W					
Dark Red Lite 50% Less Salt	½ cup	120	22	0	7
Dark Red Premium	½ cup	120	22	1	6
Water Pack	½ cup	90	16	0	7
Trappey					
Dark Red	½ cup (4.5 oz)	130	22	1	8
Light Red	½ cup (4.5 oz)	120	22	1	6
Light Red New Orleans Style With Bacon	½ cup (4.5 oz)	110	20	1	6
Light Red With Jalapeno	½ cup (4.5 oz)	110	19	1	6
With Chili Gravy	½ cup (4.5 oz)	110	20	1	6

FOOD	PORTION	CALS.	CARB.	FAT	PRO.
Van Camp's					
Dark Red	½ cup (4.6 oz)	90	20	0	6
Light Red	½ cup (4.6 oz)	90	20	0	6
DRIED					
california red cooked	1 cup	219	40	tr	16
cooked	1 cup	225	40	1	15
red cooked	1 cup	225	40	1	15
royal red cooked	1 cup	218	39	tr	17
Arrowhead					
Red	¼ cup (1.6 oz)	160	29	1	11
Hurst					
Kidney Beans	1.2 oz	120	21	1	8
SPROUTS					
cooked	1 lb	152	21	3	22
raw	½ cup	27	4	tr	4

KIWI JUICE

After The Fall					
Kiwi Bear	1 cup (8 oz)	100	24	0	1

KIWIS

California Kiwifruit	2 (4.9 oz)	90	18	1	2
fresh	1 med	46	11	tr	1
Dole					
Kiwis	2	90	18	1	1
DRIED					
Sonoma					
Dried	7-8 pieces (1 oz)	90	19	1	2

KNISH

Brand's					
Cheese 'N Blueberry	1 (7 oz)	378	40	13	24
Cheese 'N Cherry	1 (7 oz)	378	40	13	24
Everything	1 (7 oz)	221	34	8	7
Kashe	1 (7 oz)	270	45	8	7
Potato	1 (7 oz)	290	47	9	6
Potato w/ Broccoli & Cheese	1 (7 oz)	312	33	15	12
Potato w/ Spinach & Mushroom	1 (7 oz)	214	32	8	6
Joshua's					
Coney Island Potato	1 (4.6 oz)	280	52	8	1
TAKE-OUT					
cheese & blueberry	1 (7 oz)	378	40	13	24
cheese & cherry	1 (7 oz)	378	40	13	24

FOOD	PORTION	CALS.	CARB.	FAT	PRO.
everything	1 (7 oz)	221	34	8	7
kashe	1 (7 oz)	270	45	8	7
potato	1 lg (7 oz)	332	49	12	8
potato	1 med (3.5 oz)	166	25	6	4
potato	1 (7 oz)	290	47	9	6
potato w/ broccoli & cheese	1 (7 oz)	312	33	15	12
potato w/ spinach & mushroom	1 (7 oz)	214	32	8	6

KOHLRABI

raw sliced	½ cup	19	4	tr	1
sliced cooked	½ cup	24	5	tr	1

KUMQUATS

fresh	1	12	3	tr	tr

LAMB

(see also LAMB DISHES)

FRESH

cubed lean only braised	3 oz	190	0	7	29
cubed lean only broiled	3 oz	158	0	6	24
ground broiled	3 oz	240	0	17	21
leg lean & fat Choice roasted	3 oz	219	14	14	22
loin chop w/ bone lean & fat Choice broiled	1 chop (2.3 oz)	201	0	15	16
loin chop w/ bone lean only Choice broiled	1 chop (1.6 oz)	100	0	5	14
rib chop lean & fat Choice broiled	3 oz	307	0	25	19
rib chop lean only Choice broiled	3 oz	200	0	11	24
shank lean & fat Choice braised	3 oz	206	0	11	24
shank lean & fat Choice roasted	3 oz	191	0	11	22
shoulder chop w/ bone lean & fat Choice braised	1 chop (2.5 oz)	244	0	17	21
shoulder chop w/ bone lean only Choice braised	1 chop (1.9 oz)	152	0	8	19
sirloin lean & fat Choice roasted	3 oz	248	0	21	21

FROZEN

New Zealand lean & fat cooked	3 oz	259	0	19	21

FOOD	PORTION	CALS.	CARB.	FAT	PRO.
New Zealand lean only cooked	3 oz	175	0	8	25

LAMB DISHES
TAKE-OUT
curry	¾ cup	345	22	17	26
moussaka	5.6 oz	312	16	21	15
stew	¾ cup	124	11	5	10

LAMBSQUARTERS
chopped cooked	½ cup	29	5	1	3

LECITHIN
(see SOY*)*

LEEKS
chopped cooked	¼ cup	8	2	tr	tr
cooked	1 (4.4 oz)	38	9	tr	1
freeze dried	1 tbsp	1	tr	0	tr
raw	1 (4.4 oz)	76	18	tr	2
raw chopped	¼ cup	16	4	tr	tr

LEMON
FRESH
lemon	1 med	22	12	tr	1
peel	1 tbsp	0	1	tr	tr
wedge	1	5	3	tr	tr
Dole					
Lemon	1	18	4	0	0

LEMON CURD
lemon curd made w/ egg	2 tsp	29	4	1	tr
lemon curd made w/ starch	2 tsp	28	6	—	tr

LEMON JUICE
bottled	1 tbsp	3	1	tr	tr
fresh	1 tbsp	4	1	0	tr
frzn	1 tbsp	3	1	tr	tr
After The Fall					
Spicy Lemon	1 can (12 oz)	150	37	0	tr
Realemon					
Juice	1 fl oz	6	2	0	0

LEMONADE
FROZEN
as prep w/ water	1 cup	100	26	tr	tr
not prep	1 can (6 oz)	397	103	tr	1

FOOD	PORTION	CALS.	CARB.	FAT	PRO.
Bright & Early					
Lemonade	8 fl oz	120	30	0	0
Minute Maid					
Country Style	8 fl oz	120	30	0	0
Cranberry Lemonade	8 fl oz	80	30	0	0
Lemonade	8 fl oz	110	29	0	0
Pink	8 fl oz	120	30	0	0
Raspberry	8 fl oz	120	30	0	0
Seneca					
as prep	8 fl oz	110	27	0	0
MIX					
powder as prep w/ water	9 fl oz	113	29	tr	0
powder w/ nutrasweet	1 pitcher (67 oz)	40	10	0	tr
4C					
Instant as prep	8 fl oz	80	20	0	0
Country Time					
Mix	8 fl oz	82	21	0	0
Pink	8 fl oz	82	21	0	0
Pink Sugar Free	8 fl oz	4	0	0	0
Sugar Free	8 fl oz	4	0	0	0
Crystal Light					
Mix	8 fl oz	5	0	0	0
Kool-Aid					
Mix	8 fl oz	99	25	0	0
Pink	8 fl oz	99	25	0	0
Sugar Free	8 fl oz	4	0	0	0
Sugar Sweetened Pink	8 fl oz	82	21	0	0
Wylers					
Drink Mix Unsweetened	8 oz	3	1	0	0
READY-TO-DRINK					
After The Fall					
Apple Raspberry	1 bottle (10 oz)	120	29	0	1
Crystal Geyser					
Juice Squeeze Pink	1 bottle (12 fl oz)	140	34	0	0
Diet Rite					
Salt/Sodium Free	8 fl oz	2	1	0	0
Fruitopia					
Lemonade	8 fl oz	120	29	0	0
Kool-Aid					
Koolers	1 pkg (8.45 fl oz)	120	32	0	0
Minute Maid					
Chilled	8 fl oz	110	28	0	0
Cranberry Chilled	8 fl oz	120	31	0	0

FOOD	PORTION	CALS.	CARB.	FAT	PRO.
Minute Maid (CONT.)					
Juices To Go	1 bottle (16 fl oz)	110	28	0	0
Juices To Go	1 can (11.5 fl oz)	160	40	0	0
Juices To Go Cranberry Lemonade	1 bottle (16 fl oz)	110	29	0	0
Juices To Go Raspberry Lemonade	1 bottle (16 fl oz)	120	29	0	0
Pink Chilled	8 fl oz	110	28	0	0
Raspberry Chilled	8 fl oz	120	30	0	0
Mott's					
Lemonade	10 fl oz	160	41	0	0
Nehi					
Lemonade	8 fl oz	130	35	0	0
Newman's Own					
Roadside Virginia	8 fl oz	100	22	tr	tr
Ocean Spray					
Lemonade	8 fl oz	110	29	0	0
With Cranberry Juice	8 fl oz	110	26	0	0
With Raspberry Juice	8 fl oz	110	27	0	0
Odwalla					
Honey	8 fl oz	70	26	0	0
Strawberry	8 fl oz	150	40	0	0
Royal Mistic					
Lemonade Limeade	16 fl oz	230	57	0	0
Tropical Pink	16 fl oz	230	57	0	0
Snapple					
Diet Pink	8 fl oz	13	3	0	0
Lemonade	8 fl oz	110	29	0	0
Pink	8 fl oz	110	26	0	0
Strawberry	8 fl oz	110	26	0	0
Tropicana					
Lemonade	1 can (11.5 oz)	160	39	0	tr
Lemonade	8 fl oz	110	28	0	tr
Twister Orange Cranberry	8 fl oz	130	32	0	0
Twister Wild Berry	8 fl oz	120	30	0	0
Turkey Hill					
Lemonade	8 fl oz	110	29	0	0
Veryfine					
Lemonade	8 fl oz	120	30	0	0
Wylers					
Lemonade	1 can (6 fl oz)	64	17	0	0

FOOD	PORTION	CALS.	CARB.	FAT	PRO.

LENTILS
CANNED
Health Valley

FOOD	PORTION	CALS.	CARB.	FAT	PRO.
Fast Menu Hearty Lentils Garden Vegetables	7½ oz	150	16	4	13
Fast Menu Organic Lentils With Tofu Weiner	7½ oz	170	15	5	15

DRIED

FOOD	PORTION	CALS.	CARB.	FAT	PRO.
cooked	1 cup	231	40	1	18

Hurst

FOOD	PORTION	CALS.	CARB.	FAT	PRO.
Lentils	1.2 oz	120	20	1	9

FROZEN
Natural Touch

FOOD	PORTION	CALS.	CARB.	FAT	PRO.
Lentil Rice Loaf	2.5 in slice (113 g)	200	18	11	8

MIX
Casbah

FOOD	PORTION	CALS.	CARB.	FAT	PRO.
Pilaf as prep	1 cup	200	38	tr	10

SPROUTS

FOOD	PORTION	CALS.	CARB.	FAT	PRO.
raw	½ cup	40	8	tr	3

LETTUCE
(*see also* SALAD)

FOOD	PORTION	CALS.	CARB.	FAT	PRO.
bibb	1 head (6 oz)	21	4	tr	2
boston	1 head (6 oz)	21	4	tr	2
boston	2 leaves	2	tr	tr	tr
iceberg	1 leaf	3	tr	tr	tr
iceberg	1 head (19 oz)	70	11	1	5
looseleaf shredded	½ cup	5	1	tr	tr
romaine shredded	½ cup	4	1	tr	tr

Dole

FOOD	PORTION	CALS.	CARB.	FAT	PRO.
Butter	1 head	21	4	tr	2
Iceberg	⅙ med head	20	4	0	1
Leaf shredded	1½ cup	12	1	0	1
Romaine shredded	1½ cups	18	2	1	1

Western Express

FOOD	PORTION	CALS.	CARB.	FAT	PRO.
Hearts Of Romaine	6 leaves (3 oz)	20	3	1	1

LIMA BEANS
CANNED

FOOD	PORTION	CALS.	CARB.	FAT	PRO.
large	1 cup	191	36	tr	12
lima beans	½ cup	93	17	tr	6

Allen

FOOD	PORTION	CALS.	CARB.	FAT	PRO.
Green	½ cup (4.5 oz)	120	23	1	7
Green & White	½ cup (4.5 oz)	110	20	1	6

FOOD	PORTION	CALS.	CARB.	FAT	PRO.
Del Monte					
Green	½ cup (4.4 oz)	80	15	0	4
East Texas Fair					
Green	½ cup (4.5 oz)	120	23	1	7
S&W					
Small Fancy	½ cup	80	16	0	6
Seneca					
Limas	½ cup	80	15	0	4
Trappey					
Baby Green With Bacon	½ cup (4.5 oz)	120	22	1	6
DRIED					
baby cooked	1 cup	229	42	1	15
cooked	½ cup	104	20	tr	6
large cooked	1 cup	217	39	1	15
FROZEN					
cooked	½ cup	94	18	tr	6
fordhook cooked	½ cup	85	16	tr	5
Birds Eye					
Baby	½ cup	130	24	0	7
Fordhook	½ cup	100	19	0	6
Fresh Like					
Baby	3.5 oz	138	25	1	7
Green Giant					
Harvest Fresh	½ cup	80	18	0	6
In Butter Sauce	½ cup	100	17	3	6
LIME					
fresh	1	20	7	tr	tr
LIME JUICE					
bottled	1 tbsp	3	1	tr	tr
fresh	1 tbsp	4	1	tr	tr
After The Fall					
Caribbean Lime	1 can (12 oz)	170	42	0	2
Key West	1 cup (8 oz)	100	25	0	1
Lifesavers					
Lime Punch	8 fl oz	140	34	0	0
Odwalla					
Summertime Lime	8 fl oz	90	23	0	0
Realime					
Juice	1 oz	6	2	0	0
LING					
blue raw	3½ oz	83	0	1	17
fresh baked	3 oz	95	0	1	21
fresh fillet baked	5.3 oz	168	0	1	37

FOOD	PORTION	CALS.	CARB.	FAT	PRO.
LINGCOD					
baked	3 oz	93	0	1	19
fillet baked	5.3 oz	164	0	2	34
LIQUOR/LIQUEUR					
(see also BEER AND ALE, CHAMPAGNE, DRINK MIXERS, MALT, WINE, WINE COOLERS)					
aquavit	3.5 oz	229	0	0	0
bloody mary	5 oz	116	5	tr	1
bourbon & soda	4 oz	105	0	0	0
coffee liqueur	1½ oz	174	24	tr	0
coffee w/ cream liqueur	1½ oz	154	10	7	1
cognac	3.5 oz	233	1	0	0
creme de menthe	1½ oz	186	21	tr	0
daiquiri	2 oz	111	4	0	0
gin	1½ oz	110	0	0	0
gin & tonic	7.5 oz	171	16	0	0
manhattan	2 oz	128	2	0	0
martini	2½ oz	156	tr	0	0
pina colada	4½ oz	262	40	3	1
rum	1½ oz	97	0	0	0
screwdriver	7 oz	174	18	tr	1
sloe gin fizz	2½ oz	132	4	0	0
tequila sunrise	5½ oz	189	15	tr	1
tom collins	7½ oz	121	3	0	tr
vodka	1½ oz	97	0	0	0
whiskey	1½ oz	105	tr	0	0
whiskey sour	3 oz	123	5	tr	tr
whiskey sour mix not prep	1 pkg (0.6 oz)	64	16	0	tr
LIVER					
(see also PATE)					
beef braised	3 oz	137	3	4	21
beef pan-fried	3 oz	184	7	7	23
chicken stewed	1 cup (5 oz)	219	1	8	34
duck raw	1 (1.5 oz)	60	2	2	8
goose raw	1 (3.3 oz)	125	6	4	15
lamb braised	3 oz	187	2	7	26
lamb fried	3 oz	202	3	11	22
pork braised	3 oz	141	3	4	22
sheep raw	3½ oz	131	0	4	21
turkey simmered	1 cup (5 oz)	237	5	8	34
veal braised	3 oz	140	2	6	18
veal fried	3 oz	208	3	10	25

FOOD	PORTION	CALS.	CARB.	FAT	PRO.
Dakota Lean					
Beef raw	3 oz	100	8	1	14
LOBSTER					
(*see also* CRAYFISH)					
CANNED					
Progresso					
Rock Lobster Sauce	½ cup	120	11	8	4
FRESH					
northern cooked	1 cup	142	2	1	30
northern cooked	3 oz	83	1	1	17
northern raw	1 lobster (5.3 oz)	136	1	1	28
northern raw	3 oz	77	tr	1	77
spiny steamed	3 oz	122	3	2	22
spiny steamed	1 (5.7 oz)	233	5	3	43
FROZEN					
Cajun Cookin'					
Crawfish Etouffee	12 oz	390	51	10	23
TAKE-OUT					
newburg	1 cup	485	13	27	46
LOGANBERRIES					
frzn	1 cup	80	19	tr	2
LONGANS					
fresh	1	2	tr	0	tr
LOQUATS					
fresh	1	5	1	tr	tr
LOTUS					
root raw sliced	10 slices	45	14	tr	2
root sliced cooked	10 slices	59	14	tr	1
seeds dried	1 oz	94	18	1	4
LOX					
(*see* SALMON)					
LYCHEES					
fresh	1	6	2	tr	tr
Ka-Me					
Whole Pitted In Syrup	15 pieces (5 oz)	130	32	0	0
MACADAMIA NUTS					
dried	1 oz	199	4	21	2
oil roasted	1 oz	204	4	22	2
Mauna Loa					
Candy Glazed	1 oz	170	11	14	1

FOOD	PORTION	CALS.	CARB.	FAT	PRO.
Mauna Loa (CONT.)					
Chocolate Covered	1 oz	170	12	13	2
Honey Roasted	1 oz	200	8	17	2
Macadamia Nut Brittle	1 oz	150	19	8	1
Roasted & Salted	1 oz	210	4	21	2

MACARONI
(see PASTA)

MACE
ground	1 tsp	8	1	1	tr

MACKEREL
CANNED
jack	1 cup	296	0	12	44
jack	1 can (12.7 oz)	563	0	23	84
Empress					
Jack	4 oz	140	0	8	19
FRESH					
atlantic cooked	3 oz	223	0	15	20
atlantic raw	3 oz	174	0	12	16
jack baked	3 oz	171	0	9	22
jack fillet baked	6.2 oz	354	0	18	45
king baked	3 oz	114	0	2	22
king fillet baked	5.4 oz	207	0	4	40
pacific baked	3 oz	171	0	9	22
pacific fillet baked	6.2 oz	354	0	18	45
spanish cooked	3 oz	134	0	5	20
spanish cooked	1 fillet (5.1 oz)	230	0	9	34
spanish raw	3 oz	118	0	5	16

MALT
nonalcoholic	12 fl oz	32	5	0	1
Bartles & Jaymes					
Malt Cooler Berry	12 fl oz	210	32	0	0
Malt Cooler Black Cherry	12 fl oz	190	30	0	0
Malt Cooler Light Berry	12 fl oz	140	29	0	0
Malt Cooler Mandarin Lemon	12 fl oz	210	34	0	0
Malt Cooler Margarita	12 fl oz	250	44	0	0
Malt Cooler Original	12 fl oz	180	27	0	0
Malt Cooler Peach	12 fl oz	200	31	0	0
Malt Cooler Pina Colada	12 fl oz	270	48	0	0
Malt Cooler Planter's Punch	12 fl oz	220	35	0	0
Malt Cooler Red Sangria	12 fl oz	190	29	0	0

FOOD	PORTION	CALS.	CARB.	FAT	PRO.
Bartles & Jaymes (CONT.)					
Malt Cooler Strawberry	12 fl oz	200	31	0	0
Malt Cooler Strawberry Daiquiri	12 fl oz	220	35	0	0
Malt Cooler Tropical	12 fl oz	220	36	0	0
Olde English					
Malt	12 oz	163	10	0	1
Schaefer					
Malt	12 oz	165	12	0	1
Schlitz					
Malt	12 oz	177	15	0	1
MALTED MILK					
chocolate as prep w/ milk	1 cup	229	30	9	9
chocolate flavor powder	3 heaping tsp (¾ oz)	79	18	1	1
natural flavor as prep w/ milk	1 cup	237	27	10	10
natural flavor powder	3 heaping tsp (¾ oz)	87	19	2	2
Kraft					
Instant Chocolate	3 tsp (0.7 oz)	80	17	1	1
Instant Chocolate as prep w/ 2% milk	1 serv (9.5 oz)	200	29	6	9
Instant Natural	3 tsp (0.7 oz)	90	15	2	3
Instant Natural as prep w/ 2% milk	1 serv (9.5 oz)	210	27	7	11
MANGO					
fresh	1	135	35	1	1
CANNED					
Ka-Me					
Mango	4 pieces (5 oz)	102	25	0	0
DRIED					
Sonoma					
Pieces	8 pieces (2 oz)	180	44	1	0
MANGO JUICE					
After The Fall					
Hawaiian Mango	1 can (12 oz)	180	45	0	0
Mango Ginger	1 can (12 oz)	150	35	0	tr
Kern's					
Nectar	6 fl oz	100	28	0	0
Libby					
Nectar	1 can (11.5 fl oz)	210	52	0	0

FOOD	PORTION	CALS.	CARB.	FAT	PRO.
Snapple					
Diet Mango Madness	8 fl oz	13	3	0	0
Mango Madness Cocktail	8 fl oz	110	29	0	0

MARGARINE

(see also BUTTER BLENDS, BUTTER SUBSTITUTES)

FOOD	PORTION	CALS.	CARB.	FAT	PRO.
squeeze soybean & cottonseed	1 tsp	34	0	4	tr
stick corn	1 tsp	34	0	4	0
stick corn	1 stick (4 oz)	815	1	91	1
stick salted	1 tsp	39	0	4	0
stick salted	1 stick (4 oz)	815	1	91	1
stick unsalted	1 stick (4 oz)	809	1	91	1
stick unsalted	1 tsp	34	0	4	0
tub corn	1 tsp	34	0	4	0
tub corn	1 cup	1626	1	183	2
tub diet	1 tsp	17	0	2	0
tub diet	1 cup	800	1	90	1
tub safflower	1 tsp	34	0	4	0
tub safflower	1 cup	1626	1	183	2
tub salted	1 tsp	34	0	4	0
tub salted	1 cup	1626	1	183	2
tub soybean salted	1 cup	1626	1	183	2
tub soybean salted	1 tsp	34	0	4	0
tub soybean unsalted	1 cup	1626	2	182	2
tub soybean unsalted	1 tsp	34	0	4	0
tub unsalted	1 cup	1626	0	182	0
tub unsalted	1 tsp	34	0	4	0
Blue Bonnet					
Stick	1 tbsp	100	0	11	0
Tub	1 tbsp	100	0	11	0
Whipped	1 tbsp	80	0	9	0
Chiffon					
Stick	1 tbsp	100	0	11	0
Tub	1 tbsp (0.5 oz)	100	0	11	0
Whipped	1 tbsp (0.3 oz)	70	0	7	0
Fleischmann's					
Stick	1 tbsp	100	0	11	0
Stick Light Corn Oil	1 tbsp	80	0	8	0
Stick Sweet Unsalted	1 tbsp	100	0	11	0
Hain					
Stick Safflower	1 tbsp	100	0	11	0
Stick Safflower Unsalted	1 tbsp	100	0	11	0

FOOD	PORTION	CALS.	CARB.	FAT	PRO.
Hain (CONT.)					
Tub Safflower	1 tbsp	100	0	11	0
Hollywood					
Safflower	1 tbsp	100	0	11	0
Safflower Unsalted Sweet	1 tbsp	100	0	11	0
Soft Spread	1 tbsp	90	1	10	0
Land O'Lakes					
Stick	1 tbsp (0.5 oz)	90	0	10	0
Stick With Sweet Cream	1 tbsp (0.5 oz)	90	0	10	0
Stick With Sweet Cream Unsalted	1 tbsp (0.5 oz)	90	0	10	0
Tub	1 tbsp (0.5 oz)	80	0	8	0
Tub With Sweet Cream	1 tbsp (0.5 oz)	80	0	8	0
Mazola					
Stick	1 tbsp (14 g)	100	0	11	0
Stick	1 cup (229 g)	1650	3	184	1
Stick Unsalted	1 tbsp (14 g)	100	0	11	0
Stick Unsalted	1 cup (229 g)	1635	0	184	0
Tub Diet	1 cup (235 g)	815	1	93	0
Tub Diet	1 tbsp (14 g)	50	0	6	0
Tub Light Corn Oil Spread	1 tbsp (14 g)	50	0	6	0
Nucanola					
Stick	1 tbsp (14 g)	90	0	10	0
Parkay					
Squeeze	1 tbsp (0.5 oz)	80	0	9	0
Stick	1 tbsp (0.5 oz)	90	0	10	0
Stick ⅓ Less Fat	1 tbsp (0.5 oz)	70	0	7	0
Tub	1 tbsp (0.5 oz)	60	0	7	0
Tub Light	1 tbsp (0.5 oz)	50	0	6	0
Tub Soft	1 tbsp (0.5 oz)	100	0	11	0
Tub Soft Diet	1 tbsp (0.5 oz)	50	0	6	0
Whipped	1 tbsp (0.3 oz)	70	0	7	0
Smart Beat					
Tub	1 tbsp	25	0	3	0
Tub Unsalted	1 tbsp	25	0	3	0
Touch Of Butter					
Squeeze	1 tbsp (0.5 oz)	80	0	9	0
Stick	1 tbsp (0.5 oz)	90	0	10	0
Tree Of Life					
Canola Soft	1 tbsp (0.5 oz)	100	0	11	0
Stick 100% Soy	1 tbsp (0.5 oz)	100	0	11	0

FOOD	PORTION	CALS.	CARB.	FAT	PRO.
Tree Of Life (CONT.)					
Stick 100% Soy Salt Free	1 tbsp (0.5 oz)	100	0	11	0
Stick Canola Soy	1 tbsp (0.5 oz)	100	0	11	0
Stick Canola Soy Salt Free	1 tbsp (0.5 oz)	100	0	11	0
Weight Watchers					
Stick Light	1 tbsp	60	0	7	0
Tub Extra Light	1 tbsp	50	0	6	0
Tub Extra Light Sweet Unsalted	1 tbsp	50	0	6	0

MARINADE
(see SAUCE)

MARJORAM

FOOD	PORTION	CALS.	CARB.	FAT	PRO.
dried	1 tsp	2	tr	tr	tr

MARSHMALLOW

FOOD	PORTION	CALS.	CARB.	FAT	PRO.
marshmallow	1 reg (0.3 oz)	23	6	0	tr
marshmallow	1 cup (1.6 oz)	146	37	tr	1
Campfire					
Large	2	40	10	0	0
Miniature	24	40	10	0	0
Joyva					
Twists Chocolate Covered	2 (1.5 oz)	190	21	4	1
Kraft					
Funmallows	4 (1.1 oz)	110	26	0	tr
Funmallows Miniature	½ cup (1.1 oz)	100	25	0	tr
Jet-Puffed	5 (1.2 oz)	110	27	0	tr
Marshmallow Creme	2 tbsp (0.4 oz)	40	10	0	0
Miniature	½ cup (1.1 oz)	100	25	0	tr
Teddy Bear Cocoa-Flavored	½ cup (1.1 oz)	100	23	0	1

MATZO

FOOD	PORTION	CALS.	CARB.	FAT	PRO.
egg	1 (1 oz)	111	22	1	4
egg & onion	1 (1 oz)	111	22	1	3
plain	1 (1 oz)	112	24	tr	3
whole wheat	1 (1 oz)	99	22	tr	4
Goodman's					
Matzo Ball Mix 50% Less Salt	2 tbsp (0.5 oz)	50	11	0	1
Matzo Ball Mix as prep	2 tbsp (0.5 oz)	60	12	0	2

FOOD	PORTION	CALS.	CARB.	FAT	PRO.
Horowitz Margareten					
Egg Milk Chocolate Coated	1 oz	97	16	4	3
Manischewitz					
American Matzo	1	115	22	2	3
Daily Thin Tea	1	103	22	tr	3
Dietetic Thins	1	91	19	tr	3
Egg Dark Chocolate Coated	½ matzo (1 oz)	97	17	3	2
Egg n' Onion	1	112	23	tr	3
Matzo Cracker Miniatures	10	90	20	tr	2
Matzo Farfel	1 cup	180	60	1	7
Matzo Meal	1 cup	514	109	1	13
Passover	1	129	27	tr	3
Passover Egg	1	132	27	2	4
Passover Egg Matzo Crackers	10	108	20	2	3
Salted Thin	1	100	21	tr	3
Unsalted	1	110	24	tr	3
Wheat Matzo Crackers	10	90	18	1	3
Whole Wheat w/ Bran	1	110	21	1	4
Streit's					
Dietetic	1 (1 oz)	100	23	0	3
Lightly Salted	1 (1 oz)	110	23	1	3
Matzoh Meal	¼ cup (1 oz)	110	24	1	3
Passover	1 (1 oz)	110	25	1	3
Unsalted	1 (0.9 oz)	100	22	1	3
Whole Wheat	1 (1 oz)	110	24	1	5

MAYONNAISE
(*see also* MAYONNAISE TYPE SALAD DRESSING, RELISH)

FOOD	PORTION	CALS.	CARB.	FAT	PRO.
mayonnaise	1 cup	1577	6	175	2
mayonnaise	1 tbsp	99	tr	11	tr
reduced calorie	1 tbsp	34	2	3	0
reduced calorie	1 cup	556	38	46	1
sandwich spread	1 tbsp	60	3	5	tr
BAMA					
Mayonnaise	1 tbsp	100	0	11	0
Bennett's					
Mayonnaise	1 tbsp	110	1	12	0
Best Foods					
Cholesterol Free Reduced Calorie	1 tbsp (15 g)	50	1	5	0

FOOD	PORTION	CALS.	CARB.	FAT	PRO.
Best Foods (CONT.)					
Cholesterol Free Reduced Calorie	1 cup (233 g)	760	17	75	1
Light	1 cup (233 g)	760	16	78	2
Light	1 tbsp (15 g)	50	1	5	tr
Real	1 tbsp	100	tr	11	tr
Real	1 cup	1570	tr	175	2
Hain					
Canola	1 tbsp	60	2	5	0
Canola	1 tbsp	100	tr	11	0
Cold Processed	1 tbsp	110	0	12	0
Eggless No Salt Added	1 tbsp	110	0	12	0
Light Low Sodium	1 tbsp	60	2	6	0
Real No Salt Added	1 tbsp	110	0	12	0
Safflower	1 tbsp	110	0	12	0
Hellman's					
Cholesterol Free Reduced Calorie	1 tbsp (15 g)	50	1	5	0
Cholesterol Free Reduced Calorie	1 cup (233 g)	760	17	75	1
Light Reduced Calorie	1 tbsp (15 g)	50	1	5	0
Light Reduced Calorie	1 cup (233 g)	760	16	78	2
Mayonnaise	1 tbsp	100	tr	11	tr
Mayonnaise	1 cup (220 g)	1570	1	173	2
Hollywood					
Canola	1 tbsp	100	tr	11	0
Mayonnaise	1 tbsp	110	0	12	0
Safflower	1 tbsp	100	0	12	0
Kraft					
Free	1 tbsp (0.6 oz)	10	2	0	0
Light	1 tbsp (0.5 oz)	50	1	5	0
Real	1 tbsp (0.5 oz)	100	0	11	0
McIlhenny					
Spicy	1 tbsp (0.5 oz)	108	1	12	tr
Red Wing					
"H" Style	1 tbsp (0.5 oz)	110	1	11	0
Smart Beat					
Canola Oil	1 tbsp	40	1	4	0
Corn Beat	1 tbsp	40	1	4	0
Weight Watchers					
Fat Free	1 tbsp	12	4	0	0
Light	1 tbsp	50	1	5	0

FOOD	PORTION	CALS.	CARB.	FAT	PRO.
Weight Watchers (CONT.)					
Low Sodium	1 tbsp	50	1	1	0

MAYONNAISE TYPE SALAD DRESSING
(*see also* MAYONNAISE, RELISH)

FOOD	PORTION	CALS.	CARB.	FAT	PRO.
home recipe	1 tbsp	25	2	2	1
home recipe	1 cup	400	38	24	11
mayonnaise type salad dressing	1 cup	916	56	78	2
mayonnaise type salad dressing	1 tbsp	57	4	5	tr
reduced calorie w/o cholesterol	1 tbsp	68	2	7	7
reduced calorie w/o cholesterol	1 cup	1084	36	107	tr
BAMA					
Dressing	1 tbsp	50	3	4	0
Miracle Whip					
Free	1 tbsp (0.6 oz)	15	3	0	0
Light	1 tbsp (0.5 oz)	40	3	3	0
Salad Dressing	1 tbsp (0.5 oz)	70	2	7	0
Smart Beat					
Dressing	1 tbsp (15 g)	12	3	0	0
Spin Blend					
Cholesterol Free	1 tbsp	40	2	4	0
Dressing	1 tbsp	60	3	5	0
Weight Watchers					
Fat Free Whipped Dressing	1 tbsp	16	4	0	0

MEAT STICKS

FOOD	PORTION	CALS.	CARB.	FAT	PRO.
jerky beef	1 oz	96	4	4	11
jerky beef	1 lg piece (0.7 oz)	67	3	3	8
smoked	1 (0.7 oz)	109	1	10	4
smoked	1 oz	156	2	14	6
Tombstone					
Beef Jerky	1 stick (0.5 oz)	35	tr	0	6
Beef Sticks	1 (0.8 oz)	110	0	10	3
Snappy Sticks	1 (0.8 oz)	110	tr	10	4

MEAT SUBSTITUTES
(*see also* BACON SUBSTITUTES, CHICKEN SUBSTITUTES, SAUSAGE SUBSTITUTES, TURKEY SUBSTITUTES)

FOOD	PORTION	CALS.	CARB.	FAT	PRO.
simulated sausage	1 link (25 g)	64	2	5	5
simulated sausage	1 patty (38 g)	97	4	7	7

FOOD	PORTION	CALS.	CARB.	FAT	PRO.
simulated meat product	1 oz	88	11	1	11
Boca Burgers					
Original	1 patty (2.5 oz)	110	9	2	14
Green Giant					
Harvest Burgers Original	1 (3 oz)	140	8	4	18
Harvest Direct					
TVP Beef Chunks	3.5 oz	280	32	1	52
TVP Beef Chunks Flavored	3.5 oz	250	30	1	48
TVP Beef Strips	3.5 oz	280	32	1	52
TVP Ground Beef	3.5 oz	280	32	1	52
TVP Ground Beef Flavored	3.5 oz	250	30	1	48
Jaclyn's					
Salisbury Steak Style Dinner	11 oz	260	37	8	16
Sirloin Strips Style Dinner	12 oz	290	37	6	16
Ken & Robert's					
Veggie Burger	1 (62 g)	110	19	2	5
Knox Mountain Farm					
Wheat Balls Mix	1 serv (1/10 pkg)	110	9	1	14
LaLoma					
Big Franks	1 (51 g)	110	2	6	11
Corn Dogs	1 (71 g)	190	15	8	13
Dinner Cuts	2 pieces (99 g)	110	2	1	22
Griddle Steaks	1 piece (54 g)	140	4	7	14
Nuteena	1/2 in slice (65 g)	160	6	12	8
Patty Mix	1/4 cup (16 g)	50	4	0	9
Redi-Burger	1/2 in slice (68 g)	130	5	6	14
Sandwich Spread	3 tbsp (48 g)	70	4	4	4
Savory Dinner Loaf Mix not prep	1/4 cup (16 g)	50	4	0	9
Savory Meatballs	7 (70 g)	190	7	8	22
Sizzle Burger	1 patty (71 g)	220	10	12	17
Sozzle Franks	2 (68 g)	170	3	13	10
Swiss Steak	1 piece (92 g)	170	7	10	14
Tender Bits	4 pieces (57 g)	80	5	3	9
Tender Rounds	6 pieces (73 g)	120	7	4	15
Vege-Burger	1/2 cup (108 g)	110	3	2	21
Vita-Burger Chunk	1/4 cup (21 g)	70	6	0	11
Vita-Burger Granules	3 tbsp (21 g)	70	6	0	11
Lightlife					
American Grill	2.75 oz	110	8	3	13

FOOD	PORTION	CALS.	CARB.	FAT	PRO.
Lightlife (CONT.)					
Barbecue Grill	2.75 oz	130	10	6	11
Smart Deli Slices	2 slices (1.5 oz)	44	1	0	8
Smart Dogs	1 (1.5 oz)	40	1	0	8
Smart Dogs To Go	1 (5 oz)	115	19	0	13
Vegetarian Sloppy Joe	4.3 oz	130	11	6	9
Midland Harvest					
Burger n' Loaf Chili w/o Beans	0.8 oz	90	7	3	9
Burger n' Loaf Herbs & Spice	3.2 oz	140	7	5	16
Burger n' Loaf Italian	3.2 oz	140	7	5	16
Burger n' Loaf Original	3.2 oz	140	7	5	16
Burger n' Loaf Sloppy Joe w/o Sauce	0.8 oz	80	9	2	8
Burger n' Loaf Taco	2.7 oz	90	7	2	7
Morningstar Farms					
Breaded Cutlet	1 patty (71 g)	230	12	14	14
Deli Franks	1 (35 g)	90	2	6	7
Sandwich Burger Pattie w/ Cheese	1 (4.75 oz)	370	32	17	21
Sandwich Pattie Biscuit	1 (3.5 oz)	280	31	11	13
Natural Touch					
Dinner Entree	1 patty (85 g)	230	6	14	20
Garden Pattie	1 (67 g)	120	8	4	11
Loaf Mix as prep	4 oz	180	12	7	18
Okara Pattie	1 (64 g)	160	7	10	11
Stroganoff Mix as prep	4 oz	90	10	3	4
Taco Mix as prep	2 tbsp	90	6	2	10
Sovex					
Better Than Burger?	½ cup (1.9 oz)	165	25	2	20
Spring Creek					
Soysage	1 patty (1.6 oz)	63	11	tr	4
White Wave					
Meatless Healthy Franks	1 (1.5 oz)	90	6	2	13
Meatless Jumbo Franks	1 (3 oz)	170	11	3	26
Meatless Sandwich Slices Beef	2 slices (1.6 oz)	90	8	0	14
Meatless Sandwich Slices Bologna	2 slices (1.6 oz)	120	5	8	8
Meatless Sandwich Slices Pastrami	2 slices (1.6 oz)	90	8	0	14
Meatless Healthy Franks	1 (1.5 oz)	90	6	2	13
Veggie Burger	1 patty (2.5 oz)	110	16	3	5

FOOD	PORTION	CALS.	CARB.	FAT	PRO.
Worthington					
Beef Style Meatless	4 slices (70 g)	130	7	6	12
Bolono	2 slices (38 g)	60	2	2	7
Choplets	2 slices (92 g)	100	4	2	18
Corn Beef Sliced	4 slices (57 g)	120	8	6	9
Country Stew	9.5 oz (270 g)	220	23	10	10
Dinner Roast	2 oz	120	5	8	7
FriPats	1 (64 g)	180	5	12	13
Granburger not prep	6 tbsp (33 g)	110	7	1	19
Multigrain Cutlet	2 slices (92 g)	90	5	2	14
Non-Meat Balls	3 (54 g)	100	5	6	6
Numete	½ in slice (68 g)	150	7	11	7
Prime Stakes	1 piece (92 g)	160	7	10	10
Prosage Patties	2 (76 g)	210	4	14	18
Prosage Roll	2⅜ in slice (70 g)	180	4	12	13
Protose	½ in slice (76 g)	180	9	8	17
Salami Meatless	2 slices (38 g)	70	2	4	7
Savory Slices	2 slices (56 g)	100	4	6	8
Smoked Beef Slices	6 slices (56 g)	120	7	6	10
Stakelets	1 piece (71 g)	150	7	8	13
Veelets	1 patty (71 g)	230	12	14	14
Vegetable Skallops	½ cup (85 g)	90	4	2	15
Vegetable Skallops No Added Salt	½ cup (85 g)	80	4	1	13
Vegetable Steaks	2.5 pieces (90 g)	110	5	2	17
Vegetarian Burger	½ cup (113 g)	150	9	4	19
Vegetarian Burger No Added Salt	½ cup (113 g)	150	7	4	22
Vegetarian Beef Pie	1 (227 g)	360	44	16	9
Wham	3 slices (68 g)	120	3	7	12
Zoglo's					
Crispy Vegetarian Cutlets	1 (3.5 oz)	200	10	10	20
Savory Vegetarian Kebabs	1 serv (2.8 oz)	135	5	5	18
Tender Vegetarian Burgers	1 (2.6 oz)	150	5	7	17
Vegetable Patties	1 (2.6 oz)	130	10	5	11
Vegetarian Franks	1 (2.6 oz)	125	5	5	15

MELON

(see also individual names)

FROZEN

| melon balls | 1 cup | 55 | 14 | tr | 1 |

FOOD	PORTION	CALS.	CARB.	FAT	PRO.
Big Valley					
Mixed	¾ cup (4.9 oz)	40	10	0	1

MEXICAN FOOD
(*see also* SALSA, SAUCE, TORTILLA)

MILK
(*see also* CHOCOLATE, COCOA, MILK DRINKS)

CANNED

FOOD	PORTION	CALS.	CARB.	FAT	PRO.
condensed sweetened	1 oz	123	21	3	3
condensed sweetened	1 cup	982	166	27	24
evaporated	½ cup	169	13	10	9
evaporated skim	½ cup	99	14	tr	10
Carnation					
Evaporated	2 tbsp	40	3	3	2
Evaporated Lowfat	2 tbsp	25	3	1	2
Lite Evaporated Skimmed	½ cup (4 fl oz)	100	14	tr	9
Sweetened Condensed	2 tbsp	130	22	3	3
Eagle					
Sweetened Condensed	⅓ cup	320	52	9	7
Pet					
Evaporated	½ cup	170	12	10	8
Evaporated Filled	½ cup	150	12	8	8
Evaporated Light Skimmed	½ cup	100	14	tr	9

DRIED

FOOD	PORTION	CALS.	CARB.	FAT	PRO.
buttermilk	1 tbsp	25	3	tr	2
nonfat instantized	1 pkg (3.2 oz)	244	47	tr	32
Carnation					
Nonfat	⅓ cup dry	80	12	0	8
Nutra/Balance					
Lactose Reduced as prep	8 oz	80	12	tr	8
Sanalac					
As Prep	8 oz	80	12	tr	8

REFRIGERATED

FOOD	PORTION	CALS.	CARB.	FAT	PRO.
1%	1 cup	102	12	3	8
1%	1 qt	409	47	10	32
1% protein fortified	1 qt	477	54	12	39
1% protein fortified	1 cup	119	14	3	10
2%	1 cup	121	12	5	8
2%	1 qt	485	47	19	33
buffalo	3½ oz	112	5	8	4
buttermilk	1 cup	99	12	2	8

FOOD	PORTION	CALS.	CARB.	FAT	PRO.
buttermilk	1 qt	396	47	9	32
camel	3½ oz	80	5	4	5
donkey	3½ oz	43	6	1	2
goat	1 cup	168	11	10	9
goat	1 qt	672	43	40	35
human	1 cup	171	17	11	3
Indian buffalo	1 cup	236	13	17	9
low sodium	1 cup	149	11	8	8
mare	3½ oz	49	6	2	2
sheep	1 cup	264	13	17	15
skim	1 cup	86	12	tr	8
skim	1 qt	342	48	2	33
skim protein fortified	1 qt	400	55	2	39
skim protein fortified	1 cup	100	14	1	10
whole	1 cup	150	11	8	8
BodyWise					
Nonfat	8 fl oz	100	14	0	10
Borden					
Acidophilus 1%	8 fl oz	100	11	2	8
Buttermilk Lowfat Golden Churn	8 fl oz	120	11	4	8
Hi-Calcium	8 fl oz	150	11	8	8
Hi-Protein 2%	8 fl oz	140	13	5	10
Milk	8 fl oz	150	11	8	8
Skim	8 fl oz	90	12	1	8
Skim-line	8 fl oz	100	13	1	10
CaliMilk					
CalciMilk	8 fl oz	102	12	3	8
Farmland					
1%	8 fl oz	100	12	3	8
2%	8 fl oz	130	12	5	8
Cholesterol Reduced	8 oz	150	11	8	8
Easylac 1%	8 fl oz	100	11	2	8
Easylac Nonfat	8 fl oz	90	12	0	8
Skim	8 fl oz	80	12	0	8
Skim Plus	8 fl oz	100	13	tr	10
Friendship					
Buttermilk	8 fl oz	120	12	4	9
Hood					
1%	1 cup (8 oz)	110	13	3	8
Better Taste 2%	1 cup (8 oz)	130	13	5	8
Buttermilk	1 cup (8 oz)	90	13	0	9
Whole	1 cup (8 oz)	150	12	8	8

FOOD	PORTION	CALS.	CARB.	FAT	PRO.
Lactaid					
1%	8 fl oz	102	12	3	8
Nonfat	8 fl oz	86	12	tr	8
Nuform					
1%	1 cup (8 oz)	120	15	3	10
Skim	1 cup (8 oz)	100	15	0	10
Silovet					
Skim	1 cup (8 oz)	90	13	0	9
Viva					
2%	8 fl oz	120	11	5	8
Skim	8 fl oz	100	13	1	10
Weight Watchers					
Milk	1 cup	90	13	tr	9
SHELF-STABLE					
Parmalat					
1%	1 cup (8 oz)	110	13	3	9
2%	1 cup (8 oz)	130	13	5	9
Skim	1 cup (8 oz)	90	13	1	8
Whole	1 cup (8 oz)	160	13	8	9

MILK DRINKS

(*see also* BREAKFAST DRINKS, CHOCOLATE, COCOA)

FOOD	PORTION	CALS.	CARB.	FAT	PRO.
chocolate milk	1 cup	208	26	8	8
chocolate milk	1 qt	833	103	34	32
chocolate milk 1%	1 cup	158	26	3	8
chocolate milk 1%	1 qt	630	104	10	32
chocolate milk 2%	1 cup	179	26	5	8
strawberry flavor mix as prep w/ whole milk	9 oz	234	33	8	8
Body Wise					
Chocolate Nonfat Milk	1 cup (8 fl oz)	180	35	0	11
Borden					
Chocolate Lowfat Dutch Brand	8 fl oz	180	25	5	8
Bosco					
Chocolate Milk	1 cup (8 fl oz)	230	33	8	8
Hershey					
Chocolate Milk 2%	1 cup	190	29	5	8
Whole Chocolate Milk	8 oz	210	28	9	7
Hood					
Chocolate Lowfat	1 cup (8 oz)	150	27	2	8
Lactaid					
Chocolate Milk 1%	8 fl oz	158	26	3	8
Meadow Gold					
Chocolate Milk	8 fl oz	210	25	8	8

FOOD	PORTION	CALS.	CARB.	FAT	PRO.
Parmalat					
Chocolate 2%	1 box (8 oz)	180	28	5	8
Quik					
Banana Lowfat Milk	8 oz	190	30	4	8
Chocolate	2½ tsp (0.75 oz)	90	20	1	1
Chocolate Lowfat Milk	8 oz	200	29	5	8
Chocolate as prep w/ 2% milk	8 oz	210	31	5	9
Chocolate as prep w/ skim milk	8 oz	170	31	1	9
Chocolate as prep w/ whole milk	8 oz	230	31	9	9
Ready To Drink Chocolate	8 oz	230	30	9	9
Ready To Drink Lite Chocolate Lowfat	8 oz	130	13	5	9
Ready To Drink Strawberry	8 oz	230	32	8	8
Strawberry	2½ tsp (0.75 oz)	80	21	0	0
Strawberry Lowfat Milk	8 oz	200	33	4	8
Strawberry as prep w/ 2% milk	8 oz	200	32	5	8
Strawberry as prep w/ skim milk	8 oz	160	32	0	8
Strawberry as prep w/ whole milk	8 oz	220	32	8	8
Sugar Free Chocolate	1 heaping tsp (5.8 g)	18	3	tr	1
Sugar Free Chocolate as prep w/ 2% milk	8 oz	140	15	5	9
Syrup Chocolate as prep w/ 2% milk	8 oz	220	34	5	9
Syrup Chocolate as prep w/ skim milk	8 oz	220	34	9	5
Syrup Chocolate as prep w/ whole milk	8 oz	240	33	9	8
Syrup Strawberry as prep w/ 2% milk	8 oz	220	36	5	8
Syrup Strawberry as prep w/ skim milk	8 oz	180	36	0	8
Syrup Strawberry as prep w/ whole milk	8 oz	240	36	8	8

FOOD	PORTION	CALS.	CARB.	FAT	PRO.
Quik (CONT.)					
Vanilla Lowfat Milk	8 oz	200	31	4	8

MILK SUBSTITUTES
(*see also* COFFEE WHITENERS)

FOOD	PORTION	CALS.	CARB.	FAT	PRO.
imitation milk	1 cup	150	15	8	4
imitation milk	1 qt	600	60	33	17
Better Than Milk					
Carob	8 fl oz	130	20	5	2
Chocolate	8 fl oz	125	17	5	2
Light	8 fl oz	80	15	tr	2
Natural	8 fl oz	90	10	5	2
Eden					
Original	1 pkg (8.8 oz)	135	14	4	10
Original	8 fl oz	130	13	4	10
EdenBlend					
Original	8 fl oz	120	16	3	7
EdenRice					
Milk	8 fl oz	110	21	3	1
Edensoy					
Carob	8 fl oz	150	23	4	6
Extra Original	8 fl oz	130	12	5	9
Extra Original	1 pkg (8.8 oz)	140	13	5	9
Extra Vanilla	1 pkg (8.8 fl oz)	150	24	3	6
Extra Vanilla	8 fl oz	140	23	3	6
Vanilla	8 fl oz	150	23	3	6
Vanilla	1 pkg (8.8 fl oz)	150	24	3	6
Health Valley					
Soo Moo	1 cup	120	12	6	6
Rice Dream					
Carob Lite	8 fl oz	150	32	3	1
Chocolate	8 fl oz	190	44	3	1
Lite Organic Original	8 fl oz	130	28	2	1
Lite Vanilla	8 fl oz	130	30	2	1
Spring Creek					
!Honey Vanilla	1 oz	23	3	5	1
Original	1 oz	21	3	5	2
Plain	1 oz	15	1	5	2
Vegelicious					
Milk	8 fl oz	100	18	2	2
Vitasoy					
Carob Supreme	8 fl oz	150	22	4	6
Cocoa Light	8 fl oz	140	25	2	5

FOOD	PORTION	CALS.	CARB.	FAT	PRO.
Vitasoy (CONT.)					
Cocoa Rich	8 fl oz	160	24	4	6
Original Creamy	8 fl oz	100	10	5	7
Original Light	8 fl oz	90	15	2	4
Vanilla Delite	8 fl oz	150	23	4	6
Vanilla Light	8 fl oz	110	20	2	4
Westsoy					
Cocoa Lite	8 fl oz	140	25	2	4
Plain Lite	8 fl oz	100	16	2	4
Vanilla Lite	8 fl oz	110	20	2	3
MILKFISH					
baked	3 oz	162	0	7	22
MILKSHAKE					
chocolate	10 oz	360	58	11	10
strawberry	10 oz	319	53	8	10
thick shake chocolate	10.6 oz	356	63	8	9
thick shake vanilla	11 oz	350	56	10	12
vanilla	10 oz	314	51	8	10
Frostee					
Chocolate	8 fl oz	200	30	8	2
Strawberry	8 fl oz	180	27	7	2
Hood					
Shake Up Chocolate	1 cup (8 oz)	240	38	6	9
Shake Up Strawberry	1 cup (8 oz)	220	36	5	8
Shake Up Vanilla	1 cup (8 oz)	220	36	5	8
MicroMagic					
Chocolate	1 (10.5 oz)	290	46	8	7
Milky Way					
Shake	1 (10 fl oz)	390	54	16	9
Parmalat					
Shake A Shake Chocolate	1 box (6 oz)	180	29	4	8
Shake A Shake Orange Vanilla	1 box (6 oz)	110	14	3	6
Shake A Shake Vanilla	1 box (6 oz)	170	28	3	8
Weight Watchers					
Chocolate Fudge	1 pkg	70	11	tr	6
Orange Sherbet	1 pkg	70	12	tr	6
MILLET					
cooked	½ cup	143	28	1	4

FOOD	PORTION	CALS.	CARB.	FAT	PRO.
MINERAL/BOTTLED WATER					
Canada Dry					
Sparkling Water	8 fl oz	0	0	0	0
Crystal Geyser					
Sparking Natural Wild Cherry	1 bottle 12 fl oz	0	0	0	0
Sparkling Lemon	1 bottle (12 fl oz)	0	0	0	0
Sparkling Mineral	1 bottle (12 fl oz)	0	0	0	0
Sparkling Natural Cola Berry	1 bottle (12 fl oz)	0	0	0	0
Sparkling Orange	1 bottle (12 fl oz)	0	0	0	0
Evian					
Water	1 liter	0	0	0	0
San Pellegrino					
Mineral Water	1 liter (33.8 oz)	0	0	0	0
Saratoga					
Sparkling	1 liter	0	0	0	0
MISO					
miso	½ cup	284	39	8	16
Eden					
Genmai Miso Organic	1 tbsp (0.5 oz)	25	3	1	2
Hacho Miso Organic	1 tbsp (0.5 oz)	35	2	2	3
Kome Miso Organic	1 tbsp (0.6 oz)	25	3	1	2
Mugi Miso Organic	1 tbsp (0.6 oz)	25	3	1	2
Shiro Miso Organic	1 tbsp (0.6 oz)	35	5	1	2
MOLASSES					
blackstrap	1 tbsp (0.7 oz)	47	12	0	0
blackstrap	1 cup (11.5 oz)	771	199	tr	0
molasses	1 tbsp (0.7 oz)	53	14	0	0
molasses	1 cup (11.5 oz)	873	226	1	0
Brer Rabbit					
Dark	2 tbsp	110	28	0	0
Light	2 tbsp	110	29	0	0
McIlhenny					
Molasses	1 tbsp (0.7 oz)	66	16	tr	tr
Tree Of Life					
Blackstrap	1 tbsp (0.5 oz)	45	11	0	0
MONKFISH					
baked	3 oz	82	0	2	16
MOOSE					
roasted	3 oz	114	0	1	25

FOOD	PORTION	CALS.	CARB.	FAT	PRO.
MOUSSE					
FROZEN					
Pepperidge Farm					
San Francisco Chocolate Mousse	1	490	41	34	4
Sara Lee					
Chocolate	1 slice (2.7 oz)	260	23	17	3
Chocolate Light	1 (3 oz)	170	20	8	4
Weight Watchers					
Chocolate	1 (2.5 oz)	160	27	3	6
Praline Pecan	1 (2.71 oz)	180	30	4	5
HOME RECIPE					
chocolate	½ cup (7.1 oz)	447	33	33	9
orange	½ cup	87	19	5	3
MIX					
Jell-O					
Rich & Luscious Chocolate	½ cup	145	21	6	5
Rich & Luscious Chocolate Fudge	½ cup	143	20	6	5
Knorr					
Dark Chocolate as prep	½ cup	90	10	5	2
Milk Chocolate as prep	½ cup	90	11	5	2
Unflavored as prep	½ cup	80	8	5	1
White Chocolate as prep	½ cup	80	10	4	2
Royal					
Chocolate Mousse No-Bake	⅛ pie	130	21	4	3
Weight Watchers					
Chocolate	½ cup	70	7	3	3
White Chocolate Almond Mousse	½ cup	70	7	3	3
TAKE-OUT					
chocolate	½ cup (7.1 oz)	447	33	33	9
MUFFIN					
FROZEN					
Health Valley					
Almond & Date Oat Bran Fancy Fruit	1	180	31	4	4
Fat Free Apple Spice	1	140	30	tr	4
Fat Free Banana	1	130	29	tr	4
Fat Free Raisin Spice	1	140	32	tr	4
Oat Bran Fancy Fruit Blueberry	1	140	32	4	4

FOOD	PORTION	CALS.	CARB.	FAT	PRO.
Health Valley (CONT.)					
Oat Bran Fancy Fruit Raisin	1	180	5	5	4
Rice Bran Fancy Fruit Raisin	1	210	7	7	5
Pepperidge Farm					
Banana Nut	1	170	28	6	3
Blueberry	1	170	27	7	2
Cholesterol Free Multi Grain Muesli	1	200	30	8	4
Cholesterol Free Oatbran With Apple	1	190	29	7	3
Cholesterol Free Raisin Bran	1	170	30	6	4
Cinnamon Swirl	1	190	30	6	2
Corn	1	180	27	7	3
Sara Lee					
Apple Oat Bran	1	190	36	6	6
Apple Spice	1	220	36	8	4
Blueberry	1	200	34	8	3
Blueberry Free & Light	1	120	28	0	3
Cheese Streusel	1	220	27	11	4
Chocolate Chunk	1	220	33	8	3
Golden Corn	1	240	31	13	5
Oat Bran	1	210	35	8	4
Raisin Bran	1	220	37	7	4
Weight Watchers					
Banana Nut	1 (2.5 oz)	170	32	5	3
Blueberry	1 (2.5 oz)	170	32	5	3
HOME RECIPE					
blueberry as prep w/ 2% milk	1 (2 oz)	163	23	6	4
blueberry as prep w/ whole milk	1 (2 oz)	165	23	6	6
corn as prep w/ 2% milk	1 (2 oz)	180	25	7	4
corn as prep w/ whole milk	1 (2 oz)	183	25	7	4
plain as prep w/ 2% milk	1 (2 oz)	169	24	7	4
plain as prep w/ whole milk	1 (2 oz)	172	24	7	4
wheat bran as prep w/ 2% milk	1 (2 oz)	161	24	7	4
wheat bran as prep w/ whole milk	1 (2 oz)	164	24	7	4
MIX					
blueberry	1 (1¾ oz)	149	24	4	3

FOOD	PORTION	CALS.	CARB.	FAT	PRO.
corn	1 (1.75 oz)	160	25	5	4
wheat bran as prep	1 (1¾ oz)	138	23	5	5
Arrowhead					
Bran	⅓ cup (1.4 oz)	150	26	2	7
Oat Bran Wheat Free	⅓ cup (1.5 oz)	160	23	4	7
Betty Crocker					
Apple Cinnamon	1	120	18	4	2
Apple Cinnamon No Cholesterol Recipe	1	110	18	2	2
Banana Nut	1	120	17	5	2
Banana Nut No Cholesterol Recipe	1	110	17	4	2
Blueberry Streusel Bake Shop	1	210	31	8	3
Cinnamon Streusel	1	200	17	9	2
Oat Bran	1	190	25	8	4
Oat Bran No Cholesterol Recipe	1	180	25	7	4
Twice The Blueberries	1	120	18	4	2
Twice The Blueberries No Cholesterol Recipe	1	110	18	3	2
Wild Blueberry	1	120	18	4	2
Wild Blueberry Light	1	70	16	tr	1
Wild Blueberry Light No Cholesterol Recipe	1	70	16	tr	1
Wild Blueberry No Cholesterol Recipe	1	110	18	3	2
Dromedary					
Corn Muffin	1	120	20	4	3
Flako					
Corn	⅓ cup (1.4 oz)	160	29	4	3
Hain					
Oat Bran Apple Cinnamon	1	140	28	3	4
Oat Bran Banana Nut	1	140	26	4	4
Oat Bran Raspberry Spice	1	140	27	3	5
Jiffy					
Apple Cinnamon as prep	1	190	28	7	2
Banana Nut as prep	1	180	25	7	2
Blueberry as prep	1	190	28	7	2
Bran With Dates as prep	1	170	26	6	2
Corn as prep	1	180	28	4	2
Honey Date as prep	1	170	27	5	2

FOOD	PORTION	CALS.	CARB.	FAT	PRO.
Jiffy (CONT.)					
Oatmeal as prep	1	180	26	7	2
Wanda's					
Blue Corn	¼ cup mix per serv (1.2 oz)	130	25	1	4
READY-TO-EAT					
blueberry	1 (2 oz)	158	27	4	3
corn	1 (2 oz)	174	29	5	3
oat bran wheat free	1 (2 oz)	154	28	4	4
toaster type blueberry	1	103	18	3	2
toaster type corn	1	114	19	4	2
toaster type wheat bran w/ raisins	1 (36 g)	106	19	3	2
Arnold					
Bran'nola	1 (2.3 oz)	160	30	1	6
Raisin	1 (2.3 oz)	160	33	1	6
Dutch Mill					
Apple Oat Bran	1 (2 oz)	180	31	5	3
Banana Walnut	1 (2 oz)	220	33	6	3
Carrot	1 (2 oz)	190	31	7	3
Corn	1 (2 oz)	190	31	6	4
Cranberry Orange	1 (2 oz)	170	26	6	3
Raisin Bran	1 (2 oz)	230	37	5	2
Entenmann's					
Blueberry	1 (2 oz)	200	29	8	3
Freihofer's					
Corn Toasters	1 (1.3 oz)	130	18	6	2
Hostess					
Mini Apple Cinnamon	5 (2 oz)	260	28	16	3
Mini Banana Nut	5 (2 oz)	260	28	16	3
Mini Blueberry	5 (2 oz)	240	30	13	3
Mini Chocolate Chip	5 (2 oz)	260	29	15	3
Muffin Loaf Blueberry	1 (3.8 oz)	440	62	19	5
Oat Bran	1 (1.5 oz)	160	22	8	2
Oat Bran Banana Nut	1 (1.5 oz)	150	22	6	2
Weight Watchers					
Apple Cinnamon	1 (2.5 oz)	200	36	5	4
Lemon Poppy Seed	1 (2.5 oz)	200	37	5	4
MULBERRIES					
fresh	1 cup	61	14	1	2
MULLET					
striped cooked	3 oz	127	0	4	21
striped raw	3 oz	99	0	3	16

FOOD	PORTION	CALS.	CARB.	FAT	PRO.
MUNG BEANS					
DRIED					
cooked	1 cup	213	39	1	14
SPROUTS					
canned	½ cup	8	1	tr	1
cooked	½ cup	13	3	tr	1
raw	½ cup	16	3	tr	2
stir fried	½ cup	31	7	tr	3
MUNGO BEANS					
dried cooked	1 cup	190	33	1	14
MUSHROOMS					
CANNED					
chanterelle	3½ oz	12	tr	1	1
pieces	½ cup	19	4	tr	1
whole	1 (0.4 oz)	3	1	tr	tr
B In B					
Mushrooms	¼ cup	12	2	0	1
With Garlic	¼ cup	12	2	0	1
Empress					
Button	2 oz	14	2	0	1
Button Sliced	2 oz	14	2	0	1
Pieces & Stems	2 oz	14	2	0	1
Straw Broken	2 oz	10	2	0	1
Green Giant					
Oriental Straw	¼ cup	12	2	0	1
Pieces And Stems	¼ cup	12	2	0	1
Sliced	¼ cup	12	2	0	1
Whole	¼ cup	12	2	0	1
Ka-Me					
Stir Fry	½ cup (4.5 oz)	20	3	0	2
Straw Whole Peeled	½ cup (4.5 oz)	20	3	0	2
Seneca					
Mushrooms	½ cup	25	3	0	0
DRIED					
chanterelle	3½ oz	89	2	2	17
shitake	4 (½ oz)	44	11	tr	1
FRESH					
chanterelle	3½ oz	11	tr	tr	2
enoki raw	1 (4 in)	2	tr	tr	tr
morel	3½ oz	9	0	tr	2
oyster	3.5 oz	11	0	tr	2
raw	1 (½ oz)	5	1	tr	tr
raw sliced	½ cup	9	2	tr	1

FOOD	PORTION	CALS.	CARB.	FAT	PRO.
shitake cooked	4 (2.5 oz)	40	10	tr	1
sliced cooked	½ cup	21	4	tr	2
whole cooked	1 (0.4 oz)	3	1	tr	tr
FROZEN					
Empire					
Breaded	7 (2.8 oz)	90	16	1	4
Fresh Like					
Mushrooms	3.5 oz	28	4	tr	3
MUSKRAT					
roasted	3 oz	199	0	10	26
MUSSELS					
blue raw	3 oz	73	3	2	10
blue raw	1 cup	129	6	3	18
fresh blue cooked	3 oz	147	6	4	20
MUSTARD					
dry mustard seed yellow	1 tsp	15	1	1	1
yellow ready-to-use	1 tsp	5	tr	tr	tr
Blanchard & Blanchard					
Mustard	1 tsp (5 g)	0	0	0	0
Eden					
Hot Organic	1 tsp (5 g)	0	tr	0	0
Estee					
Sodium Free	1 pkg (0.5 oz)	5	tr	1	tr
Grey Poupon					
Country Dijon	1 tsp	6	0	0	0
Dijon	1 tsp	6	0	0	0
Parisian	1 tsp	6	0	0	0
Hain					
Stone Ground	1 tbsp	14	1	1	1
Stone Ground No Salt Added	1 tbsp	14	1	1	1
Heinz					
Mild Yellow	1 tbsp	8	1	tr	1
Spicy Brown	1 tbsp	14	1	1	1
Ka-Me					
Hot Mustard Powder Chinese Style	¼ tsp (1 g)	5	1	0	0
Kosciuszko					
Spicy Brown	1 tsp	5	tr	tr	tr
Kraft					
Mustard	1 tsp (0.2 oz)	0	0	0	0
McIlhenny					
Coarse Ground	1 tsp (0.2 oz)	4	tr	tr	tr

FOOD	PORTION	CALS.	CARB.	FAT	PRO.
McIlhenny (CONT.)					
Spicy	1 tsp (0.2 oz)	6	tr	tr	tr
Plochman					
Dijon	1 tsp (5 g)	7	tr	tr	tr
Spoonable Salad	1 tsp (5 g)	4	tr	tr	tr
Squeeze Salad	1 tsp (5 g)	4	tr	tr	tr
Stone Ground	1 tsp (5 g)	6	tr	tr	tr
Russer					
Deli	1 tsp (5 g)	4	0	0	0
Tree Of Life					
Dijon	1 tsp (5 g)	0	0	0	0
Dijon Imported	1 tsp (5 g)	5	tr	0	tr
Low Sodium	1 tsp (5 g)	3	tr	0	tr
Stone Ground	1 tsp (5 g)	0	0	0	0
Yellow	1 tsp (5 g)	0	0	0	0
Watkins					
Country Mill	1 tsp (7 oz)	15	2	1	0
Dusseldorf	1 tsp (7 oz)	10	1	0	0
Horseradish	1 tsp (7 oz)	10	1	0	0
Jalapeno	1 tsp (7 oz)	10	1	0	0
Onion	1 tsp (7 oz)	10	1	0	0
Parisienne	1 tsp (7 oz)	10	1	0	0

MUSTARD GREENS
CANNED
Allen

Mustard Greens	½ cup (4.1 oz)	30	5	1	1
Sunshine					
Mustard Greens	½ cup (4.1 oz)	30	5	1	1
FRESH					
chopped cooked	½ cup	11	2	tr	2
raw chopped	½ cup	7	1	tr	1
FROZEN					
chopped cooked	½ cup	14	2	tr	2

NATTO

natto	½ cup	187	13	10	16

NAVY BEANS
CANNED

navy	1 cup	296	54	1	20
Allen					
Navy Beans	½ cup (4.5 oz)	110	19	1	6
Eden					
Organic	½ cup (4.3 oz)	100	18	1	6

FOOD	PORTION	CALS.	CARB.	FAT	PRO.
Trappey					
With Bacon	½ cup (4.5 oz)	110	17	2	6
With Bacon & Jalapeno	½ cup (4.5 oz)	110	17	2	6
DRIED					
cooked	1 cup	259	48	1	16

NECTARINE

fresh	1	67	16	1	1
Dole					
Nectarine	1	70	16	1	1

NEUFCHATEL

neufchatel	1 oz	74	1	7	3
neufchatel	1 pkg (3 oz)	221	3	20	8
Philadelphia					
Neufchatel	1 oz	70	tr	6	3
Spreadery					
Classic Ranch	2 tbsp (1 oz)	60	1	7	3
Garden Vegetable	2 tbsp (1 oz)	70	2	6	3
Garlic & Herb	2 tbsp (1 oz)	80	1	7	3
With Strawberry	1 oz	70	tr	5	2
WisPride					
Garden Vegetable Cup	2 tbsp (1.1 oz)	60	2	5	3
Garlic & Herb Cup	2 tbsp (1.1 oz)	60	2	5	3

NON-DAIRY CREAMERS
(see COFFEE WHITENERS)

NON-DAIRY WHIPPED TOPPINGS
(see WHIPPED TOPPINGS)

NOODLES
(see also PASTA DINNERS)

CANNED					
Dinty Moore					
Noodles & Chicken	1 can (7.5 oz)	180	19	8	7
Micro Cup Meals					
Noodles & Chicken	1 cup (10.4 oz)	250	27	11	10
Noodles & Chicken	1 cup (7.5 oz)	180	19	8	7
Van Camp's					
Noodlee Weenee	1 can (8 oz)	230	34	8	7
DRY					
cellophane	1 cup	492	121	tr	tr
chow mein	1 cup	237	26	14	4
egg	1 cup (38 g)	145	27	2	5
egg cooked	1 cup	212	40	2	8

FOOD	PORTION	CALS.	CARB.	FAT	PRO.
japanese soba	2 oz	192	43	tr	8
japanese soba cooked	½ cup	56	12	tr	3
japanese somen	2 oz	203	42	tr	6
japanese somen cooked	½ cup	115	24	tr	4
spinach/egg	1 cup	145	27	2	6
spinach/egg cooked	1 cup	211	39	3	8
Azumaya					
Chinese	4 oz	293	60	1	11
Japanese	4 oz	289	59	1	11
Creamette					
Egg not prep	2 oz	220	40	3	8
Golden Grain					
Egg	2 oz	210	39	2	8
Hodgson Mill					
Veggie Egg not prep	2 oz	200	37	2	9
Whole Wheat Spinach Egg not prep	2 oz	190	32	2	10
Whole Wheat Egg not prep	2 oz	190	34	2	10
Ka-Me					
Chinese Egg	½ cup (2 oz)	210	40	2	7
Chinese Plain	½ cup (2 oz)	200	45	0	5
Chuka Soba Curly Noodles	2 oz	200	42	1	6
Lo Mein Wide Chinese	½ cup (2 oz)	200	45	0	5
Py Mai Fun Rice Sticks	2 oz	193	48	0	0
Sai Fun Bean Thread	1 cup (2 oz)	190	50	0	0
Soba Shin Shu Japanese Buckwheat	2 oz	200	40	1	9
Tomoshiraga Somen Noodles	2 oz	190	41	1	5
Udon Japanese Thick	2 oz	190	41	1	5
La Choy					
Chow Mein Narrow	½ cup	150	16	8	3
Chow Mein Wide	½ cup	150	16	8	3
Rice	½ cup	130	21	5	2
Mueller's					
Egg	2 oz (57 g)	220	40	3	8
Noodle Trio	2 oz (57 g)	220	40	2	8
Noodles By Leonardo					
Egg Fine not prep	1 cup (2 oz)	210	39	2	9
Egg Medium not prep	1 cup (2 oz)	210	39	2	9
Egg Wide not prep	1 cup (2 oz)	210	39	2	9

FOOD	PORTION	CALS.	CARB.	FAT	PRO.
San Giorgio					
Egg	2 oz	210	38	3	10
Shofar					
No Yolks	2 oz	210	41	0	91
FRESH					
Herb's					
Egg Fine	2 oz	220	42	2	10
Egg Medium	2 oz	220	42	2	10
Kluski Medium	2 oz	220	42	2	10
Kluski Wide	2 oz	220	42	2	10
FROZEN					
Luigino's					
Stroganoff	1 cup (7.5 oz)	290	23	16	13
Stroganoff	1 pkg (8 oz)	310	25	17	14
MIX					
Kraft					
Chicken Egg Noodle	1 cup	330	45	12	10
La Choy					
Ramen Noodles Chicken as prep	1 cup	200	29	7	6
Ramen Noodles Beef as prep	1 cup	200	33	8	6
Lipton					
Noodles & Sauce Alfredo	½ cup	131	20	3	5
Noodles & Sauce Beef	½ cup	120	22	2	5
Noodles & Sauce Butter	½ cup	142	22	4	5
Noodles & Sauce Butter & Herb	½ cup	136	22	3	5
Noodles & Sauce Carbonara Alfredo	½ cup	126	20	3	5
Noodles & Sauce Cheese	½ cup	136	24	2	5
Noodles & Sauce Chicken	½ cup	125	22	2	5
Noodles & Sauce Chicken Broccoli	½ cup	124	22	2	5
Noodles & Sauce Creamy Chicken	½ cup	125	22	2	5
Noodles & Sauce Parmesan	½ cup	138	20	4	5
Noodles & Sauce Romanoff	½ cup	136	23	3	5
Noodles & Sauce Sour Cream & Chive	½ cup	142	23	3	5
Noodles & Sauce Stroganoff	½ cup	110	19	2	4

FOOD	PORTION	CALS.	CARB.	FAT	PRO.
Lipton (CONT.)					
Noodles & Sauce Tomato Alfredo	½ cup	126	20	3	5
Minute					
Microwave Chicken Flavored	½ cup	157	23	5	6
Microwave Parmesan	½ cup	178	24	6	6
Noodle Roni					
Chicken & Mushroom	½ cup	160	25	4	6
Fettuccini	½ cup	300	29	18	7
Herb & Butter	½ cup	160	19	7	5
Parmesano	½ cup	240	23	13	7
Romanoff	½ cup	240	28	11	8
Stroganoff	½ cup	350	37	17	11
Noodles By Leonardo					
Macaroni & Cheese as prep	1 cup (2.5 oz)	250	49	1	10
Ultra Slim-Fast					
Noodles & Alfredo Sauce	2.3 oz	240	47	4	9
Noodles & Beef	2.3 oz	230	45	3	8
Noodles & Cheese	2.3 oz	230	44	4	9
Noodles & Chicken Sauce	2.3 oz	220	45	3	8
Noodles & Tomato Herb Sauce	2.3 oz	220	46	3	8
TAKE-OUT					
noodle pudding	½ cup	132	11	7	6
NOPALES					
cooked	1 cup (5.2 oz)	23	5	tr	2
raw sliced	½ cup (1.5 oz)	7	1	tr	1
raw sliced	1 cup (3 oz)	14	3	tr	1
NUTMEG					
ground	1 tsp	12	1	1	tr
Watkins					
Ground	¼ tsp (0.5 g)	0	0	0	0
NUTRITIONAL SUPPLEMENTS					
(*see also* BREAKFAST BAR, BREAKFAST DRINKS)					
DIET					
Dynatrim					
Dutch Chocolate as prep w/ 1% milk	8 oz	220	33	4	17
Strawberry Royale as prep w/ 1% milk	8 oz	220	33	4	17

FOOD	PORTION	CALS.	CARB.	FAT	PRO.
Dynatrim (CONT.)					
Vanilla as prep w/ 1% milk	8 oz	220	33	4	17
Figurines					
Chocolate	1 bar	100	11	5	2
Chocolate Caramel	1 bar	100	10	6	2
Chocolate Peanut Butter	1 bar	100	10	6	3
S'Mores	1 bar	100	11	5	2
Vanilla	1 bar	100	11	5	2
Sego					
Lite Chocolate	10 fl oz	150	20	3	11
Lite Dutch Chocolate	10 fl oz	150	20	3	11
Lite French Vanilla	10 fl oz	150	17	4	11
Lite Strawberry	10 fl oz	150	17	4	11
Lite Vanilla	10 fl oz	150	17	4	11
Very Chocolate	10 fl oz	225	43	1	11
Very Chocolate Malt	10 fl oz	225	43	1	11
Very Strawberry	10 fl oz	225	34	5	11
Very Vanilla	10 fl oz	225	34	5	11
Slim-Fast					
Powder Chocolate as prep w/ skim milk	8 oz	190	32	1	14
Powder Chocolate Malt as prep w/ skim milk	8 oz	190	32	tr	14
Powder Strawberry as prep w/ skim milk	8 oz	190	32	1	14
Powder Vanilla as prep w/ skim milk	8 oz	190	32	1	14
Sweet Success					
Chewy Bar Chocolate Brownie	1 (1.6 oz)	120	28	4	2
Chewy Bar Chocolate Peanut Butter	1 (1.6 oz)	120	23	4	2
Chewy Bar Chocolate Raspberry	1 (1.6 oz)	120	23	4	2
Chewy Bar Chocolate Chip	1 (1.6 oz)	120	23	4	2
Chewy Bar Oatmeal Raisin	1 (1.6 oz)	120	23	4	2
Chocolate Raspberry Truffle	1 can (10 fl oz)	200	38	3	12
Chocolate Raspberry as prep w/ skim milk	9 fl oz	180	30	1	14
Chocolate Mocha Supreme	1 can (10 fl oz)	200	38	3	12

FOOD	PORTION	CALS.	CARB.	FAT	PRO.
Sweet Success (CONT.)					
Chocolate Mocha Supreme as prep w/ skim milk	9 fl oz	180	30	tr	14
Classic Chocolate Chip as prep w/ skim milk	9 fl oz	180	30	1	14
Creamy Milk Chocolate	1 can (10 fl oz)	200	38	3	12
Creamy Milk Chocolate	1 carton (12 fl oz)	220	45	2	14
Creamy Milk Chocolate as prep w/ skim milk	9 fl oz	180	30	1	14
Creamy Vanilla Delight as prep w/ skim milk	9 fl oz	180	33	tr	14
Dark Chocolate Fudge	1 can (10 fl oz)	200	38	3	12
Dark Chocolate Fudge	1 carton (12 fl oz)	220	45	2	14
Dark Chocolate Fudge as prep w/ skim milk	9 fl oz	180	30	1	14
Rich Chocolate Almond	1 can (10 fl oz)	200	38	3	12
Rich Chocolate Almond	1 carton (12 fl oz)	220	45	2	14
Rich Chocolate Almond as prep w/ skim milk	9 fl oz	180	30	tr	14
Smooth Vanilla Creme	1 can (10 fl oz)	200	38	3	12
Ultra Slim-Fast					
Cafe Mocha as prep w/ skim milk	8 oz	200	38	tr	15
Chocolate Royale as prep w/ skim milk	8 oz	200	36	1	14
Crunch Bar Cocoa Almond	1	110	19	3	2
Crunch Bar Cocoa Raspberry	1	100	21	3	2
Crunch Bar Vanilla Almond	1	110	18	4	2
Dutch Chocolate as prep w/ water	8 oz	220	40	tr	14
French Vanilla as prep w/ skim milk	8 oz	190	36	tr	14
French Vanilla as prep w/ water	8 oz	220	40	tr	14
Fruit Juice Mix as prep w/ fruit juice	8 oz	200	43	tr	11
Nutrition Bar Dutch Chocolate	1	130	17	4	6
Nutrition Bar Peanut Butter	1	140	15	6	7

FOOD	PORTION	CALS.	CARB.	FAT	PRO.
Ultra Slim-Fast (CONT.)					
Pina Colada as prep w/ skim milk	8 oz	180	36	tr	14
Ready-To-Drink Chocolate Royale	11 oz	230	42	3	11
Ready-To-Drink Chocolate Royale	12 oz	250	45	1	11
Ready-To-Drink French Vanilla	11 oz	230	38	5	12
Ready-To-Drink French Vanilla	12 oz	220	38	tr	13
Ready-To-Drink Strawberry Supreme	12 oz	220	38	1	13
Strawberry Supreme as prep w/ water	8 oz	220	40	tr	14
Strawberry as prep w/ skim milk	8 oz	190	36	1	14
REGULAR					
BeneFit					
Chocolate	1 serv	120	15	2	11
Nutrition Bar	1 (2 oz)	240	33	8	9
Vanilla	1 serv	120	15	2	11
Boost					
Chocolate	1 can (8 oz)	240	40	4	10
Vanilla	8 oz	240	40	4	10
EggPro	4 oz	200	33	4	8
Fi-Bar					
Apple	1 (1 oz)	90	15	3	2
Cocoa Almond	1	130	21	4	3
Cocoa Peanut	1	130	20	4	3
Cranberry & Wild Berries	1 (1 oz)	100	13	3	2
Lemon	1 (1 oz)	90	15	3	2
Mandarin Orange	1 (1 oz)	99	15	4	2
Nuggets Almond Cappuccino Crunch	1 pkg	136	18	6	1
Nuggets Almond Butter Crunch	1 pkg	163	12	11	4
Nuggets Coconut Almond Crunch	1 pkg	136	18	6	1
Nuggets Peanut Butter Crunch	1 pkg	160	12	10	4
Raspberry	1 (1 oz)	100	13	3	2
Strawberry	1 (1 oz)	100	13	3	2
Treat Yourself Right Almond	1	152	22	6	3

FOOD	PORTION	CALS.	CARB.	FAT	PRO.
Fi-Bar (CONT.)					
Treat Yourself Right Peanutty Butter	1	152	18	5	4
Vanilla Almond	1	130	21	4	3
Vanilla Peanut	1	130	20	4	3
Gatorade					
GatorBar	1 (1.17 oz)	110	13	1	1
GatorLode	1 can (11.6 fl oz)	280	71	0	0
GatorPro	1 can (11 fl oz)	360	59	6	17
ReLode	1 pkt (0.75 oz)	80	17	0	0
Gookinaid					
Lemonade	1 cup (8 fl oz)	45	12	0	0
Meal On The Go					
Apple	1 bar (3 oz)	294	50	5	7
Banana w/ Pecans	1 bar (3 oz)	289	50	10	8
Original	1 bar (3 oz)	286	52	9	7
Nutra/Balance					
Frozen Fudding Butterscotch	4 oz	225	31	8	7
Frozen Pudding Chocolate	4 oz	225	31	8	7
Frozen Pudding Tapioca	4 oz	225	31	8	7
Frozen Pudding Vanilla	4 oz	225	31	8	7
NutraShake					
Chocolate	4 oz	200	31	6	6
Strawberry	4 oz	200	31	6	6
Vanilla	4 oz	200	31	6	6
With Fiber Strawberry	6 oz	300	60	2	11
With Fiber Vanilla	6 oz	300	60	2	11
Resource					
Fructose Sweetened	1 pkg (8 oz)	250	23	11	15
Fruit Beverage	1 pkg (8 oz)	180	36	0	9
Liquid Food	1 pkg (8 oz)	250	34	9	8
Plus Liquid Food	1 pkg (8 oz)	355	47	13	13
Sustacal					
Vanilla Sustacal	8 oz	240	33	6	15
Vita-J					
Apple Juice	11.5 fl oz	8	2	0	1
Fruit Punch	11.5 fl oz	8	2	0	1
Grapefruit Cocktail w/ Raspberry	11.5 fl oz	8	2	0	1
Orange Juice	11.5 fl oz	8	2	0	1

NUTS MIXED
(see also INDIVIDUAL NAMES)

FOOD	PORTION	CALS.	CARB.	FAT	PRO.
dry roasted w/ peanuts	1 oz	169	7	15	5

FOOD	PORTION	CALS.	CARB.	FAT	PRO.
dry roasted w/ peanuts salted	1 oz	169	7	15	5
oil roasted w/ peanuts	1 oz	175	6	16	5
oil roasted w/ peanuts salted	1 oz	175	6	16	5
oil roasted w/o peanuts	1 oz	175	6	16	4
oil roasted w/o peanuts salted	1 oz	175	6	16	4
Eagle					
Cashews & Peanuts Honey Roasted	1 oz	170	8	8	5
Mixed	1 oz	180	6	16	5
Mixed Deluxe	1 oz	180	6	17	4
Fisher					
Mixed Deluxe Lightly Salted	1 oz	180	5	16	6
Mixed Deluxe Salted	1 oz	180	5	16	6
Mixed Oil Roasted 25% More Cashews Lightly Salted	1 oz	180	5	16	6
Mixed Oil Roasted 25% More Cashews Salted	1 oz	180	5	16	6
Nut & Fruit Pina Colada	1 oz	150	13	10	4
Nut & Fruit Raisin Cranberry	1 oz	150	12	10	4
Nut & Fruit Tropical Fruit	1 oz	140	15	8	4
Nut Toppings Oil Roasted With Peanuts	1 oz	190	6	17	6
Peanuts Cashews	1 oz	170	8	13	6
Guy's					
Mixed With Peanuts	1 oz	180	3	16	7
Tasty Mix	1 oz	130	14	7	3
Planters					
Cashews & Peanuts Honey Roasted	1 oz	150	10	12	5
Deluxe Oil Roasted	1 oz	170	6	16	5
Dry Roasted	1 oz	170	7	14	6
Honey Roasted	1 oz	140	9	13	5
Lightly Salted Oil Roasted	1 oz	170	6	15	6
No Brazils Lightly Salted Oil Roasted	1 oz	170	6	15	6
No Brazils Oil Roasted	1 oz	170	6	15	5
Oil Roasted	1 oz	170	5	15	6

FOOD	PORTION	CALS.	CARB.	FAT	PRO.
Planters (CONT.)					
Select Mix Cashews Almonds & Macadamias Oil Roasted	1 oz	170	6	16	4
Select Mix Cashews Almonds & Pecans Oil Roasted	1 oz	170	7	15	4
Unsalted Oil Roasted	1 oz	170	6	15	6

OCTOPUS

FOOD	PORTION	CALS.	CARB.	FAT	PRO.
fresh steamed	3 oz	140	4	2	25

OIL

(*see also* FAT)

FOOD	PORTION	CALS.	CARB.	FAT	PRO.
almond	1 cup	1927	0	218	0
almond	1 tbsp	120	0	14	0
apricot kernel	1 cup	1927	0	218	0
apricot kernel	1 tbsp	120	0	14	0
avocado	1 tbsp	124	0	14	0
avocado	1 cup	1927	0	218	0
babassu palm	1 tbsp	120	0	14	0
butter oil	1 cup	1795	0	204	1
butter oil	1 tbsp	112	0	13	tr
canola	1 cup	1927	0	218	0
canola	1 tbsp	124	0	14	0
coconut	1 tbsp	117	0	14	0
corn	1 cup	1927	0	218	0
corn	1 tbsp	120	0	14	0
cottonseed	1 cup	1927	0	218	0
cottonseed	1 tbsp	120	0	14	0
cupu assu	1 tbsp	120	0	14	0
grapeseed	1 tbsp	120	0	14	0
hazelnut	1 cup	1927	0	218	0
hazelnut	1 tbsp	120	0	14	0
mustard	1 cup	1927	0	218	0
mustard	1 tbsp	124	0	14	0
oat	1 tbsp	120	0	14	0
olive	1 tbsp	119	0	14	0
olive	1 cup	1909	0	216	0
palm	1 tbsp	120	0	14	0
palm	1 cup	1927	0	218	0
palm kernel	1 tbsp	117	0	14	0
palm kernel	1 cup	1879	0	218	0
peanut	1 cup	1909	0	216	0

FOOD	PORTION	CALS.	CARB.	FAT	PRO.
peanut	1 tbsp	119	0	14	0
poppyseed	1 tbsp	120	0	14	0
poppyseed	3.5 fl oz	900	0	100	0
pumpkin seed	3½ oz	925	0	100	0
rice bran	1 tbsp	120	0	14	0
safflower	1 cup	1927	0	218	0
safflower	1 tbsp	120	0	14	0
sesame	1 tbsp	120	0	14	0
sheanut	1 tbsp	120	0	14	0
soybean	1 tbsp	120	0	14	0
soybean	1 cup	1927	0	218	0
sunflower	1 tbsp	120	0	14	0
sunflower	1 cup	1927	0	218	0
teaseed	1 tbsp	120	0	14	0
tomatoseed	1 tbsp	120	0	14	0
vegetable soybean & cottonseed	1 tbsp	120	0	14	0
vegetable soybean & cottonseed	1 cup	1927	0	218	0
walnut	1 tbsp	120	0	14	0
walnut	1 cup	1927	0	218	0
wheat germ	1 tbsp	120	0	14	0
Arrowhead					
Flax Seed	1 tbsp (0.5 fl oz)	120	0	14	0
Hazelnut	1 tbsp (0.5 fl oz)	120	0	14	0
Crisco					
Corn Canola	1 tbsp (0.5 fl oz)	120	0	14	0
Oil	1 tbsp (0.5 fl oz)	120	0	14	0
Puritan Canola	1 tbsp (0.5 fl oz)	120	0	14	0
Eden					
Hot Pepper Sesame	1 tbsp (0.5 oz)	130	0	14	0
Toasted Sesame	1 tbsp (0.5 oz)	130	0	14	0
Hain					
All Blend	1 tbsp	120	0	14	0
Almond	1 tbsp	120	0	14	0
Apricot Kernel	1 tbsp	120	0	14	0
Avocado	1 tbsp	120	0	14	0
Canola	1 tbsp	120	0	14	0
Canola Organic	1 tbsp	120	0	14	0
Coconut	1 tbsp	120	0	14	0
Corn	1 tbsp	120	0	14	0
Garlic & Oil	1 tbsp	120	0	14	0
Olive	1 tbsp	120	0	14	0
Peanut	1 tbsp	120	0	14	0

FOOD	PORTION	CALS.	CARB.	FAT	PRO.
Hain (CONT.)					
Rice Bran	1 tbsp	120	0	14	0
Safflower	1 tbsp	120	0	14	0
Safflower Hi-Oleic	1 tbsp	120	0	14	0
Safflower Organic	1 tbsp	120	0	14	0
Sesame	1 tbsp	120	0	14	0
Soy	1 tbsp	120	0	14	0
Sunflower	1 tbsp	120	0	14	0
Sunflower Organic	1 tbsp	120	0	14	0
Walnut	1 tbsp	120	0	14	0
Hollywood					
Canola	1 tbsp	120	0	14	0
Peanut	1 tbsp	120	0	14	0
Safflower	1 tbsp	120	0	14	0
Soy	1 tbsp	120	0	14	0
Sunflower	1 tbsp	120	0	14	0
House Of Tsang					
Hot Chili Sesame	1 tsp (5 g)	45	0	5	0
Mongolian Fire	1 tsp (5 g)	45	0	5	0
Pure Sesame	1 tsp (5 g)	45	0	5	0
Singapore Curry	1 tsp (5 g)	45	0	5	0
Wok Oil	1 tbsp (0.5 oz)	130	0	14	0
Italica					
Olive Oil	1 tbsp	120	0	9	0
Ka-Me					
Chili Hot	1 tbsp (0.5 fl oz)	130	0	14	0
Sesame	1 tbsp (0.5 fl oz)	130	0	14	0
Sesame Tempura	1 tbsp (0.5 fl oz)	130	0	14	0
Mazola					
No Stick	2.5 second spray (0.2 g)	2	0	tr	0
Oil	1 tbsp (14 g)	120	0	14	0
Oil	1 cup (221 g)	1955	0	221	0
Orville Redenbacher's	1 tbsp	120	0	14	0
Pam					
Butter	1 sec spray (0.266 g)	2	0	tr	0
Cooking Spray	1 sec spray (0.266 g)	2	0	tr	0
Olive Oil	1 sec spray (0.266 g)	2	0	tr	0
Pump	1 spray (0.43 g)	4	0	tr	0
Planters					
Peanut	1 tbsp (0.5 oz)	120	0	14	0

FOOD	PORTION	CALS.	CARB.	FAT	PRO.
Planters (CONT.)					
Popcorn	1 tbsp (0.5 oz)	120	0	14	0
Progresso					
Olive	1 tbsp	119	0	14	0
Olive Extra Light	1 tbsp	119	0	14	0
Olive Extra Virgin	1 tbsp	119	0	14	0
Smart Beat					
Canola	1 tbsp (14 g)	120	0	14	0
Oil	1 tbsp	120	0	14	0
Tree Of Life					
Almond	1 tbsp (0.5 g)	130	0	14	0
Apricot Kernel	1 tbsp (0.5 g)	130	0	14	0
Avocado	1 tbsp (0.5 g)	130	0	14	0
Macadamia Nut	1 tbsp (0.5 g)	130	0	14	0
Olive Extra Virgin Organic	1 tbsp (0.5 g)	130	0	14	0
Sesame	1 tbsp (0.5 g)	130	0	14	0
Toasted Sesame	1 tbsp (0.5 oz)	130	0	14	0
Weight Watchers					
Butter Spray	1 second spray	2	0	tr	0
Cooking Spray	1 second spray	2	0	tr	0
Wesson					
Canola	1 tbsp	120	0	14	0
Cooking Spray Lite	0.5 sec spray	0	0	0	0
Corn	1 tbsp	120	0	14	0
Olive	1 tbsp	120	0	14	0
Sunflower	1 tbsp	120	0	14	0
Vegetable	1 tbsp	120	0	14	0
FISH OIL					
cod liver	1 tbsp	123	0	14	0
herring	1 tbsp	123	0	14	0
menhaden	1 tbsp	123	0	14	0
salmon	1 tbsp	123	0	14	0
sardine	1 tbsp	123	0	14	0
shark	3½ oz	945	0	100	0
whale	3½ oz	945	0	100	0
Hain					
Cod Liver	1 tbsp	120	0	14	0
Cod Liver Cherry	1 tbsp	120	0	14	0
Cod Liver Mint	1 tbsp	120	0	14	0
OKRA					
CANNED					
Allen					
Cut	½ cup (4.4 oz)	25	6	0	1

FOOD	PORTION	CALS.	CARB.	FAT	PRO.
McIlhenny					
Pickled	2 pieces (1 oz)	7	1	tr	tr
Trappey					
Cocktail Hot	2 pieces (1 oz)	8	2	tr	tr
Cocktail Mild	1 piece (1 oz)	9	1	tr	1
Creole Gumbo	½ cup (4.2 oz)	35	6	0	2
Cut	½ cup (4.4 oz)	25	6	0	1
FRESH					
raw	8 pods	36	7	tr	2
raw sliced	½ cup	19	4	tr	1
sliced cooked	½ cup	25	6	tr	1
sliced cooked	8 pods	27	6	tr	2
FROZEN					
sliced cooked	1 pkg (10 oz)	94	21	1	5
sliced cooked	½ cup	34	8	tr	1
Fresh Like					
Cut	3.5 oz	26	6	tr	3
Whole	3.5 oz	32	7	tr	2
OLIVES					
green	3 extra lg	15	tr	2	tr
green	4 med	15	tr	2	tr
ripe	1 sm	4	tr	tr	tr
ripe	1 lg	5	tr	tr	tr
ripe	1 colossal	12	1	1	tr
ripe	1 jumbo	7	tr	1	tr
California					
Ripe	3 sm	4	tr	tr	0
Progresso					
Olive Appetizer	½ cup	180	6	21	1
Olive Condite	½ cup	130	5	14	tr
Salad Olives	½ cup	120	1	15	1
S&W					
Ripe Extra Large	3.5 oz	163	1	18	1
Ripe Pitted Large	3.5 oz	163	1	18	1
Tee Pee					
Spanish Green	2 oz	98	1	10	1
ONION					
CANNED					
chopped	½ cup	21	5	tr	1
whole	1 (2.2 oz)	12	3	tr	1
S&W					
Whole Small	½ cup	35	9	0	1

FOOD	PORTION	CALS.	CARB.	FAT	PRO.
Vlasic					
Lightly Spiced Cocktail Onions	1 oz	4	1	0	0
Watkins					
Liquid Spice	1 tbsp (0.5 oz)	120	0	14	0
DRIED					
flakes	1 tbsp	16	4	tr	tr
powder	1 tsp	7	2	tr	tr
Watkins					
Flakes	¼ tsp (1 g)	0	0	0	0
FRESH					
chopped cooked	½ cup	47	11	tr	1
raw chopped	1 tbsp	4	1	tr	tr
raw chopped	½ cup	30	7	tr	1
scallions raw chopped	1 tbsp	2	tr	tr	tr
scallions raw sliced	½ cup	16	4	tr	1
welsh raw	3½ oz	34	7	tr	2
Antioch Farms					
Vidalia	1 med	60	14	0	1
Dole					
Green Chopped	1 tbsp	2	tr	tr	tr
Medium	1	60	14	0	1
FROZEN					
chopped cooked	½ cup	30	7	tr	tr
chopped cooked	1 tbsp	4	1	tr	tr
rings	7 (2.5 oz)	285	27	19	4
rings cooked	2 (0.7 oz)	81	8	5	1
whole cooked	3½ oz	28	7	tr	tr
Birds Eye					
Polybag Whole Small	½ cup	30	8	0	1
Small With Cream Sauce	½ cup	100	12	3	2
Fresh Like					
Diced	3.5 oz	29	7	0	1
Whole	3.5 oz	37	8	tr	1
Kineret					
Rings	6 (3 oz)	200	25	10	3
Mrs. Paul's					
Crispy Onion Rings	2½ oz	190	19	12	2
Ore Ida					
Chopped	¾ cup (3 oz)	25	6	0	tr
Onion Ringers	6 pieces (3 oz)	240	26	14	3
TAKE-OUT					
fried	½ cup (7.5 oz)	176	17	11	3
rings breaded & fried	8 to 9	275	31	16	4

FOOD	PORTION	CALS.	CARB.	FAT	PRO.
OPOSSUM					
roasted	3 oz	188	0	9	26
ORANGE					
CANNED					
Del Monte					
Mandarin In Heavy Syrup	½ cup (4.4 oz)	80	19	0	0
Dole					
Mandarin Segments	½ cup	70	19	tr	0
Pineapple Mandarin Segments	½ cup	80	19	tr	0
Empress					
Mandarin	5.5 oz	100	25	0	0
Mandarin From Japan	5.5 oz	35	8	0	0
S&W					
Mandarin Natural Style	½ cup	60	15	0	0
Mandarin Selected Sections in Heavy Syrup	½ cup	76	20	0	0
Mandarin Unsweetened	½ cup	28	7	0	0
FRESH					
california valencia	1	59	14	tr	1
california navel	1	65	16	tr	1
florida	1	69	17	tr	1
peel	1 tbsp	6	2	tr	tr
sections	1 cup	85	21	tr	2
Dole					
Orange	1	50	13	0	1
ORANGE JUICE					
canned	1 cup	104	25	tr	1
chilled	1 cup	110	25	1	2
fresh	1 cup	111	26	tr	2
frzn as prep	1 cup	112	27	tr	2
frzn not prep	6 oz	339	81	tr	5
mandarin orange	3½ oz	47	10	tr	1
orange drink	6 oz	94	24	0	0
After The Fall					
Juice	1 bottle (10 oz)	110	26	0	2
Bright & Early					
Chilled	8 fl oz	120	30	0	0
Frozen	8 fl oz	120	30	0	0
Del Monte					
Juice	8 fl oz	110	27	0	2

FOOD	PORTION	CALS.	CARB.	FAT	PRO.
Hi-C					
Box	8.45 fl oz	130	33	0	0
Drink	8 fl oz	130	32	0	0
Drink	1 can (11.5 fl oz)	180	45	0	0
Hood					
From Concentrate	1 cup (8 oz)	120	30	0	0
Select	1 cup (8 oz)	120	30	0	0
With Calcium	1 cup (8 oz)	120	30	0	0
Kool-Aid					
Drink	8 oz	98	25	0	0
Koolers	1 (8.45 oz)	115	30	0	0
Sugar Sweetened	8 oz	79	20	0	0
Libby					
Juice	6 fl oz	80	20	0	1
Minute Maid					
Box	8.45 fl oz	120	28	0	0
Calcium Rich Chilled	8 fl oz	120	27	0	0r
Calcium Rich frzn	8 fl oz	120	27	0	0
Chilled	8 fl oz	110	27	0	0
Country Style Chilled	8 fl oz	110	27	0	0
Country Style frzn	8 fl oz	110	27	0	0
Juices To Go	1 can (11.5 fl oz)	140	34	0	0
Juices To Go	1 bottle (16 fl oz)	160	39	0	0
Juices To Go	1 bottle (10 fl oz)	110	27	0	0
Orange Punch Box	8.45 fl oz	130	33	0	0
Premium Choice Chilled	8 fl oz	110	27	0	0
Pulp Free Chilled	8 fl oz	110	27	0	0
Pulp Free frzn	8 fl oz	110	27	0	0
Reduced Acid frzn	8 fl oz	110	27	0	0
Mott's					
From Concentrate	10 fl oz	130	29	1	2
Ocean Spray					
Juice	8 fl oz	120	31	0	0
Odwalla					
Juice	8 fl oz	110	25	1	2
S&W					
100% Unsweetened	6 oz	83	18	0	2
Sippin' Pak					
100% Pure	8.45 fl oz	110	26	0	1
Snapple					
Juice	10 fl oz	130	29	0	0
Orangeade	8 fl oz	120	31	0	0
Tang					
Breakfast Crystals Sugar Free as prep	6 oz	5	0	0	0

FOOD	PORTION	CALS.	CARB.	FAT	PRO.
Tang (CONT.)					
Breakfast Crystals as prep	6 oz	86	22	0	0
Fruit Box	8.45 oz	127	31	0	0
Tropical Orange	8.45 fl oz	146	37	0	0
Tree Of Life					
Juice	8 fl oz	110	27	0	1
Tree Top					
Juice	6 oz	90	22	0	1
Tropicana					
Frozen as prep	6 fl oz	110	27	0	tr
Juice	1 container (8 fl oz)	110	27	0	tr
Juice	1 container (6 fl oz)	80	20	0	tr
Juice	1 container (10 fl oz)	130	33	0	tr
Juice	8 fl oz	110	27	0	tr
Season's Best	1 bottle (7 fl oz)	90	23	0	tr
Season's Best	1 can (11.5 fl oz)	140	36	0	tr
Season's Best	8 fl oz	110	27	0	tr
Season's Best	1 bottle (10 fl oz)	130	33	0	tr
Season's Best Calcium	8 fl oz	110	27	0	tr
Season's Best Homestyle	8 fl oz	110	27	0	tr
Season's Best Vitamin	8 fl oz	110	27	0	tr
Veryfine					
100%	8 oz	121	24	0	0
Orange Drink	8 oz	140	33	0	0

OREGANO

ground	1 tsp	5	1	tr	tr
Watkins					
Liquid Spice	1 tbsp (0.5 oz)	120	0	14	0

ORGAN MEATS
(*see* BRAINS, GIBLETS, GIZZARD, HEART, KIDNEY, LIVER, SWEETBREADS)

ORIENTAL FOOD
(*see also* DINNER, NOODLES, RICE)

CANNED					
chow mein chicken	1 cup	95	18	tr	7
La Choy					
Bi-Pack Beef Pepper	¾ cup	80	10	2	7
Bi-Pack Chow Mein Chicken	¾ cup	80	8	3	7
Bi-Pack Chow Mein Pork	¾ cup	80	7	4	5

FOOD	PORTION	CALS.	CARB.	FAT	PRO.
La Choy (CONT.)					
Bi-Pack Chow Mein Shrimp	¾ cup	70	6	1	7
Bi-Pack Sweet & Sour Chicken	¾ cup	120	18	2	7
Bi-Pack Teriyaki Chicken	¾ cup	85	8	2	8
Dinner Chow Mein Chicken	¾ pkg	300	29	17	12
Entree Beef Pepper Oriental	¾ cup	100	12	4	7
Entree Chow Mein Beef	¾ cup	40	5	2	5
Entree Chow Mein Chicken	¾ cup	70	2	4	5
Entree Chow Mein Meatless	¾ cup	25	5	tr	1
Entree Chow Mein Shrimp	¾ cup	35	4	1	4
Entree Sweet & Sour Chicken	¾ cup	240	47	2	8
Entree Sweet & Sour Pork	¾ cup	250	48	4	6
FRESH					
egg roll wrapper	1	83	16	tr	3
wonton wrappers	1	23	5	tr	1
Azumaya					
Won Ton Wraps	1 (8 g)	23	5	tr	1
FROZEN					
Banquet					
Chow Mein Chicken	1 pkg (9 oz)	400	28	7	9
Birds Eye					
Easy Recipe Chicken Teriyaki not prep	½ pkg	160	28	4	7
Easy Recipe Oriental Beef not prep	½ pkg	100	11	7	8
Internationals Chinese Stir Fry not prep	3.3 oz	35	6	0	2
Japanese Stir Fry International not prep	3.3 oz	30	5	0	2
Chun King					
Beef Pepper Steak	1 pkg (13 oz)	300	50	4	15
Chow Mein Chicken	1 pkg (13 oz)	370	45	14	16
Egg Rolls Chicken	8 (4.4 oz)	270	40	9	8
Egg Rolls Pork & Shrimp	8 (4.4 oz)	290	39	11	11
Egg Rolls Shrimp	8 (4.4 oz)	260	39	8	7

FOOD	PORTION	CALS.	CARB.	FAT	PRO.
Chun King (CONT.)					
Imperial Chicken	1 pkg (13 oz)	460	59	10	17
Sweet & Sour Pork	1 pkg (13 oz)	450	66	6	12
Walnut Chicken	1 pkg (13 oz)	460	56	19	19
Empire					
Large Egg Rolls	1 (3 oz)	190	28	6	6
Miniature Egg Rolls	6 (4.8 oz)	280	43	8	9
La Choy					
Egg Roll Restaurant Style Almond Chicken	1 (3 oz)	170	23	6	6
Egg Roll Restaurant Style Chicken	1 (3 oz)	170	25	5	7
Egg Roll Restaurant Style Mu Sho Pork	1 (3 oz)	190	25	7	6
Egg Roll Restaurant Style Shrimp	1 (3 oz)	150	24	4	6
Egg Roll Restaurant Style Sweet & Sour	1 (3 oz)	180	29	4	6
Egg Roll Mini Chicken	14 (7.25 oz)	430	67	11	15
Egg Roll Mini Lobster	14 (7.25 oz)	410	65	11	13
Egg Roll Mini Meat & Shrimp	15 (3.75 oz)	240	31	9	8
Egg Roll Mini Pork & Shrimp	14 (7.25 oz)	430	65	12	15
Egg Roll Mini Shrimp	14 (7.25 oz)	410	68	9	14
Restaurant Style Egg Roll Pork	1 (3 oz)	150	20	5	7
Lean Cuisine					
Chicken Chow Mein With Rice	1 meal (9 oz)	210	28	5	13
Luigino's					
Chicken & Almonds With Rice	1 pkg (8 oz)	250	33	8	12
Chop Suey Pork With Rice	1 pkg (8.5 oz)	210	34	4	10
Egg Rolls Chicken	1 pkg (6 oz)	360	48	13	12
Egg Rolls Pork & Shrimp	1 pkg (6 oz)	340	51	9	14
Egg Rolls Shrimp	1 pkg (6 oz)	350	39	11	24
Egg Rolls Sweet & Sour Chicken	1 pkg (6 oz)	400	59	12	13
Egg Rolls Sweet & Sour Pork	1 pkg (6 oz)	360	56	10	12
Egg Rolls Szechwan Vegetable	1 pkg (6 oz)	350	38	12	23

FOOD	PORTION	CALS.	CARB.	FAT	PRO.
Luigino's (CONT.)					
Lo Mein Chicken	1 pkg (8 oz)	320	35	5	13
Lo Mein Shrimp	1 pkg (8 oz)	190	31	3	8
Oriental Beef & Peppers With Rice	1 pkg (8 oz)	230	38	5	8
Pasta Favorites					
Chicken Lo Mein	1 pkg (10.5 oz)	270	43	6	11
Stouffer's					
Chicken Chow Mein With Rice	1 pkg (10.6 oz)	260	43	4	13
Chicken Oriental	1 pkg (9.75 oz)	320	45	9	14
Stir-Fry Teriyaki	1 pkg (9 oz)	260	39	5	15
Tyson					
Stir Fry Kit With Yoshida Oriental Sauce	10.6 oz	330	37	10	24
Sweet & Sour Kit With Sweet & Sour Sauce	14.85 oz	440	71	9	20
Worthington					
Vegetarian Egg Rolls	1 (85 g)	160	20	6	6
MIX					
Kikkoman					
Teriyaki Baste & Glaze	1 tbsp	24	5	tr	1
La Choy					
Dinner Classics Pepper Steak	¾ cup	180	9	9	17
Dinner Classics Egg Foo Young	2 patties + 3 oz sauce sauce	170	20	7	8
Dinner Classics Sweet & Sour	¾ cup	310	30	6	32
TAKE-OUT					
chicken teriyaki	¾ cup	399	7	27	30
chop suey w/ beef & pork	1 cup	300	13	17	26
chop suey w/ pork	1 cup	375	29	29	19
chow mein chicken	1 cup	255	10	10	31
chow mein pork	1 cup	425	21	24	32
chow mein shrimp	1 cup	221	21	10	13
chow mein vegetable	1 serv (8 oz)	90	15	3	3
egg roll lobster	1 (4.8 oz)	270	43	7	8
egg roll meat & shrimp	1 (4.8 oz)	320	41	12	10
egg roll pork & shrimp	1 (5 oz)	300	41	10	13
egg roll shrimp	1 (3 oz)	170	24	5	6
egg roll spicy pork	1 (3 oz)	200	23	9	6
egg roll vegetable	1 (3 oz)	170	28	4	5
fried rice	6.6 oz	249	48	6	4

FOOD	PORTION	CALS.	CARB.	FAT	PRO.
fried rice w/ egg	6.7 oz	395	49	20	8
oriental pepper & beef	1 serv (8 oz)	90	12	0	10
spring roll deep fried	3.5 oz	202	24	9	6
sweet & sour pork	1 serv (8 oz)	250	37	8	6
wonton fried	½ cup (1 oz)	111	8	8	2
wonton soup	1 cup	205	26	3	16

OYSTERS
CANNED

FOOD	PORTION	CALS.	CARB.	FAT	PRO.
eastern	1 cup	170	10	6	18
eastern	3 oz	58	3	2	6
Bumble Bee					
Whole	½ cup (3.5 oz)	100	6	4	10
Empress					
Whole	4 oz	100	8	4	10
S&W					
Fancy Whole	2 oz	95	4	3	12

FRESH

FOOD	PORTION	CALS.	CARB.	FAT	PRO.
eastern cooked	3 oz	117	7	4	12
eastern cooked	6 med	58	3	2	6
eastern raw	6 med	58	3	2	6
eastern raw	1 cup	170	10	6	18
pacific raw	1 med	41	2	1	5
pacific raw	3 oz	69	4	2	8
steamed	1 med	41	2	1	5
steamed	3 oz	138	8	4	16

TAKE-OUT

FOOD	PORTION	CALS.	CARB.	FAT	PRO.
battered & fried	6 (4.9 oz)	368	40	18	13
breaded & fried	6 (4.9 oz)	368	40	18	13
eastern breaded & fried	3 oz	167	10	11	7
eastern breaded & fried	6 med (88 g)	173	10	11	8
oysters rockefeller	3 oysters	66	5	2	7
stew	1 cup	278	15	18	15

PANCAKE/WAFFLE SYRUP
(*see also* SYRUP)

FOOD	PORTION	CALS.	CARB.	FAT	PRO.
low calorie	1 tbsp	12	3	0	0
maple	2 tbsp	122	32	0	0
maple	1 cup (11.1 oz)	824	212	1	tr
maple	1 tbsp (0.8 oz)	52	13	0	0
pancake syrup	1 tbsp (0.7 oz)	57	15	0	0
pancake syrup	1 cup (11 oz)	903	238	0	0
pancake syrup light	1 oz	46	13	0	0
pancake syrup w/ butter	1 cup (11 oz)	933	234	5	tr
pancake syrup w/ butter	1 tbsp (0.7 oz)	59	15	tr	tr

FOOD	PORTION	CALS.	CARB.	FAT	PRO.
Aunt Jemima					
Butter Rich	¼ cup (2.8 oz)	210	52	0	0
Butterlite	¼ cup (2.5 oz)	100	26	0	0
Lite	¼ cup (2.5 oz)	100	27	0	0
Syrup	¼ cup (2.8 oz)	210	53	0	0
Brer Rabbit					
Dark	2 tbsp	120	31	0	0
Light	2 tbsp	120	31	0	0
Estee					
Lite Maple	¼ cup (2.4 oz)	80	20	0	0
Golden Griddle					
Syrup	1 tbsp (20 g)	50	14	0	0
Syrup	1 cup (321 g)	885	229	0	0
Karo					
Syrup	1 tbsp (21 g)	60	15	0	0
Log Cabin					
Country Kitchen	1 oz	103	27	0	0
Lite	1 oz	49	13	0	0
Mrs. Richardson's					
Lite	¼ cup (2.5 oz)	100	26	0	0
Original Recipe	¼ cup (2.8 oz)	210	52	0	0
Red Wing					
Lite	¼ cup (2 oz)	100	26	0	0
Syrup	¼ cup (2 oz)	210	53	0	0
Tree Of Life					
Maple	¼ cup (2.1 oz)	200	53	0	0
Weight Watchers					
Syrup	1 tbsp	25	7	0	0
PANCAKES					
FROZEN					
buttermilk	1-4 in diam (1.3 oz)	83	16	1	2
plain	1-4 in diam (1.3 oz)	83	16	1	2
Aunt Jemima					
Blueberry	3 (3.4 oz)	210	40	4	6
Buttermilk	3 (3 oz)	180	34	3	5
Lowfat	3 (3.4 oz)	130	33	2	4
Original	3 (3.4 oz)	200	40	3	6
Downyflake					
Blueberry	3	290	48	9	5
Buttermilk	3	280	45	9	5
Pancakes And Sausages	1 pkg (5.5 oz)	430	47	23	11
Regular	3	280	45	9	5
Great Starts					
Pancakes And Sausages	6 oz	460	52	22	15

FOOD	PORTION	CALS.	CARB.	FAT	PRO.
Great Starts (CONT.)					
Pancakes With Bacon	4½ oz	400	43	20	11
Silver Dollar Pancakes And Sausage	3¾ oz	310	37	14	10
Whole Wheat Pancakes With Lite Links	5½ oz	350	39	16	15
Healthy Starts					
Pancakes w/ LeanLinks	6 oz	360	48	8	11
Jimmy Dean					
Flapstick	1 (2.5 oz)	240	22	14	6
Flapstick Blueberry	1 (2.5 oz)	260	23	15	6
Morningstar Farms					
Pancakes/Links	1 pkg (4 oz)	240	31	8	11
Pillsbury					
Buttermilk Microwave	3	260	51	4	6
Harvest Wheat Microwave	3	240	48	4	6
Microwave	3	250	49	4	5
Original Microwave	3	240	47	4	6
Quaker					
Lite Pancakes & Lite Links	1 pkg (6 oz)	310	43	10	14
Lite Pancakes & Lite Syrup	1 pkg (6 oz)	260	53	3	10
Pancakes & Sausages	1 pkg (6 oz)	420	57	16	12
Weight Watchers					
Buttermilk	2 (2.5 oz)	140	22	3	5
Pancakes With Links	4 oz	220	21	10	12
HOME RECIPE					
blueberry	1 (4 in diam)	84	11	4	2
plain	1 (4 in diam)	86	11	4	2
MIX					
buckwheat	1 (4 in diam)	62	9	2	2
buttermilk	1-4 in diam (1.3 oz)	74	14	1	2
plain	1-4 in diam (1.3 oz)	74	14	1	2
sugar free low sodium	1 (3 in diam)	44	9	tr	1
whole wheat	1 (4 in diam)	92	13	3	4
Arrowhead					
Multigrain Pancake & Waffle Mix	¼ cup (1.2 oz)	120	24	1	5
Aunt Jemima					
Buckwheat Pancake & Waffle Mix	¼ cup (1.4 oz)	120	28	1	5
Buttermilk Pancake & Waffle Mix	⅓ cup (1.9 oz)	190	38	2	6

FOOD	PORTION	CALS.	CARB.	FAT	PRO.
Aunt Jemima (CONT.)					
Original Pancake & Waffle Mix	⅓ cup (1.6 oz)	150	34	1	4
Pancake & Waffle Mix Regular	⅓ cup (1.9 oz)	190	39	2	6
Pancake & Waffle Mix Whole Wheat	¼ cup (1.4 oz)	130	28	1	6
Betty Crocker					
Buttermilk	3 (4 in diam)	280	39	10	8
Bisquick					
Apple Cinnamon Shake 'N Pour	3 (4 in diam)	240	47	3	6
Blueberry Shake 'N Pour	3 (4 in diam)	270	54	3	6
Buttermilk Shake 'N Pour	3 (4 in diam)	250	49	3	6
Original Shake 'N Pour	3 (4 in diam)	250	49	3	6
Estee					
Pancake Mix Fat Free as prep	4 (4 in diam)	180	40	0	4
Fast Shake					
Blueberry	1 serving (2.5 oz)	251	50	3	7
Buttermilk	1 serving (2.5 oz)	258	50	3	8
Original	1 serving (2.5 oz)	266	50	4	6
Health Valley					
Pancake Mix not prep	1 oz	100	20	1	4
Hodgson Mill					
Buckwheat	⅓ cup (1.8 oz)	160	35	1	5
Hungry Jack					
Bluberry	3 (4 in diam)	320	41	15	6
Buttermilk	3 (4 in diam)	240	29	11	7
Buttermilk Complete	3 (4 in diam)	180	39	1	4
Buttermilk Complete Packets	3 (4 in diam)	180	35	3	4
Extra Lights	3 (4 in diam)	210	30	7	6
Extra Lights Complete	3 (4 in diam)	190	37	2	4
Panshakes	3 (4 in diam)	250	43	6	7
Stone-Buhr					
Buckwheat	¼ cup (1.4 oz)	130	29	1	5
Oat Bran	¼ cup (1.4 oz)	130	30	0	5
Whole Wheat	¼ cup (1.4 oz)	120	25	1	5
Wanda's					
Blue Corn	⅓ cup mix per serv (1.7 oz)	170	32	2	7

FOOD	PORTION	CALS.	CARB.	FAT	PRO.
TAKE-OUT					
buckwheat	1 (4 in diam)	55	6	2	2
potato	1 (4 in diam)	78	4	6	2
w/ butter & syrup	3	519	91	14	8
PANCREAS					
(*see* SWEETBREADS)					
PAPAYA					
CANNED					
Ka-Me					
Papaya	¾ cup	120	29	0	0
DRIED					
Sonoma					
Pieces	2 pieces (2 oz)	200	41	4	0
FRESH					
cubed	1 cup	54	14	tr	1
papaya	1	117	30	tr	2
PAPAYA JUICE					
nectar	1 cup	142	36	tr	tr
Goya					
Nectar	6 oz	110	27	0	1
Kern's					
Nectar	6 fl oz	110	27	0	0
Libby					
Nectar	1 can (11.5 fl oz)	210	51	0	tr
PAPRIKA					
paprika	1 tsp	6	1	tr	tr
Watkins					
Ground	¼ tsp (0.5 oz)	0	0	0	0
PARSLEY					
dry	1 tsp	1	tr	tr	tr
dry	1 tbsp	1	tr	tr	tr
fresh chopped	½ cup	11	2	tr	1
Dole					
Chopped	1 tbsp	10	1	tr	tr
PARSNIPS					
fresh cooked	1 (5.6 oz)	130	31	tr	2
fresh sliced cooked	½ cup	63	15	tr	1
raw sliced	½ cup	50	12	tr	1
PASSION FRUIT					
purple fresh	1	18	4	tr	tr

FOOD	PORTION	CALS.	CARB.	FAT	PRO.
PASSION FRUIT JUICE					
purple	1 cup	126	34	tr	1
yellow	1 cup	149	36	tr	2
Snapple					
Passion Supreme	10 fl oz	160	39	0	0
PASTA					
(*see also* NOODLES, PASTA DINNERS, PASTA SALAD)					
DRY					
corn cooked	1 cup	176	39	1	4
elbows	1 cup	389	78	2	13
elbows cooked	1 cup	197	40	tr	7
protein-fortied cooked	1 cup	188	36	tr	9
shells	1 cup	389	78	2	13
shells cooked	1 cup	197	40	tr	7
spaghetti	2 oz	211	43	tr	7
spaghetti cooked	1 cup	197	40	tr	7
spaghetti protein fortified cooked	1 cup	229	44	tr	11
spinach spaghetti	2 oz	212	43	tr	8
spinach spaghetti cooked	1 cup	183	37	tr	6
spirals	1 cup	389	78	2	13
spirals cooked	1 cup	197	40	tr	7
vegetable	1 cup	308	63	tr	11
vegetable cooked	1 cup	171	36	tr	6
whole wheat	1 cup	365	79	1	15
whole wheat cooked	1 cup (4.9 oz)	174	37	tr	7
whole wheat spaghetti	2 oz	198	43	tr	8
whole wheat spaghetti cooked	1 cup	174	37	tr	7
Anthony					
Pasta	2 oz	210	42	1	7
Bella Via					
Angel Hair	2 oz	200	40	0	8
Artichoke Angel Hair as prep	⅝ cup	200	40	0	8
Artichoke Spaghetti as prep	⅝ cup	200	40	0	8
Elbows	2 oz	200	40	0	8
Fettucini as prep	⅝ cup	200	40	0	8
Linguini	2 oz	200	40	0	8
Penne as prep	⅝ cup	200	40	0	8
Rotelli	2 oz	200	40	0	8
Shells	2 oz	200	40	0	8

FOOD	PORTION	CALS.	CARB.	FAT	PRO.
Bella Via (CONT.)					
Spaghetti	2 oz	200	40	0	8
Ziti	2 oz	200	40	0	8
Classico					
Gnocchi Di Toscana	1 cup (2 oz)	210	42	1	7
Creamette					
Elbow Macaroni not prep	2 oz	210	42	1	7
Spaghetti not prep	2 oz	210	42	1	7
Spinach Ribbons not prep	2 oz	210	42	1	7
DeFino					
Lasagna No Boil	1 oz	102	20	tr	3
Ribbons No Boil	2 oz	204	40	2	6
Delverde					
Spaghetti Whole Wheat	2 oz	206	42	1	7
Eden					
Elbows Whole Wheat Organic	2 oz	210	39	2	10
Elbows Whole Wheat Vegetable Organic	2 oz	210	39	2	10
Kudzu And Sweet Potato Pasta	2 oz	190	47	0	0
Kudzu Kiri Pasta	2 oz	190	47	0	0
Mung Bean Pasta Harusame	2 oz	190	47	0	0
Ribbons Durum Wheat Curry Organic	2 oz	220	44	1	8
Ribbons Durum Wheat Organic	2 oz	220	44	1	8
Ribbons Durum Wheat Paella Organic	2 oz	220	44	1	8
Ribbons Durum Wheat Parsley Garlic Organic	2 oz	220	44	1	8
Ribbons Durum Wheat Pesto Organic	2 oz	220	44	1	8
Ribbons Whole Wheat Spinach Organic	2 oz	200	40	2	8
Rice Pasta Bifun	2 oz	200	44	1	5
Shells Durum Wheat Vegetable Organic	2 oz	210	42	1	7
Soba 100% Buckwheat	2 oz	200	41	0	5
Soba 40% Buckwheat	2 oz	190	37	1	8
Soba Lotus Root	2 oz	190	37	1	9
Soba Mugwort	2 oz	190	37	1	8

FOOD	PORTION	CALS.	CARB.	FAT	PRO.
Eden (CONT.)					
Soba Wild Yam Jinenjo	2 oz	190	37	1	9
Spaghetti Durum Wheat Organic	2 oz	210	42	1	7
Spaghetti Kamut Organic	2 oz	210	38	2	10
Spaghetti Parsley Garlic Organic	2 oz	210	42	1	7
Spaghetti Whole Wheat Organic	2 oz	210	39	2	10
Spirals Durum Wheat Vegetable Organic	2 oz	210	42	1	7
Spirals Kamut Organic	2 oz	210	38	2	10
Spirals Sesame Rice Organic	2 oz	200	37	2	10
Spirals Whole Wheat Vegetable Organic	2 oz	210	39	2	10
Udon	2 oz	190	37	1	8
Udon Brown Rice	2 oz	190	38	1	8
Gioia					
Pasta	2 oz	210	42	1	7
Golden Grain					
Pasta	2 oz	203	41	1	8
Health Valley					
Lasagna Whole Wheat	2 oz	170	40	1	9
Lasagna Spinach Whole Wheat	2 oz	170	40	1	9
Spaghetti Amaranth	2 oz	170	40	1	7
Spaghetti Oat Bran	2 oz	120	23	1	4
Spaghetti Spinach Whole Wheat	2 oz	170	40	1	9
Spaghetti Whole Wheat	2 oz	170	40	1	9
Hodgson Mill					
Spaghetti Whole Wheat Spinach not prep	2 oz	190	35	2	9
Veggie Bows not prep	2 oz	200	41	1	8
Veggie Rotini not prep	2 oz	200	41	1	8
Veggie Wagon Wheels not prep	2 oz	200	41	1	8
Whole Wheat Spirals not prep	2 oz	190	34	1	9
La Molisana					
Radiatori	2 oz	230	48	1	7
Lupini					
Elbow uncooked	½ cup (2 oz)	190	37	2	10

FOOD	PORTION	CALS.	CARB.	FAT	PRO.
Lupini (CONT.)					
Spaghetti Light uncooked	½ cup (2 oz)	190	37	2	10
Spaghetti With Triticale	½ pkg (2 oz)	190	38	3	9
Luxury					
Pasta	2 oz	210	42	1	7
Merlino's					
Pasta	2 oz	210	42	1	7
Mueller's					
Dinosaurs	2 oz (57 g)	210	42	1	8
Jungle Animals	2 oz (57 g)	210	42	1	8
Lasagne	2 oz (57 g)	210	42	1	8
Monsters	2 oz (57 g)	210	42	1	8
Outer Space	2 oz	210	42	1	8
Spaghetti	2 oz (57 g)	210	42	1	8
Teddy Bears	2 oz (57 g)	210	42	1	7
Twists Tri Color	2 oz (57 g)	210	41	1	8
Noodles By Leonardo					
Capellini not prep	½ cup (2 oz)	200	40	1	8
Elbows not prep	½ cup (2 oz)	200	40	1	8
Fettucini not prep	½ cup (2 oz)	200	40	1	8
Linguine not prep	½ cup (2 oz)	200	40	1	8
Rigatoni not prep	½ cup (2 oz)	200	40	1	8
Rotini not prep	½ cup (2 oz)	200	40	1	8
Shells not prep	½ cup (2 oz)	200	40	1	8
Spaghetti not prep	½ cup (2 oz)	200	40	1	8
Spaghettini not prep	½ cup (2 oz)	200	40	1	8
Vermicelli not prep	½ cup (2 oz)	200	40	1	8
Penn Dutch					
Pasta	2 oz	210	42	1	7
Pomi					
Capellini	2 oz	210	42	1	7
Prince					
Egg	2 oz	221	40	3	8
Pasta	2 oz	210	42	1	7
Rainbow	2 oz	210	42	1	8
Spinach Egg	2 oz	220	40	3	8
Red Cross					
Pasta	2 oz	210	42	1	7
Ronco					
Pasta	2 oz	210	42	1	7
Ronzoni					
Elbows	¾ cup (2 oz)	210	40	1	9
Fettucini	¾ cup (2 oz)	210	40	1	9

FOOD	PORTION	CALS.	CARB.	FAT	PRO.
Ronzoni (CONT.)					
Fusilli	¾ cup (2 oz)	210	40	1	9
Lasagne	¾ cup (2 oz)	210	40	1	9
Manicotti	¾ cup (2 oz)	210	40	1	9
Mostaccioli	¾ cup (2 oz)	210	40	1	9
Rigatoni	¾ cup (2 oz)	210	40	1	9
Rotelle uncooked	¾ cup (2 oz)	210	40	1	9
Rotini uncooked	¾ cup (2 oz)	210	40	1	9
Shells uncooked	¾ cup (2 oz)	210	40	1	9
Shells Jumbo	¾ cup (2 oz)	210	40	1	9
Spaghetti not prep	¾ cup (2 oz)	210	40	1	9
Tubettini	¾ cup (2 oz)	210	40	1	9
San Giorgio					
Bowties Egg	2 oz	210	38	3	10
Capellini	2 oz	210	40	1	9
Elbow Macaroni	2 oz	210	40	1	9
Fettuccine Egg	2 oz	210	38	3	10
Fettuccini Florentine	2 oz	210	38	3	10
Lasagne	2 oz	210	40	1	9
Linguini	2 oz	210	40	1	9
Manicotti	2 oz	210	40	1	9
Rigatoni	2 oz	210	40	1	9
Rotini	2 oz	210	40	1	9
Shells	2 oz	210	40	1	9
Spaghetti	2 oz	210	40	1	9
Spaghetti Thin	2 oz	210	40	1	9
Vermicelli	2 oz	210	40	1	9
Ziti Cut	2 oz	210	40	1	9
Tree Of Life					
Cajun as prep	⅝ cup (4.9 oz)	200	40	1	8
Confetti as prep	⅝ cup (4.9 oz)	200	40	1	8
Garlic & Parsley as prep	⅝ cup (4.9 oz)	200	40	1	8
Jamaican Spice as prep	⅝ cup (4.9 oz)	200	40	1	8
Lemon Pepper as prep	⅝ cup (4.9 oz)	200	40	1	8
Spinach as prep	⅝ cup (4.9 oz)	200	40	1	8
Tex Mex as prep	⅝ cup (4.9 oz)	200	40	1	8
Thai as prep	⅝ cup (4.9 oz)	200	40	1	8
Tomato Basil as prep	⅝ cup (4.9 oz)	200	40	1	8
Vimco					
Pasta	2 oz	210	42	1	7
Weight Watchers					
Elbow Style	2 oz	160	30	1	8
Spaghettini	2 oz	160	30	1	8

FOOD	PORTION	CALS.	CARB.	FAT	PRO.
FRESH					
plain made w/ egg cooked	2 oz	75	14	tr	3
spinach made w/ egg cooked	2 oz	74	14	tr	3
Contadina					
Angel's Hair	1¼ cup (2.8 oz)	240	43	3	10
Fettuccine	1¼ cup (2.9 oz)	250	45	4	10
Fettuccine Cholesterol Free	1 cup (2.9 oz)	240	46	3	9
Light Ravioli Cheese	1 cup (3.1 oz)	240	35	5	13
Light Ravioli Garden Vegetable	1¼ cup (3.8 oz)	290	43	6	15
Light Tortellini Garlic & Cheese	1 cup (3.6 oz)	280	50	5	15
Linguine	1¼ cup (3 oz)	260	47	4	10
Linguine Cholesterol Free	1¼ cup (3.1 oz)	250	49	3	9
Ravioli Beef And Garlic	1¼ cup (4 oz)	350	39	14	17
Ravioli Cheese	1 cup (3.1 oz)	280	31	12	13
Ravioli Chicken And Rosemary	1¼ cup (4 oz)	330	43	12	13
Tagliatelli Spinach	1¼ cup (3.1 oz)	270	46	4	12
Tortellini Spinach Three Cheese	¾ cup (3.1 oz)	280	38	5	13
Tortelloni Cheese	¾ cup (3 oz)	260	39	6	13
Tortelloni Cheese And Basil	1 cup (4 oz)	360	49	11	16
Tortelloni Chicken And Prosciutto	1 cup (3.6 oz)	360	46	13	15
Tortelloni Chicken And Vegetable	¾ cup (2.9 oz)	260	39	7	10
Tortelloni Spicy Italian Sausage And Bell Pepper	1 cup (3.6 oz)	330	47	10	13
Di Giorno					
Angel's Hair	2 oz	160	31	1	7
Fettuccine	2.5 oz	190	39	2	7
Fettuccine Spinach	2.5 oz	190	38	2	7
Linguine	2.5 oz	190	39	2	7
Linguine Herb	2.5 oz	190	39	2	7
Ravioli Italian Herb Cheese	1 cup (3.8 oz)	350	44	13	15
Ravioli Light Cheese & Garlic	1 cup (3.7 oz)	270	45	2	17

FOOD	PORTION	CALS.	CARB.	FAT	PRO.
Di Giorno (CONT.)					
Ravioli Light Tomato & Cheese	1 cup (3.7 oz)	280	49	3	14
Ravioli With Italian Sausage	¾ cup (3.6 oz)	340	41	12	16
Tortellini Cheese	¾ cup (2.8 oz)	260	37	6	12
Tortellini Mozzarella Garlic	1 cup (3.5 oz)	300	40	9	15
Tortellini Mushroom	1 cup (3.4 oz)	290	42	7	14
Tortellini Red Hot Pepper Cheese	1 cup (3.4 oz)	310	41	9	16
Tortellini With Chicken And Herbs	1 cup (3.2 oz)	260	40	5	13
Tortellini With Meat	¾ cup (3.1 oz)	290	40	9	12
Herb's					
Fettucine Bell Pepper Basil	2 oz	220	42	2	10
Fettucine Parsley Garlic	2 oz	220	42	2	10
Fettucine Spinach	2 oz	220	42	2	10
Ribbons Vegetable	2 oz	220	42	2	10
Ribbons Whole Wheat	2 oz	200	40	2	8
Rotini Mixed Vegetable	2 oz	210	42	1	7
Shells Mixed Vegetable	2 oz	210	42	1	7
Trios					
Ravioli Cracked Pepper Garlic Cheese	1 cup (4.3 oz)	340	48	9	15
HOME RECIPE					
made w/ egg cooked	2 oz	74	13	tr	3
made w/o egg cooked	2 oz	71	14	tr	2

PASTA DINNERS
(*see also* DINNER, PASTA SALAD)
CANNED
Chef Boyardee

FOOD	PORTION	CALS.	CARB.	FAT	PRO.
ABC's & 1,2,3's In Cheese Flavor Sauce	7.5 oz	180	37	1	5
ABC's & 1,2,3's w/ Mini Meatballs	7.5 oz	260	32	11	7
Beef Ravioli	7.5 oz	190	31	4	7
Beefaroni	7.5 oz	220	31	7	7
Cheese Ravioli In Meat Sauce	7.5 oz	200	37	3	6
Dinosaurs In Cheese Flavor Sauce	7.5 oz	180	36	1	6

FOOD	PORTION	CALS.	CARB.	FAT	PRO.
Chef Boyardee (CONT.)					
Dinosaurs w/ Meatballs	7.5 oz	240	32	9	8
Elbows In Beef Sauce	7.5 oz	210	29	7	8
Lasagna	7.5 oz	230	31	9	7
Lasagna In Garden Vegetable Sauce	7.5 oz	170	34	1	5
Macaroni & Cheese	7.5 oz	180	27	5	7
Microwave Main Meal Beans & Pasta	10.5 oz	200	44	1	14
Microwave Main Meal Beef Ravioli Suprema	10.5 oz	290	52	4	12
Microwave Main Meal Cheese Ravioli Suprema	10.5 oz	290	52	4	12
Microwave Main Meal Fettuccine	10.5 oz	290	46	9	13
Microwave Main Meal Lasagna	10.5 oz	290	41	8	13
Microwave Main Meal Meat Tortellini	10.5 oz	220	53	4	12
Microwave Main Meal Noodles w/ Chicken	10.5 oz	170	27	1	13
Microwave Main Meal Peas & Pasta	10.5 oz	190	39	2	9
Microwave Main Meal Spaghetti Suprema	10.5 oz	200	37	7	11
Microwave Main Meal Zesty Macaroni	10.5 oz	290	40	8	14
Microwave Main Meal Ziti In Sauce	10.5 oz	210	52	tr	8
Pasta Rings & Meatballs	7.5 oz	220	33	8	8
Rigatoni	7.5 oz	210	31	6	8
Rings & Franks	7.5 oz	190	31	5	7
Shells In Mushroom Sauce	7.5 oz	170	35	1	6
Shells In Meat Sauce	7.5 oz	210	32	6	8
Spaghetti & Meat Balls	7.5 oz	230	29	7	7
Tic Tac Toes In Cheese Flavor Sauce	7.5 oz	170	36	1	5
Tic Tac Toes w/ Mini Meatballs	7.5 oz	250	32	10	7
Turtles In Sauce	7.5 oz	160	33	1	5
Turtles w/ Meatballs	7.5 oz	210	30	8	7

FOOD	PORTION	CALS.	CARB.	FAT	PRO.
Dinty Moore					
American Classics Lasagna With Meat & Sauce	1 bowl (10 oz)	260	33	4	22
Franco-American					
Beef RavioliO's In Meat Sauce	½ can (7½ oz)	250	35	8	10
CircusO's Pasta In Tomato & Cheese Sauce	½ can (7⅜ oz)	170	33	2	5
CircusO's Pasta With Meatballs In Tomato Sauce	½ can (7⅜ oz)	210	25	8	9
Macaroni & Cheese	½ can (7⅜ oz)	170	24	6	6
Spaghetti In Tomato Sauce w/ Cheese	½ can (7⅜ oz)	180	36	2	5
Spaghetti w/ Meatballs In Tomato Sauce	½ can (7⅜ oz)	220	28	8	10
SpaghettiO's With Meatballs	½ can (7⅜ oz)	220	25	9	9
SpaghettiO's In Tomato & Cheese Sauce	½ can (7⅜ oz)	170	33	2	5
SpaghettiO's w/ Sliced Franks	½ can (7⅜ oz)	220	26	9	8
SportyO's In Tomato & Cheese Sauce	½ can (7½ oz)	170	33	2	5
SportyO's Pasta With Meatballs In Tomato Sauce	½ can (7⅜ oz)	210	25	8	9
TeddyO's In Tomato & Cheese Sauce	½ can (7½ oz)	170	33	2	5
TeddyO's Pasta With Meatballs	½ can (7⅜ oz)	210	25	8	9
Hormel					
Lasagna	1 can (7.5 oz)	250	24	14	8
Spaghetti & Meatballs	1 can (7.5 oz)	210	28	7	10
Kid's Kitchen					
Cheezy Mac & Beef	1 cup (7.5 oz)	250	34	7	15
Microwave Meals Beefy Macaroni	1 cup (7.5 oz)	190	23	6	11
Microwave Meals Macaroni & Cheese	1 cup (7.5 oz)	260	30	11	11

FOOD	PORTION	CALS.	CARB.	FAT	PRO.
Kid's Kitchen (CONT.)					
Microwave Meals Mini Ravioli	1 cup (7.5 oz)	240	35	7	10
Microwave Meals Spaghetti Ring & Meatballs	1 cup (7.5 oz)	250	35	7	11
Noodle Rings & Chicken	1 cup (7.5 oz)	150	16	5	11
Spaghetti Rings & Franks	1 cup (7.5 oz)	230	36	6	9
Micro Cup Meals					
Lasagna	1 cup (7.5 oz)	230	34	7	9
Lasagna & Beef Tomato Sauce	1 cup	359	34	19	12
Macaroni & Cheese	1 cup (7.5 oz)	260	30	11	11
Macaroni & Beef With Vegetables	1 cup	285	37	8	14
Ravioli Tomato Sauce	1 cup (7.5 oz)	260	34	10	9
Spaghetti & Meat Sauce	1 cup (7.5 oz)	220	33	5	9
Top Shelf					
Italian Lasagna	1 bowl (10 oz)	350	29	15	14
Spaghetti With Meat Sauce	1 bowl (10 oz)	240	36	5	14
Van Camp's					
Spaghetti Weenee	1 can (8 oz)	230	34	8	7
FROZEN					
Armour					
Classics Chicken Fettucini	1 meal (10 oz)	230	25	8	16
Banquet					
Family Entree Lasagna w/ Meat Sauce	1 serv (8 oz)	240	32	7	12
Family Entree Macaroni & Cheese	1 serv (8 oz)	300	39	10	14
Family Entree Macaroni & Beef	1 serv (8 oz)	230	31	7	6
Family Entree Noodle & Chicken	1 serv (8 oz)	210	24	9	10
Family Entree Noodles & Beef	1 serv (7.47 oz)	140	16	4	11
Birds Eye					
Easy Recipe Chicken Primavera not prep	½ pkg	80	14	3	4
Easy Recipe Chicken Alfredo not prep	½ pkg	160	22	7	6

FOOD	PORTION	CALS.	CARB.	FAT	PRO.
Budget Gourmet					
Cheese Ravioli	1 meal (9.5 oz)	290	34	13	12
Lasagna Italian Sausage	1 meal (10 oz)	430	34	23	20
Lasagna Vegetable	1 meal (10.5 oz)	390	36	10	16
Lasagna Three Cheese	1 meal (10 oz)	390	26	17	23
Lasagna With Meat Sauce	1 meal (9.4 oz)	290	30	11	18
Linguini With Shrimp & Clams	1 meal (9.5 oz)	280	34	10	14
Linguini With Shrimp And Clams	1 meal (10 oz)	270	35	9	12
Macaroni & Cheese With Cheddar & Parmesan	1 meal (10.5 oz)	330	49	8	19
Macaroni And Cheese	1 meal (5.75 oz)	230	22	12	9
Manicotti Cheese	1 meal (10 oz)	440	36	24	20
Pasta Alfredo With Broccoli	1 meal (5.5 oz)	210	22	10	8
Penne Pasta With Chunky Tomato Sauce & Italian Sausage	1 meal (10 oz)	320	34	9	13
Rigatoni In Cream Sauce With Broccoli & Chicken	1 meal (10.8 oz)	290	44	7	19
Spaghetti With Chunky Tomato & Meat Sauce	1 meal (10 oz)	300	44	8	18
Tortellini Cheese	1 meal (5.5 oz)	200	25	8	8
Ziti In Marinara Sauce	1 meal (6.25 oz)	200	23	9	7
Dining Light					
Cheese Cannelloni	9 oz	310	38	9	19
Formagg					
Penne Pasta Alfredo	⅔ cup (5 oz)	190	35	2	7
Penne Pasta Primavera	⅔ cup (5 oz)	190	35	2	7
Vegetable Pasta & Ceasar Italian Garden	⅔ cup (5 oz)	190	35	2	7
Green Giant					
Garden Gourmet Creamy Mushroom	1 pkg	220	29	11	6
Garden Gourmet Pasta Dijon	1 pkg	260	21	17	7
Garden Gourmet Pasta Florentine	1 pkg	230	27	9	14
Garden Gourmet Rotini Cheddar	1 pkg	230	32	10	9

FOOD	PORTION	CALS.	CARB.	FAT	PRO.
Green Giant (CONT.)					
One Serve Cheese Tortellini	1 pkg	260	37	9	8
One Serve Macaroni & Cheese	1 pkg	230	28	9	9
One Serve Pasta Marinara	1 pkg	180	29	5	5
One Serve Pasta Parmesan With Green Peas	1 pkg	170	23	5	9
Pasta Accents Creamy Cheddar	½ cup	100	12	5	4
Pasta Accents Garden Herb	½ cup	80	11	3	3
Pasta Accents Garlic Seasoning	½ cup	110	13	5	3
Pasta Accents Pasta Primavera	½ cup	110	13	5	5
Healthy Choice					
Beef Macaroni Casserole	1 meal (8.5 oz)	200	34	1	14
Cheese Ravioli Parmigiana	1 meal (9 oz)	250	44	4	11
Chicken Fettucini Alfredo	1 meal (8.5 oz)	250	34	3	20
Chicken Broccoli Alfredo	1 meal (12.1 oz)	370	53	8	23
Classics Pasta Shells Marinara	1 meal (12 oz)	360	59	3	25
Classics Turkey Fettuccine Alla Crema	1 meal (12.5 oz)	350	50	4	28
Fettucini Alfredo	1 meal (8 oz)	240	39	5	9
Lasagna Roma	1 meal (13.5 oz)	390	60	5	26
Macaroni & Cheese	1 meal (9 oz)	290	45	5	15
Spaghetti Bolognese	1 meal (10 oz)	260	43	3	14
Three Cheese Manicotti	1 meal (11 oz)	310	41	9	16
Vegetable Pasta Italiano	1 meal (10 oz)	220	44	1	8
Zucchini Lasagna	1 meal (14 oz)	330	58	2	20
Kid Cuisine					
Macaroni & Cheese	1 pkg (10.6 oz)	420	68	12	10
Mini Cheese Ravioli	1 pkg (9.82 oz)	320	63	5	7
Le Menu					
Entree LightStyle Garden Vegetables Lasagna	10½ oz	260	35	8	11
Entree LightStyle Lasagna With Meat Sauce	10 oz	290	36	8	19

FOOD	PORTION	CALS.	CARB.	FAT	PRO.
Le Menu (CONT.)					
Entree LightStyle Meat Sauce & Cheese Tortellini	8 oz	250	34	8	11
Entree LightStyle Spaghetti With Beef Sauce And Mushrooms	9 oz	280	45	6	12
LightStyle 3-Cheese Stuffed Shells	10 oz	280	34	8	17
Manicotti With Three Cheeses	11¾ oz	390	44	15	19
LightStyle Cheese Tortellini	10 oz	230	35	6	10
Lean Cuisine					
Angel Hair Pasta	1 meal (10 oz)	210	35	4	96
Cannelloni Cheese	1 meal (9.1 oz)	270	28	8	21
Cheddar Bake With Pasta	1 meal (9 oz)	220	29	6	12
Chicken Fettucini	1 pkg (9 oz)	270	33	6	22
Fettucini Alfredo	1 meal (9 oz)	270	38	7	13
Fettucini Primavera	1 meal (10 oz)	260	33	8	15
Lasagna Classic Cheese	1 meal (11.5 oz)	290	38	6	20
Lasagna Tuna	1 meal (9.75 oz)	230	29	6	14
Lasagna Zucchini	1 meal (11 oz)	240	33	4	17
Lasagna With Meat Sauce	1 pkg (10.25 oz)	270	34	6	19
Macaroni & Cheese	1 pkg (9 oz)	270	39	7	13
Macaroni & Beef	1 pkg (10 oz)	280	40	8	13
Marinara Twist	1 pkg (10 oz)	240	42	3	10
Ravioli Cheese	1 meal (8.5 oz)	250	32	8	12
Rigatoni	1 pkg (9 oz)	180	25	4	10
Spaghetti With Meat Sauce	1 meal (11.5 oz)	290	45	6	14
Spaghetti & Meatballs	1 pkg (9.5 oz)	290	40	7	17
Life Choice					
Linguini Roma	1 meal (13.2 oz)	230	48	1	8
Sun Dried Tomato Manicotti	1 meal (11.65 oz)	220	39	3	11
Vegetable Lasagna Primavera	1 meal (11.2 oz)	170	30	1	10

FOOD	PORTION	CALS.	CARB.	FAT	PRO.
Luigino's					
Cheese Tortellini & Alfredo Sauce With Broccoli	1 pkg (8 oz)	390	28	24	17
Cheese Ravioli & Alfredo With Broccoli Sauce	1 pkg (8.5 oz)	420	30	25	18
Fettuccine Alfredo	1 cup (7.5 oz)	330	36	11	13
Fettuccine Alfredo	1 pkg (9.4 oz)	390	45	14	16
Fettuccine Alfredo With Broccoli	1 pkg (9.2 oz)	360	39	16	14
Fettuccine Carbonara	1 pkg (9 oz)	360	47	13	15
Lasagna Alfredo	1 pkg (9 oz)	360	30	20	16
Lasagna Alfredo	1 cup (6.3 oz)	300	25	17	13
Lasagna Pollo	1 pkg (9 oz)	320	33	14	16
Lasagna With Meat Sauce	1 cup (7.2 oz)	240	30	8	12
Lasagna With Meat Sauce	1 pkg (9 oz)	290	36	10	15
Lasagna With Vegetables	1 pkg (9 oz)	290	35	10	14
Linguini With Red Sauce & Clams	1 pkg (9 oz)	260	41	6	11
Linguini With Clams & Sauce	1 pkg (9 oz)	270	42	6	12
Linguini With Seafood	1 pkg (9 oz)	290	45	8	10
Macaroni & Cheese	1 cup (7.2 oz)	310	37	12	11
Macaroni & Cheese	1 pkg (9 oz)	370	45	15	13
Marinara Sauce Penne Pasta Italian Sausage & Peppers	1 cup (7.4 oz)	290	27	14	15
Marinara Sauce Penne Pasta Italian Sausage & Peppers	1 pkg (9 oz)	350	32	17	18
Meat Ravioli & Pomodoro Sauce	1 pkg (8.5 oz)	320	37	13	15
Minestrone With Penne Pasta	1 cup (6.3 oz)	180	21	6	10
Penne Pollo	1 pkg (9 oz)	330	36	14	15
Penne Primavera	1 pkg (9 oz)	350	50	10	15
Rigatoni Pomodoro Italiano	1 pkg (9 oz)	290	40	8	15
Shells & Cheese With Jalapenos	1 pkg (8.5 oz)	360	41	15	14
Spaghetti Bolognese	1 pkg (9 oz)	270	38	8	13

FOOD	PORTION	CALS.	CARB.	FAT	PRO.
Luigino's (CONT.)					
Spaghetti Marinara	1 pkg (10 oz)	250	49	2	11
Spinach Ravioli & Primavera Sauce	1 pkg (8.5 oz)	360	36	17	15
Morton					
Macaroni & Cheese	1 serv (8 oz)	220	34	6	9
Mrs. Paul's					
Entrees Light Seafood Lasagne	9½ oz	290	39	8	14
Entrees Light Seafood Rotini	9 oz	240	34	6	12
Seafood Totini	9 oz	240	34	6	12
Palmazone					
Macaroni 'n Cheese	½ pkg (6 oz)	260	36	7	13
Pasta Favorites					
Chicken Pasta Primavera	1 pkg (10.5 oz)	330	40	13	13
Fettuccini Alfredo	1 pkg (10.5 oz)	370	39	18	12
Italian Sausage & Peppers	1 pkg (10.5 oz)	340	43	13	11
Lasagna	1 pkg (10.5 oz)	290	39	9	14
Macaroni & Cheese	1 pkg (10.5 oz)	350	47	12	13
Pasta Primavera	1 pkg (10.5 oz)	320	40	14	10
Spaghetti w/ Meatballs	1 pkg (10.5 oz)	370	40	16	14
Vegetable Lasagna	1 pkg (10.5 oz)	260	41	6	11
White Cheddar & Rotini	1 pkg (10.5 oz)	350	48	12	12
Senor Felix's					
Lasagna Southwestern	1 serv (6 oz)	160	15	7	8
Stouffer's					
Beef Ravioli	1 pkg (9.5 oz)	370	43	14	17
Cheese Tortellini With Alfredo Sauce	1 pkg (8.9 oz)	550	38	33	25
Cheese Tortellini With Tomato Sauce	1 pkg (9.25 oz)	290	40	6	19
Cheese Manicotti	1 pkg (9 oz)	340	32	16	18
Cheese Ravioli With Tomato Sauce	1 pkg (9.5 oz)	360	42	16	16
Cheese Shells With Tomato Sauce	1 pkg (9.25 oz)	340	29	16	19
Fettucini Alfredo	1 pkg (10 oz)	480	40	29	15
Four Cheese Lasagna	1 pkg (10.75 oz)	410	37	19	22
Homestyle Chicken Fettucini	1 pkg (10.5 oz)	380	32	15	31
Lasagna With Meat Sauce	1 cup (7 oz)	260	24	10	19

FOOD	PORTION	CALS.	CARB.	FAT	PRO.
Stouffer's (CONT.)					
Lasagna With Meat Sauce	1 pkg (10.5 oz)	360	34	13	27
Lunch Express Cheese Lasagna Casserole	1 pkg (9.5 oz)	270	38	7	14
Lunch Express Cheese Ravioli	1 pkg (8.5 oz)	310	38	12	12
Lunch Express Chicken Fettucini	1 pkg (10.25 oz)	250	32	6	16
Lunch Express Chicken Alfredo	1 pkg (9.6 oz)	360	34	17	18
Lunch Express Fettucini Primavera	1 pkg (10.25 oz)	420	33	25	15
Lunch Express Lasagna With Meat Sauce	1 pkg (10 oz)	350	42	12	18
Lunch Express Macaroni & Cheese & Broccoli	1 pkg (9.5 oz)	240	30	7	13
Lunch Express Macaroni & Cheese With Broccoli	1 pkg (10.4 oz)	360	32	19	15
Lunch Express Pasta & Chicken Marinara	1 pkg (9.1 oz)	270	38	6	15
Lunch Express Pasta & Tuna Casserole	1 pkg (9.6 oz)	280	39	6	18
Lunch Express Pasta & Turkey Dijon	1 pkg (9.9 oz)	270	37	6	16
Lunch Express Rigatoni With Meat Sauce	1 pkg (10.75 oz)	340	44	12	14
Lunch Express Spaghetti With Meat Sauce	1 pkg (9.6 oz)	320	43	10	15
Lunch Express Swedish Meatballs With Pasta	1 pkg (10.25 oz)	530	41	32	19
Macaroni & Cheese	1 cup (6 oz)	330	31	17	14
Macaroni & Beef	1 pkg (11.5 oz)	340	40	12	19
Noodles Romanoff	1 pkg (12 oz)	460	48	23	18
Spaghetti With Meat Sauce	1 pkg (12.9 oz)	430	57	13	20
Spaghetti With Meatballs	1 pkg (12.6 oz)	420	51	15	19
Tuna Noodle Casserole	1 pkg (10 oz)	330	31	14	19
Turkey Tettrazini	1 pkg (10 oz)	360	28	19	18
Vegetable Lasagna	1 cup (8 oz)	280	29	12	14
Vegetable Lasagna	1 pkg (10.5 oz)	370	31	19	18

FOOD	PORTION	CALS.	CARB.	FAT	PRO.
Swanson					
Homestyle Lasagne With Meat Sauce	10½ oz	400	39	15	26
Homestyle Macaroni & Cheese	10 oz	390	37	19	17
Homestyle Spaghetti With Italian Style Meatballs	13 oz	490	60	18	23
Macaroni & Cheese	12¼ oz	370	48	15	13
Macaroni & Cheese	7 oz	200	24	8	7
Spaghetti & Meatballs	12½ oz	390	46	17	14
Tabatchnick					
Macaroni & Cheese	7.5 oz	280	30	12	14
Tyson					
Parmigiana	1 pkg (11.25 oz)	380	37	17	19
Ultra Slim-Fast					
Pasta Primavera	12 oz	340	52	9	18
Spaghetti With Beef & Mushroom Sauce	12 oz	370	49	10	20
Weight Watchers					
Angel Hair Pasta	10 oz	200	28	4	14
Baked Cheese Ravioli	9 oz	240	27	6	18
Cheese Tortellini	9 oz	310	50	6	14
Cheese Manicotti	9.25 oz	260	31	8	17
Chicken Fettucini	8.25 oz	280	25	9	22
Fettucini Alfredo	8 oz	230	28	7	15
Garden Lasagna	11 oz	260	30	7	19
Italian Cheese Lasagna	11 oz	290	29	6	28
Lasagna	10.25 oz	240	29	6	24
Spaghetti With Meat Sauce	10 oz	240	28	7	16
HOME RECIPE					
macroni & cheese	1 cup	430	40	22	17
spaghetti w/ meatballs & tomato sauce	1 cup	330	39	12	19
MIX					
Casbah					
Pasta Fasul	1 pkg (1.6 oz)	150	10	1	11
Golden Grain					
Macaroni & Cheese	½ cup	310	36	15	8
Hain					
Pasta & Sauce Creamy Parmesan	¼ pkg	150	22	3	8
Pasta & Sauce Creamy Swiss	¼ pkg	170	26	4	6

FOOD	PORTION	CALS.	CARB.	FAT	PRO.
Hain (CONT.)					
Pasta & Sauce Fettuccine Alfredo	¼ pkg	180	27	4	5
Pasta & Sauce Italian Herb	¼ pkg	110	17	2	4
Pasta & Sauce Primavera	¼ pkg	140	20	4	7
Pasta & Sauce Tangy Cheddar	¼ pkg	180	24	6	6
Kraft					
Cheddar Cheese Egg Noodle	1 cup (8 oz)	430	46	21	12
Macaroni & Cheese Deluxe Original	1 cup (6.1 oz)	320	44	10	14
Macaroni & Cheese Dinosaurs	1 cup (6.8 oz)	390	48	17	12
Macaroni & Cheese Flintstones	1 cup (6.8 oz)	390	48	17	12
Macaroni & Cheese Milk White Cheddar	1 cup (6.8 oz)	390	48	17	11
Macaroni & Cheese Original	1 cup (6.9 oz)	390	48	17	11
Macaroni & Cheese Santa Mac	1 cup	390	48	17	12
Macaroni & Cheese Spirals	1 cup (6.8 oz)	390	48	17	12
Macaroni & Cheese Super Mario Bros	1 cup (6.8 oz)	390	48	17	12
Macaroni & Cheese Teddy Bears	1 cup (6.8 oz)	390	48	17	12
Macaroni & Cheese Thick 'N Creamy	1 cup (6.1 oz)	320	50	10	12
Spaghetti Mild American	1 cup (8.1 oz)	270	48	5	9
Spaghetti Tangy Italain	1 cup (7.9 oz)	270	46	5	10
Spaghetti With Meat Sauce	1 cup (8.2 oz)	330	46	11	12
Lipton					
Pasta & Sauce Cheddar Broccoli	½ cup	132	24	2	5
Pasta & Sauce Creamy Garlic	½ cup	146	26	2	5
Pasta & Sauce Creamy Mushroom	½ cup	143	25	3	5
Pasta & Sauce Herb Tomato	½ cup	130	26	1	5

FOOD	PORTION	CALS.	CARB.	FAT	PRO.
Minute					
Microwave Cheddar Cheese Broccoli And Pasta as prep	½ cup	160	23	5	6
Nile Spice					
Pasta'n Sauce Mediterranean	1 pkg	210	33	5	9
Pasta'n Sauce Parmesan	1 pkg	200	36	3	8
Pasta'n Sauce Primavera	1 pkg	200	34	4	9
Terrazza					
Pasta E Fagioli as prep	½ cup	150	23	3	7
Ultra Slim-Fast					
Macaroni & Cheese	2.3 oz	230	46	3	9
Uncle Ben					
Country Inn Pasta & Sauce Angel Hair Parmesan	1 serv (2.2 oz)	245	39	5	10
Country Inn Pasta & Sauce Broccoli & White Cheddar	1 serv (2.2 oz)	240	40	5	9
Country Inn Pasta & Sauce Butter & Herb	1 serv (2 oz)	230	36	6	7
Country Inn Pasta & Sauce Creamy Garlic	1 serv (2.4 oz)	261	45	5	9
Country Inn Pasta & Sauce Fettuccine Alfredo	1 serv (2.2 oz)	310	41	6	9
Country Inn Pasta & Sauce Herb Linguine	1 serv (2.2 oz)	240	43	3	9
Country Inn Pasta & Sauce Mushroom Fettuccine	1 serv (2.2 oz)	250	41	6	9
Country Inn Pasta & Sauce Vegetable Alfredo	1 serv (2.2 oz)	240	42	5	9
Velveeta					
Rotini & Cheese Broccoli	1 cup (7.2 oz)	400	46	16	18
Shells & Cheese Bacon	1 cup (6.8 oz)	360	43	14	17
Shells & Cheese Original	1 cup (6.6 oz)	360	44	13	16
Shells & Cheese Salsa	1 cup (7.5 oz)	380	47	14	17
SHELF-STABLE					
Lunch Bucket					
Elbows In Tomato Sauce	1 pkg (7.5 oz)	190	38	2	4
Lasagna With Meatsauce	1 pkg (7.5 oz)	220	38	4	8

FOOD	PORTION	CALS.	CARB.	FAT	PRO.
Lunch Bucket (CONT.)					
Light'n Healthy Italian Style Pasta	1 pkg (7.5 oz)	130	23	1	7
Light'n Healthy Pasta In Wine Sauce	1 pkg (7.5 oz)	130	21	3	5
Light'n Healthy Pasta'n Garden Vegetables	1 pkg (7.5 oz)	150	30	1	4
Macaroni'n Cheese	1 pkg (7.5 oz)	210	24	9	9
Pasta'n Chicken	1 pkg (7.5 oz)	180	22	6	9
Spaghetti'n Meatsauce	1 pkg (7.5 oz)	240	39	5	9
My Own Meal					
Cheese Tortellini	1 pkg (10 oz)	340	49	10	15
TAKE-OUT					
lasagna	1 piece (2.5 in x 2.5 in)	374	25	21	22
macaroni & cheese	1 cup	230	26	10	9
manicotti	¾ cup (6.4 oz)	273	28	12	14
rigatoni w/ sausage sauce	¾ cup	260	28	12	10
spaghetti w/ meatballs & cheese	1 cup	407	38	19	21

PASTA MACHINE MIX
Wanda's

FOOD	PORTION	CALS.	CARB.	FAT	PRO.
Dried Tomato	⅓ cup mix per serv (1.9 oz)	202	42	1	7
Durum & Semolina	⅓ cup mix per serv (1.9 oz)	199	42	1	7
Semolina Blend	⅓ cup mix per serv (1.9 oz)	202	42	1	7
Spinach	⅓ cup mix per serv (1.9 oz)	202	42	1	7
Whole Wheat & Semolina	⅓ cup mix per serv (1.9 oz)	198	41	1	7

PASTA SALAD
MIX
Kraft

FOOD	PORTION	CALS.	CARB.	FAT	PRO.
Pasta Salad Classic Ranch With Bacon	¾ cup (4.7 oz)	360	30	23	7
Pasta Salad Creamy Ceasar	¾ cup (4.8 oz)	350	30	22	7
Pasta Salad Garden Primavera	¾ cup (5 oz)	280	34	12	8
Pasta Salad Light Italian	¾ cup (5 oz)	190	34	2	8
Pasta Salad Parmesan Peppercorn	¾ cup (4.9 oz)	360	28	25	8

FOOD	PORTION	CALS.	CARB.	FAT	PRO.
Lipton					
Robust Italian	½ cup	126	25	1	5
Suddenly Salad					
Classic Pasta as prep	½ cup	160	23	6	4
Creamy Macaroni as prep	½ cup	200	21	10	4
Creamy Macaroni as prep low fat recipe	½ cup	140	21	4	4
Italian Pasta as prep	½ cup	160	22	6	4
Pasta Primavera as prep	½ cup	190	20	10	4
Pasta Primavera as prep low fat recipe	½ cup	150	21	5	4
Tortellini Italiano as prep	½ cup	160	21	7	4
TAKE-OUT					
elbow macaroni salad	3.5 oz	160	26	5	3
italian style pasta salad	3.5 oz	140	15	7	3
mustard macaroni salad	3.5 oz	190	23	10	4
pasta salad w/ vegetables	3.5 oz	140	21	4	4

PASTRY
(*see* BROWNIE, CAKE, DANISH PASTRY)

PATE
CANNED

FOOD	PORTION	CALS.	CARB.	FAT	PRO.
chicken liver	1 tbsp (13 g)	109	1	2	2
chicken liver	1 oz	238	2	4	4
goose liver smoked	1 tbsp (13 g)	60	1	6	1
goose liver smoked	1 oz	131	1	12	3
liver	1 tbsp (13 g)	41	tr	4	5
liver	1 oz	90	tr	8	4
Sells					
Liver	2.08 oz	190	4	16	8

PEACH
CANNED

FOOD	PORTION	CALS.	CARB.	FAT	PRO.
halves in heavy syrup	1 half	60	16	tr	tr
halves in light syrup	1 half	44	12	tr	tr
halves juice pack	1 half	34	9	tr	tr
halves water pack	1 half	18	5	tr	tr
spiced in heavy syrup	1 fruit	66	18	tr	tr
spiced in heavy syrup	1 cup	180	49	tr	1
Del Monte					
Halves Cling In Heavy Syrup	½ cup (4.5 oz)	100	24	0	0
Halves Cling Lite	½ cup (4.4 oz)	60	15	0	0

FOOD	PORTION	CALS.	CARB.	FAT	PRO.
Del Monte (cont.)					
Halves Cling Melba In Heavy Syrup	½ cup (4.5 oz)	100	24	0	0
Halves Freestone In Heavy Syrup	½ cup (4.5 oz)	100	24	0	0
Sliced Cling Fruit Naturals	½ cup (4.4 oz)	60	15	0	0
Sliced Cling In Heavy Syrup	½ cup (4.5 oz)	100	24	0	0
Sliced Cling Lite	½ cup (4.4 oz)	60	15	0	0
Sliced Freestone In Heavy Syrup	½ cup (4.5 oz)	100	24	0	0
Sliced Freestone Lite	½ cup (4.4 oz)	60	14	0	0
Snack Cups Diced Fruit Naturals	1 serv (4.5 oz)	60	16	0	0
Snack Cups Diced Fruit Naturals EZ-Open Lid	1 serv (4.2 oz)	60	15	0	0
Snack Cups Diced In Heavy Syrup	1 serv (4.5 oz)	100	24	0	0
Snack Cups Diced In Heavy Syrup EZ-Open Lid	1 serv (4.2 oz)	90	23	0	0
Snack Cups Diced Lite	1 serv (4.5 oz)	60	16	0	0
Snack Cups Diced Lite EZ-Open Lid	1 serv (4.2 oz)	60	15	0	0
Whole Cling In Heavy Syrup	½ cup (4.2 oz)	100	24	0	0
Hunt's					
Halves	4 oz	90	23	tr	tr
Slices	4 oz	90	23	tr	tr
Libby					
Halves Yellow Cling Lite	½ cup (4.4 oz)	60	13	0	1
Sliced Yellow Cling Lite	½ cup (4.4 oz)	60	13	0	1
S&W					
Halves Clingstone	½ cup	100	25	0	0
Halves Clingstone Diet	½ cup	30	8	0	0
Halves Clingstone Unsweetened	½ cup	30	8	0	0
Halves Freestone Diet	½ cup	30	7	0	0
Halves Freestone In Heavy Syrup	½ cup	100	26	0	0
Sliced Clingstone Diet	½ cup	30	8	0	0
Sliced Clingstone Unsweetened	½ cup	30	8	0	0

FOOD	PORTION	CALS.	CARB.	FAT	PRO.
S&W (CONT.)					
Sliced Freestone In Heavy Syrup	½ cup	100	26	0	0
Sliced Yellow Cling Natural Style	½ cup	90	20	0	0
Sliced Yellow Cling Premium In Heavy Syrup	½ cup	100	25	0	0
Slices Freestone Diet	½ cup	30	7	0	0
Whole Yellow Cling Spiced In Heavy Syrup	½ cup	90	23	0	0
Yellow Cling Natural Lite	½ cup	50	13	0	0
DRIED					
halves	10	311	80	1	5
halves	1 cup	383	98	1	6
halves cooked w/ sugar	½ cup	139	36	tr	1
halves cooked w/o sugar	½ cup	99	25	tr	1
Del Monte					
Sun Dried	⅓ cup (1.4 oz)	90	28	0	1
Sonoma					
Pieces	3-5 pieces (1.4 oz)	120	31	0	1
FRESH					
peach	1	37	10	tr	1
sliced	1 cup	73	19	tr	1
Dole					
Peach	2	70	19	0	1
FROZEN					
slices sweetened	1 cup	235	60	tr	2
Big Valley					
Freestone	⅔ cup (4.9 oz)	50	13	0	1
PEACH JUICE					
nectar	1 cup	134	35	tr	1
Goya					
Nectar	6 oz	110	27	0	tr
Kern's					
Nectar	6 fl oz	110	26	0	1
Libby					
Nectar	1 can (11.5 fl oz)	210	52	0	1
Mott's					
Fruit Basket Orchard Peach Juice Cocktail as prep	8 fl oz	130	32	0	0

FOOD	PORTION	CALS.	CARB.	FAT	PRO.
Smucker's					
Juice	8 oz	120	30	0	1
Snapple					
Dixie Peach	10 fl oz	140	39	0	0

PEANUT BUTTER

FOOD	PORTION	CALS.	CARB.	FAT	PRO.
chunky	1 cup	1520	56	129	62
chunky	2 tbsp	188	7	16	8
chunky w/o salt	2 tbsp	188	7	16	8
chunky w/o salt	1 cup	1520	56	129	62
smooth	1 cup	1517	53	128	63
smooth	2 tbsp	188	7	16	8
smooth w/o salt	2 tbsp	188	7	16	8
smooth w/o salt	1 cup	1517	53	129	63
Arrowhead					
Creamy	2 tbsp (1.1 oz)	200	6	15	9
Crunchy	2 tbsp (1.1 oz)	200	6	15	9
BAMA					
Creamy	2 tbsp	200	6	17	7
Crunchy	2 tbsp	200	6	17	7
Jelly & Peanut Butter	2 tbsp	150	20	7	3
Crazy Richard's					
Natural Creamy	2 tbsp (1.1 oz)	190	6	16	9
Erewhon					
Chunky	2 tbsp (32 g)	190	7	14	9
Chunky Unsalted	2 tbsp (32 g)	190	7	14	9
Creamy	2 tbsp (32 g)	190	7	14	9
Creamy Unsalted	2 tbsp (32 g)	190	7	14	9
Estee					
Chunky Sodium Free	2 tbsp (1 oz)	190	7	15	7
Chunky Sodium Free Sorbitol Sweetened	2 tbsp (1 oz)	190	7	15	7
Creamy Sodium Free	2 tbsp (1 oz)	190	7	15	7
Creamy Sodium Free Sorbitol Sweetened	2 tbsp (1 oz)	190	7	15	7
Health Valley					
Chunky No Salt	2 tbsp	170	6	14	8
Creamy No Salt	2 tbsp	170	6	14	8
Hollywood					
Creamy	1 tbsp	35	1	3	2
Crunchy	1 tbsp	35	1	3	2
Unsalted	1 tbsp	35	1	3	2
Jif					
Creamy	2 tbsp (1.1 oz)	190	7	16	8

FOOD	PORTION	CALS.	CARB.	FAT	PRO.
Jif (CONT.)					
Extra Crunchy	2 tbsp (1.1 oz)	190	7	16	8
Reduced Fat	2 tbsp (1.3 oz)	190	15	12	8
Simply Creamy	2 tbsp (1.1 oz)	190	6	16	8
Simply Extra Crunchy	2 tbsp (1.1 oz)	190	6	16	8
Peter Pan					
Creamy	2 tbsp	190	6	16	9
Creamy Salt Free	2 tbsp	190	5	17	9
Crunchy	2 tbsp	190	6	16	9
Crunchy Salt Free	2 tbsp	190	5	17	9
Red Wing					
Creamy	2 tbsp (1.1 oz)	200	6	16	7
Crunchy	2 tbsp (1.1 oz)	200	6	16	7
Reese's					
Peanut Butter Chips	¼ cup (1.5 oz)	230	19	13	7
Skippy					
Creamy	1 cup (263 g)	1540	38	135	78
Creamy w/ 2 slices white bread	1 sandwich	340	33	19	14
Reduced Fat Creamy	2 tbsp	190	13	12	9
Super Chunk	2 tbsp (32 g)	190	4	17	9
Super Chunk	1 cup (260 g)	1540	36	138	76
Super Chunk w/ slices white bread	1 sandwich	340	32	19	14
Smucker's					
Goober Grape	2 tbsp	180	18	10	5
Honey Sweetened	2 tbsp	200	7	16	7
Natural	2 tbsp	200	6	16	8
Natural No-Salt Added	2 tbsp	200	6	16	8
Tree Of Life					
Creamy	2 tbsp (1 oz)	190	7	15	9
Creamy No Salt	2 tbsp (1 oz)	190	7	15	9
Creamy Organic	2 tbsp (1 oz)	190	7	16	8
Creamy Organic No Salt	2 tbsp (1 oz)	190	7	16	8
Crunchy	2 tbsp (1 oz)	190	7	15	9
Crunchy No Salt	2 tbsp (1 oz)	190	7	15	9
Crunchy Organic	2 tbsp (1 oz)	190	7	16	8
Crunchy Organic No Salt	2 tbsp (1 oz)	190	7	16	8
Peanut Wonder 78% Less Fat	2 tbsp (1 oz)	100	11	4	3

PEANUTS

chocolate coated	10 (1.4 oz)	208	20	13	5
chocolate coated	1 cup (5.2 oz)	773	74	50	19

FOOD	PORTION	CALS.	CARB.	FAT	PRO.
cooked	½ cup	102	7	7	4
dry roasted	1 oz	164	6	14	7
dry roasted	1 cup	855	31	73	35
oil roasted	1 oz	163	5	14	7
oil roasted	1 cup	837	27	71	38
oil roasted w/o salt	1 oz	163	5	14	7
oil roasted w/o salt	1 cup	837	27	71	38
spanish oil roasted	1 oz	162	5	14	8
spanish oil roasted w/o salt	1 oz	162	5	14	8
unroasted	1 oz	159	5	14	7
valencia oil roasted	1 oz	165	5	14	8
valencia oil roasted	1 cup	848	23	74	39
valencia oil roasted w/o salt	1 oz	165	5	14	8
valencia oil roasted w/o salt	1 cup	848	23	74	40
virginia oil roasted	1 cup	826	28	70	37
virginia oil roasted	1 oz	161	5	14	8
Beer Nuts					
Peanuts	1 pkg (1 oz)	180	7	14	7
Eagle					
Honey Roasted	1 oz	170	7	13	7
Honey Roasted Cinnamon	1 oz	170	7	13	7
Honey Roasted Maple	1 oz	170	7	13	7
Low Salt	1 oz	170	5	15	7
Virginia Fancy	1 oz	90	3	8	4
Fisher					
Salted-In-Shell shelled	1 oz	170	6	14	7
Spanish Roasted	1 oz	180	6	16	5
Frito Lay					
Dry Roasted	1.2 oz	190	7	16	7
Salted	1 oz	170	6	15	6
Guy's					
Dry Roasted	1 oz	170	3	14	8
Spanish Salted	1 oz	170	3	14	8
Lance					
Honey Toasted	1 pkg (39 g)	230	11	17	9
Roasted w/ Shell	1 pkg (50 g)	190	8	15	9
Salted	1 pkg (32 g)	190	7	15	9
Salted Tube	1 pkg (42 g)	240	9	20	12
Little Debbie					
Salted	1 pkg (1.2 oz)	230	3	21	8
Pennant					
Oil Roasted	1 oz	170	6	14	7

FOOD	PORTION	CALS.	CARB.	FAT	PRO.
Planters					
Cocktail Lightly Salted Oil Roasted	1 oz	170	5	15	7
Cocktail Oil Roasted	1 oz	170	6	14	7
Cocktail Unsalted Oil Roasted	1 oz	170	6	14	7
Dry Roasted	1 oz	160	6	13	7
Fun Size! Oil Roasted	2 pkg (1 oz)	170	6	15	7
Heat Hot Spicy Oil Roasted	1 pkg (1.7 oz)	290	9	25	12
Heat Hot Spicy Oil Roasted	1 oz	160	5	14	7
Heat Hot Spicy Oil Roasted	1 pkg (2 oz)	330	10	29	14
Heat Mild Spicy Oil Roasted	1 oz	160	5	14	7
Honey Roasted	1 oz	160	8	13	6
Honey Roasted Dry Roasted	1 pkg (1.7 oz)	260	17	19	10
Lightly Salted Dry Roasted	1 oz	160	5	14	8
Lightly Salted Dry Roasted	1 pkg (1.75 oz)	290	9	25	13
Lightly Salted Oil Roasted	1 pkg (1.8 oz)	300	8	27	13
Munch'N Go Singles Heat Hot Spicy Oil Roasted	1 pkg (2.5 oz)	410	13	36	18
Salted Oil Roasted	1 pkg (1 oz)	170	5	15	7
Spanish Oil Roasted	1 oz	170	5	14	7
Spanish Raw	1 oz	150	6	13	7
Sweet N Crunchy	1 oz	140	16	7	4
Unsalted Dry Roasted	1 oz	160	6	14	8
Weight Watchers					
Honey Roasted	0.7 oz	100	7	6	6
PEAR					
CANNED					
halves in heavy syrup	1 cup	188	49	tr	1
halves in heavy syrup	1 half	68	15	tr	tr
halves in light syrup	1 half	45	12	tr	tr
halves juice pack	1 cup	123	32	tr	1
halves water pack	1 half	22	6	tr	tr
Del Monte					
Halves Fruit Naturals	½ cup (4.4 oz)	60	15	0	0

FOOD	PORTION	CALS.	CARB.	FAT	PRO.
Del Monte (CONT.)					
Halves In Heavy Syrup	½ cup (4.5 oz)	100	24	0	0
Halves Lite	½ cup (4.4 oz)	60	15	0	0
Sliced In Heavy Syrup	½ cup (4.5 oz)	100	24	0	0
Sliced Lite	½ cup (4.4 oz)	60	15	0	0
Snack Cups Diced In Heavy Syrup	1 serv (4.5 oz)	100	24	0	0
Snack Cups Diced In Heavy Syrup EZ-Open Lid	1 serv (4.2 oz)	90	23	0	0
Snack Cups Diced Lite	1 serv (4.5 oz)	60	15	0	0
Snack Cups Diced Lite EZ-Open Lid	1 serv (4.2 oz)	60	15	0	0
Hunt's					
Halves	4 oz	90	22	tr	tr
Libby					
Halves Lite	½ cup (4.3 oz)	60	13	0	0
Sliced Lite	½ cup (4.3 oz)	60	13	0	0
S&W					
Halves Bartlett In Heavy Syrup	½ cup	100	25	0	0
Halves Bartlett Peeled Unsweetened	½ cup	35	10	0	0
Halves Peeled Diet	½ cup	35	10	0	0
Quartered Peeled Diet	½ cup	35	10	0	0
Sliced Natural Light Bartlett	½ cup	60	15	0	0
Sliced Natural Style	½ cup	80	20	0	0
DRIED					
halves	10	459	122	1	3
halves	1 cup	472	125	1	3
halves cooked w/ sugar	½ cup	196	52	tr	1
halves cooked w/o sugar	½ cup	163	43	tr	tr
Sonoma					
Pieces	3-4 pieces (1.4 oz)	120	33	0	1
FRESH					
asian	1 (4.3 oz)	51	13	tr	1
pear	1	98	25	1	1
sliced w/ skin	1 cup	97	25	1	1
Dole					
Pear	1	100	25	1	1
PEAR JUICE					
nectar	1 cup	149	39	tr	tr

FOOD	PORTION	CALS.	CARB.	FAT	PRO.
Goya					
Nectar	6 oz	120	29	0	0
Kern's					
Nectar	6 fl oz	120	28	0	0
Libby					
Nectar	1 can (11.5 fl oz)	220	54	0	0
PEAS					
CANNED					
green	½ cup	59	11	tr	4
green low sodium	½ cup	59	11	tr	4
Allen					
Crowder	½ cup (4.5 oz)	110	19	1	6
Purple Hull	½ cup (4.4 oz)	120	21	1	7
Crest Top					
Early June	½ cup (4.5 oz)	100	20	1	5
Del Monte					
Sweet	½ cup (4.4 oz)	60	11	0	3
Sweet 50% Less Salt	½ cup (4.4 oz)	60	11	0	3
Sweet No Salt Added	½ cup (4.4 oz)	60	11	0	3
Sweet Very Young	½ cup (4.4 oz)	60	10	0	3
East Texas Fair					
Cream Peas	½ cup (4.4 oz)	120	20	1	8
Crowder	½ cup (4.5 oz)	110	19	1	6
Lady Peas With Snaps	½ cup (4.3 oz)	100	17	1	7
Peas 'n Pork	½ cup (4.5 oz)	110	19	2	6
Pepper Peas	½ cup (4.5 oz)	120	22	1	6
Purple Hull	½ cup (4.4 oz)	120	21	1	7
White Acre	½ cup (4.3 oz)	100	17	1	6
Friends					
Small Pea Beans	8 oz	360	62	4	17
Green Giant					
Sweet	½ cup	50	11	0	4
Homefolks					
Crowder	½ cup (4.5 oz)	110	19	1	6
Purple Hull	½ cup (4.4 oz)	120	21	1	7
S&W					
Petit Pois	½ cup	70	12	0	4
Sweet	½ cup	70	12	0	4
Sweet Water Pack	½ cup	40	8	0	3
Veri-Green Sweet	½ cup	70	14	0	4
Seneca					
Natural Pack	½ cup	60	9	0	4
Peas	½ cup	50	9	0	4

FOOD	PORTION	CALS.	CARB.	FAT	PRO.
Sunshine					
Field Peas	½ cup (4.4 oz)	120	21	1	7
Lady Peas	½ cup (4.3 oz)	100	17	1	6
Trappey					
Field Peas With Bacon	½ cup (4.5 oz)	90	15	1	6
Field Peas With Snaps And Bacon	½ cup (4.5 oz)	110	19	1	6
Van De Kamp's					
Baked Pea Beans	8 oz	270	50	6	14
DRIED					
split cooked	1 cup	231	41	1	16
FRESH					
edible-pod cooked	½ cup	34	6	tr	3
edible-pod raw	½ cup	30	5	tr	2
green cooked	½ cup	67	13	tr	4
green raw	½ cup	58	11	tr	4
Dole					
Sugar Peas	½ cup	30	5	tr	2
FROZEN					
edible-pod cooked	1 pkg (10 oz)	132	23	1	9
edible-pod cooked	½ cup	42	7	tr	3
green cooked	½ cup	63	11	tr	4
Birds Eye					
Green	½ cup	80	13	0	5
In Butter Sauce	½ cup	80	12	2	4
Polybag Deluxe Tender Tiny	½ cup	60	11	0	6
Polybag Green	½ cup	70	12	0	2
Sugar Snap Deluxe	½ cup	45	9	0	2
Tender Tiny Deluxe	½ cup	60	11	0	4
Chun King					
Snow Pea Pods	½ pkg (3 oz)	35	4	2	2
Fresh Like					
Green	3.5 oz	85	14	1	5
Tiny Green	3.5 oz	63	12	tr	4
Green Giant					
Harvest Fresh Early June	½ cup	60	12	1	4
Harvest Fresh Sugar Snap	½ cup	30	8	0	2
Harvest Fresh Sweet	½ cup	50	12	0	4
In Butter Sauce	½ cup	80	14	2	5
One Serve In Butter Sauce	1 pkg	90	16	2	6
Sugar Snap Sweet Select	½ cup	30	8	0	2

FOOD	PORTION	CALS.	CARB.	FAT	PRO.
Green Giant (CONT.)					
Sweet	½ cup	50	11	0	4
Le Seur					
Early In Butter Sauce	½ cup	80	14	2	5
Early Select	½ cup	60	13	0	4
Tree Of Life					
Peas	⅔ cup (3.1 oz)	70	12	0	5
SHELF-STABLE					
Green Giant					
Mini Sweet	½ cup	60	12	tr	4
SPROUTS					
raw	½ cup	77	17	tr	5
TAKE-OUT					
pea & potato curry	1 serving (7 oz)	284	19	22	5
pea curry	1 serving (4.4 oz)	438	11	42	5
PECANS					
dried	1 oz	190	5	19	19
dry roasted	1 oz	187	6	18	2
dry roasted salted	1 oz	187	6	18	2
halves dried	1 cup	721	20	73	8
oil roasted	1 oz	195	5	20	2
oil roasted salted	1 oz	195	5	20	2
Eagle					
Honey Roasted	1 oz	200	5	19	2
Planters					
Chips	1 pkg (2 oz)	390	9	40	5
Gold Measure Halves	1 pkg (2 oz)	390	9	40	5
Halves	1 oz	190	4	20	3
Honey Roasted	1 oz	180	9	16	2
Pieces	1 oz	190	4	20	3
Pieces	1 pkg (2 oz)	390	9	40	5
PECTIN					
powder	¼ pkg (0.4 oz)	39	11	0	0
powder	1 pkg (1.75 oz)	163	45	tr	tr
Slim Set					
Packet	1 pkg	208	44	0	0
Powder	1 tbsp	3	1	0	0
PEPPER					
black	1 tsp	5	1	tr	tr
cayenne	1 tsp	6	1	tr	tr
red	1 tsp	6	1	tr	tr
white	1 tsp	7	2	tr	tr

FOOD	PORTION	CALS.	CARB.	FAT	PRO.
Ac'cent					
Lemon	½ tsp	0	0	0	0
Seasoned	½ tsp	0	0	0	0
Lawry's					
Lemon	1 tsp	6	1	tr	tr
Watkins					
Black	¼ tbsp (0.5 g)	0	0	0	0
Cajun	¼ tbsp (0.5 g)	0	0	0	0
Cracked Black	¼ tbsp (0.5 g)	0	0	0	0
Dijon	¼ tbsp (0.5 g)	0	0	0	0
Garlic Peppercorn Blend	¼ tbsp (1 g)	0	0	0	0
Herb	¼ tbsp (0.5 g)	0	0	0	0
Italian	¼ tbsp (0.5 g)	0	0	0	0
Lemon	¼ tbsp (1 g)	0	0	0	0
Mexican	¼ tbsp (0.5 g)	0	0	0	0
Red Pepper Flakes	¼ tsp (0.5 oz)	0	0	0	0
Royal Pepper Blend	¼ tbsp (0.5 g)	0	0	0	0
PEPPERS					
CANNED					
chili green hot	1 (2.6 oz)	18	4	tr	1
chili green hot chopped	½ cup	17	4	tr	1
chili red hot	1 (2.6 oz)	18	4	tr	1
chili red hot chopped	½ cup	17	4	tr	1
green halves	½ cup	13	3	tr	1
jalapeno chopped	½ cup	17	3	tr	1
red halves	½ cup	13	3	tr	1
Chi-Chi's					
Chilies Diced Green	2 tbsp (1.2 oz)	10	1	0	0
Chilies Green Whole	¾ pepper (1 oz)	10	1	0	0
Jalapenos Green Wheels	1 oz	10	1	0	0
Jalapenos Green Whole	1 oz	10	2	0	0
Jalapenos Red Wheels	1 oz	10	1	0	0
Jalapenos Red Whole	1 oz	15	3	0	0
Del Monte					
Chilpotle In Spice Sauce	2 tbsp (1.1 oz)	20	4	1	tr
Hot Chili	4 (1 oz)	10	3	0	0
Jalapeno Pickled Sliced	2 tbsp (1.1 oz)	5	1	0	0
Jalapeno Pickled Whole	2 tbsp (1.1 oz)	5	1	0	0
Jalapeno Whole	1 (0.7 oz)	3	tr	0	0
Jalapeno Nacho Pickled Sliced	2 tbsp (1 oz)	5	1	0	0
Hebrew National					
Filet	¼ pepper (1 oz)	9	2	0	0

FOOD	PORTION	CALS.	CARB.	FAT	PRO.
Hebrew National (CONT.)					
Hot Cherry	⅓ pepper (1 oz)	11	2	0	0
Red Filet	¼ pepper (1 oz)	9	2	0	0
McIlhenny					
Jalapeno Nacho Slices	12 slices (1.1 oz)	7	1	tr	tr
Old El Paso					
Green Chilies Chopped	2 tbsp	5	1	0	0
Green Chilies Whole	1	10	2	0	0
Jalapenos Peeled	3	10	1	0	0
Jalapenos Slices	2 tbsp	15	1	0	0
Progresso					
Hot Cherry	½ cup	190	3	20	0
Hot Cherry Pickled	½ cup	130	3	12	0
Piccalilli	½ cup	190	4	20	tr
Roasted	½ cup	20	5	tr	tr
Sweet Fried	½ jar	37	4	tr	tr
Tuscan	½ cup	20	7	0	0
Rosoff's					
Sweet	¼ pepper (1 oz)	9	2	0	0
Schorr's					
Filet Peppers	1 oz	9	2	0	0
Trappey					
Banana Mild	3 peppers (1 oz)	6	1	tr	tr
Banana Sliced Rings	21 slices (1 oz)	6	1	tr	tr
Cherry Hot	2 peppers (1 oz)	7	1	tr	tr
Cherry Mild	2 peppers (1 oz)	10	2	tr	tr
Dulcito Italian Pepperonchini	4 peppers (1 oz)	8	2	tr	tr
In Vinegar Hot	15 peppers (1 oz)	9	2	tr	tr
Jalapeno Hot Sliced	21 slices (1 oz)	4	1	tr	tr
Jalapeno Whole	2 peppers (1 oz)	11	2	0	tr
Serano	7 peppers (1 oz)	7	1	tr	tr
Tempero Golden Greek Pepperoncini	4 peppers (1 oz)	7	1	tr	tr
Torrido Santa Fe Grande	3 peppers (1 oz)	10	2	tr	tr
Vlasic					
Hot Banana Pepper Rings	1 oz	4	1	0	0
Hot Cherry	1 oz	10	2	0	0
Jalapeno Mexican Hot	1 oz	8	2	0	0
Mexican Tiny Hot	1 oz	6	2	0	0
Mild Cherry	1 oz	8	2	0	0
Mild Greek Pepperoncini Salad Peppers	1 oz	4	1	0	0

FOOD	PORTION	CALS.	CARB.	FAT	PRO.
DRIED					
green	1 tbsp	1	tr	tr	tr
red	1 tbsp	1	tr	tr	tr
FRESH					
chili green hot raw	1	18	4	tr	1
chili green hot raw chopped	½ cup	30	7	tr	2
chili red hot raw	1 (1.6 oz)	18	4	tr	1
chili red raw chopped	½ cup	30	7	tr	2
green chopped cooked	½ cup	19	5	tr	1
green cooked	1 (2.6 oz)	20	5	tr	1
green raw	1 (2.6 oz)	20	5	tr	1
green raw chopped	½ cup	13	3	tr	tr
red chopped cooked	½ cup	19	5	tr	1
red cooked	1 (2.6 oz)	20	5	tr	1
red raw	1 (2.6 oz)	20	5	tr	1
red raw chopped	½ cup	13	3	tr	tr
yellow raw	1 (6.5 oz)	50	12	tr	2
yellow raw	10 strips	14	3	tr	1
Dole					
Medium	1	25	5	1	1
FROZEN					
green chopped not prep	1 oz	6	1	tr	tr
red chopped	1 oz	6	1	tr	tr
Old El Paso					
Jalapenos Pickled	2	5	1	0	0
PERCH					
FRESH					
cooked	1 fillet (1.6 oz)	54	0	1	11
cooked	3 oz	99	0	1	21
ocean perch atlantic cooked	1 fillet (1.8 oz)	60	0	1	12
ocean perch atlantic cooked	3 oz	103	0	2	20
ocean perch atlantic raw	3 oz	80	0	1	16
raw	3 oz	77	0	1	16
red raw	3½ oz	114	0	4	18
FROZEN					
Gorton's					
Fishmarket Fresh Ocean Perch	5 oz	140	2	3	25
Van De Kamp's					
Battered	2 pieces	310	18	21	12

FOOD	PORTION	CALS.	CARB.	FAT	PRO.
Van De Kamp's (CONT.)					
Ocean Perch Light Fillets	1 piece	280	21	14	17
Ocean Perch Natural Fillets	4 oz	130	0	5	20

PERSIMMONS

dried japanese	1	93	25	tr	tr
fresh	1	32	8	tr	tr
fresh japanese	1	118	31	tr	1
Sonoma					
Dried	6-8 pieces (1.4 oz)	140	35	0	1

PHEASANT

breast w/o skin raw	½ breast (6.4 oz)	243	0	6	44
leg w/o skin raw	1 (3.6 oz)	143	0	5	24
w/ skin raw	½ pheasant (14 oz)	723	0	37	91
w/o skin raw	½ pheasant (12.4 oz)	470	0	13	83

PHYLLO DOUGH

phyllo dough	1 oz	85	15	2	2
sheet	1	57	10	1	1
Ekizian					
Sheets	½ lb	865	151	17	23

PICKLES

dill	1 (2.3 oz)	12	3	tr	tr
dill low sodium	1 (2.3 oz)	12	3	tr	tr
dill low sodium sliced	1 slice	1	tr	tr	tr
dill sliced	1 slice	1	tr	tr	tr
gerkins	3½ oz	21	4	tr	1
kosher dill	1 (2.3 oz)	12	3	tr	tr
polish dill	1 (2.3 oz)	12	3	tr	tr
quick sour	1 (1.2 oz)	4	1	tr	tr
quick sour low sodium	1 (1.2 oz)	4	1	tr	tr
quick sour sliced	1 slice	1	tr	tr	tr
sweet	1 (1.2 oz)	41	11	tr	tr
sweet gerkin	1 sm (½ oz)	20	5	tr	tr
sweet low sodium	1 (1.2 oz)	41	11	tr	tr
sweet sliced	1 slice	7	2	tr	tr
Del Monte					
Dill Halves	¼ pickle (1 oz)	5	tr	0	0
Dill Hamburger Chips	5 pieces (1 oz)	5	1	0	0
Dill Sweet Chips	5 pieces (1 oz)	40	10	0	0
Dill Sweet Gherkin	2 pickles (1 oz)	40	10	0	0
Dill Sweet Midgets	3 pickles (1 oz)	40	10	0	0

FOOD	PORTION	CALS.	CARB.	FAT	PRO.
Del Monte (CONT.)					
Dill Sweet Whole	2 pickles (1 oz)	40	10	0	0
Dill Tiny Kosher	1½ pickle (1 oz)	5	1	0	0
Dill Whole Pickles	1½ pickle (1 oz)	5	tr	0	0
Hebrew National					
Half Sour	½ pickle (1 oz)	4	1	0	0
Kosher	⅓ pickle (1 oz)	4	1	0	0
Kosher Barrel Cured Dill	1 pkg	23	4	0	1
Kosher Barrel Cured Hot Dill	1 pkg	23	4	0	1
Kosher Chips	3 slices (1 oz)	4	1	0	0
Kosher Halves	⅓ pickle (1 oz)	4	1	0	0
Kosher Large	⅕ pickle (1 oz)	4	1	0	0
Kosher Spears	½ spear (1 oz)	4	1	0	0
Sour Garlic	⅓ pickle (1 oz)	3	1	0	0
McIlhenny					
Hot N' Sweet	4 (1 oz)	42	10	tr	tr
Rosoff's					
Half Sour	⅓ pickle (1 oz)	4	1	0	0
Half Sour Spears	½ spear (1 oz)	4	1	0	0
Kosher	⅓ pickle (1 oz)	4	1	0	0
Kosher Halves	⅓ pickle (1 oz)	4	1	0	0
Schorr's					
Garlic	⅓ pickle (1 oz)	3	1	0	0
Half Sour	½ spear (1 oz)	4	1	0	0
Half Sour	⅓ pickle (1 oz)	4	1	0	0
Kosher Deli	½ pickle (1 oz)	4	1	0	0
Kosher Halves	⅓ pickle (1 oz)	4	1	0	0
Kosher Spears	½ spear (1 oz)	4	1	0	0
Kosher Whole	⅓ pickle (1 oz)	4	1	0	0
Vlasic					
Bread & Butter Chips	1 oz	30	7	0	0
Bread & Butter Chunks	1 oz	25	6	0	0
Bread & Butter Stixs	1 oz	18	5	0	0
Deli Bread & Butter	1 oz	25	6	0	0
Deli Dill Halves	1 oz	4	1	0	0
Half-The-Salt Hamburger Dill Chips	1 oz	2	1	0	0
Half-The-Salt Kosher Crunchy Dills	1 oz	4	1	0	0
Half-The-Salt Kosher Dill Spears	1 oz	4	1	0	0
Half-The-Salt Sweet Butter Chips	1 oz	30	7	0	0

FOOD	PORTION	CALS.	CARB.	FAT	PRO.
Vlasic (CONT.)					
Hot & Spicy Garden Mix	1 oz	4	1	0	0
Kosher Baby Dills	1 oz	4	1	0	0
Kosher Crunchy Dills	1 oz	4	1	0	0
Kosher Dill Gherkins	1 oz	4	1	0	0
Kosher Dill Spears	1 oz	4	1	0	0
Kosher Snack Chunks	1 oz	4	1	0	0
No Garlic Dill Spears	1 oz	4	1	0	0
Original Dills	1 oz	2	1	0	0
Polish Snack Chunk Dills	1 oz	4	1	0	0
Zesty Crunchy Dills	1 oz	4	1	0	0
Zesty Dill Snack Chunks	1 oz	4	1	0	0
Zesty Dill Spears	1 oz	4	1	0	0

PIE

(*see also* PIE CRUST)

CANNED FILLING

FOOD	PORTION	CALS.	CARB.	FAT	PRO.
apple	1 can (21 oz)	599	156	1	1
apple	⅛ can (2.6 oz)	74	19	tr	tr
cherry	⅛ can (2.6 oz)	85	22	tr	tr
cherry	1 can (21 oz)	683	175	1	3
pumpkin pie mix	1 cup	282	71	tr	3
Libby					
Pumpkin Pie Mix	½ cup	100	25	0	<1
None Such					
Mincemeat Condensed	¼ pkg	220	50	2	1
Mincemeat Ready-to-Use	⅓ cup	200	48	1	1
Mincemeat Ready-to-Use With Brandy & Rum	⅓ cup	220	48	2	1
S&W					
Mincemeat Old Fashioned	½ cup	206	49	2	1

FROZEN

FOOD	PORTION	CALS.	CARB.	FAT	PRO.
apple	⅛ of 9 in pie (4.4 oz)	297	43	14	2
blueberry	⅛ of 9 in pie (4.4 oz)	289	44	13	2
cherry	⅛ of 9 in pie (4.4 oz)	325	50	14	3
chocolate creme	⅙ of 8 in pie (4 oz)	344	38	22	3
coconut creme	⅙ of 7 in pie (2.2 oz)	191	24	11	1

FOOD	PORTION	CALS.	CARB.	FAT	PRO.
lemon meringue	1/6 of 8 in pie (4.5 oz)	303	53	10	2
peach	1/6 of 8 in pie (4.1 oz)	261	39	12	2
Banquet					
Apple	1/5 pie (4 oz)	300	41	13	3
Banana Cream	1/3 pie (4.7 oz)	350	39	21	3
Cherry	1/5 pie (4 oz)	290	39	14	3
Chocolate Cream	1/3 pie (4.7 oz)	360	43	20	3
Coconut Cream	1/3 pie (4.7 oz)	350	39	20	3
Lemon Cream	1/3 pie (4.7 oz)	360	43	20	3
Mincemeat	1/5 pie (4 oz)	310	46	13	3
Peach	1/5 pie (4 oz)	260	36	12	3
Pumpkin	1/6 pie (4 oz)	250	40	8	4
Kineret					
Apple Homestyle	1/6 pie (4 oz)	313	41	16	2
McMillin's					
Apple	4 oz	430	51	23	4
Berry	4 oz	430	52	23	3
Cherry	4 oz	430	51	24	3
Chocolate Pudding	4 oz	420	54	21	3
Coconut Pudding	4 oz	450	50	26	4
Lemon	4 oz	450	52	25	4
Peach	4 oz	430	52	24	4
Strawberry	4 oz	400	50	20	3
Mrs. Smith's					
Apple	1/10 of 10 in pie (4.6 oz)	280	43	12	2
Apple	1/8 of 9 in pie (4.6 oz)	370	50	18	2
Apple	1/6 of 8 in pie (4.3 oz)	270	41	11	2
Apple Cranberry	1/6 of 8 in pie (4.3 oz)	280	43	11	2
Apple Lattice Ready To Serve	1/5 of 8 in pie (4.6 oz)	310	45	13	2
Banana Cream	1/4 of 8 in pie (3.4 oz)	250	40	9	2
Berry	1/6 of 8 in pie (4.3 oz)	280	44	11	2
Blackberry	1/6 of 8 in pie (4.3 oz)	280	43	11	2
Blueberry	1/6 of 8 in pie	260	39	11	2
Boston Cream	1/8 of 8 in pie (2.4 oz)	170	29	5	2

FOOD	PORTION	CALS.	CARB.	FAT	PRO.
Mrs. Smith's (CONT.)					
Cherry	1/6 of 8 in pie	270	41	11	2
Cherry	1/8 of 9 in pie (4.6 oz)	320	48	13	3
Cherry Lattice Ready To Serve	1/5 of 8 in pie (4.6 oz)	320	47	13	3
Chocolate Cream	1/4 of 8 in pie (3.4 oz)	290	37	14	2
Coconut Cream	1/4 of 8 in pie (3.4 oz)	280	36	14	2
Coconut Custard	1/5 of 8 in pie (5 oz)	280	35	12	7
Dutch Apple	1/10 of 10 in pie (4.6 oz)	320	50	12	3
Dutch Apple	1/6 of 8 in pie	310	48	13	3
Dutch Apple	1/9 of 9 in pie (4.5 oz)	300	48	12	2
French Silk Cream	1/5 of 8 in pie (4.8 oz)	410	55	21	3
Hearty Pumpkin	1/5 of 8 in pie (5.2 oz)	280	46	10	5
Lemon Cream	1/4 of 8 in pie (3.4 oz)	270	36	13	2
Lemon Meringue	1/5 of 8 in pie (4.8 oz)	300	54	8	3
Mince	1/6 of 8 in pie (4.3 oz)	300	48	11	2
Peach	1/6 of 8 in pie	260	38	11	2
Peach	1/8 of 9 in pie (4.6 oz)	310	46	13	3
Pecan	1/8 of 10 in pie (4.5 oz)	500	68	23	5
Pumpkin	1/9 of 10 in pie (5.1 oz)	250	42	8	5
Pumpkin	1/5 of 8 in pie (5.2 oz)	270	44	8	5
Red Raspberry	1/6 of 8 in pie (4.3 oz)	280	43	11	2
Strawberry Rhubarb	1/5 of 8 in pie (4.8 oz)	520	73	23	5
Strawberry Rhubarb	1/6 of 8 in pie (4.3 oz)	280	44	11	2
Pepperidge Farm					
Hyannis Boston Cream Pie	1	230	34	10	4

FOOD	PORTION	CALS.	CARB.	FAT	PRO.
Pepperidge Farm (CONT.)					
Mississippi Mud	1	310	23	23	3
Pet-Ritz					
Apple	⅙ pie (4.33 oz)	330	53	12	2
Banana Cream	⅙ pie (2.33 oz)	170	22	9	2
Blueberry	⅙ pie (4.33 oz)	370	50	12	3
Cherry	⅙ pie (4.33 oz)	300	48	12	3
Chocolate Cream	⅙ pie (2.33 oz)	190	27	8	1
Coconut Cream	⅙ pie (2.33 oz)	190	27	8	2
Egg Custard	⅙ pie (4.0 oz)	200	28	8	5
Lemon Cream	⅙ pie (2.33 oz)	190	26	9	2
Mince	⅙ pie (4.33 oz)	280	48	9	2
Neapolitan Cream	⅙ pie (2.33 oz)	180	17	10	1
Peach	⅙ pie (4.33 oz)	320	51	12	2
Pumpkin Custard	⅙ pie (4.33 oz)	250	39	9	4
Strawberry Cream	⅙ pie (2.33 oz)	170	20	9	2
Sweet Potato	⅙ pie (3.33 oz)	150	21	7	2
Sara Lee					
Apple Homestyle	1 slice (4 oz)	280	42	12	2
Apple Homestyle High	1 slice (4.9 oz)	400	46	23	3
Apple Streusel Free & Light	1 slice (2.9 oz)	170	36	2	1
Blueberry Homestyle	1 slice (4 oz)	300	45	12	2
Cherry Homestyle	1 slice (4 oz)	270	37	13	2
Cherry Streusel Free & Light	1 slice (3.6 oz)	160	34	2	2
Dutch Apple Homestyle	1 slice (4 oz)	300	45	12	2
Mince Homestyle	1 slice (4 oz)	300	43	13	3
Peach Homestyle	1 slice (3.4 oz)	280	41	12	2
Pecan Homestyle	1 slice (3.4 oz)	400	56	18	4
Pumpkin Homestyle	1 slice (4 oz)	240	34	10	4
Raspberry Homestyle	1 slice (4 oz)	280	39	13	2
Weight Watchers					
Apple	1 slice (3.5 oz)	165	30	4	2
Chocolate Mocha	1 (2.75 oz)	180	30	4	6
HOME RECIPE					
apple	⅛ of 9 in pie (5.4 oz)	411	58	19	4
banana cream	⅛ of 9 in pie (5.2 oz)	398	49	20	7
blueberry	⅛ of 9 in pie (5.2 oz)	360	49	18	4
butterscotch	⅛ of 9 in pie (4.5 oz)	355	42	18	6

FOOD	PORTION	CALS.	CARB.	FAT	PRO.
cherry	⅛ of 9 in pie (6.3 oz)	486	69	22	5
coconut creme	⅛ of 9 in pie (4.7 oz)	396	46	21	6
custard	⅛ of 9 in pie (4.5 oz)	262	34	11	7
lemon meringue	⅛ of 9 in pie (4.5 oz)	362	50	16	5
mince	⅛ of 9 in pie (5.8 oz)	477	79	18	18
pecan	⅛ of 9 in pie (4.3 oz)	502	64	27	6
pumpkin	⅛ of 9 in pie (5.4 oz)	316	41	14	7
vanilla cream	⅛ of 9 in pie (4.4 oz)	350	41	18	6
MIX					
banana cream no-bake	⅛ of 9 in pie (3.2 oz)	231	29	12	3
chocolate mousse no-bake	⅛ of 9 in pie (3.3 oz)	247	28	15	3
coconut creme no-bake	⅛ of 9 in pie (3.3 oz)	259	27	17	3
Betty Crocker					
Boston Cream Classic Dessert	⅛ pie	270	50	6	4
Jell-O					
Banana Cream as prep w/ whole milk	⅙ pie 8 in	103	18	3	3
Chocolate Mousse	⅛ pie	259	25	17	4
Coconut Cream	⅛ pie	258	27	16	3
Coconut Cream as prep w/ whole milk	⅙ pie 8 in	111	16	4	3
Lemon	⅙ pie 8 in	175	38	2	2
Pumpkin	⅛ pie	253	31	13	4
Royal					
Key Lime Pie Filling	mix for 1 serving	50	13	0	0
Lemon Pie Filling	mix for 1 serving	50	13	0	0
Lemon Meringue No-Bake	⅛ pie	210	38	5	3
READY-TO-EAT					
Entenmann's					
Apple Homestyle	1 serving (2.1 oz)	140	21	7	1
Coconut Custard	1 serving (1.8 oz)	140	16	8	3

FOOD	PORTION	CALS.	CARB.	FAT	PRO.
SNACK					
apple	1 (3 oz)	266	33	14	2
apple fried	1 (6.4 oz)	404	55	21	4
blueberry fried	1 (6.4 oz)	404	55	21	4
cherry	1 (3 oz)	266	33	14	2
cherry fried	1 (6.4 oz)	404	55	21	4
lemon	1 (3 oz)	266	33	14	2
lemon fried	1 (6.4 oz)	404	55	21	4
peach fried	1 (6.4 oz)	404	55	21	4
strawberry fried	1 (6.4 oz)	404	55	21	4
Drake's					
Apple	1 (2 oz)	210	29	10	2
Blueberry	1 (2 oz)	210	30	10	2
Cherry	1 (2 oz)	220	30	10	2
Lemon	1 (2 oz)	210	27	11	2
Lance					
Pecan	1 (38 g)	350	51	15	4
Little Debbie					
Marshmallow Banana	1 pkg (1.4 oz)	160	27	5	1
Marshmallow Banana	1 pkg (2.7 oz)	320	54	11	3
Marshmallow Banana	1 pkg (2 oz)	240	40	8	2
Marshmallow Chocolate	1 pkg (1.4 oz)	160	27	5	1
Marshmallow Chocolate	1 pkg (2.7 oz)	320	53	11	3
Marshmallow Chocolate	1 pkg (2 oz)	240	40	9	2
Oatmeal Creme	1 pkg (1.3 oz)	170	25	8	2
Oatmeal Creme	1 pkg (3 oz)	360	58	14	3
Oatmeal Creme	1 pkg (2.5 oz)	300	48	11	3
Raisin Creme	1 pkg (1.2 oz)	140	23	5	0
Raisin Creme	1 pkg (2.5 oz)	290	47	12	2
Tastykake					
Apple	1 pkg (113 g)	300	46	12	3
Banana Creme	1 pkg (120 g)	380	54	16	5
Blueberry	1 pkg (113 g)	310	55	9	3
Cherry	1 pkg (113 g)	300	49	10	3
Coconut Creme	1 pkg (113 g)	380	46	20	5
French Apple	1 pkg (120 g)	350	63	11	3
Lemon	1 pkg (113 g)	320	48	13	4
Lemon Lime	1 pkg (113 g)	320	49	13	4
Peach	1 pkg (113 g)	300	47	12	3
Pineapple Cheese	1 pkg (120 g)	340	54	13	5
Pumpkin	1 pkg (4 oz)	320	46	14	5
Strawberry	1 pkg (113 g)	340	57	11	3
Tasty Klair	1 pkg (113 g)	400	51	20	6

FOOD	PORTION	CALS.	CARB.	FAT	PRO.
TAKE-OUT					
coconut custard	⅙ of 8 in pie (3.6 oz)	271	32	14	6
custard	⅙ pie 9 in	330	36	17	9
pecan	⅙ of 8 in pie (4 oz)	452	65	21	5
pumpkin	⅙ of 8 in pie (3.8 oz)	229	30	10	4
PIE CRUST (*see also* PIE)					
FROZEN					
baked	9 in shell (4.4 oz)	647	63	41	6
baked	⅛ of 9 in pie (0.6 oz)	82	8	5	1
puff pastry baked	1 shell (1.4 oz)	223	18	15	3
Oronoque					
Deep Dish	⅙ pie (1.41 oz)	200	16	13	3
Pie Crust	⅙ pie (1.23 oz)	170	14	12	3
Pepperidge Farm					
Patty Shells	1	210	16	15	3
Puff Pastry Sheets	¼ sheet	260	22	17	4
Pet-Ritz					
Deep Dish	⅙ pie (1 oz)	130	12	8	1
Graham Cracker	⅙ pie (0.83 oz)	110	8	6	1
Regular	⅙ pie (0.83 oz)	110	11	7	1
Tart Shells	1	150	12	10	3
HOME RECIPE					
9-inch crust	1	900	79	60	11
baked	9 in shell (6.3 oz)	949	86	62	12
baked	⅛ 9 in crust (0.8 oz)	119	11	8	1
MIX					
as prep	9 in crust (5.6 oz)	801	81	49	11
as prep	⅛ of 9 in pie (0.7 oz)	100	10	6	1
Betty Crocker					
Pie Crust	1/16 pkg	120	10	8	1
Sticks	1/16 pkg	120	10	8	1
Flako					
Mix	¼ cup (0.9 oz)	130	13	8	2
Jiffy					
As prep	1/7 crust	180	19	10	2
Pillsbury					
Mix	⅙ of 2 crust pie	270	25	17	4

FOOD	PORTION	CALS.	CARB.	FAT	PRO.
Pillsbury (CONT.)					
Stick	⅛ of a 2 crust pie	270	25	17	4
READY-TO-EAT					
chocolate cookie crumb baked	9 in crust (7.7 oz)	1130	122	69	12
chocolate cookie crumb baked	⅛ of 9 in pie (1 oz)	139	15	9	1
chocolate cookie crumb chilled	9 in crust (7.8 oz)	1127	121	69	12
chocolate cookie crumb chilled	⅛ of 9 in pie (1 oz)	142	15	9	1
graham cracker baked	9 in crust (8.4 oz)	1181	156	60	10
graham cracker baked	⅛ of 9 in pie (1 oz)	148	20	8	1
graham cracker chilled	9 in crust (8.6 oz)	1182	155	60	10
graham cracker chilled	⅛ of 9 in pie (1 oz)	150	20	8	1
vanilla wafer cracker crumbs baked	9 in crust (6.1 oz)	937	89	64	7
vanilla wafer cracker crumbs baked	⅛ of 9 in pie (0.8 oz)	119	11	8	1
vanilla wafer cracker crumbs chilled	9 in crust (6.2 oz)	934	88	64	7
vanilla wafer cracker crumbs chilled	⅛ of 9 in pie (0.8 oz)	117	11	8	1
Generic Label					
Graham	⅛ pie (0.7 oz)	110	14	5	1
Honey Maid					
Graham	⅙ crust (1 oz)	140	18	7	1
Nabisco					
Nilla	⅙ crust (1 oz)	140	18	8	1
Oreo					
Crumb Crust	⅙ crust (1 oz)	140	18	11	1
Ready Crust					
Chocolate	⅛ pie 9 in	100	14	5	1
Chocolate	1 (3 in diam)	110	15	5	1
Graham	1 (3 in diam)	110	15	5	1
Graham	⅛ pie 9 in	100	13	5	1
REFRIGERATED					
Pillsbury					
All Ready	⅛ of 2 crust pie	240	24	15	2

PIEROGI

FROZEN
Empire

Potato Cheese	3 (4.6 oz)	260	40	6	11

FOOD	PORTION	CALS.	CARB.	FAT	PRO.
Empire (CONT.)					
Potato Onion	3 (4.6 oz)	250	43	5	10
Golden					
Potato Cheese	3 (4 oz)	250	38	8	8
Potato Onion	3 (4 oz)	210	36	6	6
Mrs. T's					
Potato And Cheddar Cheese	1 (1.3 oz)	60	11	tr	2
Potato And Onion	1 (1.3 oz)	50	10	tr	2
TAKE-OUT					
pierogi	¾ cup (4.4 oz)	307	24	19	11

PIG'S EARS AND FEET

FOOD	PORTION	CALS.	CARB.	FAT	PRO.
ears, frzn, simmered	1 ear (3.7 oz)	183	0	12	18
feet pickled	1 oz	58	tr	5	4
feet pickled	1 lb	923	tr	73	61
feet, simmered	2.5 oz	138	0	9	14
Hormel					
Pickled Feet	2 oz	80	0	6	7
Pickled Hocks	2 oz	110	0	8	9

PIGEON

FOOD	PORTION	CALS.	CARB.	FAT	PRO.
w/ skin & bone	3.5 oz	169	0	10	21

PIGEON PEAS

FOOD	PORTION	CALS.	CARB.	FAT	PRO.
dried cooked	½ cup	102	20	tr	6
dried cooked	1 cup	204	39	1	11

PIGNOLIA
(*see* PINE NUTS)

PIKE

FOOD	PORTION	CALS.	CARB.	FAT	PRO.
northern cooked	½ fillet (5.4 oz)	176	0	1	38
northern cooked	3 oz	96	0	1	21
northern raw	3 oz	75	0	1	16
roe raw	3½ oz	130	2	2	24
walleye baked	3 oz	101	0	1	21
walleye fillet baked	4.4 oz	147	0	2	30

PIMIENTOS

FOOD	PORTION	CALS.	CARB.	FAT	PRO.
canned	1 tbsp	3	1	tr	tr
canned	1 slice	0	tr	0	tr
Dromedary					
Pimientos	1 oz	10	2	0	0

PINE NUTS

FOOD	PORTION	CALS.	CARB.	FAT	PRO.
pignolia dried	1 oz	146	4	14	7
pignolia dried	1 tbsp	51	1	5	2
pinyon dried	1 oz	161	5	17	3

FOOD	PORTION	CALS.	CARB.	FAT	PRO.
PINEAPPLE					
CANNED					
chunks in heavy syrup	1 cup	199	52	tr	1
chunks juice pack	1 cup	150	39	tr	1
crushed in heavy syrup	1 cup	199	52	tr	1
slices in heavy syrup	1 slice	45	12	tr	tr
slices in light syrup	1 slice	30	8	tr	tr
slices juice pack	1 slice	35	9	tr	tr
slices water pack	1 slice	19	5	tr	tr
tidbits in heavy syrup	1 cup	199	52	tr	1
tidbits in juice	1 cup	150	19	tr	1
tidbits in water	1 cup	79	20	tr	1
Del Monte					
Chunks In Heavy Syrup	½ cup (4.3 oz)	90	24	0	0
Chunks In Its Own Juice	½ cup (4.4 oz)	70	17	0	0
Crushed In Heavy Syrup	½ cup (4.4 oz)	90	24	0	0
Crushed In Its Own Juice	½ cup (4.3 oz)	70	17	0	0
Sliced In Heavy Syrup	½ cup (4.1 oz)	90	23	0	0
Sliced In Its Own Juice	½ cup (4 oz)	60	16	0	0
Snack Cups Tidbits In Juice	1 serv (4.5 oz)	70	18	0	1
Snack Cups Tidbits In Juice EZ-Open Lid	1 serv (4.2 oz)	60	17	0	0
Spears In Its Own Juice	½ cup (4.3 oz)	70	17	0	0
Tidbits In Its Own Juice	½ cup (4.3 oz)	70	17	0	0
Wedges In Its Own Juice	½ cup (4.3 oz)	70	17	0	0
Dole					
All Cuts Juice Pack	½ cup	70	18	tr	0
All Cuts Syrup Pack	½ cup	90	23	0	0
Empress					
Chunk	4 oz	70	18	0	0
Crushed	4 oz	70	18	0	0
Sliced	4 oz	70	18	0	0
Libby					
Crushed	1 cup with juice	140	35	0	1
Sliced In Unsweetened Juice	1 cup with juice	140	35	0	1
S&W					
Hawaiian Slice In Heavy Syrup	½ cup	90	23	0	0
Hawaiian Slice Juice Pack	½ cup	70	17	0	0

FOOD	PORTION	CALS.	CARB.	FAT	PRO.
S&W (CONT.)					
Sliced Unsweetened	½ cup	60	15	0	0
DRIED					
Sonoma					
Pieces	2 pieces (1.4 oz)	140	30	2	0
FRESH					
diced	1 cup	77	19	tr	1
slice	1 slice	42	10	tr	tr
Dole					
Pineapple	2 slices	90	21	1	1
FROZEN					
chunks sweetened	½ cup	104	27	tr	tr
PINEAPPLE JUICE					
canned	1 cup	139	34	tr	1
frzn as prep	1 cup	129	32	tr	1
frzn not prep	6 oz	387	96	tr	3
After The Fall					
Mandarin Pineapple	1 can (12 oz)	150	37	0	1
Bright & Early					
Frozen	8 fl oz	120	30	0	0
Del Monte					
Juice	8 fl oz	110	26	0	tr
Juice	6 fl oz	80	20	0	tr
Juice	1 serv (11.5 oz)	190	45	0	1
Dole					
100% frzn as prep	8 fl oz	130	30	0	1
Chilled	6 fl oz	90	22	0	0
Minute Maid					
Box	8.45 fl oz	130	33	0	0
Frozen	8 fl oz	130	31	0	0
Frozen	8 fl oz	110	28	0	0
S&W					
Unsweentened	6 oz	100	25	0	0
Tree Top					
Juice	6 oz	100	24	0	1
Veryfine					
100%	8 oz	125	31	0	0
PINK BEANS					
CANNED					
Goya					
Spanish Style	7.5 oz	140	32	tr	10
DRIED					
cooked	1 cup	252	47	1	15

FOOD	PORTION	CALS.	CARB.	FAT	PRO.
PINTO BEANS					
CANNED					
pinto	1 cup	186	35	1	11
Allen					
Pinto Beans	½ cup (4.5 oz)	110	20	1	5
Brown Beauty					
Pinto Beans	½ cup (4.5 oz)	110	20	1	5
East Texas Fair					
Pinto Beans	½ cup (4.5 oz)	110	20	1	5
Eden					
Organic	½ cup (4.4 oz)	90	17	1	5
Gebhardt					
Pinto Beans	4 oz	100	19	tr	6
Goya					
Spanish Style	7.5 oz	140	31	1	11
Green Giant					
Picante	½ cup	100	21	1	7
Pinto Beans	½ cup	90	20	1	6
Old El Paso					
Pinto Beans	½ cup	100	19	0	6
Progresso					
Pinto Beans	½ cup	110	21	tr	8
Trappey					
Jalapinto With Bacon	½ cup (4.5 oz)	120	22	1	6
With Bacon	½ cup (4.5 oz)	120	20	1	6
DRIED					
cooked	1 cup	235	44	1	14
Arrowhead					
Dried	¼ cup (1.5 oz)	150	27	1	10
Bean Cuisine					
Dried	½ cup	115	—	1	8
Hurst					
Pinto Beans	1.2 oz	120	22	1	7
With Spanish Seasoning	1.3 oz	120	22	1	7
FROZEN					
cooked	3 oz	152	29	tr	9
PINYON					
(*see* PINE NUTS)					
PISTACHIOS					
dried	1 oz	164	7	14	6
dried	1 cup	739	32	62	26
dry roasted	1 oz	172	8	15	4
dry roasted salted	1 oz	172	8	15	4

FOOD	PORTION	CALS.	CARB.	FAT	PRO.
dry roasted salted	1 cup	776	35	68	19
Dole					
Shelled	1 oz	163	7	14	6
Shells On	1 oz	90	3	7	3
Fisher					
Red Tint	1 oz	170	6	15	5
Lance					
Pistachios	1 pkg (32 g)	100	4	8	3
Planters					
Munch'N Go Singles Shelled Dry Roasted	1 pkg (2 oz)	330	14	29	11
Red Salted Dry Roasted	1 pkg	160	7	14	5
Uncolored Dry Roasted	½ cup	160	7	14	5
Sonoma					
Salted Shelled	¼ cup (1 oz)	190	9	14	6
PITANGA					
fresh	1 cup	57	13	1	1
fresh	1	2	1	tr	tr
PIZZA					
DOUGH					
Boboli					
Shell + Sauce	⅛ lg shell (2.6 oz)	170	28	3	7
Shell + Sauce	⅙ sm shell (2.6 oz)	170	29	3	7
House of Pasta					
Frozen	⅛ of 14 in pie (1.9 oz)	140	27	1	4
Jiffy					
As prep	¼ crust	180	33	3	4
Sassafras					
Cornmeal Pizza Crust	1 slice (1.4 oz)	140	30	0	4
Italian Pizza Crust Mix	1 slice (1.4 oz)	140	30	0	4
Wanda's					
Crust Mix Oregano & Basil	⅒ pie (1.4 oz)	149	32	0	4
Crust Mix Oregano & Basil Whole Wheat	⅒ pie (1.4 oz)	141	30	1	6
Watkins					
Crust Mix	⅛ pkg (1.8 oz)	180	36	1	6
FROZEN					
Celeste					
Italian Bread Deluxe	1 (5.1 oz)	290	36	11	16
Italian Bread Garlic & Herb Zesty Chicken	1 (5 oz)	260	34	8	17

FOOD	PORTION	CALS.	CARB.	FAT	PRO.
Celeste (CONT.)					
Italian Bread Pepperoni	1 (5 oz)	320	37	13	17
Italian Bread Zesty Four Cheese	1 (4.6 oz)	300	32	12	15
Large Cheese	¼ pie (4.4 oz)	320	32	16	14
Large Deluxe	¼ pie (5.5 oz)	350	35	18	14
Large Pepperoni	¼ pie (4.7 oz)	350	33	20	13
Large Suprema With Meat	⅓ pie (4.6 oz)	290	27	16	13
Large Zesty Four Cheese	¼ pie (4.4 oz)	330	34	16	14
Small Cheese	1 (7.5 oz)	540	60	25	23
Small Deluxe	1 (8.2 oz)	540	53	29	21
Small Hot & Zesty Four Cheese	1 (7 oz)	530	50	27	24
Small Original Four Cheese	1 (7 oz)	540	47	30	25
Small Pepperoni	1 (6.7 oz)	520	53	27	19
Small Sausage	1 (7.5 oz)	530	52	27	23
Small Suprema Vegetable	1 (7.5 oz)	480	52	23	20
Small Suprema With Meat	1 (9 oz)	580	56	31	25
Small Zesty Four Cheese	1 (7 oz)	530	50	27	24
Croissant Pocket					
Stuffed Sandwich Pepperoni Pizza	1 piece (4.5 oz)	350	39	15	16
Empire					
3 Pack	1 (3 oz)	210	23	9	10
Bagel	1 (2 oz)	150	15	5	7
English Muffin	1 (2 oz)	130	15	5	7
Pizza	½ pie (5 oz)	340	38	13	18
Fox					
Deluxe Golden Topping	½ pizza	240	25	11	9
Deluxe Hamburger	½ pizza	260	26	12	11
Deluxe Pepperoni	½ pizza	250	26	13	8
Deluxe Sausage	½ pizza	260	26	13	10
Deluxe Sausage & Pepperoni	½ pizza	260	26	13	10
Healthy Choice					
French Bread Cheese	1 (5.6 oz)	310	49	4	20
French Bread Pepperoni	1 (6 oz)	360	48	9	22
French Bread Sausage	1 (6 oz)	330	52	4	20
French Bread Supreme	1 (6.35 oz)	340	49	6	22

FOOD	PORTION	CALS.	CARB.	FAT	PRO.
Hot Pocket					
Stuffed Sandwich Pepperoni & Sausage Pizza	1 (4.5 oz)	340	38	16	12
Stuffed Sandwich Pepperoni Pizza	1 (4.5 oz)	350	38	17	13
Jeno's					
4-Pack Cheese	1 pizza	160	17	8	6
4-Pack Combination	1 pizza	180	17	9	7
4-Pack Hamburger	1 pizza	180	17	9	8
4-Pack Pepperoni	1 pizza	170	17	9	6
4-Pack Sausage	1 pizza	180	17	9	7
Crisp 'n Tasty Canandian Bacon	½ pizza	250	27	11	11
Crisp 'n Tasty Cheese	½ pizza	270	28	14	10
Crisp 'n Tasty Hamburger	½ pizza	290	28	15	12
Crisp 'n Tasty Pepperoni	½ pizza	280	27	15	10
Crisp 'n Tasty Sausage	½ pizza	300	28	16	11
Crisp 'n Tasty Sausage & Pepperoni	½ pizza	300	27	16	10
Microwave Pizza Rolls Pepperoni & Cheese	6	240	23	13	7
Microwave Pizza Rolls Sausage & Cheese	6	250	24	13	8
Pizza Rolls Cheese	6	240	23	12	8
Pizza Rolls Hamburger	6	240	21	13	9
Pizza Rolls Pepperoni & Cheese	6	230	22	13	7
Pizza Rolls Sausage & Pepperoni	6	230	22	13	7
Kid Cuisine					
Cheese	1 (8 oz)	430	71	11	12
Hamburger	1 (8.30 oz)	400	61	11	14
Kineret					
Bagel Pizza	2 (4 oz)	300	39	10	15
Slice	1 (4.9 oz)	490	93	9	14
Lean Cuisine					
French Bread Cheese	1 pkg (6 oz)	350	48	8	22
French Bread Deluxe	1 pkg (6.1 oz)	350	45	6	23
French Bread Pepperoni	1 pkg (5.25 oz)	330	46	7	20
Lean Pockets					
Stuffed Sandwich Pizza Deluxe	1 (4.5 oz)	270	37	8	12

FOOD	PORTION	CALS.	CARB.	FAT	PRO.
MicroMagic					
Deep Dish Combination	1 (6.5 oz)	605	60	34	14
Deep Dish Pepperoni	1 (6.5 oz)	615	65	32	15
Deep Dish Sausage	1 (6.5 oz)	590	62	31	15
Mrs. P's					
Combination	½ pizza	260	26	13	10
Golden Topping	½ pizza	240	25	11	9
Hamburger	½ pizza	260	26	12	11
Pepperoni	½ pizza	250	26	13	8
Sausage	½ pizza	260	26	13	10
Old El Paso					
Pizza Burrito Cheese	1	320	27	9	13
Pizza Burrito Pepperoni	1	260	31	10	12
Pizza Burrito Sausage	1	260	32	9	11
Pappalo's					
French Bread Cheese	1 pizza	360	40	15	16
French Bread Combination	1 pizza	430	41	21	19
French Bread Pepperoni	1 pizza	410	41	20	16
French Bread Sausage	1 pizza	410	41	18	18
Pan Combination	⅙ pizza	340	34	15	17
Pan Hamburger	⅙ pizza	310	34	12	17
Pan Pepperoni	⅙ pizza	330	34	14	16
Pan Sausage	⅙ pizza	360	34	18	14
Thin Crust Combination	⅙ pizza	260	29	10	13
Thin Crust Hamburger	⅙ pizza	240	28	8	14
Thin Crust Pepperoni	⅙ pizza	270	28	11	13
Thin Crust Sausage	⅙ pizza	250	28	9	12
Pepperidge Farm					
Croissant Pastry Cheese	1	430	41	23	15
Croissant Pastry Deluxe	1	440	43	23	16
Croissant Pastry Pepperoni	1	420	43	22	14
Pillsbury					
Microwave Cheese	½ pizza	240	28	10	10
Microwave Combination	½ pizza	310	29	15	14
Microwave French Bread	1 pizza	370	41	15	18
Microwave French Bread Pepperoni	1 pizza	430	46	19	19
Microwave French Bread Sausage	1 pizza	410	48	16	18
Microwave French Bread Sausage & Pepperoni	1 pizza	450	47	21	19
Microwave Pepperoni	½ pizza	300	29	15	13

FOOD	PORTION	CALS.	CARB.	FAT	PRO.
Pillsbury (CONT.)					
Microwave Sausage	½ pizza	280	29	13	13
Small World					
Four Cheese	1 (4 oz)	240	38	6	10
Special Delivery					
Organic	⅓ pizza (5.3 oz)	320	46	9	13
Organic Soy Kaas	⅓ pizza (5.3 oz)	320	47	7	16
Stouffer's					
French Bread Bacon Cheddar	1 piece (5.8 oz)	440	44	22	16
French Bread Cheese	1 piece (5.2 oz)	350	42	14	15
French Bread Cheeseburger	1 piece (6 oz)	440	31	26	21
French Bread Deluxe	1 piece (6.2 oz)	440	42	22	19
French Bread Double Cheese	1 piece (5.9 oz)	420	44	19	19
French Bread Garden Vegetable	1 piece (5.8 oz)	340	45	12	12
French Bread Pepperoni	1 piece (5.6 oz)	420	42	20	18
French Bread Pepperoni & Mushroom	1 piece (6.1 oz)	430	43	21	17
French Bread Sausage	1 piece (6 oz)	420	41	20	19
French Bread Sausage & Pepperoni	1 piece (6.25 oz)	460	45	25	22
French Bread Vegetable Deluxe	1 piece (6.4 oz)	380	43	17	18
French Bread White Pizza	1 piece (5.1 oz)	460	43	28	17
Lunch Express Deluxe	1 pkg (6.6 oz)	460	40	25	21
Lunch Express Double Cheese	1 pkg (5.9 oz)	420	41	19	21
Lunch Express Pepperoni	1 pkg (5.75 oz)	440	39	23	19
Lunch Express Sausage	1 pkg (6.5 oz)	460	40	25	21
Lunch Express Sausage & Pepperoni	1 pkg (6.4 oz)	500	41	27	24
Tombstone					
12 in Canadian Bacon	⅕ pie (5.5 oz)	360	36	15	20
12 in Cheese & Hamburger	⅕ pie (4.4 oz)	320	29	16	15
12 in Cheese & Pepperoni	⅕ pie (4.4 oz)	340	29	18	15
12 in Cheese & Sausage	⅕ pie (4.4 oz)	320	29	16	15

FOOD	PORTION	CALS.	CARB.	FAT	PRO.
Tombstone (CONT.)					
12 in Cheese Sausage & Mushroom	⅕ pie (4.5 oz)	320	29	16	15
12 in Deluxe	⅕ pie (4.7 oz)	320	29	16	15
12 in Extra Cheese	⅕ pie (5.1 oz)	370	36	17	18
12 in Sausage & Pepperoni	⅕ pie (4.4 oz)	340	29	18	16
12 in Special Order Four Cheese	⅕ pie (5.2 oz)	400	37	19	20
12 in Special Order Four Meat	⅙ pie (4.7 oz)	350	31	18	17
12 in Special Order Pepperoni	⅙ pie (4.5 oz)	360	31	19	16
12 in Special Order Super Supreme	⅙ pie (4.8 oz)	350	31	18	17
12 in Special Order Three Sausage	⅙ pie (4.6 oz)	340	31	17	16
12 in Supreme	⅕ pie (4.6 oz)	330	29	17	15
12 in ThinCrust Italian Style Three Cheese	¼ pie (4.8 oz)	380	25	22	20
9 in Cheese & Hamburger	⅓ pie (4.1 oz)	310	28	16	14
9 in Cheese & Pepperoni	⅓ pie (4.1 oz)	340	28	19	15
9 in Cheese & Sausage	⅓ pie (4.1 oz)	310	28	16	14
9 in Deluxe	⅓ pie (4.5 oz)	320	28	16	15
9 in Extra Cheese	⅓ pie (5.6 oz)	420	42	19	20
9 in Pepperoni & Sausage	⅓ pie (4.4 oz)	360	28	21	16
9 in Special Order Four Meat	⅓ pie (5.3 oz)	400	35	20	19
9 in Special Order Pepperoni	⅓ pie (5.1 oz)	400	35	21	19
9 in Special Order Super Supreme	⅓ pie (5.5 oz)	400	36	21	19
9 in Special Order Three Sausage	⅓ pie (5.2 oz)	390	35	19	19
Double Top Pepperoni With Double Cheese	⅙ pie (4.5 oz)	350	25	20	19
Double Top Sausage & Pepperoni With Double Cheese	⅙ pie (4.7 oz)	360	25	20	20
Double Top Sausage With Double Cheese	⅙ pie (4.7 oz)	350	25	19	20
For One ½ Less Fat Cheese	1 pie (6.5 oz)	360	45	10	23

FOOD	PORTION	CALS.	CARB.	FAT	PRO.
Tombstone (CONT.)					
For One ½ Less Fat Pepperoni	1 pie (6.7 oz)	400	45	13	26
For One ½ Less Fat Supreme	1 pie (7.7 oz)	400	45	13	27
For One ½ Less Fat Vegetable	1 pie (7.2 oz)	360	46	10	22
For One Cheese & Pepperoni	1 pie (7 oz)	580	41	35	25
For One Extra Cheese	1 pie (7 oz)	540	41	30	27
For One Italian Sausage	1 pie (7 oz)	560	40	33	25
For One Sausage & Pepperoni	1 pie (7 oz)	590	40	37	25
For One Supreme	1 pie (7.5 oz)	570	41	34	24
Light Supreme	⅕ pie (4.8 oz)	270	30	9	25
Light Vegetable	⅕ pie (4.6 oz)	240	31	7	25
ThinCrust Italian Style Four Meat Combo	¼ pie (5.1 oz)	410	25	25	20
ThinCrust Italian Style Pepperoni	¼ pie (5 oz)	420	25	27	20
ThinCrust Italian Style Sausage	¼ pie (5.1 oz)	400	25	24	19
ThinCrust Italian Style Supreme	¼ pie (5.3 oz)	400	26	24	18
ThinCrust Mexican Style Supreme Taco	¼ pie (5.1 oz)	380	26	23	16
Totino's					
Microwave Cheese	1 pizza	250	34	8	10
Microwave Pepperoni	1 pizza	280	34	12	10
Microwave Sausage	1 pizza	320	33	16	11
Microwave Sausage Pepperoni Combination	1 pizza	310	31	15	12
My Classic Deluxe Cheese	⅙ pizza	210	23	9	10
My Classic Deluxe Combination	⅙ pizza	270	23	14	13
My Classic Deluxe Pepperoni	⅙ pizza	260	23	13	12
Pan Pepperoni	⅙ pizza	330	34	14	16
Pan Sausage	⅙ pizza	320	34	13	16
Pan Sausage & Pepperoni Combination	⅙ pizza	340	34	15	16

FOOD	PORTION	CALS.	CARB.	FAT	PRO.
Totino's (CONT.)					
Pan Three Cheese	⅙ pizza	290	33	10	15
Party Bacon	½ pizza	370	35	20	11
Party Canadian Bacon	½ pizza	310	35	14	13
Party Cheese	½ pizza	340	34	17	13
Party Combination	½ pizza	380	35	21	13
Party Hamburger	½ pizza	370	35	19	15
Party Mexican Style	½ pizza	380	35	21	13
Party Pepperoni	½ pizza	370	35	20	13
Party Sausage	½ pizza	390	35	21	14
Party Vegetable	½ pizza	300	36	13	11
Slices Cheese	1	170	20	7	7
Slices Combination	1	200	20	10	7
Slices Pepperoni	1	190	20	9	7
Slices Sausage	1	200	20	10	7
Weight Watchers					
Cheese	1 (6.03 oz)	300	36	7	24
Deluxe Combination	1 (7.32 oz)	320	36	9	25
Deluxe French Bread	1 (5.94 oz)	260	29	7	20
Pepperoni	1 (6.08 oz)	320	36	8	25
Sausage	1 (6.43 oz)	340	37	10	26
SAUCE					
Boboli					
Sauce	1 pkg (1.2 oz)	20	4	0	1
Sauce	¼ cup (2.5 oz)	40	9	0	1
Contadina					
Flavored With Pepperoni	¼ cup	40	6	2	1
Pizza Sauce	¼ cup	35	6	2	1
Squeeze	¼ cup	35	6	2	1
With Italian Cheeses	¼ cup	40	6	2	1
Eden					
Pizza Pasta Sauce	½ cup (4.4 oz)	80	12	3	3
Muir Glen					
Organic	¼ cup (2.2 oz)	40	6	1	1
Ragu					
Quick Traditional	3 tbsp (1.7 oz)	35	3	2	1
Tree Of Life					
Sauce	¼ cup (1.9 oz)	30	5	1	1
TAKE-OUT					
cheese	12 in pie	1121	164	26	61
cheese	⅛ pie 12 in	140	21	3	8
cheese deep dish individual	1 (5.5 oz)	460	47	24	15
cheese meat & vegetables	12 in pie	1472	170	43	104
cheese meat & vegetables	⅛ pie 12 in	184	21	5	13

FOOD	PORTION	CALS.	CARB.	FAT	PRO.
pepperoni	⅛ pie 12 in	181	20	7	10
pepperoni	12 in pie	1445	157	56	81

PLANTAINS
fresh uncooked	1 (6.3 oz)	218	57	1	2
sliced cooked	½ cup	89	24	tr	1
Top Banana					
All Natural Plantain Chips	1 oz	150	17	8	1
TAKE-OUT					
ripe fried	2.8 oz	214	38	7	1

PLUMS
CANNED					
purple in heavy syrup	3	119	31	tr	tr
purple in heavy syrup	1 cup	320	60	tr	1
purple in light syrup	3	83	22	tr	tr
purple in light syrup	1 cup	158	41	tr	1
purple juice pack	3	55	14	tr	tr
purple juice pack	1 cup	146	38	tr	1
purple water pack	1 cup	102	27	tr	1
purple water pack	3	39	10	tr	tr
S&W					
Halves Purple Fancy Unpeeled In Extra Heavy Syrup	½ cup	135	35	0	0
Whole Purple Fancy Unpeeled In Extra Heavy Syrup	½ cup	135	35	0	0
Whole Unpeeled Diet	½ cup	52	13	0	0
FRESH					
plum	1	36	9	tr	1
sliced	1 cup	91	21	1	1
Dole					
Plums	2	70	17	1	1

POI
poi	½ cup	134	33	tr	tr

POKEBERRY SHOOTS
cooked	½ cup	16	3	tr	2
raw	½ cup	18	3	tr	2
Allen					
Pokeberry Shoots	½ cup (4.1 oz)	35	5	1	2

POLENTA
(see CORNMEAL)

POLLACK
atlantic fillet baked	5.3 oz	178	0	2	38

FOOD	PORTION	CALS.	CARB.	FAT	PRO.
atlantic baked	3 oz	100	0	1	21
FROZEN					
Mrs. Paul's					
Fillets Light	1 fillet (4.5 oz)	240	18	11	18
POMEGRANATES					
pomegranate	1	104	26	tr	1
POMPANO					
florida cooked	3 oz	179	0	10	20
florida raw	3 oz	140	0	8	16
POPCORN					
(*see also* CHIPS, POPCORN CAKES, PRETZELS, SNACKS)					
air-popped	1 cup (0.3 oz)	31	6	tr	1
air-popped	1 oz	108	22	1	3
caramel coated	1 oz	122	22	4	1
caramel coated	1 cup (1.2 oz)	152	28	5	1
caramel coated w/ peanuts	⅔ cup (1 oz)	114	23	2	2
cheese	1 oz	149	15	9	3
cheese	1 cup (0.4 oz)	58	6	4	1
oil popped	1 oz	142	16	8	3
oil popped	1 cup (0.4 oz)	55	6	3	1
Barrel O' Fun					
Baked Curl	1 oz	150	17	9	2
Caramel Corn	1 oz	115	25	1	1
Corn Pop	1 oz	190	10	16	0
Popcorn	1 oz	160	13	12	2
White Cheddar Pops	1 oz	170	11	13	2
Cape Cod					
Light	½ oz	60	8	3	1
Popcorn	½ oz	80	6	5	2
Cheetos					
Cheddar Cheese	0.5 oz	80	6	6	1
Chesters					
Cheddar Cheese	0.5 oz	80	7	5	1
Microwave	3 cups	110	13	7	1
Microwave Butter	3 cups	120	13	7	2
Microwave Cheese	3 cups	110	11	8	2
Popcorn	0.5 oz	70	9	3	1
Cracker Jack					
Original	1 oz	120	22	3	2
Eagle					
Popcorn	½ oz	80	6	6	2
Estee					
No Sugar Added Caramel	1 cup (1 oz)	120	26	2	1

FOOD	PORTION	CALS.	CARB.	FAT	PRO.
Greenfield					
Caramel	1 cup (1 oz)	120	22	2	2
Jiffy Pop					
Bag Butter	3 cups	90	11	5	2
Bag Lite	3 cups	70	11	3	2
Bag Regular	3 cups	100	11	6	2
Glazed Popcorn Clusters	1 oz	120	25	2	0
Microwave Butter	4 cups	140	17	7	3
Microwave Regular	4 cups	140	17	7	3
Pan Butter	4 cups	130	16	6	3
Pan Regular	4 cups	130	16	6	3
Lance					
Cheese	1 pkg (25 g)	130	13	8	2
Plain	1 pkg (25 g)	140	13	9	2
White Cheddar Cheese	1 pkg (25 g)	140	12	9	2
Louise's					
Fat-Free Apple Cinnamon	1 oz	100	24	0	1
Fat-Free Buttery Toffee	1 oz	100	24	0	1
Fat-Free Caramel	1 oz	100	24	0	1
Newman's Own					
Oldstyle Picture Show	3 ⅓ cups	80	16	1	3
Oldstyle Picture Show Microwave Natural Butter	3 cups	150	18	8	2
Oldstyle Picture Show Microwave No Salt	3 cups	150	18	8	2
Oldstyle Picture Show Microwave Light Butter	3 cups	90	18	3	2
Oldstyle Picture Show Microwave Light Natural	3 cups	90	18	3	2
Orville Redenbacher's					
Gourmet Hot Air	3 cups	40	10	tr	1
Gourmet Original	3 cups	80	10	4	1
Gourmet White	3 cups	80	10	4	1
Microwave Gourmet	3 cups	100	11	6	2
Microwave Gourmet Butter Toffee	2½ cups	210	26	12	2
Microwave Gourmet Caramel	2½ cups	240	29	14	2
Microwave Gourmet Cheddar Cheese	3 cups	130	14	8	2

FOOD	PORTION	CALS.	CARB.	FAT	PRO.
Orville Redenbacher's (CONT.)					
Microwave Gourmet Salt Free	3 cups	100	11	6	2
Microwave Gourmet Salt Free Butter	3 cups	100	11	6	2
Microwave Gourmet Sour Cream 'n Onion	3 cups	160	12	12	2
Microwave Gourmet Butter	3 cups	100	11	6	2
Microwave Gourmet Frozen	3 cups	100	11	6	2
Microwave Gourmet Frozen Butter	3 cups	100	11	6	2
Microwave Gourmet Light	3 cups	70	8	3	2
Microwave Gourmet Light Butter	3 cups	70	8	3	2
Pillsbury					
Microwave Butter	3 cups	210	20	13	3
Microwave Original	3 cups	210	20	13	3
Microwave Salt Free	3 cups	170	23	7	3
Pop Secret					
Butter Flavor	3 cups	100	11	6	2
Butter Flavor Singles	6 cups	250	23	16	3
Light Butter Flavor	3 cups	70	12	3	2
Light Butter Flavor Singles	6 cups	140	23	6	3
Light Natural Flavor	3 cups	70	12	3	2
Light Natural Flavor Singles	6 cups	150	23	6	4
Natural Flavor	3 cups	100	11	6	2
Natural Flavor Salt Free	3 cups	100	11	6	2
Pop Chips	1½ cups (1 oz)	130	23	4	2
Pop Qwiz Butter Flavor	3 cups	100	11	6	2
Pop Qwiz Natural Flavor	3 cups	100	11	6	2
Smartfood					
Cheddar Cheese	0.5 oz	80	7	5	1
Light Butter	0.5 oz	70	9	3	1
Snyder's					
Butter	1 oz	140	13	9	2
Ultra Slim-Fast					
Lite N' Tasty	½ oz	60	10	2	2
Weight Watchers					
Microwave	1 oz	100	22	1	4
Ready-To-Eat Butter	0.7 oz	90	13	3	2

FOOD	PORTION	CALS.	CARB.	FAT	PRO.
Weight Watchers (CONT.)					
Ready-To-Eat White Cheddar Cheese	0.7 oz	90	11	4	2
Wise					
Tender Eating	0.5 oz	70	4	6	1
With Real Premium White Cheddar Cheese	0.5 oz	70	4	5	1

POPCORN CAKES

popcorn cake	1 (0.3 oz)	38	8	tr	1
Lundberg					
Organic Lightly Salted	1	60	12	1	1
Organic Unsalted	1	60	12	1	1
Rye With Caraway Lightly Salted	1	59	14	0	1
Mother's					
Butter Flavor	1 (0.3 oz)	35	7	0	1
Unsalted	1 (0.3 oz)	35	7	0	1
Quaker					
Blueberry Crunch	1 (0.5 oz)	50	11	0	1
Butter Popped	1 (0.3 oz)	35	7	0	1
Caramel	1 (0.5 oz)	50	12	0	1
Monterey Jack	1 (0.4 oz)	40	8	0	1
Strawberry Crunch	1 (0.5 oz)	50	11	0	1
White Cheddar	1 (0.4 oz)	40	8	0	1

POPOVER

home recipe as prep w/ 2% milk	1 (1.4 oz)	87	11	3	4
home recipe as prep w/ whole milk	1 (1.4 oz)	90	11	3	4
mix as prep	1 (1.2 oz)	67	10	2	3

POPPY SEEDS

poppy seeds	1 tsp	15	1	1	1

PORK

(*see also* BACON, BACON SUBSTITUTES, CANADIAN BACON, DELI MEAT/ COLD CUTS, HAM, SAUSAGE)

The values for cooked pork may differ slightly from values for raw pork. When meat is cooked some moisture and fat is lost, changing the nutritive value slightly. As a rule of thumb, it can be assumed that a 4 oz raw portion will equal a 3 oz cooked portion of meat.

CANNED

Hormel					
Pickled Tidbits	2 oz	100	0	8	8

FOOD	PORTION	CALS.	CARB.	FAT	PRO.
FRESH					
blade chop, roasted	1 (3.1 oz)	321	0	27	19
center loin chop, broiled	1 (3.1 oz)	275	0	24	24
center loin, roasted	3 oz	259	0	18	22
loin w/ fat, roasted	3 oz	271	0	21	20
shoulder arm picnic cured lean only roasted	3 oz	145	0	6	21
shoulder blade roll cured lean & fat	3 oz	304	0	25	19
shoulder whole, roasted	3 oz	277	0	22	19
spareribs, braised	3 oz	338	0	26	26
spleen braised	3 oz	127	0	3	24
tenderloin lean only, roasted	3 oz	141	0	4	24
Oscar Mayer					
Sweet Morsel Smoked Boneless Pork Shoulder	3 oz	180	0	15	11
TAKE-OUT					
pork roast	2 oz	70	0	3	10
PORK DISHES					
FROZEN					
Jimmy Dean					
BBQ Pork Rib Sandwich	1 (5.4 oz)	440	36	23	24
TAKE-OUT					
tourtiere	1 piece (4.9 oz)	451	21	34	15
POSOLE					
(*see* HOMINY)					
POT PIE					
FROZEN					
Award Brand					
Beef	1 (7 oz)	350	37	18	7
Chicken	1 (7 oz)	350	39	19	9
Banquet					
Family Entree Chicken Pie	1 serv (8 oz)	450	39	30	14
Macaroni & Cheese	1 pkg (6.5 oz)	200	35	3	7
Vegetable & Cheese	1 (7 oz)	390	49	18	8
Vegetable Pie w/ Beef	1 (7 oz)	330	38	15	9
Vegetable Pie w/ Chicken	1 (7 oz)	350	36	18	10
Vegetable Pie w/ Turkey	1 (7 oz)	370	38	20	10
Empire					
Chicken	1 (8.1 oz)	440	41	21	23

FOOD	PORTION	CALS.	CARB.	FAT	PRO.
Empire (CONT.)					
Turkey	1 (8.1 oz)	470	46	23	21
Great Value					
Beef	1 (7 oz)	390	38	19	15
Chicken	1 (7 oz)	380	39	20	10
Turkey	1 (7 oz)	400	42	22	9
Morton					
Beef	1 (7 oz)	310	34	17	7
Chicken	1 (7 oz)	320	32	18	8
Macaroni & Cheese	1 (6 oz)	160	30	3	6
Turkey	1 (7 oz)	300	29	18	8
Ozark Valley					
Chicken	1 (7 oz)	330	32	19	8
Macaroni & Cheese	1 (6.5 oz)	160	29	3	6
Turkey	1 (7 oz)	280	29	16	6
Stouffer's					
Beef Pie	1 pkg (10 oz)	450	36	26	19
Chicken Pie	1 pkg (10 oz)	520	37	33	18
Chicken Pie	½ pkg (8 oz)	460	35	30	15
Turkey	1 cup (8 oz)	500	36	31	20
Turkey	1 pkg (10 oz)	530	36	33	21
Swanson					
Beef	7 oz	370	36	19	12
Beef Hungry Man	16 oz	610	58	31	24
Chicken	7 oz	380	35	22	11
Chicken Homestyle	8 oz	410	41	21	15
Hungry Man Chicken	16 oz	630	57	35	22
Hungry Man Turkey	16 oz	650	57	36	24
Turkey	7 oz	380	36	21	11
TAKE-OUT					
beef	⅓ pie 9 in (7.4 oz)	515	39	30	21
chicken	⅓ pie 9 in (8.1 oz)	545	42	31	23

POTATO
(see also CHIPS, KNISH)

FOOD	PORTION	CALS.	CARB.	FAT	PRO.
CANNED					
potatoes	½ cup	54	12	tr	1
Allen					
Refried Potatoes	½ cup (4.5 oz)	150	24	3	7
Butterfield					
Diced	⅔ cup (5.7 oz)	100	22	0	2
Sliced	½ cup (5.7 oz)	100	22	0	2
Whole	2½ pieces (5.6 oz)	90	20	0	2
Del Monte					
New Sliced	⅔ cup (5.4 oz)	60	13	0	1

FOOD	PORTION	CALS.	CARB.	FAT	PRO.
Del Monte (CONT.)					
New Whole	⅔ cup (5.5 oz)	60	13	0	1
Hormel					
Au Gratin & Bacon	1 can (7.5 oz)	250	23	14	8
Scalloped & Ham	1 can (7.5 oz)	260	20	16	7
Hunt's					
Whole New	4 oz	70	15	tr	2
Micro Cup Meals					
Scalloped Potatoes & Ham	1 cup (10.4 oz)	360	28	23	10
Scalloped Potatoes With Ham	1 cup (7.5 oz)	260	20	16	7
S&W					
New Potatoes Extra Small	½ cup	45	9	0	2
Seneca					
Potatoes	½ cup	80	15	0	3
Sunshine					
Whole	2½ pieces (5.6 oz)	90	20	0	2
FRESH					
baked skin only	1 skin (2 oz)	115	27	tr	2
baked w/ skin	1 (6½ oz)	220	51	tr	5
baked w/o skin	1 (5 oz)	145	34	tr	3
baked w/o skin	½ cup	57	13	tr	1
boiled	½ cup	68	16	tr	1
microwaved	1 (7 oz)	212	49	tr	5
microwaved w/o skin	½ cup	78	18	tr	2
raw w/o skin	1 (3.9 oz)	88	20	tr	2
FROZEN					
french fries	10 strips	111	17	4	2
french fries thick cut	10 strips	109	17	4	2
hashed brown	½ cup	170	22	9	2
potato puffs	½ cup	138	19	7	2
potato puffs as prep	1	16	2	1	tr
Budget Gourmet					
Baked With Broccoli And Cheese	1 pkg (10.5 oz)	300	40	10	13
Cheddared Potatoes	1 pkg (5.5 oz)	260	22	16	7
Cheddared Potatoes With Broccoli	1 pkg (5 oz)	150	14	7	6
Three Cheese Potatoes	1 pkg (5.75 oz)	220	23	11	7
Empire					
Crinkle Cut French Fries	½ cup (3 oz)	90	18	2	1
Latkes Potato Pancakes	1 (2 oz)	80	15	2	1

FOOD	PORTION	CALS.	CARB.	FAT	PRO.
Empire (CONT.)					
Latkes Mini Potato Pancakes	2 (2 oz)	90	16	3	1
Golden					
Potato Pancakes	1 (1.33 oz)	71	10	3	2
Green Giant					
One Serve Au Gratin	1 pkg	200	20	10	7
One Serve Potatoes & Broccoli In Cheese Sauce	1 pkg	130	19	5	4
Healthy Choice					
Cheddar Broccoli Potatoes	1 meal (10.5 oz)	310	53	5	13
Garden Potato Casserole	1 meal (9.25 oz)	200	30	4	11
Kineret					
Crinkle Cut	18 pieces (3 oz)	120	20	4	2
Kugel	1 piece (2.5 oz)	150	13	10	2
Latkes	1 (1.5 oz)	90	9	5	2
Latkes Mini	10 (3 oz)	160	18	9	1
Lean Cuisine					
Deluxe Cheddar	1 pkg (10.4 oz)	270	30	10	14
MicroMagic					
French Fries	1 pkg (3 oz)	290	40	13	3
Skinny Fries	1 pkg (3 oz)	350	49	15	4
Oh Boy!					
Stuffed With Cheddar Cheese	1 (6 oz)	130	20	4	4
Stuffed With Real Bacon	1 (6 oz)	120	20	3	4
Ore Ida					
Cheddar Browns	1 patty (3 oz)	90	14	3	3
Cottage Fries	14 pieces (3 oz)	130	21	4	2
Crispers!	17 pieces (3 oz)	220	24	13	2
Crispers! Nacho	10 pieces (3 oz)	170	21	9	2
Crispers! Texas	3 oz	170	19	10	3
Crispy Crowns!	12 pieces (3 oz)	100	21	11	2
Crispy Crunchies	12 pieces (3 oz)	160	18	9	2
Deep Fries Crinkle Cuts	18 pieces (3 oz)	160	23	7	2
Deep Fries French Fries	22 pieces (3 oz)	160	22	7	2
Dinner Fries Country Style	8 pieces (3 oz)	110	19	3	2
Fast Fries	23 pieces (3 oz)	140	20	6	2
Fast Fries Ranch	22 pieces (3 oz)	150	21	7	2
Golden Crinkles	16 pieces (3 oz)	120	20	4	2
Golden Fries	16 pieces (3 oz)	120	20	4	2

FOOD	PORTION	CALS.	CARB.	FAT	PRO.
Ore Ida (CONT.)					
Golden Patties	1 (2.5 oz)	140	16	7	1
Golden Twirls	28 pieces (3 oz)	160	22	7	2
Hash Browns Country Style	1 cup (2.6 oz)	60	13	0	2
Hash Browns Shredded	1 patty (3 oz)	70	15	0	2
Hash Browns Southern Style	¾ cup (3 oz)	70	17	0	2
Hot Tots	9 pieces (3 oz)	150	21	6	2
Mashed Natural Butter	½ cup (2.1 oz)	80	14	2	2
Microwave Crinkle Cuts	1 pkg (3.5 oz)	180	26	8	3
Microwave Hash Browns	1 patty (2 oz)	110	13	6	1
Microwave Tater Tots	1 pkg (3.75 oz)	190	26	10	2
O'Brien Potatoes	¾ cup (3 oz)	60	13	0	1
Pixie Crinkles	33 pieces (3 oz)	140	21	5	2
Shoestrings	38 pieces (3 oz)	150	22	5	2
Snackin' Fries	1 pkg (5 oz)	180	36	20	4
Snackin' Fries Extra Zesty	1 pkg (5 oz)	180	35	20	4
Tater ABC's	10 pieces (3 oz)	190	20	11	2
Tater Tots	9 pieces (3 oz)	160	21	8	2
Tater Tots Bacon	9 pieces (3 oz)	150	20	7	2
Tater Tots Onion	9 pieces (3 oz)	150	20	7	2
Toaster Hash Browns	2 patties (3.5 oz)	190	21	12	2
Topped Broccoli & Cheese	½ (6 oz)	150	24	4	5
Topped Salsa & Cheese	½ (5.5 oz)	160	25	5	5
Topped Vegetable Primavera	1 (6.13 oz)	160	23	5	6
Twice Baked Butter	1 (5 oz)	200	27	9	4
Twice Baked Cheddar Cheese	1 (5 oz)	190	27	8	4
Twice Baked Ranch	1 (5 oz)	180	27	6	5
Twice Baked Sour Cream & Chives	1 (5 oz)	180	28	6	4
Waffle Fries	15 pieces (3 oz)	140	22	5	2
Wedges With Skin	9 pieces (3 oz)	110	19	3	2
Zesties!	12 pieces (3 oz)	160	21	9	2
Stouffer's					
Au Gratin	½ cup (2.25 oz)	130	15	6	4
Baked Broccoli & Cheese	1 pkg (10.1 oz)	320	30	15	15
Baked Cheddar Cheese & Bacon	1 pkg (9.4 oz)	380	31	22	15
Lunch Express Baked Broccoli & Cheese	1 pkg (10.25 oz)	250	28	9	13

FOOD	PORTION	CALS.	CARB.	FAT	PRO.
Stouffer's (CONT.)					
Scalloped	½ cup (2.25 oz)	130	17	6	4
Weight Watchers					
Baked Broccoli & Cheese	10.5 oz	270	43	6	10
Baked Broccoli & Ham	11.5 oz	280	39	17	19
Baked Chicken Divan	11.25 oz	280	38	7	17
Baked Homestyle Turkey	11.75 oz	250	26	7	20
HOME RECIPE					
au gratin	½ cup	160	14	9	6
mashed	½ cup	111	18	4	2
scalloped	½ cup	105	13	5	4
MIX					
au gratin as prep	4½ oz	127	18	6	3
instant mashed flakes as prep w/ whole milk & butter	½ cup	118	16	6	2
instant mashed flakes not prep	½ cup	78	18	tr	2
instant mashed granules as prep w/ whole milk & butter	½ cup	114	15	5	2
instant mashed granules not prep	½ cup	372	86	1	8
scalloped as prep	4½ oz	127	18	6	3
Betty Crocker					
Au Gratin as prep	½ cup	140	21	5	3
Cheddar 'N Bacon as prep	½ cup	140	21	5	3
Cheesy Scalloped as prep	½ cup	140	20	5	3
Hash Browns as prep	½ cup	160	24	6	2
Hash Browns as prep w/o salt	½ cup	160	24	6	2
Homestyle American Cheese as prep	½ cup	140	20	5	3
Homestyle Broccoli Au Gratin as prep	½ cup	130	19	5	3
Homestyle Cheddar Cheese as prep	½ cup	140	20	5	4
Homestyle Cheesy Scalloped as prep	½ cup	140	20	5	3
Julienne as prep	½ cup	130	18	5	3
Potato Buds as prep	½ cup	130	17	6	3
Potato Buds as prep w/o salt	½ cup	130	17	6	3

FOOD	PORTION	CALS.	CARB.	FAT	PRO.
Betty Crocker (CONT.)					
Scalloped as prep	½ cup	140	20	5	3
Scalloped & Ham as prep	½ cup	160	22	6	4
Smokey Cheddar as prep	½ cup	140	21	5	3
Sour Cream 'N Chive as prep	½ cup	140	21	5	3
Twice Baked Bacon & Cheddar as prep	½ cup	210	21	11	6
Twice Baked Cheddar With Mild Onion as prep	½ cup	190	20	10	5
Twice Baked Herbed Butter as prep	½ cup	220	20	13	5
Twice Baked Sour Cream & Chive as prep	½ cup	200	19	11	5
Country Store					
Mashed not prep	⅓ cup	70	15	0	2
French's					
Cheddar & Bacon Casserole	½ cup	130	18	5	4
Creamy Stroganoff	½ cup	130	20	4	3
Creamy Italian Scalloped	½ cup	120	19	3	4
Crispy top Scalloped With Savory Onion	½ cup	140	20	5	3
Real Cheese Scalloped	½ cup	140	19	5	4
Real Sour Cream & Chives	½ cup	150	19	7	3
Spuds Mashed	½ cup	140	17	7	3
Tangy Au Gratin	½ cup	130	20	5	4
Hungry Jack					
Mashed Flakes	½ cup	40	17	7	3
Kraft					
Potatoes & Cheese Au Gratin	½ cup	130	19	5	4
Potatoes & Cheese Broccoli Au Gratin	½ cup	120	20	5	5
Potatoes & Cheese Scalloped	½ cup	140	20	5	4
Potatoes & Cheese Scalloped With Ham	½ cup	150	20	5	5
REFRIGERATED					
Simply Potatoes					
Au Gratin	¼ pkg (3 oz)	130	13	8	3

FOOD	PORTION	CALS.	CARB.	FAT	PRO.
Simply Potatoes (CONT.)					
Hash Browns	⅕ pkg (4 oz)	100	23	tr	3
Hash Browns Onion	⅕ pkg (4 oz)	120	26	tr	3
Hash Browns Southwest Style	⅕ pkg (4 oz)	100	23	tr	3
Mashed	⅕ pkg (4 oz)	90	15	2	2
Scalloped	¼ pkg (3 oz)	100	11	5	2
SHELF-STABLE					
Lunch Bucket					
Scalloped	1 pkg (7.5 oz)	160	20	7	4
Pantry Express					
Augratin	½ cup	120	17	5	3
TAKE-OUT					
au gratin w/ cheese	½ cup	178	17	10	7
baked topped w/ cheese sauce	1	475	47	29	15
baked topped w/ cheese sauce & bacon	1	451	44	26	18
baked topped w/ cheese sauce & broccoli	1	402	47	14	14
baked topped w/ cheese sauce & chili	1	481	56	22	23
baked topped w/ sour cream & chives	1	394	50	22	7
curry	1 serving (6 oz)	292	36	16	4
french fried in beef tallow	1 reg	237	29	12	3
french fried in beef tallow	1 lg	358	44	19	5
french fried in vegetable oil	1 reg	235	29	12	3
french fried in vegetable oil	1 lg	355	44	19	5
hash brown	½ cup	163	17	11	2
mashed w/ whole milk & margarine	⅓ cup	66	13	tr	2
mustard potato salad	3.5 oz	120	16	6	1
o'brien	1 cup	157	30	3	5
potato dumpling	3½ oz	334	74	1	7
potato pancakes	1 (1.3 oz)	101	11	7	2
potato salad	⅓ cup	108	13	6	1
potato salad	½ cup	179	14	10	3
potato salad w/ vegetables	3.5 oz	120	20	3	2
scalloped	½ cup	127	18	5	4
POTATO STARCH					
potato starch	3½ oz	335	83	tr	1
Manischewitz					
Potato Starch	1 cup	570	137	0	tr

FOOD	PORTION	CALS.	CARB.	FAT	PRO.
POUT					
ocean baked	3 oz	86	0	1	18
ocean fillet baked	4.8 oz	139	0	2	29
PRESERVE					
(see JAM/JELLY/PRESERVE)					
PRETZELS					
(see also CHIPS, POPCORN, SNACKS)					
chocolate covered	1 (0.4 oz)	50	8	2	1
chocolate covered	1 oz	130	20	5	2
dutch twist	4 (2.1 oz)	229	48	2	6
pretzels	1 oz	108	23	1	3
rods	4 (2 oz)	229	48	2	6
sticks	10	10	2	tr	tr
sticks	120 (2 oz)	229	48	2	6
twist	1 (½ oz)	65	13	1	2
twists	10 (2.1 oz)	229	48	2	6
whole wheat	2 med (2 oz)	205	46	2	6
whole wheat	2 sm (1 oz)	103	23	1	3
A & Eagle					
Beer	1 oz	110	22	2	3
Pretzels	1 oz	110	22	2	3
Barrel O' Fun					
Mini	1 oz	110	23	1	3
Sticks	1 oz	110	23	1	3
Twists	1 oz	110	23	1	3
Estee					
Dutch Unsalted	2 (1.1 oz)	130	26	1	3
Nuggets Ranch Reduced Sodium	23 (1 oz)	130	24	2	3
Nuggets Reduced Sodium	30 (1 oz)	120	24	2	3
Unsalted	23 (1 oz)	120	25	1	3
Formagg					
Pretzel Nuts	1 oz	120	21	4	2
J&J					
Soft	1 (2.25 oz)	170	37	0	6
Soft Bites	5 bites	110	23	0	4
Lance					
Twist	1 pkg (42 g)	150	30	1	4
Manischewitz					
Bagel Pretzels Original	4 (1 oz)	110	22	0	0
Mister Salty					
Chips	16 (1 oz)	110	21	3	2

FOOD	PORTION	CALS.	CARB.	FAT	PRO.
Mister Salty (CONT.)					
Dutch	2 (1.1 oz)	120	25	1	3
Fat Free Chips	16 (1 oz)	100	22	0	2
Mini	22 (1 oz)	110	22	1	3
Sticks Fat Free	47 (1 oz)	110	23	0	3
Twist Fat Free	9 (1 oz)	110	23	0	3
Mr. Phipps					
Chipps Original	16 (1 oz)	120	21	3	2
Chips Lower Sodium	16 (1 oz)	120	21	3	2
Chips Original Fat Free	16 (1 oz)	100	22	0	2
Planters					
Twists	1 pkg (1.5 oz)	160	35	1	4
Twists	1 oz	100	23	1	3
Quinlan					
Beers	1 oz	110	22	2	2
Hard Sourdough	1 oz	110	22	2	2
Logs	1 oz	110	22	2	2
Nuggets	1 oz	110	22	2	2
Rods	1 oz	110	22	2	2
Sticks	1 oz	110	22	2	2
Thins	1 oz	110	22	2	2
Rold Gold					
Bavarian	3 pieces (1 oz)	120	22	2	3
Pretzel Chips	1 oz	110	22	1	3
Pretzel Chips Cheese	1 oz	120	22	3	3
Rods	3 pieces (1 oz)	110	23	2	3
Snack Mix	½ cup (1 oz)	140	18	6	3
Sour Dough	1½ pieces (1 oz)	110	22	2	3
Sticks	50 pieces (1 oz)	110	23	2	3
Thin Twist	10 pieces (1 oz)	110	23	1	2
Tiny Twist	15 pieces (1 oz)	110	23	1	3
Seyfart's					
Butter Rods	1 oz	110	21	1	3
Snyder's					
Logs	1 oz	310	22	0	3
Minis	1 oz	310	22	0	3
Minis Unsalted	1 oz	310	22	0	3
Nibblers	1 oz	310	22	0	3
Oat Bran	1 oz	120	14	1	2
Old Fashioned Hard	1 oz	111	23	0	3
Old Fashioned Hard Unsalted	1 oz	100	23	0	3
Old Tyme	1 oz	310	22	0	3
Old Tyme Unsalted	1 oz	110	22	0	3

FOOD	PORTION	CALS.	CARB.	FAT	PRO.
Snyder's (CONT.)					
Rods	1 oz	310	22	0	3
Sourdough Hard Buttermilk Ranch	1 oz	130	19	5	2
Sourdough Hard Cheddar Cheese	1 oz	160	13	7	4
Sourdough Hard Honey Mustard & Onion	1 oz	130	19	5	2
Stix	1 oz	310	22	0	3
Very Thins	1 oz	310	22	0	3
Sunshine					
California Pretzels	1 oz	110	22	2	3
Ultra Slim-Fast					
Lite N' Tasty	1 oz	100	21	tr	2
Wege					
Sourdough	1 oz	102	23	tr	3
Unsalted	1 oz	102	23	tr	3
Whole Wheat	1 oz	109	21	1	3
PRICKLY PEAR					
fresh	1	42	10	1	1
PRUNE JUICE					
canned	1 cup	181	45	tr	2
Del Monte					
Juice	8 fl oz	170	43	0	1
S&W					
Unsweetened	6 oz	120	31	0	1
PRUNES					
CANNED					
in heavy syrup	5	90	24	tr	1
in heavy syrup	1 cup	245	65	tr	2
Sonoma					
Pitted	3-4 (1.4 oz)	110	26	0	1
DRIED					
cooked w/ sugar	½ cup	147	39	tr	1
cooked w/o sugar	½ cup	113	30	tr	1
dried	1 cup	385	101	1	4
dried	10	201	53	tr	2
Del Monte					
Pitted	¼ cup (1.4 oz)	120	29	0	1
Unpitted	⅓ cup (1.4 oz)	110	12	0	1
Sonoma					
Pitted	¼ cup (1.4 oz)	120	29	0	1

FOOD	PORTION	CALS.	CARB.	FAT	PRO.
Sunsweet					
Orange Essence Pitted Prunes	6 (1.4 oz)	100	26	0	1

PUDDING
(see also CUSTARD, PUDDING POPS)

HOME RECIPE

FOOD	PORTION	CALS.	CARB.	FAT	PRO.
bread pudding	½ cup (4.4 oz)	212	31	7	7
bread w/ raisins	½ cup	180	31	5	5
chocolate as prep w/ 2% milk	½ cup (5.5 oz)	206	41	4	5
chocolate as prep w/ whole milk	½ cup (5.5 oz)	221	40	6	5
corn	⅔ cup	181	21	9	7
cornstarch	½ cup (4.4 oz)	137	20	5	5
rice	½ cup (5.3 oz)	217	40	4	6
yorkshire as prep w/ skim milk	3.5 oz	93	12	4	3
yorkshire as prep w/ whole milk	3.5 oz	104	12	5	3
MIX					
lemon	½ cup (5.1 oz)	163	36	2	1
MIX WITH 2% MILK					
chocolate	½ cup (5 oz)	150	28	3	5
chocolate instant	½ cup (5.2 oz)	149	28	3	3
coconut cream	½ cup (4.9 oz)	148	25	4	4
coconut cream instant	½ cup (5.2 oz)	157	28	3	4
lemon instant	½ cup (5.2 oz)	155	30	4	4
rice	½ cup (5.1 oz)	161	30	2	5
tapioca	½ cup (5 oz)	147	28	2	4
vanilla	½ cup (4.9 oz)	141	26	2	4
vanilla instant	½ cup (5 oz)	147	28	2	2
MIX WITH WHOLE MILK					
chocolate	½ cup (5 oz)	158	26	5	5
chocolate instant	½ cup (5.2 oz)	164	28	5	5
coconut cream	½ cup (4.9 oz)	160	25	4	4
coconut cream instant	½ cup (5.2 oz)	172	28	5	4
lemon instant	½ cup (5.2 oz)	169	30	4	4
rice	½ cup (5.1 oz)	175	30	4	5
tapioca	½ cup (5 oz)	161	28	4	4
vanilla	½ cup (4.9 oz)	155	26	4	2
vanilla instant	½ cup (5 oz)	181	28	4	4
READY-TO-USE					
chocolate	1 pkg (5 oz)	189	32	6	4

FOOD	PORTION	CALS.	CARB.	FAT	PRO.
lemon	1 pkg (5 oz)	177	36	4	tr
rice	1 pkg (5 oz)	231	31	11	3
tapioca	1 pkg (5 oz)	169	28	5	3
vanilla	1 pkg (4 oz)	146	25	4	3
TAKE-OUT					
blancmange	1 serving (4.7 oz)	154	25	5	4
bread pudding	½ cup (4.4 oz)	212	31	7	7
rice pudding	1 serving (3 oz)	110	17	4	3
rice w/ raisins	½ cup	246	42	6	7
tapioca	½ cup (5.3 oz)	189	26	7	7
vanilla	½ cup (4.3 oz)	130	20	4	4

PUDDING POPS

(see also ICE CREAM AND FROZEN DESSERTS, PUDDING)

FOOD	PORTION	CALS.	CARB.	FAT	PRO.
chocolate	1 (1.6 oz)	72	12	2	2
vanilla	1 (1.6 oz)	75	13	2	2
Jell-O					
Chocolate	1 pop	79	13	2	2
Chocolate Caramel Swirl	1 pop	74	12	2	2
Chocolate Fudge	1 pop	79	13	2	2
Chocolate Peanut Butter Swirl	1 bar	78	12	3	2
Chocolate Swirl	1 pop	80	13	2	2
Chocolate Vanilla Swirl	1 pop	78	13	2	2
Deluxe Chocolate Covered	1 pop	201	27	10	3
Deluxe Peanuts And Chocolate	1 bar	185	24	9	3
Milk Chocolate	1 pop	80	13	2	2
Vanilla	1 pop	77	13	2	2

PUMMELO

FOOD	PORTION	CALS.	CARB.	FAT	PRO.
fresh	1	228	59	tr	5
sections	1 cup	71	18	tr	1

PUMPKIN

CANNED

FOOD	PORTION	CALS.	CARB.	FAT	PRO.
pumpkin	½ cup	41	10	tr	1
Libby					
Solid Pack	½ cup	60	15	1	2
FRESH					
cooked mashed	½ cup	24	6	tr	1
flowers cooked	½ cup	10	2	tr	1
flowers raw	1	0	tr	0	tr
leaves cooked	½ cup	7	1	tr	1

FOOD	PORTION	CALS.	CARB.	FAT	PRO.
leaves raw	½ cup	4	tr	tr	1
raw cubed	½ cup	15	4	tr	1
SEEDS					
dried	1 oz	154	5	13	7
roasted	1 cup	1184	31	96	75
roasted	1 oz	148	4	12	9
salted & roasted	1 cup	1184	31	96	75
salted & roasted	1 oz	148	4	12	9
whole roasted	1 oz	127	15	6	5
whole roasted	1 cup	285	34	12	12
whole salted roasted	1 cup	285	34	12	12
whole salted roasted	1 oz	127	15	6	5
PURSLANE					
cooked	1 cup	21	4	tr	2
raw	1 cup	7	1	tr	1
QUAHOGS					
(see CLAMS)					
QUAIL					
breast w/o skin raw	1 (2 oz)	69	0	2	13
w/ skin raw	1 quail (3.8 oz)	210	0	13	21
w/o skin raw	1 quail (3.2 oz)	123	0	4	20
QUICHE					
HOME RECIPE					
lorraine	⅛ pie 8 in	600	29	48	13
TAKE-OUT					
cheese	1 slice (3 oz)	283	16	20	11
lorraine	1 slice (3 oz)	352	18	25	15
mushroom	1 slice (3 oz)	256	17	18	9
QUINCE					
fresh	1	53	14	tr	tr
QUINOA					
quinoa	½ cup	318	59	5	11
Arrowhead					
Quinoa	¼ cup (1.4 oz)	140	25	2	5
Eden					
Not Prep	¼ cup (1.6 oz)	170	31	3	6
RABBIT					
domestic w/o bone roasted	3 oz	167	0	7	25
wild w/o bone stewed	3 oz	147	0	3	28
RACCOON					
roasted	3 oz	217	0	12	25

FOOD	PORTION	CALS.	CARB.	FAT	PRO.
RADICCHIO					
leaf	3.5 oz	18	3	tr	1
raw shredded	½ cup	5	1	tr	tr
RADISHES					
DRIED					
chinese	½ cup	157	37	tr	5
daikon	½ cup	157	37	tr	5
FRESH					
chinese raw	1 (12 oz)	62	14	tr	2
chinese raw sliced	½ cup	8	2	tr	tr
chinese sliced cooked	½ cup	13	3	tr	tr
daikon raw	1 (12 oz)	62	14	tr	2
daikon raw sliced	½ cup	8	2	tr	tr
daikon sliced cooked	½ cup	13	3	tr	tr
red raw	10	7	2	tr	tr
red sliced	½ cup	10	2	tr	tr
white icicle raw	1 (½ oz)	2	tr	tr	tr
white icicle raw sliced	½ cup	7	1	tr	1
Dole					
Radishes	7	20	3	0	0
SPROUTS					
raw	½ cup	8	1	tr	1
RAISINS					
chocolate coated	1 cup (6.7 oz)	741	130	28	8
chocolate coated	10 (0.4 oz)	39	7	2	tr
golden seedless	1 cup	437	115	1	5
seedless	1 cup	434	115	1	5
seedless	1 tbsp	27	7	tr	tr
sultanas	1 oz	88	23	0	1
Del Monte					
Golden	¼ cup (1.4 oz)	130	31	0	0
Raisins	1 box (1.5 oz)	140	33	0	0
Raisins	¼ cup (1.4 oz)	130	31	0	0
Raisins	1 box (1 oz)	90	22	0	0
Raisins	1 box (0.5 oz)	45	11	0	0
Yogurt Raisins Strawberry	1 pkg (0.9 oz)	110	20	3	2
Yogurt Raisins Vanilla	1 pkg (0.9 oz)	110	20	3	2
Yogurt Raisins Vanilla	1 pkg (1 oz)	120	22	3	2
Yogurt Raisins Vanilla	3 tbsp (1 oz)	130	23	3	2
Dole					
Golden	½ cup	250	66	0	3

FOOD	PORTION	CALS.	CARB.	FAT	PRO.
Dole (CONT.)					
Seedless	½ cup	250	66	0	3
Sonoma					
Monukka Thompson	¼ cup (1.4 oz)	130	31	0	1
Tree Of Life					
Organic	¼ cup (1.4 oz)	130	31	0	1

RASPBERRIES

FOOD	PORTION	CALS.	CARB.	FAT	PRO.
CANNED					
in heavy syrup	½ cup	117	30	tr	1
FRESH					
raspberries	1 cup	61	14	1	1
raspberries	1 pint	154	36	2	3
Dole					
Raspberries	1 cup	45	10	0	1
FROZEN					
sweetened	1 cup	256	65	tr	2
sweetened	1 pkg (10 oz)	291	74	tr	2
Big Valley					
Raspberries	⅔ cup (4.9 oz)	80	18	0	1
Birds Eye					
Whole In Lite Syrup	½ cup	100	25	1	1

RASPBERRY JUICE

FOOD	PORTION	CALS.	CARB.	FAT	PRO.
After The Fall					
Raspberry Ginger Ale	1 can (12 oz)	150	36	0	1
Crystal Geyser					
Juice Squeeze Mountain Raspberry	1 bottle (12 fl oz)	135	32	0	1
Kool-Aid					
Sugar Free	8 oz	2	0	0	0
Smucker's					
Juice	8 oz	120	30	0	0
Juice Sparkler	10 oz	130	32	tr	1

RED BEANS

FOOD	PORTION	CALS.	CARB.	FAT	PRO.
CANNED					
Allen					
Red Beans	½ cup (4.5 oz)	160	19	1	6
B&M					
Small Baked	8 oz	223	36	5	9
Green Giant					
Red Beans	½ cup	90	19	1	6
Hunt's					
Small	4 oz	90	18	tr	6

FOOD	PORTION	CALS.	CARB.	FAT	PRO.
Van Camp's					
Red Beans	½ cup (4.6 oz)	90	20	0	6
DRIED					
Bean Cuisine					
Dried	½ cup	115	—	1	8
MIX					
Bean Cuisine					
Pasta & Beans Barcelona	½ cup	170	170	4	60
Red With Radiatore					
Mahatma					
Red Beans & Rice	1 cup	190	40	1	8
RELISH					
cranberry orange	½ cup	246	64	tr	tr
hamburger	1 tbsp	19	5	tr	tr
hamburger	½ cup	158	42	1	1
hot dog	1 tbsp	14	4	tr	tr
hot dog	½ cup	111	28	1	2
piccalilli	1.4 oz	13	2	tr	tr
sweet	1 tbsp	19	5	tr	tr
sweet	½ cup	159	43	1	tr
Del Monte					
Hamburger	1 tbsp (0.5 oz)	20	6	0	0
Hot Dog	1 tbsp (0.5 oz)	15	4	0	0
Sweet Pickle	1 tbsp (0.5 oz)	20	5	0	0
Hellman's					
Sandwich Spred	1 tbsp (15 g)	55	2	5	tr
Old El Paso					
Jalapeno	2 tbsp	5	1	0	0
Vlasic					
Dill	1 oz	2	1	0	0
Hamburger	1 oz	40	9	0	0
Hot Dog	1 oz	40	8	1	0
Hot Piccalilli	1 oz	35	8	0	0
India	1 oz	30	8	0	0
Sweet	1 oz	30	8	0	0
RHUBARB					
fresh	½ cup	13	3	tr	1
frzn	½ cup	60	3	tr	tr
frzn as prep w/ sugar	½ cup	139	37	tr	tr
RICE					
(*see also* BRAN, CEREAL, FLOUR, RICE CAKES, WILD RICE)					
BROWN					
long-grain cooked	½ cup	109	23	tr	3

FOOD	PORTION	CALS.	CARB.	FAT	PRO.
medium-grain cooked	½ cup	109	23	tr	2
Arrowhead					
Basmati	¼ cup (1.5 oz)	150	33	1	3
Quick Regular	⅓ cup (1.5 oz)	150	32	1	3
Quick Spanish Style	¼ pkg (1.4 oz)	150	30	1	4
Quick Vegetable Herb	¼ pkg (1.4 oz)	150	30	1	4
Quick Wild Rice & Herb	¼ pkg (1.3 oz)	140	28	1	4
Minute					
Precooked as prep	½ cup	121	26	1	3
Near East					
Pilaf as prep	1 cup	220	41	5	6
S&W					
Quick Natural Long Grain	3.5 oz	110	25	0	2
Quick Natural Long Grain cooked	3.5 oz	119	26	0	3
Uncle Ben					
Brown Rice	1 serv (1.6 oz)	158	34	1	4
CANNED					
Old El Paso					
Spanish	½ cup	130	28	1	3
Van Camp's					
Spanish	1 cup (9 oz)	180	37	3	3
FROZEN					
Birds Eye					
Rice & Broccoli Au Gratin	½ pkg	150	24	4	5
Budget Gourmet					
Oriental Rice With Vegetables	1 pkg (5.75 oz)	230	28	12	4
Rice Pilaf With Green Beans	1 pkg (5.5 oz)	230	30	11	4
Chun King					
Fried Rice	1 pkg (8 oz)	290	48	6	11
Fried Rice With Chicken	1 pkg (8 oz)	270	44	6	9
Green Giant					
Garden Gourmet Asparagus Pilaf	1 pkg	190	37	4	5
Garden Gourmet Sherry Wild Rice	1 pkg	210	40	4	6
One Serve Rice 'N Broccoli In Cheese Sauce	1 pkg	180	25	6	5

FOOD	PORTION	CALS.	CARB.	FAT	PRO.
Green Giant (CONT.)					
One Serve Rice Peas & Mushrooms With Sauce	1 pkg	130	27	2	4
Rice Originals Italian Rice & Spinach In Cheese Sauce	½ cup	140	22	4	4
Rice Originals Pilaf	½ cup	110	21	1	2
Rice Originals Rice 'N Broccoli In Cheese Sauce	½ cup	120	18	4	3
Rice Originals Rice Medley	½ cup	100	19	1	3
Rice Originals White & Wild	½ cup	130	24	2	3
Luigino's					
Fried Rice Chicken	1 pkg (8 oz)	250	38	5	11
Fried Rice Pork	1 pkg (8 oz)	250	37	7	11
Fried Rice Pork & Shrimp	1 pkg (8 oz)	250	39	5	10
Fried Rice Shrimp	1 pkg (8 oz)	220	38	4	9
Risotto Parmesano	1 pkg (8 oz)	360	30	20	14
MIX					
Casbah					
Jambalaya	1 pkg (1.4 oz)	130	27	0	4
La Fiesta	1 pkg (1.59 oz)	170	34	1	6
Nutted Pilaf as prep	1 cup	220	40	3	6
Pilaf as prep	1 cup	200	44	tr	6
Spanish Pilaf as prep	1 cup	200	44	1	6
Thai Yum	1 pkg (1.7 oz)	180	33	3	5
Goodman's					
Rice & Vermicelli For Beef	¾ cup	160	33	1	4
Rice & Vermicelli For Chicken	¾ cup	160	33	1	4
Hain					
Rice Almondine	½ cup	130	17	5	3
Rice Oriental 3-Grain Goodness	½ cup	120	15	5	4
Kitchen Del Sol					
Mediterranean Paella Costa Brave as prep	½ cup (1.2 oz)	130	23	2	3
Mediterranean Sunny Lemon Pilaf as prep	½ cup (1.2 oz)	110	22	1	3

FOOD	PORTION	CALS.	CARB.	FAT	PRO.
Kitchen Del Sol (CONT.)					
Mediterranean Tomato & Basil With Pine Nuts	½ cup (1 oz)	110	18	4	2
Knorr					
Risotto Milanese With Saffron	½ cup	130	24	3	2
Risotto Tomato	½ cup	110	23	tr	2
Risotto With Mushrooms	½ cup	110	24	tr	2
Risotto With Onion	½ cup	110	24	tr	2
Risotto With Peas And Corn	½ cup	110	23	1	2
La Choy					
Chinese Fried Rice	¾ cup	190	41	1	4
Lipton					
Golden Saute Fried Rice Beef	½ cup	124	24	2	3
Golden Saute Fried Rice Chicken	½ cup	129	24	2	4
Golden Saute Fried Rice Oriental	½ cup	127	24	2	4
Rice & Sauce Beef	½ cup	119	26	1	3
Rice & Sauce Cajun	½ cup	123	26	tr	4
Rice & Sauce Cheddar Broccoli	½ cup	125	25	1	3
Rice & Sauce Chicken	½ cup	124	25	1	3
Rice & Sauce Chicken Broccoli	½ cup	129	25	2	5
Rice & Sauce Creamy Chicken	½ cup	142	27	2	3
Rice & Sauce Herbs & Butter	½ cup	123	24	2	3
Rice & Sauce Long Grain & Wild Rice Original	½ cup	121	26	tr	4
Rice & Sauce Mushroom	½ cup	123	26	1	3
Rice & Sauce Pilaf	½ cup	122	26	1	4
Rice & Sauce Skillet Style Spanish	½ cup	104	21	1	3
Rice & Sauce Spanish	½ cup	118	25	1	3
Rice Asparagus With Hollandaise	½ cup	123	25	1	4
Mahatma					
Broccoli & Cheese	1 cup	200	41	2	5

FOOD	PORTION	CALS.	CARB.	FAT	PRO.
Mahatma (CONT.)					
Jambalaya	1 cup (2 oz)	190	43	1	4
Long Grain & Wild	1 cup (2 oz)	190	41	1	5
Pilaf	1 cup (2 oz)	190	43	0	5
Spanish	1 cup (2 oz)	180	42	1	4
Yellow Rice Mix	1 cup	190	43	0	4
Minute					
Fried Rice With Vermicelli as prep	½ cup	158	25	5	3
Microwave Broccoli Almondin	½ cup	143	24	4	3
Microwave Cheddar Cheese Broccoli	½ cup	164	26	5	4
Microwave French Pilaf	½ cup	133	24	3	2
Microwave Long Grain Brown And Wild	½ cup	140	25	3	3
Microwave Rice With Savory Cheese Sauce as prep	½ cup	162	26	5	4
Rice Drumstick With Vermicelli as prep	½ cup	153	25	4	3
Rice Rib Roast With Vermicelli as prep	½ cup	151	25	4	3
Near East					
Barley Pilaf as prep	1 cup	220	41	4	6
Beef Pilaf as prep	1 cup	220	42	5	5
Curry Rice as prep	1 cup	220	42	4	5
Lentil Pilif as prep	1 cup	210	37	4	10
Long Grain & Wild as prep	1 cup	220	42	5	6
Pilaf Chicken as prep	1 cup	220	42	5	5
Pilaf Kosher as prep	1 cup	220	42	5	6
Spanish Pilaf as prep	1 cup	230	42	6	5
Old El Paso					
Mexican	½ cup	140	28	2	2
Rice-A-Roni					
Beef	½ cup	140	24	4	4
Beef & Mushroom	½ cup	150	26	3	4
Chicken	½ cup	150	26	3	3
Chicken & Broccoli	½ cup	150	25	3	3
Chicken & Mushroom	½ cup	180	26	7	4
Chicken & Vegetables	½ cup	140	25	3	3
Fried Rice	½ cup	110	21	5	3
Herb & Butter	½ cup	130	22	4	2

FOOD	PORTION	CALS.	CARB.	FAT	PRO.
Rice-A-Roni (CONT.)					
Long Grain & Wild Chicken w/ Almonds	½ cup	140	24	4	3
Long Grain & Wild Original	½ cup	130	23	3	3
Long Grain & Wild Pilaf	½ cup	130	23	3	3
Pilaf	½ cup	150	25	4	4
Risotto	½ cup	200	32	6	4
Spanish	½ cup	150	25	4	4
Stroganoff	½ cup	200	27	8	4
Yellow Rice	½ cup	140	25	4	2
Success					
Beef Oriental	½ cup	190	43	1	5
Broccoli & Cheese	½ cup	200	41	2	6
Brown & Wild	½ cup	190	40	1	6
Classic Chicken	½ cup	150	32	1	4
Long Grain & Wild	½ cup	190	42	0	5
Pilaf	½ cup	200	44	0	5
Spanish	½ cup	190	43	1	5
Ultra Slim-Fast					
Oriental Style	2.3 oz	240	58	1	5
Rice & Chicken Sauce	2.3 oz	240	56	1	5
Uncle Ben					
Brown & Wild Fast Cooking	1 serv (1.3 oz)	120	26	1	4
Country Inn Broccoli Almondine	1 serv (1.2 oz)	124	25	2	4
Country Inn Broccoli & White Cheddar	1 serv (1.2 oz)	131	24	3	4
Country Inn Broccoli Au Gratin	1 serv (1.1 oz)	116	22	2	4
Country Inn Chicken With Wild Rice	1 serv (1.1 oz)	108	23	1	3
Country Inn Creamy Chicken & Mushroom	1 serv (1.3 oz)	138	24	3	4
Country Inn Creamy Chicken & Wild Rice	1 serv (1.3 oz)	135	27	1	4
Country Inn Green Bean Almondine	1 serv (1.2 oz)	128	25	2	4
Country Inn Herbed Au Gratin	1 serv (1.2 oz)	119	24	2	3
Country Inn Homestyle Chicken & Vegetables	1 serv (1.3 oz)	139	24	3	4
Country Inn Rice Florentine	1 serv (1.2 oz)	212	24	2	4

FOOD	PORTION	CALS.	CARB.	FAT	PRO.
Uncle Ben (CONT.)					
Country Inn Vegetable Pilaf	1 serv (1.2 oz)	115	25	1	3
Country Inn Chicken Stock	1 serv (1.2 oz)	123	24	1	4
Long Grain & Wild Chicken Stock Sauce	1 serv (1.3 oz)	133	25	2	4
Long Grain & Wild Fast Cooking	1 serv (1 oz)	101	22	tr	3
Long Grain & Wild Garden Vegetable Blend	1 serv (1.3 oz)	128	26	1	4
Long Grain & Wild Original	1 serv (1 oz)	96	21	tr	3
Watkins					
Brown & Wild	¼ cup (1.6 oz)	160	34	0	4
Calico Medley	¼ cup (1.6 oz)	160	37	0	4
East/West Medley	¼ cup (1.6 oz)	160	33	0	6
Heartland Medley	¼ cup (1.6 oz)	160	35	0	5
Minnesota Medley	¼ cup (1.6 oz)	160	34	0	5
White & Wild	¼ cup (1.6 oz)	160	34	0	4
TAKE-OUT					
pilaf	½ cup	84	11	3	4
risotto	6.6 oz	426	65	18	6
spanish	¾ cup	363	19	27	11
WHITE					
glutinous cooked	½ cup	116	25	tr	2
long-grain cooked	½ cup	131	28	tr	3
long-grain instant cooked	½ cup	80	17	tr	2
long-grain parboiled cooked	½ cup	100	22	tr	2
medium-grain cooked	½ cup	132	29	tr	2
short-grain cooked	½ cup	133	29	tr	2
starch	3½ oz	343	85	0	1
Arrowhead					
Basmati	¼ cup (1.5 oz)	150	34	0	4
Casbah					
Basmati as prep	1 cup	158	36	tr	3
Minute					
Boil In Bag Long Grain as prep	½ cup	94	21	0	2
Long Grain as prep	⅔ cup	150	27	3	3
Rice as prep	⅔ cup	141	27	2	3
Rice Long Grain & Wild as prep	½ cup	149	25	4	3

FOOD	PORTION	CALS.	CARB.	FAT	PRO.
S&W					
Long Grain cooked	3.5 oz	106	23	0	2
Superfino					
Arborio Rice	½ cup	100	22	0	2
Uncle Ben					
Boil-In-Bag	1 serv (0.9 oz)	94	22	tr	2
Converted	1 serv (1.2 oz)	123	27	tr	3
In An Instant	1 serv (1.1 oz)	111	25	tr	2

RICE CAKES
(see also POPCORN CAKES)

FOOD	PORTION	CALS.	CARB.	FAT	PRO.
brown rice	1 (0.3 oz)	35	7	tr	1
brown rice & buckwheat	1 (0.3 oz)	34	7	tr	1
brown rice & buckwheat unsalted	1 (0.3 oz)	34	7	tr	1
brown rice & corn	1 (0.3 oz)	35	7	tr	1
brown rice & rye	1 (0.3 oz)	35	7	tr	1
brown rice & sesame seed	1 (0.3 oz)	35	7	tr	1
brown rice multigrain	1 (0.3 oz)	35	7	tr	1
brown rice multigrain unsalted	1 (0.3 oz)	35	7	tr	1
brown rice unsalted	1 (0.3 oz)	35	7	tr	1
Hain					
5-Grain	1	40	8	tr	tr
Mini Apple Cinnamon	½ oz	60	12	tr	1
Mini Barbeque	½ oz	70	10	3	1
Mini Cheese	½ oz	60	10	2	1
Mini Honey Nut	½ oz	60	11	tr	1
Mini Nacho Cheese	½ oz	70	10	2	1
Mini Plain	½ oz	60	12	tr	1
Mini Plain No Salt Added	½ oz	60	12	tr	1
Mini Ranch	½ oz	70	9	3	1
Mini Teriyaki	½ oz	50	12	tr	1
Plain	1	40	8	tr	tr
Plain No Salt Added	1	40	8	tr	tr
Sesame	1	40	8	tr	tr
Sesame No Salt	1	40	8	tr	tr
Ka-Me					
Cheese	16 pieces (1 oz)	120	24	2	3
Onion	16 pieces (1 oz)	120	25	1	3
Plain	16 pieces (1 oz)	120	25	2	3
Seaweed	16 pieces (1 oz)	120	25	2	3
Sesame	16 pieces (1 oz)	120	24	2	3
Unsalted	16 pieces (1 oz)	120	26	1	3

FOOD	PORTION	CALS.	CARB.	FAT	PRO.
Lundberg					
Organic Lightly Salted	1	60	14	1	1
Organic Unsalted	1	60	14	1	1
Premium Lightly Salted	1	60	14	1	1
Premium Unsalted	1	60	14	1	1
Sesame Lightly Salted	1	59	16	0	1
Mother's					
Mini Apple	5 (0.5 oz)	50	12	0	1
Mini Caramel	5 (0.5 oz)	50	12	0	1
Mini Cinnamon	5 (0.5 oz)	50	12	0	1
Mini Plain Unsalted	7 (0.5 oz)	60	12	0	1
Multigrain Lightly Salted	1 (0.3 oz)	35	7	0	1
Rye Unsalted	1 (0.3 oz)	35	7	0	1
Wheat Unsalted	1 (0.3 oz)	35	7	0	1
Quaker					
Apple Cinnamon	1 (0.5 oz)	50	11	0	1
Banana Crunch	1 (0.5 oz)	50	11	0	1
Cinnamon Crunch	1 (0.5 oz)	50	11	0	1
Mini Apple Cinnamon	5 (0.5 oz)	50	12	0	1
Mini Banana Nut	5 (0.5 oz)	50	12	0	1
Mini Butter Popped Corn	6 (0.5 oz)	50	12	0	1
Mini Caramel Corn	5 (0.5 oz)	50	12	0	1
Mini Chocolate Crunch	5 (0.5 oz)	50	12	0	1
Mini Cinnamon Crunch	5 (0.5 oz)	50	12	0	1
Mini Honey Nut	5 (0.5 oz)	50	12	0	1
Mini Monterey Jack	6 (0.5 oz)	50	11	0	1
Mini White Cheddar	6 (0.5 oz)	50	11	0	1
Salt-Free	1 (0.3 oz)	35	7	0	1
Salted	1 (0.3 oz)	35	7	0	1
Tree Of Life					
Fat Free Mini Apple Cinnamon	15	60	13	0	1
Fat Free Mini Caramel	15	60	13	0	1
Fat Free Mini Honey Nut	15	60	13	0	1
Fat Free Mini Jalapeno	15	60	13	0	1
Fat Free Mini Plain	15	50	12	0	1

ROCKFISH

FOOD	PORTION	CALS.	CARB.	FAT	PRO.
pacific cooked	1 fillet (5.2 oz)	180	0	3	36
pacific cooked	3 oz	103	0	2	20
pacific raw	3 oz	80	0	1	16

ROE
(see also individual fish names)

FOOD	PORTION	CALS.	CARB.	FAT	PRO.
fish	3.5 oz	39	tr	2	6

FOOD	PORTION	CALS.	CARB.	FAT	PRO.
fresh baked	1 oz	58	1	2	8
fresh baked	3 oz	173	2	7	24

ROLL

(*see also* BISCUIT, CROISSANT, ENGLISH MUFFIN, MUFFIN, POPOVER, SCONE)

FROZEN

Pepperidge Farm

Cinnamon Roll	1 (2¼ oz)	220	34	14	4

Sara Lee

All Butter Cinnamon Roll w/ Icing	1	280	43	11	3
All Butter Cinnamon Roll w/o Icing	1	230	31	11	3

Weight Watchers

Cinnamon Rolls	1 (2.1 oz)	180	31	5	4

HOME RECIPE

dinner as prep w/ 2% milk	1 (2½ in)	111	19	3	3
dinner as prep w/ whole milk	1 (2½ in)	112	19	3	3
raisin & nut	1 (2 oz)	196	30	7	4

MIX

Dromedary

Hot Roll Mix	2	239	41	5	6

Natural Ovens

German Hard	1 (2.1 oz)	138	36	1	5
Gourmet Dinner	1 (1 oz)	50	15	1	3
Hearty Sandwich	1 (1.8 oz)	110	30	1	5

Pillsbury

Hot Roll Mix	2	240	42	4	7

READY-TO-EAT

brown & serve	1 (1 oz)	85	14	2	2
cheese	1 (2.3 oz)	238	29	12	5
cinnamon raisin	1 (2¾ in)	223	31	10	4
dinner	1 (1 oz)	85	14	2	2
egg	1 (2½ in)	107	18	2	3
french	1 (1.3 oz)	105	19	2	3
hamburger	1 (1½ oz)	123	22	2	4
hamburger multi-grain	1 (1½ oz)	113	19	2	4
hamburger reduced calorie	1 (1½ oz)	84	18	1	4
hard	1 (3½ in)	167	30	2	6
hot cross bun	1	202	38	4	5
hotdog	1 (1½ oz)	123	22	2	4
hotdog multi-grain	1 (1½ oz)	113	19	2	4

FOOD	PORTION	CALS.	CARB.	FAT	PRO.
hotdog reduced calorie	1 (1½ oz)	84	18	1	4
kaiser	1 (3½ in)	167	30	2	6
oat bran	1 (1.2 oz)	78	13	2	3
rye	1 (1 oz)	81	15	1	3
submarine	1 (4.7 oz)	155	30	2	5
wheat	1 (1 oz)	77	13	2	2
whole wheat	1 (1 oz)	75	15	1	3
Alvarado St. Bakery					
Burger Buns	1 (2.2 oz)	140	27	2	7
Hot Dog Buns	1 (2.2 oz)	140	28	2	7
Arnold					
8-inch Francisco	1 (2.5 oz)	210	39	3	7
Augusto Pan Cubano	1	230	43	3	7
Bakery Light	1 (1.5 oz)	80	21	<2	4
Bran'nola Buns	1 (1.5 oz)	100	20	1	5
Deli Kaiser	1	170	34	2	5
Deli Onion	1	170	34	2	5
Dinner Plain	1 (0.7 oz)	50	9	1	2
Dinner Sesame	1 (0.7 oz)	50	9	1	2
Dutch Egg	1	130	21	3	4
French Francisco	1 (2.5 oz)	210	39	3	7
French Mini Francisco	1	130	24	2	4
Hamburger	1	120	20	2	4
Hot Dog	1 (1.5 oz)	110	21	2	4
Hot Dog Bran'nola	1 (1.5 oz)	110	18	2	4
Hot Dog New England Style	1	110	20	2	4
Italian 8-inch Savoni	1	210	38	3	8
Kaiser Francisco	1 (2 oz)	180	34	—	6
Onion Premium	1 (2.6 oz)	180	38	1	7
Onion Soft	1	140	28	—	5
Party Petite	2	70	10	2	2
Potato	1	140	25	2	5
Sandwich Soft Sesame	1	130	23	3	4
Sourdough Brown N' Serve	1 (1 oz)	100	19	1	3
Sourdough Francisco	1 (1 oz)	100	19	1	3
Wheat Old Fashioned	2	80	11	3	2
August Bros.					
Dinner	1	90	18	1	6
Kaiser	1	170	35	1	6
Onion	1	160	33	1	6
Sesame Cubano	1	170	35	1	6

FOOD	PORTION	CALS.	CARB.	FAT	PRO.
Bread Du Jour					
Bavarian Cracked Wheat	1 (1.2 oz)	90	17	1	3
Crusty Italian	1 (1.2 oz)	80	16	1	4
French Petite	1 (3.5 oz)	230	47	2	10
Rye	1 (1.2 oz)	90	16	2	3
Sourdough	1 (2.2 oz)	140	29	2	6
Dicarlo's					
Extra Sourdough	1 (1.6 oz)	100	20	1	3
French	1 (1 oz)	70	14	1	3
Home Pride					
Dinner Wheat	1 (1.9 oz)	160	26	4	5
Hamburger Potato Bun	1 (1.9 oz)	130	27	2	5
Hot Dog Potato Bun	1 (1.9 oz)	130	27	2	5
Sandwich Roll Wheat	1 (1.9 oz)	160	26	4	5
White	2 (1.6 oz)	130	22	4	4
Levy					
Sub Old Country	1	180	34	2	6
Martin's					
Big Marty Poppy	1	170	31	2	11
Big Marty Sesame	1	170	31	2	11
Hoagie	1	240	41	3	16
Hoagie Sesame	1	240	41	3	16
Potato Dinner	1	100	18	1	5
Potato Long	1	140	27	1	8
Potato Party	1	50	10	1	3
Potato Sandwich	1	140	26	1	8
Sandwich Whole Wheat 100% Stoneground	1	160	28	2	11
Matthew's					
Salad Roll	1	110	19	2	5
Sandwich	1	110	19	2	5
Pepperidge Farm					
Brown 'N Serve Club	1	100	19	1	3
Brown 'N Serve French	½ roll	180	36	2	6
Brown 'N Serve Hearth	1	50	10	1	2
Dinner	1	60	8	2	2
Dinner Country Style Classic	1	50	9	1	2
Finger Poppy Seed	1	50	8	2	2
Finger Sesame Seed	1	60	9	2	2
Frankfurter Dijon	1	160	23	5	5
Frankfurter Side Sliced	1	140	24	3	5
Frankfurter w/ Poppy Seeds	1	130	23	2	6

FOOD	PORTION	CALS.	CARB.	FAT	PRO.
Pepperidge Farm (CONT.)					
Frankfurter Top Sliced	1	140	24	3	5
French Style	1	100	20	1	4
Hamburger	1	130	22	2	5
Hamburger	1	130	22	2	5
Heat & Serve Butter Crescent	1	110	13	6	2
Heat & Serve Golden Twist	1	110	14	5	2
Hoagie Soft	1	210	34	5	8
Old Fashioned	1	50	7	2	2
Parker House	1	60	9	1	2
Party	1	30	5	1	1
Potato Sandwich	1	160	28	4	4
Sandwich Onion w/ Poppy Seeds	1	150	26	3	5
Sandwich Salad	1	110	16	4	4
Sandwich w/ Sesame Seeds	1	140	23	3	5
Soft Family	1	100	18	2	4
Sourdough French	1	100	19	1	4
Roman Meal					
Brown & Serve	2 (2 oz)	140	24	3	5
Dinner	2 (2 oz)	136	24	2	6
Hamburger	1 (1.6 oz)	111	19	2	5
Hotdog	1 (1.5 oz)	103	18	2	4
Sandwich	1 (2.7 oz)	181	31	3	7
Sandwich	1 (2.7 oz)	181	31	3	7
San Francisco					
Sourdough	1 (1.8 oz)	180	37	0	6
The Baker					
Honey Cinnamon Raisin	1 (2 oz)	150	31	2	4
Wonder					
Brown 'N Serve Wheat	1 (1 oz)	70	14	1	2
Brown 'N Serve White	1 (1 oz)	70	14	1	2
Brown N' Serve Buttermilk	1 (1 oz)	70	13	1	3
Dinner White Light	1 (1 oz)	60	9	1	3
Hamburger	1 (1.5 oz)	110	21	2	4
Hamburger Light	1 (1.5 oz)	80	13	2	5
Hamburger Wheat	1 (2.2 oz)	170	31	3	6
Hot Dog	1 (1.5 oz)	110	21	2	4
Hot Dog Light	1 (1.5 oz)	80	13	2	5
Tea Dinner Rolls	1 (1.5 oz)	80	19	1	4

FOOD	PORTION	CALS.	CARB.	FAT	PRO.
REFRIGERATED					
cinnamon w/ frosting	1	109	17	4	2
crescent	1 (1 oz)	98	14	4	2
Pillsbury					
Best Quick Cinamon Rolls w/ Icing	1	110	17	5	1
Butterflake	1	140	20	5	3
Crescent	1	100	11	6	2
ROMAN BEANS					
Progresso					
Roman Beans	½ cup	110	18	tr	7
ROSE HIP					
fresh	3½ oz	91	19	0	4
ROUGHY					
orange baked	3 oz	75	0	1	16
RUTABAGA					
CANNED					
Sunshine					
Diced	½ cup (4.2 oz)	30	7	0	tr
FRESH					
cooked mashed	½ cup	41	9	tr	1
raw cubed	½ cup	25	6	tr	1
SABLEFISH					
baked	3 oz	213	0	17	15
fillet baked	5.3 oz	378	0	30	26
smoked	1 oz	72	0	6	5
smoked	3 oz	218	0	17	15
SAFFLOWER					
seeds dried	1 oz	147	10	11	5
SALAD					
(*see also* LETTUCE, PASTA SALAD)					
MIX					
Dole					
Caesar Salad	⅓ pkg (3.5 oz)	170	9	14	3
Classic Blend	3.5 oz	25	4	1	1
Coleslaw Blend	3.5 oz	30	5	1	1
French Blend	3.5 oz	25	4	1	1
Italian Blend	3.5 oz	25	3	1	1
Salad-In-A-Minute Oriental	3.5 oz	110	12	7	2
Salad-In-A-Minute Spinach	3.5 oz	180	19	9	5

FOOD	PORTION	CALS.	CARB.	FAT	PRO.
Fresh Express					
American Salad	1½ cups (3 oz)	20	3	0	1
Caesar Salad	1½ cups (3 oz)	140	8	11	3
European Salad	1½ cups (3 oz)	20	3	0	1
Garden Salad	1½ cups (3 oz)	20	3	0	1
Italian Salad	1½ cups (3 oz)	20	3	0	1
Oriental Salad	1½ cups (3 oz)	120	11	8	3
Rivera Salad	1½ cups (3 oz)	10	2	0	1
Spinach Salad	1½ cups (3 oz)	130	23	3	3
Suddenly Salad					
Caesar as prep	½ cup	170	20	8	4
Ranch & Bacon as prep	½ cup	210	22	11	6
Ranch & Bacon as prep low fat recipe	½ cup	160	23	5	6
TAKE-OUT					
chef w/o dressing	1½ cups	386	9	28	24
tossed w/o dressing	¾ cup	16	3	0	1
tossed w/o dressing	1½ cups	32	7	tr	3
tossed w/o dressing w/ cheese & egg	1½ cups	102	5	6	9
tossed w/o dressing w/ chicken	1½ cups	105	4	2	17
tossed w/o dressing w/ pasta & seafood	1½ cups (14.6 oz)	380	32	21	16
tossed w/o dressing w/ shrimp	1½ cups	107	7	2	15
waldorf	½ cup	79	6	6	1
SALAD DRESSING					
HOME RECIPE					
french	1 tbsp	88	1	10	0
vinegar & oil	1 tbsp	72	tr	8	0
MIX					
Good Seasons					
Blue Cheese & Herbs as prep	1 tbsp	72	1	8	0
Buttermilk Farm as prep	1 tbsp	58	1	6	1
Cheese Garlic as prep	1 tbsp	72	1	8	0
Cheese Italian as prep	1 tbsp	72	1	8	0
Classic Dill	1 pkg	28	5	tr	1
Garlic & Herbs as prep	1 tbsp	71	1	8	0
Italian as prep	1 tbsp	71	1	8	0
Italian Lite as prep	1 tbsp	27	1	3	0
Italian No Oil as prep	1 tbsp	7	2	0	0

FOOD	PORTION	CALS.	CARB.	FAT	PRO.
Good Seasons (CONT.)					
Lemon & Herbs as prep	1 tbsp	71	1	8	0
Lite Cheese Italian as prep	1 tbsp	27	1	3	0
Lite Ranch as prep	1 tbsp	29	2	2	1
Lite Zesty Italian as prep	1 tbsp	26	1	3	0
Mild Italian as prep	1 tbsp	73	1	8	0
Ranch as prep	1 tbsp	57	1	6	1
Zesty Italian as prep	1 tbsp	71	1	8	0
Hain					
No Oil 1000 Island	1 tbsp	12	3	0	0
No Oil Bleu Cheese	1 tbsp	14	1	1	1
No Oil Buttermilk	1 tbsp	11	1	tr	1
No Oil Caesar	1 tbsp	6	1	tr	0
No Oil French	1 tbsp	12	3	0	0
No Oil Garlic & Cheese	1 tbsp	6	1	tr	tr
No Oil Herb	1 tbsp	2	1	0	0
No Oil Italian	1 tbsp	2	1	0	0
READY-TO-USE					
blue cheese	1 tbsp	77	1	8	1
french	1 tbsp	67	3	6	tr
french reduced calorie	1 tbsp	22	4	1	0
italian	1 tbsp	69	2	7	tr
italian reduced calorie	1 tbsp	16	1	2	tr
russian	1 tbsp	76	2	8	tr
russian reduced calorie	1 tbsp	23	5	1	tr
sesame seed	1 tbsp	68	1	7	1
thousand island	1 tbsp	59	2	6	tr
thousand island reduced calorie	1 tbsp	24	3	2	tr
Estee					
Blue Cheese	2 tbsp (1 oz)	15	1	1	tr
Creamy French	2 tbsp (1 oz)	10	2	0	0
Creamy French Fat Free	1 pkg (0.5 oz)	5	1	0	0
Creamy Garlic	2 tbsp (1 oz)	60	2	6	0
Creamy Garlic Fat Free	1 pkg (0.5 oz)	5	1	0	0
Creamy Italian	2 tbsp (1 oz)	15	2	1	0
Fat Free Thousand Island	1 pkg (0.5 oz)	5	1	0	0
Italian	2 tbsp (1 oz)	5	1	0	0
Italian Fat Free	1 pkg (0.5 oz)	0	tr	0	0
Low Fat Blue Cheese	1 pkg (0.5 oz)	5	tr	0	0
Thousand Island	2 tbsp (1 oz)	10	2	0	0
Hain					
1000 Island	1 tbsp	50	0	5	0

FOOD	PORTION	CALS.	CARB.	FAT	PRO.
Hain (CONT.)					
Canola Garden Tomato	1 tbsp	60	1	6	0
Canola Italian	1 tbsp	50	1	5	0
Canola Spicy French Mustard	1 tbsp	50	1	5	1
Canola Tangy Citrus	1 tbsp	50	1	5	0
Creamy Caesar	1 tbsp	60	1	6	0
Creamy Caesar Low Salt	1 tbsp	60	1	6	0
Creamy French	1 tbsp	60	1	6	0
Creamy Italian	1 tbsp	80	0	8	0
Creamy Italian No Salt Added	1 tbsp	80	1	8	0
Cucumber Dill	1 tbsp	80	0	8	0
Dijon Vinaigrette	1 tbsp	50	0	5	0
Garlic & Sour Cream	1 tbsp	70	0	7	0
Honey & Sesame	1 tbsp	60	2	5	0
Italian Cheese Vinaigrette	1 tbsp	55	0	6	0
Old Fashioned Buttermilk	1 tbsp	70	0	7	0
Poppyseed Rancher's	1 tbsp	60	0	7	0
Savory Herb No Salt Added	1 tbsp	90	0	10	0
Swiss Cheese Vinaigrette	1 tbsp	60	0	7	0
Traditional Italian	1 tbsp	80	0	8	0
Traditional Italian No Salt Added	1 tbsp	60	1	6	0
Healthy Sensation					
Blue Cheese	1 tbsp	19	4	1	tr
French	1 tbsp	21	4	1	0
Honey Dijon	1 tbsp	26	5	1	tr
Italian	1 tbsp	7	1	tr	tr
Ranch	1 tbsp	15	3	tr	tr
Thousand Island	1 tbsp	20	4	tr	0
Hollywood					
Caesar	1 tbsp	70	2	7	1
Creamy French	1 tbsp	70	2	7	0
Creamy Italian	1 tbsp	90	2	9	0
Dijon Vinaigrette	1 tbsp	60	2	6	0
Italian	1 tbsp	90	1	9	0
Italian Cheese	1 tbsp	80	2	8	0
Old Fashion Buttermilk	1 tbsp	75	1	8	0

FOOD	PORTION	CALS.	CARB.	FAT	PRO.
Hollywood (CONT.)					
Poppy Seed Rancher's	1 tbsp	75	1	8	0
Thousand Island	1 tbsp	60	3	6	0
Kraft					
Bacon & Tomato	2 tbsp (1.1 oz)	140	2	14	tr
Buttermilk Ranch	2 tbsp (1 oz)	150	2	16	0
Caesar	2 tbsp (1.1 oz)	130	2	13	tr
Caesar Ranch	2 tbsp (1 oz)	140	1	15	tr
Catalina With Honey	2 tbsp (1.2 oz)	140	8	12	0
Catalina French	2 tbsp (1.2 oz)	140	8	11	0
Chunky Blue Cheese	2 tbsp (1.2 oz)	90	5	7	1
Coleslaw	2 tbsp (1.2 oz)	150	8	12	0
Creamy Caesar	2 tbsp (1 oz)	140	1	15	tr
Creamy Garlic	2 tbsp (1.1 oz)	110	2	11	0
Creamy Italian	2 tbsp (1.1 oz)	110	3	11	0
Cucumber Ranch	2 tbsp (1.1 oz)	150	2	15	0
Deliciously Right Bacon & Tomato	2 tbsp (1.1 oz)	60	3	5	tr
Deliciously Right Caesar	2 tbsp (1.1 oz)	50	2	5	tr
Deliciously Right Catalina French	2 tbsp (1.2 oz)	80	9	4	0
Deliciously Right Creamy Italian	2 tbsp (1.1 oz)	50	3	5	0
Deliciously Right Cucumber Ranch	2 tbsp (1.1 oz)	60	2	5	0
Deliciously Right French	2 tbsp (1.2 oz)	50	6	3	0
Deliciously Right Italian	2 tbsp (1.1 oz)	70	3	7	0
Deliciously Right Ranch	2 tbsp (1.1 oz)	110	2	11	0
Deliciously Right Thousand Island	2 tbsp (1.2 oz)	70	8	4	0
Free Blue Cheese	2 tbsp (1.2 oz)	50	12	0	tr
Free Catalina	2 tbsp (1.2 oz)	45	11	0	0
Free French	2 tbsp (1.2 oz)	50	12	0	0
Free Honey Dijon	2 tbsp (1.2 oz)	50	11	0	tr
Free Italian	2 tbsp (1.1 oz)	10	2	0	0
Free Peppercorn Ranch	2 tbsp (1.2 oz)	50	11	0	tr
Free Ranch	1 tbsp (1.2 oz)	50	11	0	tr
Free Red Wine Vinegar	2 tbsp (1.1 oz)	15	3	0	0
Free Thousand Island	2 tbsp (1.2 oz)	45	11	0	0
French	2 tbsp (1.1 oz)	120	4	12	0
Honey Dijon	2 tbsp (1.1 oz)	150	4	15	0
House Italian	2 tbsp (1.1 oz)	120	3	12	0
Oil-Free Italian	2 tbsp (1.1 oz)	5	2	0	0

FOOD	PORTION	CALS.	CARB.	FAT	PRO.
Kraft (CONT.)					
Peppercorn Ranch	2 tbsp (1 oz)	170	1	18	tr
Pesto Italian	2 tbsp (1.1 oz)	140	2	15	0
Ranch	2 tbsp (1 oz)	170	2	18	0
Roka Blue Cheese	2 tbsp (1.2 oz)	90	5	7	1
Russian	2 tbsp (1.2 oz)	130	10	10	0
Salsa Ranch	2 tbsp (1 oz)	130	1	13	0
Salsa Zesty Garden	2 tbsp (1.1 oz)	70	3	6	0
Sour Cream & Onion Ranch	2 tbsp (1 oz)	170	1	18	0
Thousand Island	2 tbsp (1.1 oz)	110	5	10	0
Thousand Island With Bacon	2 tbsp (1 oz)	120	5	12	0
Zesty Italian	2 tbsp (1.1 oz)	110	2	11	0
Marzetti					
Bacon Spinach Salad	2 tbsp	80	16	15	0
Blue Cheese	2 tbsp	160	0	17	1
Buttermilk Parmesan Pepper	2 tbsp	170	1	18	0
Buttermilk Parmesan Ranch	2 tbsp	160	1	17	0
Buttermilk Veggie Dip	2 tbsp	170	1	18	0
Buttermilk & Herb	2 tbsp	180	1	20	0
Buttermilk Bacon Ranch	2 tbsp	180	1	19	0
Buttermilk Blue Cheese	2 tbsp	160	1	18	1
Buttermilk Ranch	2 tbsp	180	1	20	0
Caesar	2 tbsp	150	1	16	0
Caesar Ranch	2 tbsp	190	2	20	0
California French	2 tbsp	160	11	13	0
Celery Seed	2 tbsp	160	10	13	0
Chunky Blue Cheese	2 tbsp	150	1	16	1
Classic Caesar Ranch	2 tbsp	190	2	20	0
Country French	2 tbsp	150	7	13	0
Cracked Peppercorn	2 tbsp	140	1	14	1
Creamy Garlic Italian	2 tbsp	160	1	17	0
Creamy Italian	2 tbsp	150	1	16	0
Crispy Celery Seed	2 tbsp	160	11	13	0
Dijon Honey Mustard	2 tbsp	140	6	13	0
Dijon Ranch	2 tbsp	170	2	18	0
Dutch Sweet'N Sour	2 tbsp	160	10	13	0
Fat Free California French	2 tbsp	45	11	0	0
Fat Free Honey Dijon	2 tbsp	60	14	0	0
Fat Free Honey French	2 tbsp	45	11	0	0

FOOD	PORTION	CALS.	CARB.	FAT	PRO.
Marzetti (CONT.)					
Fat Free Italian	2 tbsp	15	3	0	0
Fat Free Peppercorn Ranch	2 tbsp	30	7	0	0
Fat Free Ranch	2 tbsp	30	7	0	0
Fat Free Raspberry	2 tbsp	70	18	0	0
Fat Free Slaw	2 tbsp	45	11	0	0
Fat Free Sweet & Sour	2 tbsp	45	14	0	0
Fat Free Thousand Island	2 tbsp	35	9	0	0
Garden Ranch	2 tbsp	180	1	19	0
Gusto Italian	2 tbsp	120	1	13	0
Honey Dijon	2 tbsp	140	6	13	0
Honey Dijon Ranch	2 tbsp	150	2	15	0
Honey French	2 tbsp	160	11	14	0
Honey French Blue Cheese	2 tbsp	160	11	13	1
House Caesar	2 tbsp	150	1	16	0
Italian With Olive Oil	2 tbsp	120	1	13	0
Light Blue Cheese	2 tbsp	60	4	6	2
Light Buttermilk Ranch	2 tbsp	90	3	9	0
Light California French	2 tbsp	80	8	6	0
Light Chunky Blue Cheese	2 tbsp	80	4	7	1
Light French	2 tbsp	40	6	2	0
Light French	2 tbsp	40	6	2	0
Light Honey French	2 tbsp	80	12	4	1
Light Italian	2 tbsp	60	3	5	0
Light Ranch	2 tbsp	90	7	8	0
Light Red Wine Vinegar & Oil	2 tbsp	20	3	1	0
Light Slaw	2 tbsp	60	10	7	0
Light Sweet & Sour	2 tbsp	100	11	6	0
Light Thousand Island	2 tbsp	70	6	5	0
Old Fashioned Poppyseed	2 tbsp	140	10	11	0
Olde Venice Italain	2 tbsp	130	2	13	0
Olde World Caesar	2 tbsp	150	1	16	0
Parmesan Pepper	2 tbsp	160	1	17	0
Peppercorn Ranch	2 tbsp	180	1	19	0
Poppyseed	2 tbsp	160	10	13	0
Potato Salad Dressing	2 tbsp	120	7	13	0
Ranch	2 tbsp	180	1	20	0
Red Wine Vinegar & Oil	2 tbsp	130	2	14	0
Romano Cheese Caesar	2 tbsp	150	1	16	0

FOOD	PORTION	CALS.	CARB.	FAT	PRO.
Marzetti (CONT.)					
Romano Italian	2 tbsp	160	1	17	0
Savory Italian	2 tbsp	110	3	12	0
Slaw	2 tbsp	170	6	16	0
Southern Slaw	2 tbsp	100	14	11	0
Sweet & Saucy	2 tbsp	140	9	12	0
Sweet & Sour	2 tbsp	160	10	13	0
Thousand Island	2 tbsp	150	5	15	0
Vintage Champagne	2 tbsp	150	2	16	0
Wilde Raspberry	2 tbsp	150	12	12	0
Newman's Own					
Italian Light	1 tbsp (0.5 fl oz)	10	tr	tr	tr
Olive Oil & Vinegar	1 tbsp (0.5 fl oz)	80	tr	9	tr
Ranch	1 tbsp (0.5 fl oz)	90	1	9	tr
Pfeiffer					
1000 Island	2 tbsp	140	4	14	0
California French	2 tbsp	140	9	12	0
French	2 tbsp	150	7	13	0
Honey Dijon	2 tbsp	140	6	13	0
Lite Italian	2 tbsp	50	3	5	0
Ranch	2 tbsp	180	1	20	0
Savory Italian	2 tbsp	110	3	12	0
Red Wing					
"K" Dressing	1 tbsp (0.5 oz)	70	4	7	0
Chunky Blue Cheese	2 tbsp (1 oz)	130	3	13	0
Creamy Ranch	2 tbsp (1 oz)	150	2	15	0
French Traditional	2 tbsp (1 oz)	130	8	11	0
Italian Traditional	2 tbsp (1 oz)	100	4	9	0
Spicy Sweet French	2 tbsp (1 oz)	130	8	11	0
Thousand Island Thick & Rich	2 tbsp (1 oz)	110	8	9	0
S&W					
Blue Cheese Low Calorie	1 tbsp	25	2	2	0
Creamy Cucumber Low Calorie	1 tbsp	25	2	2	0
Creamy Italian Low Calorie	1 tbsp	10	1	1	0
French Low Calorie	1 tbsp	18	3	0	0
Italian No-Oil	1 tbsp	2	0	0	0
Russian Low Calorie	1 tbsp	25	4	1	0
Thousand Island Low Calorie	1 tbsp	25	2	2	0
Seven Seas					
Creamy Italian	2 tbsp (1.1 oz)	110	2	12	0

FOOD	PORTION	CALS.	CARB.	FAT	PRO.
Seven Seas (CONT.)					
Free Italian	2 tbsp (1.1 oz)	10	2	0	0
Free Ranch	2 tbsp (1.2 oz)	50	12	0	tr
Free Red Wine Vinegar	2 tbsp (1.1 oz)	15	3	0	0
Green Goddess	2 tbsp (1 oz)	120	1	13	0
Herbs & Spices	2 tbsp (1.1 oz)	120	1	12	0
Ranch	2 tbsp (1 oz)	150	2	16	0
Red Wine Vinegar & Oil	2 tbsp (1.1 oz)	110	2	11	0
Reduced Calorie Creamy Italian	2 tbsp (1.1 oz)	60	2	5	0
Reduced Calorie Italian With Olive Oil	2 tbsp (1.1 oz)	50	2	5	0
Reduced Calorie Ranch	2 tbsp (1.1 oz)	100	5	9	0
Reduced Calorie Red Wine Vinegar & Oil	2 tbsp (1.1 oz)	60	2	5	0
Two Cheese Italian	2 tbsp (1.1 oz)	70	3	7	0
Viva Buttermilk	2 tbsp (1.1)	150	3	16	0
Viva Caesar	2 tbsp (1.1 oz)	120	2	12	tr
Viva Italian	2 tbsp (1.1 oz)	110	2	11	0
Viva Reduced Calorie Italian	2 tbsp (1.1 oz)	45	2	4	0
Tree Of Life					
Cafe Venice	2 tbsp (1 oz)	100	2	12	0
Fat Free Blue Cheese	2 tbsp (1 oz)	15	2	1	0
Fat Free Honey French	2 tbsp (1 oz)	35	8	0	0
Fat Free Italian Garlic	2 tbsp (1 oz)	20	4	0	0
Fat Free Oriental Ginger	2 tbsp (1 oz)	15	3	0	0
Frisco's Raspberry	2 tbsp (1 oz)	120	5	11	0
Maison Caesar	2 tbsp (1 oz)	70	1	6	2
Shanghai Palace	2 tbsp (1 oz)	80	3	7	1
Ultra Slim-Fast					
French	1 tbsp	20	4	tr	0
Italian	1 tbsp	6	1	tr	0
W.J. Clark					
Ginger Orange Vinaigrette	1 tbsp	73	tr	7	0
Herbs & Romano	1 tbsp	67	2	6	0
Lemon Peppercorn	1 tbsp	72	tr	7	0
Lime Cilantro Vinaigrette	1 tbsp	73	tr	8	0
Poppy Seed	1 tbsp	75	3	6	0
Sweet Pepper Basil	1 tbsp	69	2	7	0
Tarragon Honey Mustard	1 tbsp	66	2	6	0
Walden Farms					
Bleu Cheese Fat Free	2 tbsp (1 oz)	25	4	0	0
Creamy Italian With Parmesan Fat Free	1 tbsp (1 oz)	25	4	0	1

FOOD	PORTION	CALS.	CARB.	FAT	PRO.
Walden Farms (CONT.)					
Fat Free Balsamic Vinaigrette	2 tbsp (1 oz)	15	3	0	0
Fat Free Caesar	2 tbsp (1 oz)	25	4	0	1
Fat Free Italian	2 tbsp (1 oz)	10	2	0	0
Fat Free Raspberry Vinaigrette	2 tbsp (1 oz)	20	4	0	0
Fat Free Russian	2 tbsp (1 oz)	30	6	0	0
French Style Fat Free	2 tbsp (1 oz)	25	4	0	1
Honey Dijon Fat Free	2 tbsp (1 oz)	25	6	0	0
Italian Sodium Free Fat Free	2 tbsp (1 oz)	10	2	0	0
Italian Sugar Free Fat Free	2 tbsp (1 oz)	0	0	0	0
Italian With Sun Dried Tomato	2 tbsp (1 oz)	15	3	0	0
Ranch Fat Free	2 tbsp (1 oz)	25	4	0	1
Ranch With Sun Dried Tomato	2 tbsp (1 oz)	25	4	0	1
Thousand Island Fat Free	2 tbsp (1 oz)	35	7	0	0
Weight Watchers					
Caesar	1 tbsp	4	1	0	0
Caesar	1 pkg (¾ oz)	6	1	0	0
Cucumber Creamy	1 tbsp	18	4	0	tr
Italian	1 pkg (¾ oz)	8	2	tr	tr
Italian	1 tbsp	6	1	tr	tr
Italian Creamy	1 tbsp	12	3	0	0
Ranch Creamy	1 pkg (¾ oz)	35	8	tr	tr
Ranch Creamy	1 tbsp	25	6	tr	tr
Russian	1 tbsp	50	2	5	0
Thousand Island	1 tbsp	50	2	5	0
Wishbone					
Blue Cheese Chunky Lite	1 tbsp	40	2	4	tr
Blue Cheese Chunky	1 tbsp	73	1	8	tr
Classic Olive Oil Italian	1 tbsp	33	2	3	0
Classic Lite Dijon Vinaigrette	1 tbsp	30	1	3	tr
Classic Lite Olive Oil Italian	1 tbsp	20	1	2	tr
Creamy Italian	1 tbsp	54	1	6	tr
Deluxe French	1 tbsp	57	2	5	tr
Dijon Vinaigrette Classic	1 tbsp	57	1	6	tr
French Fat Free	1 tbsp	6	1	tr	0
French Lite	1 tbsp	30	4	tr	tr
French Sweet 'N Spicy Lite	1 tbsp	17	4	tr	0

FOOD	PORTION	CALS.	CARB.	FAT	PRO.
Wishbone (CONT.)					
French Red	1 tbsp	64	4	6	tr
French Sweet 'N Spicy	1 tbsp	613	3	6	tr
Italian	1 tbsp	45	1	5	0
Italian Lite	1 tbsp	6	1	tr	0
Italian Cream Lite	1 tbsp	26	2	2	tr
Lite Caesar With Olive Oil	1 tbsp	28	1	3	tr
Lite French Red	1 tbsp	17	3	tr	tr
Lite Olive Oil Vinaigrette	1 tbsp	16	2	1	0
Lite Red Wine Vinaigrette Olive Oil	1 tbsp	20	1	2	tr
Olive Oil Vinaigrette	1 tbsp	30	2	3	0
Ranch	1 tbsp	76	1	8	tr
Ranch Lite	1 tbsp	42	3	4	tr
Red Wine Olive Oil Vinaigrette	1 tbsp.	34	2	3	0
Robusto Italian	1 tbsp	46	2	5	tr
Russian	1 tbsp	54	7	3	tr
Russian Lite	1 tbsp	21	5	tr	tr
Thousand Island	1 tbsp	66	3	6	tr
Thousand Island Lite	1 tbsp	22	5	1	tr

SALMON
CANNED

FOOD	PORTION	CALS.	CARB.	FAT	PRO.
chum w/ bone	1 can (13.9 oz)	521	0	20	79
chum w/ bone	3 oz	120	0	5	18
pink w/ bone	3 oz	118	0	5	17
pink w/ bone	1 can (15.9 oz)	631	0	27	90
sockeye w/ bone	1 can (12.9 oz)	566	0	27	76
sockeye w/ bone	3 oz	130	0	6	17
Bumble Bee					
Keta	3.5 oz	160	0	8	20
Pink	3.5 oz	160	0	8	20
Pink Skinless & Boneless	3.25 oz	120	0	5	17
Red	3.5 oz	180	0	10	20
Red Skinless & Boneless	3.25 oz	130	0	6	17
Deming's					
Alaska Keta	½ cup	140	0	5	22
Alaska Pink	½ cup	140	0	6	20
Alaska Red Sockeye	½ cup	170	0	9	20
Double Q					
Alaska Pink	½ cup	140	0	6	20

FOOD	PORTION	CALS.	CARB.	FAT	PRO.
Humpty Dumpty					
Alaska Chum	½ cup	140	0	2	22
S&W					
Bluepack Fancy Diet	½ cup	188	0	11	22
Red Fancy Sockeye Bluepack	½ cup	190	0	10	25
FRESH					
atlantic baked	3 oz	155	0	7	22
chinook baked	3 oz	196	0	11	22
chum baked	3 oz	131	0	4	22
coho cooked	3 oz	157	0	6	23
coho cooked	½ fillet (5.4 oz)	286	0	12	42
coho raw	3 oz	124	0	5	18
pink baked	3 oz	127	0	4	22
roe raw	3.5 oz	207	1	10	25
sockeye cooked	3 oz	183	0	9	23
sockeye cooked	½ fillet (5.4 oz)	334	0	17	42
sockeye raw	3 oz	143	0	7	18
SMOKED					
chinook	1 oz	33	0	1	5
chinook	3 oz	99	0	4	16
TAKE-OUT					
salmon cake	1 (3 oz)	241	6	15	18

SALSA

(*see also* KETCHUP, MEXICAN FOOD, SAUCE)

FOOD	PORTION	CALS.	CARB.	FAT	PRO.
Casa Fiesta					
Chili Salsa	1 oz	9	2	tr	tr
Chi-Chi's					
Hot	2 tbsp (1 oz)	10	1	0	0
Medium	1 tbsp (1 oz)	10	1	0	0
Mild	2 tbsp (1 oz)	10	1	0	0
Verde Medium	2 tbsp (1.2 oz)	15	3	0	0
Verde Mild	2 tbsp (1.2 oz)	15	3	0	0
Del Monte					
Mexicana	2 tbsp (1.1 oz)	5	2	0	0
Taquera	2 tbsp (1.1 oz)	5	2	0	0
Verde	2 tbsp (1.1 oz)	10	2	0	0
Frito Lay					
Hot	1 oz	12	2	0	0
Medium	1 oz	12	2	0	0
Mild	1 oz	12	2	0	0
Hain					
Hot	¼ cup	22	4	0	1

FOOD	PORTION	CALS.	CARB.	FAT	PRO.
Hain (CONT.)					
Mild	¼ cup	20	4	0	1
Heluva Good Cheese					
Cheese & Salsa	2 tbsp (1.1 oz)	80	3	6	3
Thick & Chunky Hot	2 tbsp (1.2 oz)	10	2	0	0
Thick & Chunky Mild	2 tbsp (1.2 oz)	10	2	0	0
Hot Cha Cha					
Medium	2 tbsp (1 oz)	5	2	0	0
Louise's					
Fat Free BBQ Black Bean	1 oz	10	2	0	0
Fat Free Black Bean	1 oz	10	2	0	0
Fat Free Medium	1 oz	10	3	0	0
Fat Free Mild	1 oz	10	3	0	0
Fat Free Nacho Queso	1 oz	15	3	0	1
Muir Glen					
Organic Fat Free Hot	2 tbsp (1.1 oz)	10	2	0	tr
Organic Fat Free Medium	2 tbsp (1.1 oz)	10	2	0	tr
Organic Fat Free Mild	2 tbsp (1.1 oz)	10	2	0	tr
Newman's Own					
Bandito Hot	1 tbsp (0.7 oz)	6	tr	tr	tr
Bandito Medium	1 tbsp (0.7 oz)	6	tr	tr	tr
Bandito Mild	1 tbsp (0.7 oz)	6	tr	tr	tr
Old El Paso					
Homestyle Chunky Mild	2 tbsp	5	1	0	0
Medium	2 tbsp	5	1	0	0
Picante Salsa Hot	2 tbsp	10	2	tr	tr
Picante Salsa Medium	2 tbsp	10	2	tr	tr
Picante Salsa Mild	2 tbsp	10	2	tr	tr
Thick'n Chunky Green Chili	2 tbsp	3	1	0	0
Thick'n Chunky Hot	2 tbsp	10	2	0	0
Thick'n Chunky Medium	2 tbsp	10	2	0	0
Thick'n Chunky Mild	2 tbsp	10	2	0	0
Thick'n Chunky Salsa Verde	2 tbsp	10	2	tr	0
Ortega					
Hot Green Chili	1 tbsp	6	2	0	0
Medium Green Chili	1 tbsp	6	1	0	0
Mild Green Chili	1 tbsp	8	2	0	0
Pace					
Thick & Chunky	2 tbsp (1 fl oz)	12	2	0	tr
Roserita					
Chunky Hot	3 tbsp (1.5 oz)	25	6	tr	1
Chunky Medium	3 tbsp (1.5 oz)	25	6	tr	1

FOOD	PORTION	CALS.	CARB.	FAT	PRO.
Roserita (CONT.)					
Chunky Mild	3 tbsp (1.5 oz)	25	6	tr	1
Taco Salsa Chunky Medium	3 tbsp (1.5 oz)	25	6	tr	1
Taco Salsa Chunky Mild	3 tbsp (1.5 oz)	25	6	tr	1
Tree Of Life					
Hot	2 tbsp (1 oz)	10	2	0	0
Medium	2 tbsp (1 oz)	10	2	0	0
Mild	2 tbsp (1 oz)	10	2	0	0
No Salt	2 tbsp (1 oz)	10	2	0	0
Watkins					
Salsa Seasoning Blend	1/8 tsp (0.5 g)	0	0	0	0
Tropical	2 tbsp (1 oz)	60	13	0	0

SALT SUBSTITUTES
Papa Dash

Lite Lite Lite Salt	1/4 tsp (0.5 g)	1	tr	0	0
Salt Lover's Blend	1/4 tsp (0.7 g)	tr	tr	0	0

SALT/SEASONED SALT
(*see also* SALT SUBSTITUTES)

salt	1 tbsp (18 g)	0	0	0	0
salt	1 tsp (6 g)	0	0	0	0
Hain					
Sea Salt	1 tsp	0	0	0	0
Sea Salt Iodized	1 tsp	0	0	0	0
Watkins					
Bacon Cheese Salt	1/4 tbsp (1 g)	0	0	0	0
Butter Salt	1/4 tbsp (1 g)	0	0	0	0
Cheese Salt	1/4 tbsp (1 g)	0	0	0	0
Garlic Salt	1/4 tsp (1 g)	0	0	0	0
Salt & Vinegar Seasoning	1/4 tsp (1 g)	0	0	0	0
Seasoning Salt	1/4 tsp (1 g)	0	0	0	0
Sour Cream & Onion Salt	1/4 tbsp (1 g)	0	0	0	0

SAPODILLA

fresh	1	140	34	2	1
fresh cut up	1 cup	199	48	3	1

SAPOTES

fresh	1	301	76	1	5

SARDINES
CANNED

atlantic in oil w/ bone	2	50	0	3	6

FOOD	PORTION	CALS.	CARB.	FAT	PRO.
atlantic in oil w/ bone	1 can (3.2 oz)	192	0	11	23
pacific in tomato sauce w/ bone	1 can (13 oz)	658	0	44	61
pacific in tomato sauce w/ bone	1	68	0	5	6
Del Monte					
In Tomato Sauce	1 fish (1.4 oz)	50	1	3	5
Empress					
Skinless & Boneless Olive Oil	1 can (3.8 oz)	420	2	38	18
Skinless & Boneless Soy Oil	1 can (4.4 oz)	500	2	45	22
Port Clyde					
In Louisiana Hot Sauce	1 can (3.75 oz)	170	1	9	19
In Mustard Sauce	1 can (3.75 oz)	150	1	9	18
In Soybean Oil Select Small	1 can (3.3 oz)	220	0	17	19
In Soybean Oil With Hot Chilies	1 can (3.3 oz)	155	0	9	21
In Soybean Oil drained	1 can (3.3 oz)	220	0	17	19
In Spring Water	1 can (3.3 oz)	170	0	10	18
In Tomato Sauce	1 can (3.75 oz)	150	0	9	17
S&W					
Norwegian Brisling	1.5 oz	130	0	10	10
Underwood					
Brisling In Olive Oil	3.75 oz	260	1	20	19
In Mustard Sauce	3.75 oz	220	2	16	16
In Sild Oil drained	3.75 oz	460	1	42	19
In Soya Oil drained	3 oz	230	1	18	16
In Tomato Sauce	3.75 oz	220	2	16	16
With Tabasco Pepper Sauce drained	3 oz	220	1	16	16
Viking's Delight					
Brisling In Olive Oil	1 can (3.75 oz)	460	1	42	19
Brisling In Olive Oil drained	1 can (3.75 oz)	260	1	20	19
FRESH					
raw	3½ oz	135	0	5	19

SAUCE

(*see also* BARBECUE SAUCE, GRAVY, PIZZA, SALSA, SPAGHETTI SAUCE, TOMATO)

FOOD	PORTION	CALS.	CARB.	FAT	PRO.
DRY					
bearnaise as prep w/ milk & butter	1 cup	701	18	68	8
cheese as prep w/ milk	1 cup	307	23	17	16
curry as prep w/ milk	1 cup	270	26	15	11
mushroom as prep w/ milk	1 cup	228	24	10	11
sourcream as prep w/ milk	1 cup	509	45	30	19
stroganoff as prep	1 cup	271	34	11	12
sweet & sour as prep	1 cup	294	73	tr	1
teriyaki as prep	1 cup	131	28	1	4
white as prep w/ milk	1 cup	241	21	13	10
Cajun King					
Etoufee Seasoning Mix	3.5 oz	383	70	6	12
Jambalaya Seasoning Mix	3.5 oz	375	61	9	12
Knorr					
Au Jus as prep	2 oz	8	1	tr	tr
Bearnaise as prep	2 oz	170	5	17	2
Classic Brown Gravy as prep	2 oz	25	3	1	tr
Demi-Glace as prep	2 oz	30	4	1	tr
Hollandaise as prep	2 oz	170	5	18	2
Hunter as prep	2 oz	25	4	tr	tr
Lyonnaise as prep	2 oz	20	3	tr	tr
Mushroom as prep	2 oz	60	5	3	3
Napoli as prep	4 oz	100	17	3	3
Pepper as prep	2 oz	20	3	1	tr
JARRED					
teriyaki	1 oz	30	6	0	2
teriyaki	1 tbsp	15	3	0	1
Armour					
Chili Hot Dog	¼ cup (2.2 oz)	120	6	9	4
Meatless Sloppy Joe Sauce	¼ cup (2.2 oz)	30	7	0	0
Best Foods					
Tartar	1 tbsp (14 g)	70	tr	8	tr
Casa Fiesta					
Taco Mild	1 oz	9	2	tr	tr
Chi-Chi's					
Taco Thick & Chunky	1 tbsp (0.5 oz)	10	1	0	0
Contadina					
Sweet 'n Sour	2 tbsp	40	8	1	0
Del Monte					
Cocktail	¼ cup (2.7 oz)	100	24	0	1

FOOD	PORTION	CALS.	CARB.	FAT	PRO.
Del Monte (CONT.)					
Sloppy Joe Hickory Flavor	¼ cup (2.4 oz)	70	18	0	1
Sloppy Joe Italian Style	¼ cup (2.4 oz)	70	16	0	1
Sloppy Joe Original	¼ cup (2.4 oz)	70	16	0	1
El Molino					
Taco Red Mild	2 tbsp	10	2	0	0
Escoffier					
Diable	1 tbsp	20	4	0	0
Gebhardt					
Enchilada Sauce	3 tbsp (1.5 oz)	25	2	1	tr
Hot Dog Chili Sauce	2 tbsp	30	4	1	1
Hot Sauce	½ tsp	tr	tr	tr	tr
Gold's					
Rib	1 oz	60	14	0	0
Golden Dipt					
Cajun Style	1 oz	90	5	8	0
Creole	1 oz	20	2	1	0
Dijonaisse	1 oz	52	2	4	0
French White	1 oz	55	3	4	0
Ginger Teriyaki Marinade	1 oz	120	12	7	1
Lemon Butter Dill	1 oz	100	4	9	0
Lemon Herb Marinade	1 oz	130	2	14	0
Seafood Cocktail	1 tbsp	20	5	0	0
Seafood Cocktail Extra Hot	1 tbsp	20	5	0	0
Tartar	1 tbsp	70	2	7	0
Tartar Lite	1 tbsp	50	4	4	0
Guiltless Gourmet					
Picante Hot	1 oz	6	1	0	0
Picante Medium	1 oz	6	1	0	0
Heinz					
Worcestershire	1 tbsp	6	1	0	0
Hellman's					
Tartar	1 tbsp (14 g)	70	tr	8	tr
Heluva Good Cheese					
Cocktail	¼ cup (1.6 oz)	40	10	0	0
Hormel					
Not-So-Sloppy-Joe Sauce	¼ cup (2.2 oz)	70	15	0	1
House Of Tsang					
Bangkok Padang	1 tbsp (0.6 oz)	45	4	3	1
Hoisin	1 tsp (6 g)	15	3	0	0
Mandarin Marinade	1 tbsp (0.6 oz)	25	6	0	0

FOOD	PORTION	CALS.	CARB.	FAT	PRO.
House Of Tsang (cont.)					
Saigon Sizzle	1 tbsp (0.6 oz)	40	8	1	0
Spicy Brown Bean	1 tsp (6 g)	15	3	0	0
Stir Fry Sweet & Sour	1 tbsp (0.6 oz)	35	8	0	0
Stir Fry Szechuan Spicy	1 tbsp (0.6 oz)	20	4	1	0
Stir Fry Classic	1 tbsp (0.6 oz)	25	4	1	0
Sweet & Sour Concentrate	1 tsp (6 g)	10	3	0	0
Teriyaki Korean	1 tbsp (0.6 oz)	30	6	1	0
Just Rite					
Hot Dog	2 oz	60	6	3	2
Ka-Me					
Black Bean Sauce	1 tbsp (0.5 oz)	10	2	0	1
Chili Sauce Hot Garlic	1 tbsp (0.5 oz)	15	4	0	0
Duck Sauce	2 tbsp (1 oz)	80	20	0	0
Fish Sauce	1 tbsp (0.5 fl oz)	10	1	0	1
Hoisin Sauce	2 tbsp (1 oz)	45	10	0	1
Hot Sauce	1 tsp (5 g)	0	1	0	0
Lemon Sauce	1 tbsp (0.5 oz)	45	11	0	0
Mandarin Orange Sauce	2 tbsp (1 oz)	80	21	0	0
Oyster Sauce	1 tbsp (0.5 fl oz)	10	3	0	0
Plum	2 tbsp (1 fl oz)	80	19	0	0
Stir Fry Sauce	1 tbsp	10	1	0	1
Sweet & Sour	2 tbsp (1 fl oz)	50	13	0	0
Szechuan	1 tbsp (0.5 oz)	20	2	1	1
Tamari	1 tbsp (0.5 fl oz)	10	1	1	2
Tempura Sauce	2 tbsp (1 fl oz)	15	3	0	1
Teriyaki Sauce	1 tbsp (0.5 fl oz)	10	2	0	0
Kikkoman					
Stir-Fry	1 tbsp	16	3	tr	1
Sweet & Sour	1 tbsp	19	4	tr	tr
Teriyaki	1 tbsp	15	3	0	1
Knorr					
Grilling And Broiling Chardonnay	1.6 oz	50	4	4	tr
Grilling And Broiling Tequilla Lime	1.6 oz	50	6	3	1
Grilling And Broiling Spicy Plum	1.7 oz	60	11	2	tr
Grilling And Broiling Tuscan Herb	1.6 oz	50	5	4	tr
Microwave Hollandaise	1 oz	50	1	5	tr
Microwave Mandarin Ginger	1.6 oz	50	5	4	tr

FOOD	PORTION	CALS.	CARB.	FAT	PRO.
Knorr (CONT.)					
Microwave Parmesano	1.6 oz	50	3	4	1
Microwave Vera Cruz	3.3 oz	70	9	3	1
Kraft					
Sandwich Spread & Burger Sauce	1 tbsp (0.5 oz)	50	3	5	0
Sweet'n Sour	2 tbsp (1.3 oz)	80	19	1	0
Tartar Sauce Nonfat	2 tbsp (1.1 oz)	25	5	0	0
La Choy					
Duck Sauce Sweet & Sour	1 tbsp	25	7	tr	tr
Sweet & Sour	1 tbsp	25	7	tr	tr
Lawry's					
Marinade Lemon Pepper	1 tbsp (0.5 oz)	10	1	1	0
Teriyaki Marinade	2 tbsp	72	11	tr	6
Lea & Perrins					
Steak	1 oz	40	10	tr	tr
Worcestershire	1 tsp	5	1	tr	tr
Worcestershire White Wine	1 tsp	4	1	tr	tr
Manwich					
Mexican	2.5 oz	35	9	1	1
Sloppy Joe	2.5 oz	40	10	tr	1
Marzetti					
Teriyaki Stir-Fry	2 tbsp	80	14	2	2
McIlhenny					
7 Spice Chili	2 tbsp (1.1 fl oz)	16	3	tr	1
Sauce	2 tbsp (1.1 oz)	48	7	2	1
Tabasco	1 tsp	1	tr	tr	tr
Mrs. Dash					
Steak	1 tbsp	17	4	tr	tr
Newman's Own					
Bandito Diavalo Spicy	4 oz	70	11	2	2
Old El Paso					
Enchilada Green	2 tbsp	11	3	1	tr
Enchilada Hot	¼ cup	30	4	1	tr
Enchilada Mild	¼ cup	25	4	1	tr
Picante Thick'n Chunky Hot	2 tbsp	10	2	0	0
Picante Thick'n Chunky Medium	2 tbsp	10	2	0	0
Picante Thick'n Chunky Mild	2 tbsp	10	2	0	0
Taco Hot	1 tbsp	5	1	0	0

FOOD	PORTION	CALS.	CARB.	FAT	PRO.
Old El Paso (CONT.)					
Taco Medium	1 tbsp	5	1	0	0
Taco Mild	1 tbsp	5	1	0	0
Tomatoes & Jalapenos	¼ cup	11	3	0	1
Tomatoes & Green Chilies	¼ cup	10	2	0	0
Ortega					
Taco Thick & Smooth Hot	1 tbsp	8	2	0	0
Taco Thick & Smooth Mild	1 tbsp	8	2	0	0
Pace					
Picante	2 tbsp (1 fl oz)	7	2	0	tr
Progresso					
Alfredo	½ cup	340	6	30	13
Primavera Creamy	½ cup	190	8	17	5
Red Wing					
Chili Sauce	1 tbsp (0.6 oz)	20	5	0	0
Seafood Cocktail	¼ cup (2 oz)	90	22	1	0
Sauce Arturo					
Original	¼ cup (2.2 fl oz)	50	8	1	1
Sauceworks					
Cocktail	¼ cup (2.3 oz)	60	13	1	1
Sweet'n Sour	2 tbsp (1.2 oz)	60	14	0	0
Tartar	2 tbsp (1.1 oz)	100	4	10	0
Tartar Natural Lemon & Herb	2 tbsp (1 oz)	150	tr	16	0
Simmer Chef					
Golden Honey Mustard	½ cup (4 fl oz)	150	30	2	1
Hearty Onion & Mushroom	½ cup (4 fl oz)	50	9	1	1
Snow's					
Newburg With Sherry	⅓ cup	120	10	8	3
Welsh Rarebit Cheese	½ cup	170	10	11	9
Tabasco					
Picante	2 tbsp (1.5 oz)	17	3	tr	1
Trappey					
Indi-Pep West Indian Style Pepper Sauce	1 tsp (0.1 oz)	1	tr	tr	tr
Mexi Pep Louisiana Hot Sauce	1 tsp (0.1 oz)	tr	tr	tr	tr
Pepper Sauce	1 tsp (0.2 oz)	1	tr	tr	tr
Red Devil Buffalo Style Hot Sauce	1 tsp (0.1 oz)	1	tr	tr	tr

FOOD	PORTION	CALS.	CARB.	FAT	PRO.
Trappey (CONT.)					
Red Devil Cayenne Pepper Sauce	1 tsp (0.1 oz)	1	tr	tr	tr
Worcestershire Chef Magic	1 tsp (0.1 oz)	3	1	tr	tr
Watkins					
Beef Marinade	¼ tbsp (2 g)	5	1	0	0
Calypso Hot Pepper Sauce	1 tsp (5 g)	10	3	0	0
Carribean Red Pepper Sauce	1 tsp (5 g)	10	3	0	0
Chicken & Pork Marinade	¼ tbsp (2 g)	5	2	0	0
Fish & Seafood Marinade	¼ tbsp (2 g)	10	1	0	0
Inferno Hot Pepper Sauce	2 tbsp (1 oz)	35	8	0	0
Meat Magic	1 tsp (6 g)	10	2	0	0
Steak Sauce	1 tbsp (0.5 oz)	20	4	0	0
Weight Watchers					
Tartar	1 tbsp	35	3	3	0
Wise					
Picante	2 tbsp	12	3	0	0
Wolf Brand					
Hot Dog	1.25 oz	44	4	2	2
SHELF-STABLE					
Cheez Whiz					
Cheese Sauce With Mild Salsa Zap-A-Pack	2 tbsp (1.2 oz)	90	3	8	3
Zap-A-Pack	2 tbsp (1.2 oz)	90	3	8	3
Fresh Gourmet					
Stir 'n Sauce Italian	1 tbsp (0.5 oz)	30	5	1	0
SAUERKRAUT					
canned	½ cup	22	5	tr	1
Del Monte	½ cup (4.2 oz)	15	4	0	1
Eden					
Organic	½ cup (3.9 oz)	25	4	0	2
Hebrew National					
Gallon Kraut	½ cup	25	4	0	0
New Kraut	½ cup (3.1 oz)	50	11	1	1
Rosoff's					
Sauerkraut	½ cup (3.2 oz)	50	11	1	1
S&W					
Canned	½ cup	25	5	0	1

FOOD	PORTION	CALS.	CARB.	FAT	PRO.
Schorr's					
New Kraut	½ cup (3.2 oz)	50	11	1	1
Seneca					
Canned	2 tbsp	5	0	0	0
SnowFloss					
Kraut	4 oz	28	4	0	1
Kraut Bavarian Style	4 oz	64	12	0	1
Vlasic					
Old Fashioned	1 oz	4	1	0	0

SAUERKRAUT JUICE
S&W

Juice	4 oz	14	3	0	1

SAUSAGE
(*see also* HOT DOG, SAUSAGE SUBSTITUTES)

bierschinken	3.5 oz	174	tr	11	18
bierwurst	3.5 oz	258	0	21	16
blutwurst uncooked	3½ oz	424	0	39	13
bockwurst	3.5 oz	276	0	25	12
bockwurst pork & veal raw	1 link (2.3 oz)	200	tr	18	9
bratwurst pork, cooked	1 link (3 oz)	256	2	22	12
brotwurst pork	1 oz	92	1	8	4
brotwurst pork & beef	1 link (2.5 oz)	226	2	19	10
country-style pork, cooked	1 link (½ oz)	48	tr	4	3
country-style pork, cooked	1 patty (1 oz)	100	tr	8	5
fleischwurst	3.5 oz	305	0	29	12
gelbwurst uncooked	3½ oz	363	0	33	12
italian pork, cooked	1 (2.4 oz)	216	1	17	13
italian pork, cooked	1 (3 oz)	268	1	21	17
jagdwurst	3.5 oz	211	0	16	16
kielbasa pork	1 oz	88	1	8	8
knockwurst pork & beef	1 (2.4 oz)	209	1	19	8
knockwurst pork & beef	1 oz	87	1	8	3
mettwurst uncooked	3½ oz	483	0	45	13
plockwurst uncooked	3½ oz	312	0	45	19
polish pork	1 (8 oz)	739	4	65	32
polish pork	1 oz	92	tr	8	4
pork & beef, cooked	1 link (½ oz)	52	tr	5	2
pork & beef, cooked	1 patty (1 oz)	107	1	10	4
pork cooked	1 patty (1 oz)	100	tr	8	5
pork, cooked	1 link (½ oz)	48	tr	4	3
regensburger uncooked	3½ oz	354	0	31	13
smoked pork	1 link (2.4 oz)	265	1	22	15
smoked pork	1 sm link (½ oz)	62	tr	5	4

FOOD	PORTION	CALS.	CARB.	FAT	PRO.
smoked pork & beef	1 link (2.4 oz)	229	1	21	9
smoked pork & beef	1 sm link (½ oz)	54	tr	5	2
vienna canned	1 (½ oz)	45	tr	4	2
vienna canned	7 (4 oz)	315	2	28	12
weisswurst uncooked	3½ oz	305	0	27	11
zungenwurst (tongue)	3.5 oz	285	0	24	17
Aidells					
Andouille Cajun Cooked	1 (3.5 oz)	220	1	17	16
Burmese Curry Cooked	1 (3.5 oz)	220	3	15	18
Chicken & Apple Fresh	1 (1.9 oz)	110	1	8	9
Chicken & Apple Smoked	1 (3.5 oz)	220	0	16	16
Chicken & Turkey New Mexico Smoked	1 (3.5 oz)	220	2	16	15
Chicken & Turkey Thai Fresh	1 (3.5 oz)	200	0	16	15
Chicken & Turkey Thai Smoked	1 (3.5 oz)	220	0	16	18
Chicken & Turkey With Sun-Dried Tomatoes & Basil Fresh	1 (3.5 oz)	200	1	15	15
Chicken & Turkey With Sun-Dried Tomatoes & Basil Smoked	1 (3.5 oz)	200	0	14	19
Creole Hot Cooked	1 (3.5 oz)	220	2	16	17
Duck & Turkey Smoked	1 (3.5 oz)	220	1	16	17
Hunter's Cooked	1 (3.5 oz)	240	0	19	17
Italian Hot Fresh	1 (3.5 oz)	230	0	18	16
Italian Mild Fresh	1 (3.5 oz)	230	0	18	16
Lamb & Beef With Rosemary Fresh	1 (3.5 oz)	220	2	16	16
Lemon Chicken Cooked	1 (3.5 oz)	220	1	16	15
Mexican Chorizo Beef Fresh	1 (3.5 oz)	400	3	37	13
Whiskey Fennel Cooked	1 (3.5 oz)	230	1	18	17
Armour					
Vienna Sausage 25% Less Fat	3 (1.9 oz)	130	1	11	6
Vienna Sausage In BBQ Sauce	3 (2.1 oz)	160	4	14	5
Vienna Sausage In Beef Stock	3 (1.9 oz)	170	1	16	5

FOOD	PORTION	CALS.	CARB.	FAT	PRO.
Armour (CONT.)					
Vienna Sausage In Hot Sauce	3 (2.1 oz)	170	3	15	5
Vienna Sausage Smoked	3 (1.9 oz)	170	1	16	5
Banner					
Sausage Tripe	2 oz	90	2	5	9
Bilinski's					
Chicken & Vegetable	1 (3 oz)	80	2	2	14
Chicken Italian With Peppers & Onions	1 (3 oz)	120	1	4	19
Golden Brown					
Beef	1	80	tr	7	4
Mild	1	100	tr	10	3
Spicy	1	100	tr	9	3
Healthy Choice					
Low Fat Smoked	2 oz	70	4	2	8
Low Fat Smoked Polska Kielbasa	2 oz	70	4	2	8
Hebrew National					
Beef Knocks	1 (3 oz)	260	—	25	10
Polish Beef	1 link	240	—	22	12
Hillshire					
Beer Bratwurst	1 (2 oz)	190	2	17	7
Bratwurst Fresh	1 (2 oz)	190	1	17	7
Bratwurst Light Fresh	1 (2 oz)	150	1	11	9
Bratwurst Spicy	1 (2 oz)	180	1	17	8
Flavorseal Kielbasa Polska	2 oz	190	2	17	7
Flavorseal Kielbasa Polska Beef	2 oz	190	2	17	7
Flavorseal Kielbasa Polska Lite	2 oz	130	1	11	8
Flavorseal Kielbasa Polska Mild	2 oz	190	2	17	7
Flavorseal Kielbasa Polska Turkey	2 oz	90	2	5	9
Flavorseal Smoked	2 oz	190	2	17	7
Flavorseal Smoked Beef	2 oz	180	2	16	7
Flavorseal Smoked Beef & Cheddar	2 oz	190	1	15	8
Flavorseal Smoked Country Recipe	2 oz	180	2	16	7
Flavorseal Smoked Hot	2 oz	180	2	16	7
Flavorseal Smoked Lite	2 oz	130	1	11	8

FOOD	PORTION	CALS.	CARB.	FAT	PRO.
Hillshire (CONT.)					
Flavorseal Smoked Turkey	2 oz	90	2	5	9
Flavorseal Smoked w/ Italian Seasoning	2 oz	200	1	18	7
Italian Mild	1 (2 oz)	190	1	17	7
Italian Mild Light	1 (2 oz)	150	2	11	9
Italian Hot	1 (2 oz)	180	1	17	7
Italian Hot Light	1 (2 oz)	150	2	11	9
Kielbasa Fresh Polska	1 (2 oz)	190	1	17	7
Kielbasa Fresh Polska Lower Fat	1 (2 oz)	150	2	11	9
Links 80% Fat Fre Smokies	2 oz	130	2	10	8
Links 80% Fat Free Cheddar Hots	2 oz	150	1	12	9
Links 80% Fat Free Kielbasa	2 oz	130	2	10	8
Links Brats Fully Cooked	2 oz	170	1	16	7
Links Bratwurst Smoked	2 oz	190	1	17	8
Links Bun Size Cheddarwurst	2 oz	200	1	18	8
Links Bun Size Kielbasa	2 oz	180	2	16	8
Links Bun Size Smoked	2 oz	180	2	16	8
Links Bun Size Smoked Beef	2 oz	180	2	16	8
Links Cheddarwurst	2 oz	190	1	17	8
Links Cheddarwurst Lite	1 link (2.7 oz)	190	2	15	12
Links Hot	2 oz	190	2	16	8
Links Hot Beef	2 oz	190	1	17	8
Links Hot Lite	1 link (2.7 oz)	190	2	15	11
Links Kielbasa Polska	2 oz	190	2	17	7
Links Kielbasa Polska Lite	1 link (2.7 oz)	190	2	15	11
Links Knockwurst Lite	2 oz	180	1	16	7
Links Lit'l Polskas	2 oz	180	2	16	6
Links Lit'l Smokies	2 oz	180	2	16	8
Links Lit'l Smokies Beef	2 oz	180	2	16	8
Links Lit'l Smokies Cheddar	2 oz	180	2	16	8
Links Lit'l Smokies Light	2 oz	120	1	8	8
Links Polish	2 oz	190	2	17	7
Links Smoked	2 oz	190	1	18	8
Mexican Style	1 (2 oz)	190	1	17	7

FOOD	PORTION	CALS.	CARB.	FAT	PRO.
Hillshire (CONT.)					
Mexican Style Lower Fat	1 (2 oz)	150	2	11	9
Hormel					
Light & Lean 97 Dinner Smoked	2 oz	60	2	2	8
Pickled Hot	6 (2 oz)	140	1	11	8
Pickled Smoked	6 (2 oz)	140	1	11	8
Vienna	2 oz	140	1	13	6
Vienna Chicken	2 oz	90	1	10	6
Jimmy Dean					
Brick Sausage	2.5 oz	270	0	25	10
Bulk	2.5 oz	300	0	28	9
Hickory Smoked Dinner Sausage	2 oz	170	2	14	7
Pattie Pre-Cooked	1 (1.9 oz)	230	0	22	7
Polska Kielbaska	2 oz	170	1	15	7
Sage Pattie	1 (2 oz)	200	0	19	7
Sausage Pattie Raw	1 (2 oz)	200	0	19	7
Skinless Link	4 (2 oz)	200	0	19	6
Skinless Link	2 (2 oz)	200	0	19	7
Jones					
Brown & Serve Bacon	1	90	tr	8	3
Brown & Serve Beef	1	90	tr	9	3
Brown & Serve Light	1	60	1	5	3
Brown & Serve Regular	1	100	tr	10	3
Cello Beef	1 slice (1 oz)	130	tr	13	3
Cello Hot Country	1 slice (1 oz)	110	tr	10	4
Cello Original	1 slice (1 oz)	100	tr	10	4
Dinner Link	1	280	tr	28	6
Golden Brown Light Links	1	60	1	5	3
Golden Brown Mild Pattie	1	150	tr	14	5
Italian	1	160	tr	14	8
Light Link	1	70	1	6	4
Little Link	1	140	tr	14	3
Patties	1	150	tr	14	6
Scrapple	1 slice	90	5	6	4
Scrapple	1 slice (1½ oz)	90	5	6	4
Little Sizzlers					
Brown & Serve	2 patties (1.4 oz)	190	1	18	7
Brown & Serve	3 links (2.1 oz)	190	1	22	8
Cooked	3 links (1.4 oz)	210	0	20	8
Cooked	2 patties (2 oz)	250	0	23	10

FOOD	PORTION	CALS.	CARB.	FAT	PRO.
Little Sizzlers (CONT.)					
Heat & Serve Pork cooked	3 links (1.4 oz)	210	0	20	8
Louis Rich					
Polska Kielbasa	2 oz	80	1	5	9
Smoked Sausage With Cheese cooked	1 (1 oz)	47	1	3	5
Turkey	2.5 oz	110	3	6	11
Turkey & Cheese Smoked	2 oz	90	2	5	10
Turkey Links	2 (2 oz)	90	0	6	11
Turkey Smoked	2 oz	90	2	5	9
Mr. Turkey					
Breakfast	2.5 oz	130	0	9	12
Hearty Blend Polish Kielbasa	1 oz	70	1	6	4
Hearty Blend Smoked	1 oz	70	1	6	4
Hot Smoked	1 oz	45	2	3	4
Italian Smoked	1 oz	45	2	3	4
Polish Kielbasa	1 oz	45	2	3	4
Smoked	1 oz	45	2	3	4
Old Smokehouse					
Summer Sausage	1 oz	110	1	10	4
Oscar Mayer					
Pork cooked	2 links (1.7 oz)	170	1	15	9
Smokies Beef	1 (1.5 oz)	120	1	11	6
Smokies Cheese	1 (1.5 oz)	130	1	12	6
Smokies Links	1 (1.5 oz)	130	1	12	5
Smokies Little	6 (2 oz)	170	1	16	7
Perdue					
Breakfast Links Turkey cooked	1 (1.3 oz)	40	tr	3	4
Breakfast Patties Turkey cooked	1 (1.3 oz)	61	tr	4	6
Hot Italian Turkey cooked	1 (2 oz)	94	0	6	10
Sweet Italian Turkey cooked	1 (2 oz)	94	0	6	10
Rudy's Farm					
Italian Mild	2.5 oz	240	0	22	10
Italian Hot	2.5 oz	240	0	22	10
Italian Mild Natural Casing	1 (2 oz)	190	0	17	8
Morning Right Link	3 (2.9 oz)	150	0	10	15

FOOD	PORTION	CALS.	CARB.	FAT	PRO.
Rudy's Farm (CONT.)					
Morning Right Pattie	2 (2.9 oz)	150	0	10	15
Pattie Pre-Cooked	1 (1.4 oz)	100	0	6	13
Smoked	4 (2.1 oz)	200	1	18	7
Sweet Link	1 (3.9 oz)	380	1	35	16
Shofar					
Knockwurst Beef	1 (3 oz)	260	tr	23	11
Tyson					
Country Pork	3.5 oz	320	1	29	13
Wampler Longacre					
Breakfast Links	1 (2.8 oz)	170	2	12	15
Italian Links	1 (2.8 oz)	170	2	12	15
Tinderlings Garlic & Pepper	1 (3.5 oz)	143	3	5	23
Turkey	1 pattie (2 oz)	120	4	8	10
Turkey	1 link (1 oz)	60	1	4	5
TAKE-OUT					
pork	1 link (.5 oz)	48	tr	4	3
pork	1 patty (1 oz)	100	tr	8	5

SAUSAGE DISHES
FROZEN
Jimmy Dean

Italian Sausage & Mozzarella Sandwich	1 (4.5 oz)	380	28	22	17
Ovenstuffs					
French Roll Italian Sausage	1 (4.75 oz)	390	29	22	17
French Roll Pepperoni	1 (4.75 oz)	370	30	20	17
TAKE-OUT					
sausage roll	1 (2.3 oz)	311	22	24	5

SAUSAGE SUBSTITUTES
Knox Mountain Farm

No-So-Sausage	1 serv (1/10 pkg)	120	6	1	14
LaLoma					
Linketts	2 (71 g)	140	2	8	15
Little Links	2 (46 g)	90	2	5	9
Lightlife					
Lean Links Breakfast	1.25 oz	69	4	3	4
Lean Links Italian	1.5 oz	83	5	3	5
Morningstar Farms					
Breakfast Links	2 (45 g)	90	3	5	8
Breakfast Patties	2 (76 g)	190	7	12	15
Country Crisp Patties	1 (71 g)	220	13	15	8

FOOD	PORTION	CALS.	CARB.	FAT	PRO.
Morningstar Farms (CONT.)					
Grillers	1 (64 g)	180	5	12	13
White Wave					
Meatless Healthy Links	2 (1.6 oz)	140	5	10	8
Worthington					
Leanies	1 link (40 g)	100	2	6	8
Prosage Links	2 (45 g)	130	3	9	9
Saucettes	2 links (67 g)	150	3	11	10
Super-Links	1 (48 g)	100	3	7	7
Veja-Links	2 (62 g)	140	4	10	8

SCALLOP
FRESH
raw	3 oz	75	2	1	14

FROZEN
Mrs. Paul's
Fried	2 oz	160	18	7	8

HOME RECIPE
breaded & fried	2 lg	67	3	3	6

TAKE-OUT
breaded & fried	6 (5 oz)	386	38	19	16

SCONE
Finnegan's
Irish Raisin	1 (2.7 oz)	90	20	2	2

HOME RECIPE
apricot scone	1	232	39	7	5

TAKE-OUT
cheese	1 (1.75 oz)	182	22	9	5
fruit	1 (1.75 oz)	158	27	5	4
plain	1 (1.75 oz)	181	27	7	4

SCROD
FROZEN
Gorton's
Microwave Entree Baked	1 pkg	320	18	18	17

SCUP
fresh baked	3 oz	115	0	3	21

SEA BASS
(*see* BASS)

SEATROUT
(*see* TROUT)

SEAWEED
agar dried	1 oz	87	23	tr	2

FOOD	PORTION	CALS.	CARB.	FAT	PRO.
agar fresh	1 oz	tr	2	tr	tr
irishmoss fresh	1 oz	14	4	tr	tr
kelp fresh	1 oz	12	3	tr	tr
kombu fresh	1 oz	12	3	tr	tr
laver fresh	1 oz	10	1	tr	2
nori fresh	1 oz	10	1	tr	2
spirulina dried	1 oz	83	7	2	16
spirulina fresh	1 oz	7	1	tr	2
tangle fresh	1 oz	12	3	tr	tr
wakame fresh	1 oz	13	3	tr	1
Eden					
Agar Agar Bars	1 tbsp (2.5 oz)	10	2	0	0
Agar Agar Flakes	1 tbsp (2.5 oz)	10	2	0	0
Arame	½ cup (0.3 oz)	30	7	0	1
Hiziki	½ cup (0.3 oz)	30	6	0	tr
Kombu	3.5 in piece (3.3 g)	10	2	0	0
Nori	1 sheet (2.5 g)	10	1	0	1
Sushi Nori	1 sheet (2.5 g)	10	1	0	1
Wakame	½ cup (0.3 oz)	25	4	0	2
Wakame Flakes	½ cup (0.3 oz)	25	4	0	2
Maine Coast					
Alaria	⅓ cup (7 g)	18	3	0	1
Dulse	⅓ cup (7 g)	18	3	0	2
Dulse Flakes	1 oz	75	13	1	6
Kelp	⅓ cup (7 g)	17	3	0	1
Kelp Crunch	1 bar (1 oz)	129	14	6	3
Kelp Crunch Peanut-Raisin	1 bar (1 oz)	129	14	6	3
Laver	⅓ cup (7 g)	22	3	0	4
Sea Seasoning Dulse	1 g	3	1	0	0
Sea Seasoning Dulse With Celery	1 g	3	1	0	0
Sea Seasoning Dulse With Garlic	1 g	3	1	0	0
Sea Seasoning Dulse With Sesame	1 g	3	1	0	0
Sea Seasoning Kelp	1 g	3	1	0	0
Sea Seasoning Kelp With Cayenne	1 g	3	1	0	0
Sea Seasoning Nori	1 g	3	1	0	0
Sea Seasoning Nori With Ginger	1 g	3	1	0	0

SEITAN
(*see* WHEAT)

SEMOLINA

dry	½ cup	303	61	tr	11

FOOD	PORTION	CALS.	CARB.	FAT	PRO.
SESAME					
seeds	1 tsp	16	tr	2	1
seeds dried	1 tbsp	52	2	5	2
seeds dried	1 cup	825	34	72	26
seeds roasted & toasted	1 oz	161	7	14	14
sesame butter	1 tbsp	95	4	8	3
sesame crunch candy	20 pieces (1.2 oz)	181	18	12	4
sesame crunch candy	1 oz	146	14	9	3
sesame sticks	1 oz	153	13	10	3
sesame sticks unsalted	1 oz	153	13	10	3
tahini from roasted & toasted kernels	1 tbsp	89	3	8	3
tahini from stone ground kernels	1 tbsp	86	4	7	3
tahini from unroasted kernels	1 tbsp	85	3	8	3
Arrowhead					
Sesame Tahini	1 oz	170	4	17	6
Casbah					
Tahini Sauce Mix as prep	¼ cup	160	10	13	4
Eden					
Sesame Shake	½ tsp (1.5 g)	10	0	1	0
Sesame Shake Garlic	½ tsp (1.5 g)	10	0	1	0
Sesame Shake Organic Seaweed	½ tsp (1.5 g)	10	0	1	0
Erewhon					
Sesame Butter	2 tbsp (32 g)	190	3	17	7
Sesame Tahini	2 tbsp (32 g)	200	3	18	6
Joyva					
Tahini	2 tbsp (1 oz)	200	3	18	5
Planters					
Nut Mix	1 oz	150	9	12	5
Stone-Buhr					
Seeds Raw	4 tsp (1 oz)	180	3	16	8
SESBANIA					
flower	1	1	tr	0	tr
SHAD					
american baked	3 oz	214	0	15	18
roe baked w/ butter & lemon	3.5 oz	126	2	3	22
roe raw	3½ oz	130	2	2	24
SHALLOTS					
dried	1 tbsp	3	1	0	tr
raw chopped	1 tbsp	7	2	tr	tr

FOOD	PORTION	CALS.	CARB.	FAT	PRO.
SHARK					
batter-dipped & fried	3 oz	194	5	12	16
raw	3 oz	111	0	4	18
SHEEPSHEAD FISH					
cooked	1 fillet (6.5 oz)	234	0	3	48
cooked	3 oz	107	0	1	22
raw	3 oz	92	0	2	17
SHELLFISH					
(see individual names, SHELLFISH SUBSTITUTES)					
SHELLFISH SUBSTITUTES					
crab imitation	3 oz	87	1	1	10
scallop imitation	3 oz	84	9	tr	11
shrimp imitation	3 oz	86	8	1	11
surimi	1 oz	28	2	tr	4
surimi	3 oz	84	6	1	13
Louis Kemp					
Crab Delights Chunk Style	2 oz	54	5	tr	6
Lobster Delights	2 oz	60	6	tr	8
Maryland Style Cakes	2.5 oz	154	10	9	8
Ocean Magic					
Imitation King Crab	3 oz	80	11	tr	8
SHELLIE BEANS					
canned	½ cup	37	8	tr	2
SHERBET					
(see also ICES AND ICE POPS)					
orange	½ cup (4 fl oz)	132	29	2	1
orange	½ gal	2158	469	31	17
orange	1 bar (2.75 fl oz)	91	20	1	1
orange home recipe	½ cup	120	24	2	2
Borden					
Orange	½ cup	110	25	1	1
Bresler's					
All Flavors	3.5 oz	140	30	2	1
Hood					
Lime Orange Lemon	½ cup (3.1 oz)	120	26	1	1
Orange	½ cup (3.1 oz)	120	26	1	1
Rainbow Swirl	½ cup (3.1 oz)	120	26	1	1
Raspberry Orange Lime	½ cup (3.1 oz)	120	26	1	1
Sealtest					
Lime	½ cup (3 oz)	130	28	1	1

FOOD	PORTION	CALS.	CARB.	FAT	PRO.
Sealtest (CONT.)					
Orange	½ cup (3 oz)	130	28	1	1
Rainbow Orange Red Raspberry Lime	½ cup (3 oz)	130	28	1	1
Red Raspberry	½ cup (3 oz)	130	28	1	1
SHRIMP					
CANNED					
canned	3 oz	102	1	2	20
canned	1 cup	154	1	3	30
S&W					
Deveined Medium Whole Shrimp	2 oz	65	1	0	13
FRESH					
cooked	3 oz	84	0	1	18
cooked	4 large	22	0	tr	5
raw	4 large	30	tr	tr	6
raw	3 oz	90	1	1	17
FROZEN					
Cajun Cookin'					
Shrimp Creole	12 oz	390	55	11	17
Shrimp Etouffee	17 oz	360	52	9	19
Shrimp Jambalaya	12 oz	450	43	20	20
Gorton's					
Butterfly Shrimp	4 oz	160	16	tr	19
Microwave Crunchy Shrimp	5 oz	380	35	20	14
Microwave Entree Shrimp Scampi	1 pkg	390	21	30	10
Shrimp Crisps	4 oz	280	26	15	9
Mrs. Paul's					
Entrees Light Seafood & Clams With Linguini	10 oz	240	36	5	12
READY-TO-USE					
American Original Foods					
Fried	4 oz	253	23	12	12
TAKE-OUT					
breaded & fried	4 large	73	3	4	6
breaded & fried	3 oz	206	10	10	18
breaded & fried	6 to 8 (6 oz)	454	40	25	19
jambalaya	¾ cup	188	26	5	11
SMELT					
rainbow cooked	3 oz	106	0	3	19
rainbow raw	3 oz	83	0	2	15

FOOD	PORTION	CALS.	CARB.	FAT	PRO.
SNACKS					
(*see also* CHIPS, FRUIT SNACKS, NUTS MIXED, POPCORN, PRETZELS)					
oriental mix	1 oz	155	9	12	6
pork skins	½ oz	77	0	4	9
pork skins	1 oz	154	0	9	17
pork skins barbecue	1 oz	152	1	9	16
pork skins barbecue	½ oz	76	tr	5	8
trail mix	1 oz	131	13	8	4
trail mix	1 cup (5.3 oz)	693	67	44	21
trail mix tropical	1 oz	115	19	5	2
trail mix w/ chocolate chips	1 cup (5.1 oz)	707	66	47	21
trail mix w/ chocolate chips	1 oz	137	13	9	4
Bakem-ets					
Hot'N Spicy	21 pieces (1 oz)	150	1	9	17
Bugles					
Nacho Cheese	1 oz	160	17	9	2
Ranch	1 oz	150	16	9	2
Snacks	1 oz	150	18	8	2
Cheetos					
Cheddar Valley	26 pieces (1 oz)	160	16	9	2
Crunchy	26 pieces (1 oz)	150	17	9	1
Curls	15 pieces (1 oz)	150	17	9	1
Flamin' Hot	26 pieces (1 oz)	150	16	9	2
Light	38 pieces (1 oz)	140	19	6	2
Paws	16 pieces (1 oz)	160	15	10	1
Puffed Ball	38 pieces (1 oz)	160	16	10	2
Puffs	33 pieces (1 oz)	160	16	9	1
Cheez Doodles					
Crunchy	1 oz	160	16	10	2
Puffed	1 oz	150	16	9	2
Cheez Waffies					
Snacks	1 oz	140	14	8	3
Chex					
Snack Mix Barbeque	½ cup (1.1 oz)	130	20	5	3
Snack Mix Cool Sour Cream And Onion	½ cup (1 oz)	130	21	4	3
Snack Mix Golden Cheddar	½ cup (1 oz)	130	20	4	3
Snack Mix Traditional	⅔ cup (1.2 oz)	150	23	5	3
Combos					
Cheddar Cheese Cracker	1 pkg (1.7 oz)	250	28	13	5
Cheddar Cheese Cracker	1 oz	140	16	8	3
Cheddar Cheese Pretzel	1 pkg (1.8 oz)	240	33	9	5

FOOD	PORTION	CALS.	CARB.	FAT	PRO.
Combos (CONT.)					
Cheddar Cheese Pretzel	1 oz	130	18	5	3
Chili Cheese w/ Corn Shell	1 oz	140	17	6	2
Chili Cheese w/ Corn Shell	1 pkg (1.7 oz)	230	29	11	4
Mustard Pretzel	1 pkg (1.8 oz)	230	35	8	4
Mustard Pretzel	1 oz	130	19	4	2
Nacho Cheese Pretzel	1 pkg (1.7 oz)	230	34	8	5
Nacho Cheese Pretzel	1 oz	130	19	5	3
Nacho Cheese w/ Tortilla Shell	1 oz	140	17	6	2
Nacho Cheese w/ Tortilla Shell	1 pkg (1.7 oz)	230	30	11	4
Peanut Butter Cracker	1 oz	140	15	8	4
Pepperoni & Cheese Pizza	1 oz	140	17	7	2
Pepperoni & Cheese Pizza	1 pkg (1.7 oz)	240	30	11	4
Pizzeria Pretzel	1 pkg (1.8 oz)	230	35	8	5
Pizzeria Pretzel	1 oz	130	19	5	3
Tortilla Ranch	1 bag (1.7 oz)	240	29	12	4
Tortilla Ranch	1 oz	140	17	7	2
Cornnuts					
Barbecue	1 oz	120	22	4	2
Nacho Cheese	1 oz	120	22	4	2
Original	1 oz	120	22	4	2
Original	1 pkg (2 oz)	260	40	8	5
Picante	1 oz	120	22	4	2
Ranch	1 oz	120	20	4	2
Doo Dads					
Snacks	1 oz	130	17	6	3
Eagle					
Cheese Crunch	1 oz	160	16	10	2
Energy Food Factory					
Poprice Cheddar Cheese	½ oz	60	8	3	2
Poprice Herb & Garlic	½ oz	50	10	2	1
Poprice Lite	½ oz	50	9	2	1
Poprice Original No Salt	½ oz	45	11	0	1
Estee					
Snack Crisps Apple Cinnamon	1 pkg (0.66 oz)	90	16	2	1
Snack Crisps Apple Cinnamon	27 crisps (1 oz)	130	24	3	2

FOOD	PORTION	CALS.	CARB.	FAT	PRO.
Estee (CONT.)					
Snack Crisps Chocolate	30 crisps (1 oz)	130	23	3	2
Snack Crisps Chocolate	1 pkg (0.66 oz)	90	15	2	2
Snack Crisps Lemon	1 pkg (0.66 oz)	90	16	2	2
Snack Crisps Lemon	30 (1 oz)	130	23	3	2
Snack Crisps Ranch	30 (1 oz)	130	22	3	3
Snack Crisps Ranch	1 pkg (0.6 oz)	90	15	2	2
Snack Crisps White Cheddar	1 pkg (0.6 oz)	90	14	2	2
Snack Crisps With Cheddar	27 crisps (1 oz)	130	22	3	3
Frito Lay					
Corn Nuggets Toasted	1.38 oz	170	29	5	3
Funyums					
Onion Rings	11 pieces (1 oz)	140	18	7	2
Handi-Snacks					
Peanut Butter'n Crackers	1 pkg (1.1 oz)	180	12	12	5
Peanut Butter'n Grahamsticks	1 pkg (1.1 oz)	170	14	10	5
Hapi					
Chili Bits	½ cup (1 oz)	110	25	0	3
Health Valley					
Cheddar Lites	0.75 oz	40	4	2	1
Cheddar Lites With Green Onion	0.75 oz	40	4	2	1
Lance					
Cheese Balls	1 pkg (32 g)	190	16	13	2
Crunchy Cheese Twists	1 pkg (42 g)	260	25	16	3
Gold-N-Cheese	1 pkg (39 g)	180	23	9	4
Pork Skins	1 pkg (14 g)	80	0	5	9
Pork Skins BBQ	1 pkg (14 g)	80	0	5	9
Mr. Peanut					
Peanut Butter Crisps Graham	12 pieces (1.1 oz)	150	18	8	4
Munchos					
Snack	16 pieces (1 oz)	160	15	10	1
Planters					
Cheez Balls	1 pkg (1 oz)	150	15	10	2
Cheez Balls	1 oz	150	15	10	2
Cheez Curls	1 oz	150	15	10	2
Cheez Curls	1 pkg (1.2 oz)	190	19	12	2
Heat Snack Mix	1 oz	140	13	8	5
Snyder's					
Cheddar Cheese Twists	1 oz	150	17	8	2

FOOD	PORTION	CALS.	CARB.	FAT	PRO.
Snyder's (CONT.)					
Kruncheez	1 oz	160	15	10	2
Onion Toasters	1 oz	150	17	8	2
Snack Mix	1 oz	170	11	8	2
Sopaipillas Apple & Cinnamon	1 oz	150	18	8	2
Ultra Slim-Fast					
Lite N' Tasty Cheese Curls	1 oz	110	20	3	2
Weight Watchers					
Cheese Curls	½ oz	70	10	2	1

SNAIL

cooked	3 oz	233	13	1	41
raw	3 oz	117	7	tr	20

SNAP BEANS
CANNED

green	½ cup	13	3	tr	1
green low sodium	½ cup	13	3	tr	1
italian	½ cup	13	3	tr	1
italian low sodium	½ cup	13	3	tr	1
yellow	½ cup	13	3	tr	1
yellow low sodium	½ cup	13	3	tr	1
FRESH					
green cooked	½ cup	22	5	tr	1
green raw	½ cup	17	4	tr	1
yellow cooked	½ cup	22	5	tr	1
yellow raw	½ cup	17	4	tr	1
FROZEN					
green cooked	½ cup	18	4	tr	1
italian cooked	½ cup	18	4	tr	1
yellow cooked	½ cup	18	4	tr	1

SNAPPER

cooked	1 fillet (6 oz)	217	0	3	45
cooked	3 oz	109	0	1	22
raw	3 oz	85	0	1	17

SODA
(*see also* DRINK MIXERS, MINERAL/BOTTLED WATER)

club	12 oz	0	0	0	0
cola	12 oz	151	39	tr	tr
cream	12 oz	191	49	0	0
diet cola	12 oz	2	tr	0	tr
diet cola w/ equal	12 oz	2	tr	0	tr

FOOD	PORTION	CALS.	CARB.	FAT	PRO.
diet cola w/ saccharin	12 oz	2	tr	0	tr
ginger ale	12 oz can	124	32	0	tr
grape	12 oz	161	42	0	0
lemon lime	12 oz	149	38	0	0
orange	12 oz	177	46	0	0
pepper type	12 oz	151	38	tr	0
quinine	12 oz	125	32	0	0
root beer	12 oz	152	39	0	tr
tonic water	12 oz	125	32	0	0
Barrelhead					
Root Beer	8 fl oz	110	27	0	0
Canada Dry					
Birch Beer Brown	8 fl oz	110	27	0	0
Club Sodium Free	8 fl oz	0	0	0	0
Diet Ginger Ale	8 fl oz	0	0	0	0
Diet Tonic Water	8 fl oz	0	0	0	0
Ginger Ale	8 fl oz	100	25	0	0
Seltzer	8 fl oz	0	0	0	0
Seltzer Cherry	8 fl oz	0	0	0	0
Seltzer Cranberry Lime	8 fl oz	0	0	0	0
Seltzer Grapefruit	8 fl oz	0	0	0	0
Seltzer Lemon Lime	8 fl oz	0	0	0	0
Seltzer Mandarin Orange	8 fl oz	0	0	0	0
Seltzer Peach	8 fl oz	0	0	0	0
Seltzer Raspberry	8 fl oz	0	0	0	0
Seltzer Strawberry	8 fl oz	0	0	0	0
Seltzer Tropical	8 fl oz	0	0	0	0
Tonic Water	8 fl oz	100	24	0	0
Tonic Water Twist Of Lime	8 fl oz	100	24	0	0
Coca-Cola					
Cherry	8 fl oz	104	28	0	0
Classic	8 fl oz	97	27	0	0
Classic Caffeine-Free	8 fl oz	97	27	0	0
Diet	8 fl oz	1	tr	0	0
Diet Cherry	8 fl oz	1	tr	0	0
Diet Coke Caffeine-free	8 fl oz	1	tr	0	0
Crush					
Pineapple	8 fl oz	140	35	0	0
Tropical Fruit Punch	1 bottle (10 fl oz)	180	44	0	0
Diet Rite					
Cola	8 fl oz	1	tr	0	0
Cola Salt/Sodium Free	8 fl oz	1	tr	0	0

FOOD	PORTION	CALS.	CARB.	FAT	PRO.
Dr. Nehi					
Soda	8 fl oz	100	26	0	0
Fresca					
Soda	8 fl oz	3	tr	0	0
Health Valley					
Ginger Ale	12 oz	153	35	1	1
Sarsaparilla Rootbeer	12 oz	153	35	1	1
Hires					
Cream	8 fl oz	130	0	0	0
Cream Soda Diet	8 fl oz	0	0	0	0
Root Beer	8 fl oz	130	31	0	0
Root Beer Diet	8 fl oz	0	0	0	0
Kick					
Soda	8 fl oz	120	32	0	0
Lucozade					
Soda	7 oz	136	36	0	0
Manischewitz					
Seltzer No Salt Added No Calories	8 fl oz	0	0	0	0
Mello Yellow					
Diet	8 fl oz	4	tr	0	0
Soda	8 fl oz	119	32	0	0
Mountain Dew					
Diet	8 fl oz	2	tr	0	tr
Soda	8 fl oz	118	30	0	tr
Mr. PiBB					
Diet	8 fl oz	1	tr	0	0
Soda	6 oz	97	26	0	0
Mug					
Cream	8 fl oz	122	32	0	tr
Diet Cream	8 fl oz	2	0	0	tr
Diet Root Beer	8 fl oz	1	tr	0	tr
Root Beer	8 fl oz	141	29	0	tr
Orangina					
Sparkling Citrus	6 fl oz	80	19	0	0
Pepsi					
Caffeine Free	8 fl oz	105	27	0	tr
Diet	8 fl oz	1	tr	0	tr
Diet Caffeine Free	8 fl oz	1	tr	0	tr
Regular	8 fl oz	105	27	0	tr
Ramblin' Root Beer	8 fl oz	120	33	0	0
Royal Crown					
Caffeine Free Cola	8 fl oz	110	29	0	0
Cola	8 fl oz	100	28	0	0

FOOD	PORTION	CALS.	CARB.	FAT	PRO.
Royal Crown (CONT.)					
Diet	8 fl oz	1	tr	0	0
Diet	8 fl oz	1	tr	0	0
Diet Caffeine Free	8 fl oz	1	tr	0	0
Royal Mistic					
'N Juice Tropical Supreme	12 fl oz	152	38	0	0
'N Juice Wild Berry	12 fl oz	156	38	0	0
Caribbean Fruit Punch	16 fl oz	230	57	0	0
Sparkling Diet With Lime Kiwi	11.1 fl oz	0	0	0	0
Sparkling Diet With Raspberry Boysenberry	11.1 fl oz	0	0	0	0
Sparkling Diet With Wild Cherry	11.1 fl oz	0	0	0	0
Sparkling With Lime Kiwi	11.1 fl oz	112	28	0	0
Sparkling With Mandarin Orange Pineappple	11.1 fl oz	120	30	0	0
Sparking With Raspberry Boysenberry	11.1 fl oz	112	28	0	0
Sparkling With Royal Peach	11.1 fl oz	112	28	0	0
Schweppes					
Bitter Lemon	8 fl oz	110	28	0	0
Ginger Ale	8 fl oz	90	22	0	0
Ginger Ale Dry Grape	8 fl oz	100	26	0	0
Tonic Water Diet	8 fl oz	0	0	0	0
Slice					
Diet Lemon Lime	8 fl oz	5	tr	0	tr
Lemon Lime	8 fl oz	100	26	0	tr
Snapple					
Amazin' Grape	8 fl oz	120	28	0	0
Cherry Lime Ricky	8 fl oz	110	27	0	0
Kiwi Peach	8 fl oz	120	29	0	0
Mango Madness	8 fl oz	130	33	0	0
Passion Supreme	8 fl oz	120	29	0	0
Sprite					
Diet	8 fl oz	3	0	0	0
Soda	8 fl oz	100	26	0	0
Sunkist					
Diet Citrus	8 fl oz	0	0	0	0

FOOD	PORTION	CALS.	CARB.	FAT	PRO.
Sunkist (CONT.)					
Diet Orange	8 fl oz	5	0	0	0
Fruit Punch	8 fl oz	130	33	0	0
Orange	8 fl oz	140	35	0	0
Strawberry	8 fl oz	140	34	0	0
TAB					
Soda	8 fl oz	1	tr	0	0
Upper 10					
Diet	8 fl oz	3	1	0	0
Diet Salt/Sodium Free	8 fl oz	3	1	0	0
Salt Free	8 fl oz	100	29	0	0
Soda	8 fl oz	100	28	0	0
Wink					
Diet	8 fl oz	5	1	0	0
Soda	8 fl oz	130	31	0	0
Yoo-Hoo					
Original	9 fl oz	150	31	tr	3

SOLDIER BEANS
DRIED

Bean Cuisine					
Dried	½ cup	115	—	1	8

SOLE
FRESH

cooked	3 oz	99	0	1	21
cooked	1 fillet (4.5 oz)	148	0	2	31
lemon raw	3½ oz	85	0	1	17
raw	3½ oz	90	0	1	18

FROZEN

Gorton's					
Fishmarket Fresh	5 oz	110	1	1	24
Microwave Entree In Lemon Butter	1 pkg	380	17	24	25
Microwave Entree In Wine Sauce	1 pkg	180	3	8	25
Mrs. Paul's					
Light Fillets	1 fillet	240	20	10	16
Van De Kamp's					
Light Fillets	1 piece	250	18	12	17
Natural Fillets	4 oz	100	0	2	22

TAKE-OUT

battered & fried	3.2 oz	211	15	11	13
breaded & fried	3.2 oz	211	15	11	13

FOOD	PORTION	CALS.	CARB.	FAT	PRO.
SORBET					
(*see* ICES AND ICE POPS)					
SORGHUM					
sorghum	½ cup	325	72	3	11
SOUFFLE					
HOME RECIPE					
cheese	3.5 oz	253	10	20	11
grand marnier	1 cup	109	14	4	5
lemon chilled	1 cup	176	34	tr	9
raspberry chilled	1 cup	173	34	tr	10
spinach	1 cup	218	3	18	11
SOUP					
CANNED					
asparagus cream of as prep w/ milk	1 cup	161	16	8	6
asparagus cream of as prep w/ water	1 cup	87	11	4	1
beef broth ready-to-serve	1 can (14 oz)	27	tr	1	5
beef broth ready-to-serve	1 cup	16	tr	1	3
beef noodle as prep w/water	1 cup	84	9	3	5
black bean turtle soup	1 cup	218	40	1	14
black bean as prep w/water	1 cup	116	20	2	6
celery cream of as prep w/ milk	1 cup	165	15	10	6
celery cream of as prep w/ water	1 cup	90	9	6	2
celery cream of not prep	1 can (10¾ oz)	219	21	14	4
cheese as prep w/ milk	1 cup	230	16	15	9
cheese as prep w/ water	1 cup	155	11	10	5
cheese not prep	1 can (11 oz)	377	26	25	13
chicken broth as prep w/ water	1 cup	39	1	1	5
chicken cream of as prep w/ milk	1 cup	191	15	11	7
chicken cream of as prep w/ water	1 cup	116	9	7	3
chicken gumbo as prep w/water	1 cup	56	8	1	3
chicken noodle as prep w/ water	1 cup	75	9	2	4
chicken rice as prep w/ water	1 cup	251	7	2	4

FOOD	PORTION	CALS.	CARB.	FAT	PRO.
clam chowder manhattan as prep w/ water	1 cup	77	12	2	2
clam chowder new england as prep w/ water	1 cup	95	12	3	5
clam chowder new england as prep w/ milk	1 cup	163	17	7	9
consomme w/ gelatin not prep	1 can (10½ oz)	71	4	0	13
consomme w/ gelatin as prep w/ water	1 cup	29	2	0	5
escarole ready-to-serve	1 cup	27	2	2	2
french onion as prep w/ water	1 cup	57	8	2	4
gazpacho ready-to-serve	1 cup	57	1	2	9
minestrone as prep w/water	1 cup	83	11	3	4
mushroom cream of as prep w/ milk	1 cup	203	15	14	6
mushroom cream of as prep w/ water	1 cup	129	9	9	2
oyster stew as prep w/ milk	1 cup	134	10	8	6
oyster stew as prep w/ water	1 cup	59	4	4	2
pepperpot as prep w/ water	1 cup	103	9	5	6
potato cream of as prep w/ milk	1 cup	148	17	6	6
potato cream of as prep w/ water	1 cup	73	11	2	2
scotch broth as prep w/ water	1 cup	80	9	3	5
split pea w/ ham as prep w/ water	1 cup	189	28	4	10
tomato as prep w/ milk	1 cup	160	22	6	6
tomato as prep w/water	1 cup	86	17	2	2
vegetarian vegetable as prep w/ water	1 cup	72	12	2	2
vichyssoise	1 cup	148	17	6	6
American Original Foods					
New England Chowder	4 oz	64	8	1	5
New England Chowder as prep w/ milk	4 oz	145	14	6	9
Campbell					
Asparagus Cream Of as prep	8 oz	80	10	4	2

FOOD	PORTION	CALS.	CARB.	FAT	PRO.
Campbell (CONT.)					
Bean Homestyle as prep	8 oz	130	25	1	6
Bean With Bacon as prep	8 oz	140	21	4	6
Beef as prep	8 oz	80	10	2	5
Beef Broth as prep	8 oz	16	1	0	3
Beef Noodle Homestyle as prep	8 oz	80	7	4	5
Beef Noodle as prep	8 oz	70	7	3	4
Beefy Mushroom as prep	8 oz	60	5	3	4
Broccoli Cream Of as prep	8 oz	80	8	5	1
Broccoli Cream Of as prep w/ 2% milk	8 oz	140	14	7	5
Celery Cream Of as prep	8 oz	100	8	7	2
Cheddar Cheese as prep	8 oz	110	10	6	4
Chicken Alphabet as prep	8 oz	80	10	3	3
Chicken & Stars as prep	8 oz	60	7	2	3
Chicken 'n Dumplings as prep	8 oz	80	9	3	4
Chicken Barley as prep	8 oz	70	10	2	3
Chicken Broth as prep	8 oz	30	2	2	1
Chicken Broth & Noodles as prep	8 oz	45	8	1	1
Chicken Cream Of as prep	8 oz	110	9	7	2
Chicken Gumbo as prep	8 oz	60	8	2	2
Chicken Mushroom Creamy as prep	8 oz	120	8	8	3
Chicken Noodle Homestyle as prep	8 oz	70	8	3	3
Chicken Noodle as prep	8 oz	60	8	2	3
Chicken Noodle-O's as prep	8 oz	70	9	2	3
Chicken Vegetable as prep	8 oz	70	8	3	3
Chicken With Rice as prep	8 oz	60	7	3	2
Chili Beef as prep	8 oz	140	20	5	5
Chunky Chicken Nuggets w/ Vegetables & Noodles	10¾ oz	190	24	6	11

FOOD	PORTION	CALS.	CARB.	FAT	PRO.
Campbell (CONT.)					
Clam Chowder Manhattan Style as prep	8 oz	70	10	2	2
Clam Chowder New England as prep	8 oz	80	12	3	3
Clam Chowder New England as prep w/ whole milk	8 oz	150	17	7	7
Consomme as prep	8 oz	25	2	0	4
Curly Noodle With Chicken as prep	8 oz	80	11	3	3
French Onion as prep	8 oz	60	9	2	2
Green Pea as prep	8 oz	160	25	3	8
Healthy Request Bean With Bacon as prep	8 oz	140	22	4	6
Healthy Request Chicken Noodle as prep	8 oz	60	8	2	3
Healthy Request Chicken With Rice as prep	8 oz	60	7	3	2
Healthy Request Cream Of Chicken	8 oz	70	11	2	2
Healthy Request Cream Of Mushroom as prep	8 oz	60	9	2	1
Healthy Request Hearty Chicken Vegetable	8 oz	120	16	2	7
Healthy Request Ready-To-Serve Chicken Broth	8 oz	10	1	0	1
Healthy Request Ready-To-Serve Hearty Chicken Noodle	8 oz	80	7	2	9
Healthy Request Ready-To-Serve Hearty Chicken Rice	8 oz	110	15	2	7
Healthy Request Ready-To-Serve Hearty Minestrone	8 oz	90	13	3	4
Healthy Request Ready-To-Serve Hearty Vegetable	8 oz	110	17	3	3
Healthy Request Ready-To-Serve Hearty Vegetable Beef	8 oz	120	15	3	9

FOOD	PORTION	CALS.	CARB.	FAT	PRO.
Campbell (CONT.)					
Healthy Request Tomato as prep	8 oz	90	17	2	1
Healthy Request Tomato as prep w/ skim milk	8 oz	130	22	2	5
Healthy Request Vegetable as prep	8 oz	90	14	2	3
Healthy Request Vegetable Beef as prep	8 oz	70	9	2	5
Home Cookin' Bean & Ham	10¾ oz	210	29	4	14
Home Cookin' Beef With Vegetables & Pasta	10¾ oz	140	18	2	12
Home Cookin' Chicken Minestrone	10¾ oz	180	17	6	15
Home Cookin' Chicken Gumbo With Sausages	10¾ oz	140	15	4	11
Home Cookin' Chicken Rice	10¾ oz	150	10	6	14
Home Cookin' Chicken With Noodles	10¾ oz	140	12	4	13
Home Cookin' Country Vegetable	10¾ oz	120	20	2	4
Home Cookin' Garden Tomato	10¾ oz	150	29	3	2
Home Cookin' Hearty Lentil	10¾ oz	170	28	2	11
Home Cookin' Minestrone	10¾ oz	140	22	3	4
Home Cookin' Split Pea With Ham	10¾ oz	230	38	1	16
Home Cookin' Vegetable Beef	10¾ oz	140	17	3	13
Minestrone as prep	8 oz	80	13	2	3
Mushroom Cream Of as prep	8 oz	100	8	7	2
Mushroom Golden as prep	8 oz	70	9	3	2
Nacho Cheese as prep	8 oz	110	8	8	4
Nacho Cheese as prep w/ milk	8 oz	180	13	12	8
Noodles & Ground Beef as prep	8 oz	90	10	4	4

FOOD	PORTION	CALS.	CARB.	FAT	PRO.
Campbell (CONT.)					
Onion Cream Of as prep	8 oz	100	12	5	2
Onion Cream Of as prep w/ whole milk & water	8 oz	140	15	7	4
Oyster Stew as prep	8 oz	70	5	5	2
Oyster Stew as prep w/ whole milk	8 oz	140	10	9	6
Pepper Pot as prep	8 oz	90	9	4	5
Potato Cream Of as prep	8 oz	80	12	3	1
Potato Cream Of as prep w/ whole milk & water	8 oz	120	15	4	3
Ready-To-Serve Chunky Beef	10¾ oz	200	24	5	15
Ready-To-Serve Chunky Beef Stroganoff	10¾ oz	320	28	16	15
Ready-To-Serve Chunky Chicken Corn Chowder	10¾ oz	340	23	21	14
Ready-To-Serve Chunky Chicken Noodle	10¾ oz	200	20	7	14
Ready-To-Serve Chunky Chicken Vegetable	9½ oz	170	19	6	10
Ready-To-Serve Chunky Chicken With Rice	9½ oz	140	16	4	10
Ready-To-Serve Chunky Chili Beef	11 oz	290	37	7	21
Ready-To-Serve Chunky Creamy Chicken Mushroom	10½ oz	270	13	19	12
Ready-To-Serve Chunky Creole Style	10¾ oz	240	31	8	11
Ready-To-Serve Chunky Ham 'n Butter Bean	10¾ oz	280	34	10	12
Ready-To-Serve Chunky Manhattan Style Clam Chowder	10¾ oz	160	24	4	7
Ready-To-Serve Chunky Mediterranean Vegetable	9½ oz	170	24	6	4
Ready-To-Serve Chunky New England Clam Chowder	10¾ oz	290	26	17	9
Ready-To-Serve Chunky Old Fashioned Chicken	10¾ oz	180	21	5	12

FOOD	PORTION	CALS.	CARB.	FAT	PRO.
Campbell (CONT.)					
Ready-To-Serve Chunky Old Fashioned Vegetable Beef	10¾ oz	190	20	6	13
Ready-To-Serve Chunky Old Fashioned Bean w/ Ham	11 oz	290	38	9	14
Ready-To-Serve Chunky Pepper Steak	10¾ oz	180	24	3	14
Ready-To-Serve Chunky Sirloin Burger	10¾ oz	220	23	9	12
Ready-To-Serve Chunky Split Pea w/ Ham	10¾ oz	230	33	6	12
Ready-To-Serve Chunky Steak & Potato	10¾ oz	200	24	5	14
Ready-To-Serve Chunky Turkey Vegetable	9⅜ oz	150	16	6	9
Ready-To-Serve Chunky Vegetable	10¾ oz	160	28	4	4
Ready-To-Serve Low Sodium Chicken Vegetable Beef	10¾ oz	180	19	5	14
Ready-To-Serve Low Sodium Chicken Broth	10½ oz	30	2	1	3
Ready-To-Serve Low Sodium Chicken With Noodles	10¾ oz	170	17	5	13
Ready-To-Serve Low Sodium Mushroom Cream Of	10½ oz	210	18	14	3
Ready-To-Serve Low Sodium Split Pea	10¾ oz	230	37	4	12
Ready-To-Use Low Sodium Tomato With Tomato Pieces	10½ oz	190	30	6	4
Reardy-To-Serve Chunky Minestrone	9½ oz	160	24	4	6
Scotch Broth as prep	8 oz	80	9	3	4
Shrimp Cream Of as prep	8 oz	90	8	6	2
Shrimp Cream Of as prep w/ whole milk	8 oz	160	13	10	5
Split Pea With Bacon as prep	8 oz	160	24	4	9

FOOD	PORTION	CALS.	CARB.	FAT	PRO.
Campbell (CONT.)					
Teddy Bear as prep	8 oz	70	11	2	3
Tomato as prep	8 oz	90	17	2	1
Tomato as prep w/ 2% milk	8 oz	150	22	4	5
Tomato Bisque as prep	8 oz	120	22	3	2
Tomato Homestyle Cream Of as prep	8 oz	110	20	3	1
Tomato Homestyle Cream Of as prep w/ whole milk	8 oz	180	25	7	5
Tomato Rice Old Fashioned as prep	8 oz	110	22	2	1
Tomato Zesty as prep	8 oz	100	20	2	1
Turkey Vegetable as prep	8 oz	70	8	3	2
Turkey Noodle as prep	8 oz	70	9	2	3
Vegetable Homestyle as prep	8 oz	60	9	2	2
Vegetable as prep	8 oz	90	14	2	3
Vegetable Beef as prep	8 oz	70	10	2	4
Vegetable Old Fashioned as prep	8 oz	60	9	2	2
Vegetarian Vegetable as prep	8 oz	80	13	2	2
Won Ton as prep	8 oz	40	5	1	2
College Inn					
Beef Broth	½ can (7 oz)	16	1	0	3
Chicken Broth	½ can (7 oz)	35	0	3	1
Chicken Broth Lower Salt	½ can (7 oz)	20	0	2	1
Gold's					
Borscht	8 oz	100	21	0	4
Borscht Lo-Cal	8 oz	20	5	tr	1
Schav	8 oz	25	4	0	2
Gorton's					
New England Clam Chowder as prep w/ whole milk	¼ can	140	17	5	7
Goya					
Black Bean	7.5 oz	160	29	4	11
Hain					
Chicken Broth	8¾ fl oz	70	0	6	2
Chicken Broth No Salt Added	8¾ fl oz	60	0	5	3

FOOD	PORTION	CALS.	CARB.	FAT	PRO.
Hain (CONT.)					
Chicken Noodle	9½ fl oz	120	11	4	9
Chicken Noodle No Salt Added	9½ fl oz	120	12	4	9
Creamy Mushroom	9¼ fl oz	110	16	4	4
Italian Vegetable Pasta	9½ fl oz	160	25	5	4
Italian Vegetable Pasta Low Sodium	9½ fl oz	140	22	6	4
Minestrone	9½ fl oz	170	27	2	8
Minestrone No Salt Added	9½ fl oz	160	28	4	7
Mushroom Barley	9½ fl oz	100	17	2	4
New England Clam Chowder	9¼ fl oz	180	26	4	8
Split Pea	9½ fl oz	170	28	1	11
Split Pea No Salt Added	9½ fl oz	170	29	1	11
Turkey Rice	9½ fl oz	100	10	3	8
Turkey Rice No Salt Added	9½ fl oz	120	13	4	7
Vegetable Broth	9½ fl oz	45	10	0	1
Vegetable Broth Low Sodium	9½ fl oz	40	8	tr	1
Vegetable Chicken	9½ fl oz	120	14	4	8
Vegetable Chicken No Salt Added	9½ fl oz	130	14	4	8
Vegetable Split Pea	9½ fl oz	170	28	1	11
Vegetable Split Pea No Salt Added	9½ fl oz	170	27	1	13
Vegetarian Lentil	9½ fl oz	160	25	3	9
Vegetarian Lentil No Salt Added	9½ fl oz	160	24	3	9
Vegetarian Vegetable	9½ fl oz	140	22	4	4
Vegetarian Vegetable No Salt Added	9½ fl oz	150	23	5	5
Health Valley					
Beef Broth	7.5 oz	10	2	tr	1
Beef Broth No Salt Added	7.5 oz	10	2	tr	1
Black Bean	7.5 oz	150	24	2	7
Black Bean No Salt Added	7.5 oz	150	24	2	7
Chicken Broth	7.5 oz	35	1	2	4
Chicken Broth No Salt Added	7.5 oz	35	1	2	4

FOOD	PORTION	CALS.	CARB.	FAT	PRO.
Health Valley (CONT.)					
Chunky Chicken Vegetable	7.5 oz	125	20	2	7
Chunky Five Bean Vegetable	7.5 oz	110	21	2	4
Chunky Five Bean Vegetable No Salt Added	7.5 oz	110	21	2	4
Chunky Vegetable Chicken No Salt Added	7.5 oz	125	20	2	7
Green Split Pea	7.5 oz	180	34	tr	11
Green Split Pea No Salt Added	7.5 oz	180	34	tr	11
Lentil	7.5 oz	220	33	4	13
Lentil No Salt Added	7.5 oz	220	4	4	13
Manhattan Clam Chowder	7.5 oz	110	15	2	6
Manhattan Clam Chowder No Salt Added	7.5 oz	110	15	2	6
Minestrone	7.5 oz	130	19	3	6
Minestrone No Salt Added	7.5 oz	130	19	3	6
Mushroom Barley	7.5 oz	100	2	2	5
Mushroom Barley No Salt Added	7.5 oz	100	16	2	5
Potato Leek	7.5 oz	130	23	2	4
Potato Leek No Salt Added	7.5 oz	130	23	2	4
Tomato	7.5 oz	130	21	3	3
Tomato No Salt Added	7.5 oz	130	21	3	3
Vegetable	7.5 oz	110	20	1	4
Vegetable No Salt Added	7.5 oz	110	20	1	4
Healthy Choice					
Bean & Ham	1 cup (8.7 oz)	180	34	3	10
Beef & Potato	1 cup (8.5 oz)	120	18	2	10
Chicken Corn Chowder	1 cup (8.8 oz)	150	27	3	7
Chicken With Pasta	1 cup (8.6 oz)	120	18	3	7
Chicken With Rice	1 cup (8.4 oz)	100	13	3	7
Chili Beef	1 cup (9 oz)	190	33	1	15
Country Vegetable	1 cup (8.6 oz)	100	22	1	4
Garden Vegetable	1 cup (8.6 oz)	110	22	1	5
Hearty Chicken	1 cup (8.7 oz)	140	20	3	9

FOOD	PORTION	CALS.	CARB.	FAT	PRO.
Healthy Choice (CONT.)					
Lentil	1 cup (8.7 oz)	140	30	1	7
Minestrone	1 cup (8.6 oz)	110	21	2	6
New England Clam Chowder	1 cup (8.8 oz)	130	19	3	9
Old Fashioned Chicken Noodle	1 cup (8.8 oz)	130	21	2	10
Split Pea With Ham	1 cup (8.8 oz)	160	26	2	11
Tomato Garden	1 cup (8.6 oz)	110	19	2	5
Turkey With White & Wild Rice	1 cup (8.4 oz)	110	18	3	6
Vegetable Beef	1 cup (8.8 oz)	170	32	2	9
Hormel					
Bean & Ham	1 cup (7.5 oz)	190	28	4	9
Beef Vegetable	1 cup (7.5 oz)	90	14	1	6
Broccoli Cheese With Ham	1 cup (7.5 oz)	170	10	13	4
Chicken & Rice	1 cup (7.5 oz)	110	17	3	5
Chicken Noodle	1 cup (7.5 oz)	110	13	3	7
New England Clam Chowder	1 cup (7.5 oz)	130	16	5	5
Potato Cheese With Ham	1 cup (7.5 oz)	190	16	13	4
Manischewitz					
Borscht Low Calorie	8 fl oz	20	4	0	1
Borscht With Beets	8 fl oz	80	20	0	1
Old El Paso					
Black Bean With Bacon	1 cup	160	26	2	11
Chicken Vegetable	1 cup	110	13	3	9
Chicken With Rice	1 cup	90	10	3	8
Garden Vegetable	1 cup	110	17	3	5
Hearty Beef	1 cup	120	14	3	10
Hearty Chicken Noodle	1 cup	110	10	3	9
Progresso					
Beef	1 can (10.5 fl oz)	180	17	6	15
Beef Barley	1 can (10.5 fl oz)	150	16	5	13
Beef Minestrone	1 can (10.5 fl oz)	180	18	6	15
Beef Noodle	9.5 fl oz	170	18	4	15
Beef Vegetable	1 can (10.5 fl oz)	170	18	3	17
Chickarina	9.5 fl oz	130	13	5	8
Chicken Barley	9.25 fl oz	100	12	2	10
Chicken Broth	4 fl oz	8	0	0	2
Chicken Cream Of	9.5 fl oz	190	12	11	10
Chicken Minestrone	1 can (10.5 fl oz)	140	14	4	12
Chicken Noodle	1 can (10.5 fl oz)	120	8	4	12

FOOD	PORTION	CALS.	CARB.	FAT	PRO.
Progresso (CONT.)					
Chicken Rice	1 can (10.5 fl oz)	120	12	4	9
Chicken Vegetable	1 can (10.5 fl oz)	150	18	4	10
Corn Chowder	9.25 fl oz	200	22	10	5
Escarole In Chicken Broth	9.25 fl oz	30	2	1	2
Green Split Pea	1 can (10.5 fl oz)	201	31	3	12
Ham & Bean	9.5 fl oz	140	28	2	11
Hearty Minestrone	9.25 fl oz	110	16	2	7
Hearty Beef	9.5 fl oz	160	15	4	15
Hearty Chicken	1 can (10.5 fl oz)	130	9	4	14
Homestyle Chicken	9.5 fl oz	110	12	3	11
Lentil	1 can (10.5 fl oz)	140	24	4	10
Lentil With Sausage	9.5 fl oz	170	21	8	8
Macaroni & Bean	1 can (10.5 fl oz)	150	27	4	9
Manhattan Clam Chowder	9.5 fl oz	120	13	2	13
Minestrone	1 can (10.5 fl oz)	120	25	3	7
Mushroom Cream Of	9.25 fl oz	160	14	10	4
New England Style Clam Chowder	1 can (10.5 fl oz)	220	21	12	7
Seasoned Beef Broth	4 fl oz	40	tr	tr	2
Split Pea With Ham	1 can (10.5 fl oz)	160	24	5	11
Tomato	9.5 fl oz	120	20	3	4
Tomato Beef With Rotini	9.5 fl oz	170	18	6	12
Tomato Tortellini	9.5 fl oz	130	16	5	5
Tortellini	9.5 fl oz	90	11	3	5
Tortellini Creamy	9.25 fl oz	240	17	16	5
Vegetable	1 can (10.5 fl oz)	80	15	2	4
Zesty Minestrone	9.5 fl oz	150	19	8	7
Snow's					
Manhattan Clam Chowder as prep w/ water	7.5 fl oz	70	9	2	3
New England Clam Chowder as prep w/ milk	7.5 fl oz	140	13	6	8
New England Corn Chowder as prep w/ milk	7.5 fl oz	150	18	6	5
New England Fish Chowder as prep w/ milk	7.5 fl oz	130	11	6	9

FOOD	PORTION	CALS.	CARB.	FAT	PRO.
Snow's (CONT.)					
New England Seafood Chowder as prep w/ milk	7.5 fl oz	130	11	6	8
Swanson					
Beef Broth	7¼ oz	18	1	1	2
Chicken Broth	7¼ oz	30	2	2	2
Natural Goodness Clear Chicken Broth	7¼ oz	20	1	1	2
Vegetable Broth	7.25 fl oz	20	3	1	0
Weight Watchers					
Chicken Noodle	10.5 oz	80	9	2	6
Mushroom Cream Of	10.5 oz	90	14	2	3
DRY					
asparagus cream of as prep w/ water	1 cup	59	9	2	2
beef broth	1 pkg (0.2 oz)	14	1	1	1
beef broth as prep w/ water	1 cup	19	2	1	1
beef broth cube	1 cube (3.6 g)	6	1	tr	1
beef broth cube as prep w/water	1 cup	8	1	tr	1
celery cream of as prep w/ water	1 cup	63	10	2	3
chicken broth	1 pkg (0.2 oz)	16	1	1	1
chicken broth as prep w/water	1 cup	21	1	1	1
chicken broth cube	1 cube (4.8 g)	9	1	tr	1
chicken broth cube as prep w/ water	1 cup	13	2	tr	1
chicken cream of as prep w/ water	1 cup	107	13	5	2
chicken noodle as prep w/ water	1 cup	53	7	1	3
french onion not prep	1 pkg (1.4 oz)	115	21	2	5
leek as prep w/ water	1 cup	71	11	2	2
onion as prep w/ water	1 cup	28	5	1	1
tomato as prep w/ water	1 cup	102	19	2	2
4C					
Noodle	8 oz	50	7	2	2
Onion Reduced Salt	8 oz	30	5	1	1
Armour					
Bouillon Cubes Beef	1 (4 g)	5	1	0	0
Bouillon Cubes Chicken	1 (4 g)	5	1	0	0

FOOD	PORTION	CALS.	CARB.	FAT	PRO.
Arrowhead					
Bean & Barley	¼ cup (1.9 oz)	170	35	0	12
Bean Cuisine					
Bean Bouillabaisse	1 cup (7.5 fl oz)	174	18	tr	6
Island Black Bean	1 cup (8.6 fl oz)	202	24	tr	7
Lots of Lentil	1 cup (7.7 oz)	166	19	tr	6
Mesa Maize	1 cup (9.2 fl oz)	179	21	tr	6
Rocky Mountain Red Bean	1 cup (8.6 oz)	202	24	tr	7
Sante Fe Corn Chowder	1 cup (9.2 oz)	179	21	tr	6
Thick As Fog Split Pea	1 cup (8.6 fl oz)	189	21	tr	8
Ultima Pasta E Fagioli	1 cup (8.6 fl oz)	179	22	tr	7
White Bean Provencal	1 cup (7.7 fl oz)	166	19	tr	6
Campbell					
Bean With Bacon 'n Ham Microwave	7½ oz	230	38	5	8
Chicken Noodle Microwave	7½ oz	100	11	4	5
Chicken Noodle as prep	8 oz	100	16	2	5
Chicken With Rice Microwave	7½ oz	100	14	4	3
Chili Beef Microwave	7½ oz	190	32	4	7
Hearty Noodle as prep	8 oz	90	15	1	4
Noodle as prep	8 oz	110	19	2	5
Onion as prep	8 oz	30	7	0	1
Vegetable as prep	8 oz	40	8	0	1
Vegetable Beef Microwave	7½ oz	100	16	2	5
Campbell's Cup					
Beef Noodle	1 (1.35 oz)	130	23	2	6
Chicken Noodle	1 (1.35 oz)	140	22	3	7
Chicken Noodle w/ White Meat as prep	6 oz	90	12	2	6
Creamy Chicken w/ White Meat as prep	6 oz	90	12	4	3
Hearty Noodles With Vegetables	1 (1.7 oz)	180	32	2	7
Noodle With Chicken Broth as prep	6 oz	90	15	2	4
Casbah					
Black Bean	1 pkg (1.7 oz)	170	30	2	9
Split Pea	1 pkg (2.3 oz)	230	40	1	15
Sweet Corn Chowder	1 pkg (1.2 oz)	125	26	1	4
Vegetarian Chili	1 pkg (1.8 oz)	170	31	2	10

FOOD	PORTION	CALS.	CARB.	FAT	PRO.
Cup-A-Ramen					
Beef With Vegetables Low Fat as prep	8 oz	220	44	2	7
Beef With Vegetables as prep	8 oz	270	38	10	6
Chicken With Vegetables Low Fat as prep	8 oz	220	44	2	7
Chicken With Vegetables as prep	8 oz	270	38	10	6
Oriental With Vegetables Low Fat as prep	8 oz	220	44	2	7
Oriental With Vegetables as prep	8 oz	270	38	10	6
Shrimp With Vegetables Low Fat as prep	8 oz	230	45	2	7
Shrimp With Vegetables as prep	8 oz	280	40	10	6
Cup-A-Soup					
Chicken Broth	6 oz	19	3	1	tr
Chicken Vegetable	6 oz	47	8	1	3
Creamy Broccoli And Cheese	6 oz	70	10	3	2
Green Pea	6 oz	113	14	4	4
Hearty Chicken And Noodles	6 oz	110	20	2	4
Hearty Creamy Chicken Lots-A-Noodles	7 oz	179	21	8	5
Mushroom Cream Of	6 oz	71	9	3	1
Onion	6 oz	27	5	1	1
Tomato	6 oz	103	21	1	3
Emes					
Beef Base	1 tsp	18	2	tr	3
Chicken Base	1 tsp	18	2	tr	3
Fantastic					
Cha-Cha Chili Low Fat	1 pkg	220	37	1	18
Golden Dipt					
Lobster Bisque	¼ pkg	30	5	1	1
Manhattan Clam Chowder	¼ pkg	80	13	2	2
New England Clam Chowder	¼ pkg	24	12	2	2
Seafood Chowder	¼ pkg	70	12	2	2
Shrimp Bisque	¼ pkg	30	5	1	1
Goodman's					
Cup Of Soup Beef	1 pkg (1½ cups)	180	32	3	7

FOOD	PORTION	CALS.	CARB.	FAT	PRO.
Goodman's (CONT.)					
Cup Of Soup Chicken Noodle	1 pkg (1½ cups)	180	31	3	7
Cup Of Soup Vegetable	1 pkg (1½ cups)	180	32	3	8
Matzo Ball & Soup	1 cup	40	9	1	2
Matzo Ball & Soup 50% Less Salt	1 serv	50	10	1	2
Noodleman	1 cup	45	9	1	2
Noodleman Low Sodium	1 cup	50	9	1	2
Onion	1 cup	30	5	1	1
Onion Low Sodium	1 cup	30	6	1	1
Hain					
Cheese & Broccoli	¾ cup	310	19	22	7
Cheese Savory	¾ cup	250	20	16	6
Savory Lentil	¾ cup	130	20	2	4
Savory Minestrone	¾ cup	110	20	1	4
Savory Mushroom	¾ cup	210	11	15	4
Savory Mushroom No Salt Added	¾ cup	250	15	20	5
Savory Onion	¾ cup	50	6	2	2
Savory Onion No Salt Added	¾ cup	50	9	1	1
Savory Potato Leek	¾ cup	260	20	18	4
Savory Split Pea	¾ cup	310	16	10	4
Savory Tomato	¾ cup	220	19	14	3
Savory Vegetable	¾ cup	80	13	1	2
Savory Vegetable No Salt Added	¾ cup	80	13	1	2
Herb-Ox					
Beef Bouillon	1 cube (3.5 g)	10	1	0	0
Beef Instant Bouillon Powder	1 tsp (4 g)	10	1	0	0
Beef Instant Broth & Seasoning Pack	1 pkg (4.5 g)	10	1	0	0
Beef Instant Broth & Seasoning Pack Low Sodium	1 pkg (4 g)	15	2	0	0
Chicken Bouillon	1 cube (4 g)	10	1	0	0
Chicken Instant Bouillon Powder	1 tsp (4 g)	10	1	0	0
Chicken Instant Broth & Seasoning Pack	1 pkg (5 g)	10	1	0	0
Chicken Instant Broth & Seasoning Pack Low Sodium	1 pkg (4 g)	15	1	0	0

FOOD	PORTION	CALS.	CARB.	FAT	PRO.
Herb-Ox (cont.)					
Vegetable Bouillon	1 cube (4 g)	10	1	0	0
Hodgson Mill					
13 Bean not prep	1.5 oz	100	14	1	9
Hurst					
15 Bean Soup Beef	1 serv (1.7 oz)	160	27	1	11
15 Bean Soup Cajun	1 serv (1.7 oz)	160	27	1	11
15 Bean Soup Chicken	1 serv (1.7 oz)	160	27	1	11
15 Bean Soup Chili	1 serv (1.7 oz)	160	27	1	11
15 Bean Soup Ham	1 serv (1.7 oz)	160	26	1	11
Spanish-American Black Bean	1 serv (1.3 oz)	120	22	1	7
Ka-Me					
Won Ton Chicken not prep	1 pkg (1.25 oz)	180	18	11	4
Won Ton Pork not prep	1 pkg (1.25 oz)	180	18	11	4
Knorr					
Black Bean Cup-A-Soup as prep	1 pkg	200	37	1	11
Broccoli as prep	8 fl oz	160	16	8	6
Cauliflower as prep	8 fl oz	100	13	3	5
Chef's Series Wild Mushroom as prep	8 fl oz	100	14	3	3
Chick 'N Pasta as prep	8 fl oz	90	16	2	4
Chicken Bouillon as prep	8 fl oz	16	tr	1	tr
Chicken Flavored Noodle as prep	8 fl oz	100	18	2	4
Chicken Noodle Instant as prep	6 fl oz	25	4	tr	1
Fine Herb as prep	8 fl oz	130	15	6	4
Fish Bouillon as prep	8 fl oz	10	tr	tr	1
French Onion as prep	8 fl oz	50	9	1	1
Hearty Minestrone Cup-A-Soup as prep	1 pkg	150	29	1	5
Lentil Cup-A-Soup as prep	1 pkg	220	40	0	13
Mushroom as prep	8 fl oz	100	12	4	4
Navy Bean Cup-A-Soup as prep	1 pkg	140	27	0	7
Oriental Hot And Sour as prep	8 fl oz	50	9	1	1
Oxtail Hearty Beef as prep	8 fl oz	70	10	2	2
Potato Leek Cup-A-Soup as prep	1 pkg	120	24	0	4

FOOD	PORTION	CALS.	CARB.	FAT	PRO.
Knorr (CONT.)					
Spinach as prep	8 fl oz	100	11	5	3
Spring Vegetable With Herbs as prep	8 fl oz	30	6	tr	1
Tomato Basil as prep	8 fl oz	90	14	3	2
Tortellini In Brodo as prep	8 fl oz	60	11	1	2
Vegetable Cup-A-Soup as prep	1 pkg	100	21	0	3
Vegetable as prep	8 fl oz	35	7	1	1
Vegetarian Vegetable Bouillon as prep	8 fl oz	16	1	1	tr
Kojel					
Hearty Potato With Vegetables Instant	1 serv (6 fl oz)	60	15	0	1
Noodle Soup Chicken Flavor Instant	1 serv (6 fl oz)	70	11	1	4
Split Pea Instant	1 serv (6 fl oz)	60	14	tr	3
Tomato Instant	1 serv 6 fl oz	50	15	0	1
Vegetable Chicken Couscous Instant	1 serv (6 fl oz)	80	18	1	4
Lipton					
Beef Mushroom	8 oz	38	7	1	2
Beefy Onion	8 oz	27	5	1	1
Chicken Noodle	8 oz	82	12	2	4
Chicken Noodle Hearty	8 oz	81	14	1	4
Country Vegetable	8 oz	80	16	1	3
Giggle Noodle	8 oz	72	12	2	2
Hearty Noodles With Vegetables	8 oz	75	12	2	3
Instant Oriental Noodle Beef	8 oz	177	34	1	8
Instant Oriental Noodle Chicken	8 oz	180	33	2	8
Onion	8 oz	20	4	tr	1
Onion Golden	8 oz	62	11	2	1
Onion Mushroom	8 oz	41	7	1	1
Ring-O-Noodle	8 oz	67	11	2	2
Vegetable	8 oz	37	7	1	2
Lite Line					
Beef Bouillon Instant Low Sodium	1 tsp	12	2	tr	tr
Chicken Bouillon Instant Low Sodium	1 tsp	12	2	tr	tr

FOOD	PORTION	CALS.	CARB.	FAT	PRO.
Manischewitz					
Minestrone as prep	6 fl oz	50	9	tr	3
Split Pea as prep	6 fl oz	45	9	tr	3
Vegetable as prep	6 fl oz	50	9	tr	3
Maruchan					
Instant Lunch Oriental Noodles Beef	1 pkg (2.25 oz)	290	37	13	6
Instant Lunch Oriental Noodles Chicken	1 pkg (2.25 oz)	290	36	13	6
Instant Lunch Oriental Noodles Chicken Mushroom	1 pkg (2.25 oz)	280	34	13	6
Instant Lunch Oriental Noodles Mushroom	1 pkg (2.25 oz)	290	35	13	6
Instant Lunch Oriental Noodles Pork	1 pkg (2.25 oz)	290	35	13	6
Instant Lunch Oriental Noodles Shrimp	1 pkg (2.25 oz)	290	37	13	7
Instant Lunch Oriental Noodles Toast Onion	1 pkg (2.25 oz)	270	34	12	6
Instant Lunch Oriental Noodles Vegetable Beef	1 pkg (2.25 oz)	290	34	12	6
Instant Wonton Chicken	1 pkg (1.49 oz)	200	19	12	5
Instant Wonton Hot & Sour	1 pkg (1.49 oz)	200	21	11	4
Instant Wonton Oriental	1 pkg (1.49 oz)	190	19	12	5
Instant Wonton Pork	1 pkg (1.49 oz)	200	19	12	5
Instant Wonton Shrimp	1 pkg (1.49 oz)	200	19	12	6
Oriental Noodle Picante Style Beef	1 pkg (2.25 oz)	290	37	15	7
Oriental Noodle Picante Style Chicken	1 pkg (2.25 oz)	290	38	15	7
Oriental Noodle Picante Style Shrimp	1 pkg (2.25 oz)	300	36	16	7
Ramen Beef	½ pkg (1.5 oz)	190	26	9	5
Ramen Chicken	½ pkg (1.5 oz)	190	20	8	5
Ramen Chicken Mushroom	½ pkg (1.5 oz)	190	25	8	4
Ramen Chili	½ pkg (1.5 oz)	190	26	9	5
Ramen Mushroom	½ pkg (1.5 oz)	190	25	9	5
Ramen Oriental	½ pkg (1.5 oz)	190	26	9	5
Ramen Pork	½ pkg (1.5 oz)	190	25	9	5
Ramen Shrimp	½ pkg (1.5 oz)	190	26	9	5

FOOD	PORTION	CALS.	CARB.	FAT	PRO.
Maruchan (CONT.)					
Wonton Beef	⅓ pkg (0.68 oz)	90	8	5	2
Wonton Chicken	⅓ pkg (0.67 oz)	90	8	5	2
Wonton Pork	⅓ pkg (0.68 oz)	90	9	5	2
Wonton Vegetable	⅓ pkg (0.7 oz)	90	9	6	2
Nile Spice					
Couscous Almondine	1 pkg	200	37	3	7
Couscous Garbanzo	1 pkg	220	39	3	9
Couscous Lentil Curry	1 pkg	200	36	2	10
Couscous Minestrone	1 pkg	180	34	2	8
Couscous Parmesan	1 pkg	200	34	3	8
Homestyle Black Bean	1 pkg	190	34	2	11
Homestyle Chicken Flavored Vegetable	1 pkg	120	20	2	4
Homestyle Lentil	1 pkg	180	31	2	12
Homestyle Minestrone	1 pkg	160	29	2	8
Homestyle Red Beans & Rice	1 pkg	190	36	2	9
Homestyle Split Pea	1 pkg	200	35	2	13
Homestyle Sweet Corn Chowder	1 pkg	120	20	3	3
Italian Tomato	1 pkg	140	21	4	4
Potato Leek	1 pkg	150	21	6	4
Potato Romano	1 pkg	140	19	5	5
Ramen Noodle					
Beef Low Fat as prep	8 oz	160	32	1	5
Beef as prep	8 oz	190	26	8	5
Chicken Low Fat as prep	8 oz	160	32	1	5
Chicken as prep	8 oz	190	26	8	5
Oriental Low Fat as prep	8 oz	150	31	1	5
Oriental as prep	8 oz	190	26	8	5
Pork Low Fat as prep	8 oz	150	31	1	4
Pork as prep	8 oz	200	26	8	5
Ultra Slim-Fast					
Beef Noodle	6 oz	45	7	tr	4
Chicken Leek	6 oz	50	7	tr	5
Chicken Noodle	6 oz	45	6	tr	5
Creamy Broccoli	6 oz	75	14	tr	5
Creamy Tomato	6 oz	60	10	tr	5
Hearty Vegetable	6 oz	50	7	tr	5
Onion	6 oz	45	7	tr	4
Potato Leek	6 oz	80	15	tr	5
Weight Watchers					
Beef Broth Instant	1 pkg	8	1	0	1

FOOD	PORTION	CALS.	CARB.	FAT	PRO.
Weight Watchers (CONT.)					
Chicken Broth Instant	1 pkg	8	1	0	1
Chicken Noodle	7.5 oz	90	13	1	8
Chunky Beef Stew	7.5 oz	120	14	2	14
New England Clam Chowder	7.5 oz	90	16	0	5
Vegetable Beef	7.5 oz	90	13	1	8
Wylers					
Beef Bouillon Instant	1 tsp	6	1	tr	tr
Beef Bouillon Instant Cube	1	6	1	tr	tr
Chicken Bouillon Instant	1 tsp	8	1	tr	tr
Chicken Bouillon Instant Cube	1	8	1	tr	tr
Onion Bouillon Instant	1 tsp	10	1	tr	tr
Vegetable Bouillon Instant	1 tsp	6	1	tr	tr
FROZEN					
Jaclyn's					
Barley & Mushroom	7.5 fl oz	90	16	1	2
Split Pea	7.5 fl oz	180	31	2	11
Vegetable	7.5 fl oz	90	18	1	4
Kettle Ready					
Asparagus Cream Of	6 oz	62	5	5	1
Black Bean With Ham	6 oz	154	23	6	8
Boston Clam Chowder	6 oz	131	13	7	4
Broccoli Cream Of	6 oz	94	6	7	1
Cauliflower Cream Of	6 oz	93	6	7	2
Cheddar Broccoli Cream Of	6 oz	137	5	11	4
Chicken Cream Of	6 oz	98	5	6	6
Chicken Gumbo	6 oz	94	12	4	4
Chicken Noodle	6 oz	94	12	3	5
Chili	6 oz	161	14	7	12
Corn & Broccoli Chowder	6 oz	102	13	5	1
Creamy Cheddar	6 oz	158	7	13	4
French Onion	6 oz	42	5	2	1
Garden Vegetable	6 oz	85	12	3	3
Hearty Minestrone	6 oz	104	15	4	3
Hearty Beef Vegetable	6 oz	85	11	3	4
Manhattan Clam Chowder	6 oz	69	8	3	4
Mushroom Cream Of	6 oz	85	6	6	1

FOOD	PORTION	CALS.	CARB.	FAT	PRO.
Kettle Ready (CONT.)					
New England Clam Chowder	6 oz	116	11	7	3
Potato Cream Of	6 oz	121	17	5	2
Savory Bean With Ham	6 oz	113	20	4	7
Split Pea With Ham	6 oz	155	25	4	11
Tomato Florentine	6 oz	106	15	4	3
Tortellini In Tomato	6 oz	122	15	5	4
Tabatchnick					
Barley Mushroom	1 serv (7.5 oz)	70	13	0	2
Barley Mushroom No Salt Added	1 serv (7.5 oz)	70	13	0	2
Broccoli Cream Of	1 serv (7.5 oz)	90	12	4	3
Cabbage	1 serv (7.5 oz)	60	14	0	1
Chicken With Dumplings	1 serv (7.5 oz)	70	13	2	1
Corn Chowder	1 serv (7.5 oz)	150	22	6	3
Minestrone	1 serv (7.5 oz)	150	27	1	9
New England Potato	1 serv (7.5 oz)	150	21	6	4
New York Chicken	1 serv (7.5 oz)	35	6	0	2
Old Fashion Potato	1 serv (7.5 oz)	70	16	0	2
Pea	1 serv (7.5 oz)	180	31	2	12
Pea No Salt Added	1 serv (7.5 oz)	180	31	2	12
Spinach Cream Of	1 serv (7.5 oz)	90	11	4	3
Vegetable	1 serv (7.5 oz)	110	20	1	5
Vegetable No Salt Added	1 serv (7.5 oz)	110	20	1	5
Wisconsin Cheddar Vegetable	1 serv (7.5 oz)	140	12	9	4
Yankee Bean	1 serv (7.5 oz)	160	27	2	10
SHELF-STABLE					
Lunch Bucket					
Chicken Noodle	1 pkg (7.25 oz)	90	13	2	4
Country Vegetable	1 pkg (7.25 oz)	70	15	1	1
TAKE-OUT					
beef stew soup	1 cup (8.8 oz)	221	20	5	23
black bean turtle soup	1 cup	241	45	1	15
brunswick stew soup	1 cup (8.5 oz)	232	17	6	27
corn & cheese chowder	¾ cup	215	21	12	9
gazpacho	1 cup	46	5	tr	1
greek	¾ cup	63	7	2	4
hot & sour	1 serv (14 oz)	173	8	8	15
oxtail	5 oz	64	7	3	4
pasta e fagioli	1 cup (8.8 oz)	194	30	5	9
ratatouille	1 cup (7.5 oz)	266	12	25	2

FOOD	PORTION	CALS.	CARB.	FAT	PRO.
SOUR CREAM					
(see also SOUR CREAM SUBSTITUTES)					
sour cream	1 cup	493	10	48	7
sour cream	1 tbsp	26	1	3	tr
Breakstone					
Free	2 tbsp (1.1 oz)	35	6	0	2
Half & Half	2 tbsp (1.1 oz)	45	2	4	1
Sour Cream	2 tbsp (1 oz)	60	1	5	1
Cabot					
Light	1 oz	33	2	2	1
Sour Cream	1 oz	60	1	6	1
Friendship					
Light	2 tbsp (1 oz)	35	2	3	1
Sour Cream	2 tbsp (1 oz)	60	2	5	1
Heluva Good Cheese					
Fat-Free	2 tbsp (1.1 oz)	20	3	0	1
Light	2 tbsp (1.1 oz)	40	3	3	1
Sour Cream	2 tbsp (1.1 oz)	60	2	5	1
Hood					
Fat Free	2 tbsp (1 oz)	20	3	0	1
Light	2 tbsp (1 oz)	40	2	3	1
Sour Cream	2 tbsp (1 oz)	60	2	5	1
Knudsen					
Free	2 tbsp (1.1 oz)	35	6	0	2
Hampshire	2 tbsp (1 oz)	60	1	6	1
Light	2 tbsp (1.1 oz)	40	2	3	2
Naturally Yours					
No Fat	2 tbsp (1 fl oz)	15	1	0	3
Sealtest					
Free	2 tbsp (1.1 oz)	35	6	0	2
Light	2 tbsp (1.1 oz)	40	2	3	2
Sour Cream	2 tbsp (1 oz)	60	1	5	tr
Weight Watchers					
Light Sour	2 tbsp	35	2	2	2
SOUR CREAM SUBSTITUTES					
nondairy	1 cup	479	15	45	6
nondairy	1 oz	59	2	6	1
Pet					
Imitation	1 tbsp	25	tr	2	tr
Tofutti					
Better Than Sour Cream	1 oz	50	1	5	1
Sour Supreme					

FOOD	PORTION	CALS.	CARB.	FAT	PRO.

SOY
(see also ICE CREAM AND FROZEN DESSERTS, MILK SUBSTITUTES, MISO, SOY SAUCE, SOYBEANS, TEMPEH AND TOFU)

FOOD	PORTION	CALS.	CARB.	FAT	PRO.
lecithin	1 tbsp	104	0	14	0
roasted & toasted	1 cup	490	33	26	40
soy milk	1 cup	79	4	5	7
soya cheese	1.4 oz	128	tr	11	7
Eden					
Tamari Organic Domestic	1 tbsp (0.5 oz)	15	2	0	2
Tamari Organic Imported	1 tbsp (0.5 oz)	15	2	0	2
LaLoma					
Soyagen All Purpose	¼ cup	130	14	6	6
Soyagen Carob	¼ cup	140	16	6	6
Soyagen No Sucrose	¼ cup	130	14	6	6
Tree Of Life					
Shoyu	1 tbsp (0.5 oz)	15	1	0	2
Tamari Reduced Sodium	1 tbsp (0.5 oz)	20	1	0	2
Tamari Wheat Free	1 tbsp (0.5 oz)	15	1	0	2
Worthington					
Soyamel	1 oz	130	11	7	6

SOY SAUCE
(see also SAUCE, SOY)

FOOD	PORTION	CALS.	CARB.	FAT	PRO.
shoyu	1 tbsp	9	2	tr	1
soy sauce	1 tbsp	7	1	tr	tr
tamari	1 tbsp	11	1	tr	2
Eden					
Shoyu Organic	1 tbsp (0.5 oz)	15	2	0	2
Shoyu Traditional	1 tbsp (0.5 oz)	15	2	0	2
House Of Tsang					
Dark	1 tbsp (0.6 oz)	10	1	0	1
Ginger Flavored Low Sodium	1 tbsp (0.6 oz)	10	2	0	0
Ginger Flavored	1 tbsp (0.6 oz)	20	4	0	1
Light	1 tbsp (0.6 oz)	5	0	0	1
Low Sodium	1 tbsp (0.6 oz)	5	0	0	0
Mushroom Flavored Low Sodium	1 tbsp (0.6 oz)	10	2	0	0
Ka-Me					
Chinese Dark	1 tbsp (0.5 fl oz)	10	3	0	0
Chinese Light	1 tbsp (0.5 fl oz)	5	1	0	0
Dark	1 tbsp (0.5 fl oz)	10	3	0	0
Japanese	1 tbsp (0.5 fl oz)	5	1	0	0

FOOD	PORTION	CALS.	CARB.	FAT	PRO.
Ka-Me (CONT.)					
Light	1 tbsp (0.5 oz)	5	1	0	0
Mild	1 tbsp (0.5 fl oz)	5	0	0	1
Kikkoman					
Lite	1 tbsp	13	2	0	1
Soy Sauce	1 tbsp	12	2	0	1
La Choy					
Lite	½ tsp	1	tr	tr	tr
Soy Sauce	½ tsp	2	tr	tr	tr
Trappey					
Chef Magic	1 tbsp (0.5 oz)	23	4	tr	1

SOYBEANS

(see also MILK SUBSTITUTES, MISO, SOY, TEMPEH, AND TOFU)

FOOD	PORTION	CALS.	CARB.	FAT	PRO.
dried cooked	1 cup	298	17	15	29
dry-roasted	½ cup	387	28	19	34
roasted	½ cup	405	29	22	30
roasted & toasted	1 oz	129	9	7	11
roasted & toasted salted	1 cup	490	33	26	40
roasted & toasted salted	1 oz	129	9	7	11
sprouts raw	½ cup	43	3	2	5
sprouts steamed	½ cup	38	3	2	4
sprouts stir fried	1 cup	125	9	7	13
FRESH					
green cooked	½ cup	127	10	6	11

SPAGHETTI

(see PASTA, PASTA DINNERS, PASTA SALAD, SPAGHETTI SAUCE)

SPAGHETTI SAUCE

(see also PIZZA, TOMATO)

FOOD	PORTION	CALS.	CARB.	FAT	PRO.
JARRED					
marinara sauce	1 cup	171	25	8	4
spaghetti sauce	1 cup	272	40	12	12
Classico					
Beef & Pork	4 fl oz	80	7	4	3
Four Cheese	4 fl oz	70	7	4	2
Spicy Red Pepper	4 fl oz	50	6	2	2
Sweet Peppers & Onions	4 fl oz	50	7	4	1
Tomato & Basil	4 fl oz	60	6	3	2
Ripe Olives & Mushrooms	4 fl oz	50	7	2	2
Contadina					
Italian	¼ cup	15	4	0	tr
Sauce	¼ cup	20	4	0	tr

FOOD	PORTION	CALS.	CARB.	FAT	PRO.
Contadina (CONT.)					
Thick & Zesty	¼ cup	15	4	0	tr
Del Monte					
Traditional	½ cup (4.4 oz)	80	15	1	2
Traditional No Sugar Added	½ cup (4.4 oz)	60	11	1	2
With Garlic & Onion	½ cup (4.4 oz)	70	15	1	2
With Green Peppers & Mushrooms	½ cup (4.4 oz)	70	13	1	2
With Meat	½ cup (4.4 oz)	40	13	2	3
With Mushrooms	½ cup (4.4 oz)	80	15	2	2
Eden					
Organic	½ cup (4.4 oz)	80	12	3	3
Organic No Salt Added	½ cup (4.4 oz)	80	12	3	3
Enrico's					
Fat Free Organic Basil	½ cup (4 oz)	50	8	0	5
Fat Free Organic Garlic	½ cup (4 oz)	50	9	0	3
Fat Free Organic Hot Pepper	½ cup (4 oz)	50	8	0	4
Fat Free Organic Mushroom	½ cup (4 oz)	60	10	0	3
Fat Free Organic Traditional	½ cup (4 oz)	45	4	0	7
Healthy Choice					
Extra Chunky Garlic & Onions	½ cup (4.4 oz)	50	11	1	2
Extra Chunky Italian Style Vegetable	½ cup (4.4 oz)	50	11	1	2
Extra Chunky Mushrooms	½ cup (4.4 oz)	50	10	1	2
Original Garlic & Herbs	½ cup (4.4 oz)	50	10	1	2
Original Mushrooms	½ cup (4.4 oz)	50	10	1	2
Original Traditional	½ cup (4.4 oz)	50	10	1	2
Original With Meat	½ cup (4.4 oz)	50	8	1	2
Super Chunky Mushrooms & Sweet Peppers	½ cup (4.4 oz)	50	11	1	2
Super Chunky Vegetable Primavera	½ cup (4.4 oz)	50	11	1	2
Hunt's					
Chunky	¼ cup (2.2 fl oz)	30	4	1	tr
Classic Italian With Parmesan	½ cup (4.4 fl oz)	50	8	2	2
Homestyle Traditional No Sugar Added	½ cup (4.4 fl oz)	60	7	3	2

FOOD	PORTION	CALS.	CARB.	FAT	PRO.
Hunt's (CONT.)					
Traditional	4 oz	70	12	2	2
Traditional Light	½ cup (4 oz)	40	7	1	2
With Meat	4 oz	70	12	2	2
With Mushrooms	4 oz	70	12	2	2
Mama Rizzo's					
Mushroom Onion	½ cup (4.3 oz)	60	9	2	2
Pepper Mushroom Onion	½ cup (4.3 oz)	60	9	2	2
Pepper Primavera Vegetable	½ cup (4.2 oz)	50	8	2	2
Pepper Tomato Basil Garlic	½ cup (4.7 oz)	60	10	2	2
Primavera Vegetable	½ cup (4.2 oz)	50	8	2	2
Tomato Basil Garlic	½ cup (4.6 oz)	60	8	2	2
Muir Glen					
Organic Cabernet Marinara	½ cup (4.4 oz)	45	10	0	2
Organic Chunky Style	½ cup (4.5 oz)	80	13	2	2
Organic Fat Free Tomato Basil	½ cup (4.3 oz)	50	10	0	2
Organic Garlic Onion	½ cup (4.3 oz)	50	11	0	2
Organic Garlic Roasted Garlic	½ cup (4.4 oz)	45	10	0	2
Organic Green Pepper & Mushroom	½ cup (4.5 oz)	70	10	2	2
Organic Italian Herb	½ cup (4.5 oz)	60	13	0	2
Organic Romano Cheese	½ cup (4.5 oz)	90	14	3	2
Organic Sun Dried Tomato	½ cup (4.4 oz)	40	9	0	2
Organic Sweet Pepper Onion	½ cup (4.4 oz)	40	8	0	2
Organic Tomato Basil	½ cup (4.3 oz)	50	10	0	2
Newman's Own					
Marinara	4 oz	70	11	2	2
Marinara With Mushrooms	4 oz	70	11	2	2
Sockarooni	4 oz	70	11	2	2
Prego					
Chunky Sausage & Green Peppers	4 oz	160	19	8	3
Extra Chunky Garden Combination	4 oz	80	14	2	2
Extra Chunky Mushroom & Tomato	4 oz	110	14	5	1

FOOD	PORTION	CALS.	CARB.	FAT	PRO.
Prego (CONT.)					
Extra Chunky Mushroom & Green Pepper	4 oz	100	14	4	2
Extra Chunky Mushroom & Onion	4 oz	100	13	4	2
Extra Chunky Mushroom With Extra Spice	4 oz	100	17	3	2
Extra Chunky Tomato & Onion	4 oz	110	14	5	2
Marinara	4 oz	100	10	6	2
Meat Flavored	4 oz	140	20	6	2
Mushroom	4 oz	130	20	5	2
Onion & Garlic	4 oz	110	16	4	1
Regular	4 oz	130	20	5	2
Three Cheese	4 oz	100	17	2	3
Tomato & Basil	4 oz	100	18	2	2
Progresso					
Bolognese	½ cup	150	12	12	10
Marinara	½ cup	90	9	5	4
Meat Flavored	½ cup	110	13	5	4
Mushroom	½ cup	110	13	5	3
Sauce	½ cup	110	13	5	3
Sicilian	½ cup	30	2	3	tr
Ragu					
Fino Italian Garden Medley	½ cup (4.5 oz)	90	14	3	2
Fino Italian Garlic & Basil	½ cup (4.5 oz)	90	15	3	2
Fino Italian Parmesan	½ cup (4.5 oz)	100	15	3	3
Fino Italian Sliced Mushroom	½ cup (4.5 oz)	90	14	3	2
Fino Italian Tomato & Herb	½ cup (4.5 oz)	90	15	3	2
Fino Italian Zesty Tomato	½ cup (4.5 oz)	90	14	3	2
Gardenstyle Chunky Garden Combination	½ cup (4.5 oz)	120	18	4	2
Gardenstyle Chunky Green & Red Pepper	½ cup (4.5 oz)	120	19	4	2
Gardenstyle Chunky Mushroom & Green Pepper	½ cup (4.5 oz)	120	18	4	2
Gardenstyle Chunky Mushroom & Onion	½ cup (4.5 oz)	120	19	4	2

FOOD	PORTION	CALS.	CARB.	FAT	PRO.
Ragu (CONT.)					
Gardenstyle Chunky Tomato Garlic & Onion	½ cup (4.5 oz)	120	19	4	2
Gardenstyle Super Mushroom	½ cup (4.5 oz)	120	19	4	3
Gardenstyle Super Vegetable Primavera	½ cup (4.5 oz)	110	17	4	2
Homestyle Mushroom	½ cup (4.5 oz)	120	18	4	3
Homestyle Tomato & Herb	½ cup (4.5 oz)	120	18	4	3
Homestyle With Meat	½ cup (4.5 oz)	130	18	4	3
Light Chunky Mushroom	½ cup (4.4 oz)	50	10	0	2
Light Garden Harvest	½ cup (4.4 oz)	50	11	0	2
Light No Sugar Added	½ cup (4.4 oz)	60	9	0	3
Light Tomato & Herb	½ cup (4.4 oz)	50	10	0	2
Old World Style Marinara	½ cup (4.4 oz)	90	9	5	2
Old World Style Mushrooms	½ cup (4.4 oz)	80	10	3	2
Old World Style Traditional	½ cup (4.4 oz)	80	10	3	2
Old World Style With Meat	½ cup (4.4 oz)	90	9	5	3
Sauce	4 fl oz	80	9	4	2
Thick & Hearty Mushroom	½ cup (4.5 oz)	120	19	3	3
Thick & Hearty Spaghetti Sauce	4 oz	100	15	3	2
Thick & Hearty Tomato & Herb	½ cup (4.5 oz)	120	19	3	3
Thick & Hearty With Meat	1.2 cup (4.5 oz)	130	19	5	4
Tree Of Life					
Pasta Sauce	½ cup (4 oz)	50	9	2	2
Pasta Sauce Calabrese	½ cup (3.9 oz)	60	9	3	2
Pasta Sauce Fat Free Classic	½ cup (3.9 oz)	40	8	0	2
Pasta Sauce Fat Free Mushroom & Basil	½ cup (3.9 oz)	30	7	0	1
Pasta Sauce Fat Free Onion & Garlic	½ cup (3.9 oz)	30	7	0	1
Pasta Sauce Fat Free Sweet Pepper	½ cup (3.9 oz)	30	7	0	1
Pasta Sauce No Salt	½ cup (3.9 oz)	50	9	2	2

FOOD	PORTION	CALS.	CARB.	FAT	PRO.
Weight Watchers					
With Meat	⅓ cup	45	7	1	2
With Mushrooms	⅓ cup	35	7	0	1
REFRIGERATED					
Contadina					
Alfredo	½ cup (4.2 fl oz)	400	8	38	7
Four Cheese Sauce With White Wine & Shallots	½ cup (4.2 fl oz)	320	8	25	8
Light Alfredo	½ cup (4.2 fl oz)	190	10	13	8
Light Chunky Tomato	½ cup (4.4 fl oz)	45	8	0	2
Light Garden Vegetable	½ cup (4.4 fl oz)	45	8	1	2
Marinara	½ cup (4.4 fl oz)	80	8	4	2
Pesto With Basil	¼ cup (2 oz)	310	5	30	6
Pesto With Sun Dried Tomatoes	¼ cup (2 oz)	250	6	24	3
Plum Tomato With Basil	½ cup (4.4 fl oz)	70	8	3	2
Spicy Italian Sausage & Bell Pepper	½ cup (4.4 fl oz)	100	9	5	4
Di Giorno					
Alfredo	¼ cup (2.2 oz)	230	2	22	4
Four Cheese	¼ cup (2.2 oz)	200	2	19	5
Light Chunky Tomato With Basil	½ cup (4.5 oz)	70	16	0	2
Light Reduced Fat Alfredo	¼ cup (2.4 oz)	170	16	10	5
Marinara	½ cup (4.5 oz)	100	12	5	3
Olive Oil & Garlic With Grated Cheese	¼ cup (2.1 oz)	370	3	36	9
Pesto	¼ cup (2.2 oz)	320	3	31	8
Plum Tomato & Mushroom	½ cup (4.4 oz)	70	15	0	2
Traditional Meat	½ cup (4.5 oz)	120	12	6	6
TAKE-OUT					
bolognese	5 oz	195	4	15	11

SPANISH FOOD

(*see also* BEANS, CHIPS, DINNER, PEPPERS, SALSA, SNACKS, SAUCE, TORTILLA)

FOOD	PORTION	CALS.	CARB.	FAT	PRO.
CANNED					
Casa Fiesta					
Picante Mild	1 oz	9	2	tr	tr
Chi-Chi's					
Picante Hot	2 tbsp (1 oz)	10	2	0	0
Picante Medium	2 tbsp (1 oz)	10	2	0	0

FOOD	PORTION	CALS.	CARB.	FAT	PRO.
Chi-Chi's (CONT.)					
Picante Mild	2 tbsp (1 oz)	10	2	0	0
Pico De Gallo	2 tbsp (1.2 oz)	10	2	0	0
Derby					
Tamales	2	160	15	7	8
El Molino					
Enchilada Sauce Hot	2 tbsp	16	2	1	0
Green Chili Sauce Mild	2 tbsp	10	2	0	0
Gebhardt					
Enchiladas	2	310	20	24	5
Tamales	2	290	19	22	5
Tamales Jumbo	2	400	26	30	7
Guiltless Gourmet					
Picante Mild	1 oz	6	1	0	0
Queso Mild Cheddar	1 oz	22	5	tr	tr
Hormel					
Tamales Beef	3 (7.5 oz)	280	20	21	6
Tamales Chicken	3 (7.5 oz)	210	23	10	7
Tamales Hot Spicy Beef	3 (7.5 oz)	280	20	21	6
Tamales Jumbo Beef	2 (6.9 oz)	270	18	20	5
Tamales Beef	1 can (7.5 oz)	290	20	21	5
Old El Paso					
Tamales	2	190	16	12	5
Rosarita					
Enchilada Sauce Mild	2.5 oz	25	3	1	tr
Picante Chunky Hot	3 tbsp (2 fl oz)	18	4	tr	tr
Picante Chunky Medium	3 tbsp (2 fl oz)	16	4	tr	tr
Picante Chunky Mild	3 tbsp (2 oz)	25	5	tr	1
Van Camp's					
Tamales	2 (5.1 oz)	210	20	13	6
Wolf Brand					
Tamales	7.5 oz	328	25	25	8
FROZEN					
Amy's Organic					
Enchilada Cheese	1 (4.7 oz)	210	16	9	11
Banquet					
Beef Enchilada	1 pkg (11 oz)	320	54	12	15
Chimichanga Meal	1 pkg (9.5 oz)	470	56	23	13
Enchilada Cheese	1 pkg (11 oz)	350	56	6	15
Enchilada Chicken	1 pkg (11 oz)	360	54	10	15
Family Entree Beef Enchilada w/ Cheese	1 serv (4.67 oz)	130	19	4	45
Healthy Choice					
Beef Burrito Ranchero Medium	1 (5.4 oz)	290	44	7	13

FOOD	PORTION	CALS.	CARB.	FAT	PRO.
Healthy Choice (CONT.)					
Beef Burrito Ranchero Mild	1 (5.4 oz)	300	45	7	13
Beef Enchilada Rio Grande	1 meal (13.4 oz)	410	70	8	14
Burrito Chicken Con Queso	1 (5.4 oz)	280	43	6	12
Chicken Enchilada Supreme	1 meal (13.4 oz)	390	60	9	17
Enchiladas Suiza Chicken	1 meal (10 oz)	270	43	4	14
Feista Chicken Fajitas	1 meal (7 oz)	260	36	4	21
Jimmy Dean					
Burrito Breakfast Bacon	1 (4 oz)	260	37	8	11
Burrito Breakfast Sausage	1 (4 oz)	250	36	8	10
Le Menu					
Entree LightStyle Enchilada Chicken	8 oz	280	32	8	21
Lean Cuisine					
Enchanadas Chicken	1 meal (9.9 oz)	220	29	6	13
Enchilada Suiza Chicken	1 meal (9 oz)	290	48	5	12
Life Choice					
Burrito Black Bean	1 meal (13.2 oz)	410	86	2	12
Vegetable Enchilada Sonora	1 meal (14 oz)	420	89	2	12
Lightlife					
Vegetarian Taco	2 oz	51	4	1	5
Old El Paso					
Burrito Beef & Bean Hot	1	320	45	10	12
Burrito Beef & Bean Medium	1	320	46	10	12
Burrito Beef & Bean Mild	1	330	48	9	12
Burrito Beef & Cheese	1	290	44	9	12
Chimichangas Beef	1	310	37	20	9
Chimichangas Chicken	1	350	39	16	11
Patio					
Burrito Bean & Cheese	1 (5 oz)	270	46	5	9
Burrito Chicken	1 (5 oz)	260	44	4	12
Burrito Red Chili	1 (5 oz)	270	42	6	11
Burritos Beef & Bean	1 (5 oz)	280	45	7	10
Burritos Beef & Bean Green Chili	1 (5 oz)	260	44	5	11
Burritos Beef & Bean Red Chili	1 (5 oz)	260	42	5	11

FOOD	PORTION	CALS.	CARB.	FAT	PRO.
Patio (CONT.)					
Enchilada Beef Dinner	1 meal (12 oz)	320	52	8	12
Enchilada Cheese Dinner	1 meal (12 oz)	330	52	8	13
Enchilada Chicken	1 pkg (12 oz)	380	58	9	14
Family Entree Beef Enchilada	2 (5.7 oz)	170	27	4	6
Family Entree Enchilada Beef	2 (5.3 oz)	250	35	7	12
Family Entree Enchilada Beef & Cheese	2 (5.3 oz)	250	35	6	12
Family Entree Enchilada Cheese	2 (5.7 oz)	170	26	4	6
Fiesta Dinner	1 meal (12 oz)	340	51	9	13
Mexican Dinner	1 meal (13.25 oz)	440	59	15	15
Salis Con Queso	1 pkg (11 oz)	390	33	20	18
Patio Britos					
Beef & Bean	10 (6 oz)	420	51	19	11
Nacho Beef	10 (6 oz)	410	48	18	13
Nacho Cheese	10 (6 oz)	360	52	13	10
Spicy Chicken	10 (6 oz)	400	52	16	13
Rudy's Farm					
Burrito Beef/Bean	1 (5 oz)	326	43	12	12
Burrito Hot Beef/Bean	1 (5 oz)	305	44	9	12
Senor Felix's					
Burrito Black Bean	1 (10 oz)	540	70	18	26
Burrito Black Bean Soy	1 (5 oz)	240	36	7	12
Burrito Charbroiled Chicken	1 + 4 tsp sauce (6.7 oz)	320	40	11	15
Burrito Chicken	1 (10 oz)	520	51	20	32
Burrito Hot Potato	1 (10 oz)	560	67	24	19
Burrito Soy Hot	1 (10 oz)	520	70	20	18
Burritos Sonora Style	1 + 4 tsp sauce (6.7 oz)	280	45	8	10
Burritos Yucatan Style	1 + 4 tsp sauce (6.7 oz)	310	46	9	14
Empanadas Chicken	1 (4.7 oz)	340	41	15	11
Empanadas Corn & Rice	1 (4.7 oz)	280	37	13	9
Empanadas Pumpkin & Mushroom	1 (4.7 oz)	260	32	11	10
Empanadas Spinach & Ricotta	1 (4.7 oz)	260	32	12	10
Enchilada Red Pepper	1 (10 oz)	420	51	19	18
Enchilada Soy Verda	1 (10 oz)	430	41	24	14
Enchilada Supreme Soy Cheese	1 (10 oz)	460	48	23	20

FOOD	PORTION	CALS.	CARB.	FAT	PRO.
Senor Felix's (CONT.)					
Enchilada Verde	1 (5 oz)	423	41	23	16
Tamales Blue Corn & Soy Cheese	2 + 4 tsp sauce (5.7 oz)	240	28	10	8
Tamales Chicken	2 + 4 tsp sauce (5.7 oz)	240	30	9	10
Tamales Gourmet Vegetarian	2 + 4 tsp sauce	240	30	9	10
Taquitos Blue Corn Soy	3 + 4 tsp sauce (5.2 oz)	230	27	11	7
Taquitos Chicken	2 + 4 tsp sauce (5.7 oz)	240	28	10	8
Stouffer's					
Cheese Enchilada	1 pkg (9.75 oz)	370	48	14	12
Chicken Enchilada	1 pkg (10 oz)	370	45	14	16
Swanson					
Enchiladas Beef	13¾ oz	480	55	21	17
Mexican Style Combination	14¼ oz	490	62	18	19
Mexican Style Hungry Man	20¼ oz	820	88	41	25
Today's Tamales					
Cheese & Chili	1 pkg (7 oz)	390	38	21	12
Del Sol	1 pkg (6.5 oz)	310	40	15	5
Original Bean	1 pkg (7 oz)	330	49	11	9
Spicy Taco	1 pkg (7 oz)	310	41	15	12
Tyson					
Fajita Kit Beef	3.84 oz	160	21	4	9
Fajita Kit Chicken	4 oz	80	2	2	7
Weight Watchers					
Enchiladas Ranchero Beef	9.12 oz	190	18	5	18
Enchiladas Ranchero Cheese	8.87 oz	260	25	10	18
Enchiladas Suiza Chicken	9 oz	230	25	7	16
Fajitas Chicken	6.75 oz	210	24	5	17
MIX					
Gebhardt					
Menudo Mix	1 tsp	5	1	tr	tr
Hain					
Taco Seasoning Mix	¹⁄₁₀ pkg	10	2	0	1
Old El Paso					
Burrito Seasoning Mix	⅛ pkg	17	3	0	1

FOOD	PORTION	CALS.	CARB.	FAT	PRO.
Old El Paso (CONT.)					
Burrito Dinner (with filling)	1 serv	299	36	13	11
Enchilada Seasoning Mix	1/18 pkg	6	1	0	0
Guacamole Seasoning Mix	1/7 pkg	7	2	0	0
Taco Seasoning Mix	1/12 pkg	8	2	tr	tr
Ortega					
Taco Meat Seasoning Mix Mild	1 filled taco	90	18	1	2
Quaker					
Masa Harina De Maiz	2 tortillas	137	28	2	4
Masa Trigo	2 tortillas	149	25	4	4
READY-TO-USE					
taco shell baked	1 med (1/2 oz)	61	8	3	1
taco shell baked w/o salt	1 med (1/2 oz)	61	8	3	1
Casa Fiesta					
Taco Shells	3.5 oz	480	60	23	9
Chi-Chi's					
Taco Shells White Corned	2 (1 oz)	130	17	6	2
Gebhardt					
Taco Shells	1	50	7	3	1
Old El Paso					
Taco Shells	1	55	6	3	0
Taco Shells Mini	3	70	7	4	1
Taco Shells Super	1	100	11	6	1
Taco Shells White Corn	1	60	6	3	1
Tastaco Shells	1	100	11	5	1
Tostada Shells	1	55	6	3	tr
Rosarita					
Taco Shells	1 shell (11 g)	50	7	2	1
Tostada Shells	1 shell (14 g)	60	8	3	1
TAKE-OUT					
burrito w/ apple	1 lg (5.4 oz)	484	73	20	5
burrito w/ apple	1 sm (2.6 oz)	231	35	10	3
burrito w/ beans	2 (7.6 oz)	448	71	14	14
burrito w/ beans & cheese	2 (6.5 oz)	377	55	12	15
burrito w/ beans & chili peppers	2 (7.2 oz)	413	58	15	16
burrito w/ beans & meat	2 (8.1 oz)	508	66	18	22
burrito w/ beans cheese & beef	2 (7.1 oz)	331	40	13	15
burrito w/ beans cheese & chili peppers	2 (11.8 oz)	663	85	23	33

FOOD	PORTION	CALS.	CARB.	FAT	PRO.
burrito w/ beef	2 (7.7 oz)	523	59	21	27
burrito w/ beef & chili peppers	2 (7.1 oz)	426	49	17	22
burrito w/ beef cheese & chili peppers	2 (10.7 oz)	634	64	25	41
burrito w/ cherry	1 sm (2.6 oz)	231	35	10	3
burrito w/ cherry	1 lg (5.4 oz)	484	73	20	5
chimichanga w/ beef	1 (6.1 oz)	425	43	20	20
chimichanga w/ beef & cheese	1 (6.4 oz)	443	39	23	20
chimichanga w/ beef & red chili peppers	1 (6.7 oz)	424	46	19	18
chimichanga w/ beef cheese & red chili peppers	1 (6.3 oz)	364	38	18	15
enchilada w/ cheese	1 (5.7 oz)	320	29	19	10
enchilada w/ cheese & beef	1 (6.7 oz)	324	30	18	12
enchirito w/ cheese beef & beans	1 (6.8 oz)	344	34	16	18
frijoles w/ cheese	1 cup (5.9 oz)	226	29	8	11
nachos w/ cheese	6 to 8 (4 oz)	345	36	19	9
nachos w/ cheese & jalapeno peppers	6 to 8 (7.2 oz)	607	60	34	17
nachos w/ cheese beans ground beef & peppers	6 to 8 (8.9 oz)	568	56	31	20
nachos w/ cinnamon & sugar	6 to 8 (3.8 oz)	592	63	36	7
taco	1 sm (6 oz)	370	27	21	21
taco salad	1½ cups	279	24	15	13
taco salad w/ chili con carne	1½ cups	288	27	13	17
tostada w/ beans & cheese	1 (5.1 oz)	223	27	10	10
tostada w/ beans beef & cheese	1 (7.9 oz)	334	30	17	16
tostada w/ beef & cheese	1 (5.7 oz)	315	23	16	19
tostada w/ guacamole	2 (9.2 oz)	360	32	23	12

SPARE RIBS
(see PORK)

SPELT
Arrowhead
| Spelt | 1 oz | 83 | 20 | 1 | 4 |

SPINACH
CANNED
| spinach | ½ cup | 25 | 4 | 1 | 3 |

FOOD	PORTION	CALS.	CARB.	FAT	PRO.
Del Monte					
50% Less Salt	½ cup (4 oz)	30	4	0	2
Chopped	½ cup (4 oz)	30	4	0	2
No Salt Added	½ cup (4 oz)	30	4	0	2
Whole Leaf	½ cup (4 oz)	30	4	0	2
Popeye					
Chopped	½ cup (4.1 oz)	40	6	1	2
Leaf	½ cup (4.2 oz)	45	7	1	2
Low Sodium	½ cup (4.2 oz)	35	4	1	2
S&W					
Northwest Premium	½ cup	25	3	0	2
Sunshine					
Chopped	½ cup (4.1 oz)	40	6	1	2
FRESH					
cooked	½ cup	21	3	tr	3
mustard chopped cooked	½ cup	14	3	tr	2
mustard raw chopped	½ cup	17	3	tr	2
new zealand chopped cooked	½ cup	11	2	tr	1
new zealand raw	½ cup	4	1	tr	tr
raw chopped	½ cup	6	1	tr	1
raw chopped	1 pkg (10 oz)	46	7	1	6
Dole					
Spinach	3 oz	9	tr	tr	3
Fresh Express					
Spinach	1½ cups (3 oz)	40	10	0	2
FROZEN					
cooked	½ cup	27	5	tr	3
Birds Eye					
Chopped	½ cup	20	3	0	3
Creamed	½ cup	90	9	5	3
Leaf	½ cup	20	4	0	3
Budget Gourmet					
Au Gratin	1 pkg (5.5 oz)	160	9	11	5
Fresh Like					
Cut Leaf	3.5 oz	21	4	tr	3
Green Giant					
Creamed	½ cup	70	10	3	3
Cut Leaf In Butter Sauce	½ cup	40	6	2	3
Harvest Fresh	½ cup	25	5	0	4
Spinach	½ cup	25	6	0	3
Stouffer's					
Creamed	½ cup (2.25 oz)	150	8	12	4
Souffle	½ cup (4 oz)	150	9	10	6

FOOD	PORTION	CALS.	CARB.	FAT	PRO.
Tabatchnick					
Creamed	7.5 oz	60	8	2	2
SPINACH JUICE					
juice	3½ oz	7	1	0	1
SPORTS DRINKS					
(*see also* NUTRITIONAL SUPPLEMENTS)					
Gatorade					
Citrus Cooler	1 cup (8 oz)	50	14	0	0
Fruit Punch	1 cup (8 oz)	50	14	0	0
Grape	1 cup (8 oz)	50	14	0	0
Iced Tea Cooler	1 cup (8 oz)	50	14	0	0
Lemon-Lime	1 cup (8 oz)	50	14	0	0
Lemonade	1 cup (8 oz)	50	14	0	0
Orange	1 cup (8 fl oz)	50	14	0	0
Tropical Fruit	1 cup (8 oz)	50	14	0	0
PowerAde					
Fruit Punch	8 fl oz	72	19	0	0
Grape	8 fl oz	73	19	0	0
Lemon-Lime	8 fl oz	72	19	0	0
Orange	8 fl oz	72	19	0	0
Slice					
All Sport Diet Lemon Lime	8 fl oz	1	0	0	tr
All Sport Lemon Lime	8 fl oz	72	19	0	tr
All Sport Orange	8 fl oz	74	19	0	tr
All Sport Punch	8 fl oz	81	22	0	tr
Snapple					
Sport Fruit	1 bottle	80	20	0	0
Sport Lemon	1 bottle	80	20	0	0
Sport Lemon Lime	1 bottle	80	20	0	0
Sport Orange	1 bottle	80	20	0	0
SPOT					
baked	3 oz	134	0	5	20
SQUAB					
breast w/o skin raw	1 (3.5 oz)	135	0	5	22
w/ skin raw	1 squab (6.9 oz)	584	0	47	37
w/o skin raw	1 squab (5.9 oz)	239	0	13	29
SQUASH					
(*see also* ZUCCHINI)					
CANNED					
crookneck sliced	½ cup	14	3	tr	1

FOOD	PORTION	CALS.	CARB.	FAT	PRO.
Allen					
Yellow	½ cup (4.2 oz)	25	5	0	0
Sunshine					
Yellow	½ cup (4.2 oz)	25	5	0	0
FRESH					
acorn cooked mashed	½ cup	41	11	tr	1
acorn cubed baked	½ cup	57	15	tr	1
butternut baked	½ cup	41	11	tr	1
crookneck raw sliced	½ cup	12	3	tr	1
crookneck sliced cooked	½ cup	18	4	tr	1
hubbard baked	½ cup	51	11	tr	3
hubbard cooked mashed	½ cup	35	8	tr	2
scallop raw sliced	½ cup	12	3	tr	1
scallop sliced cooked	½ cup	14	3	tr	1
spaghetti cooked	½ cup	23	5	tr	1
Nature's Pasta					
Spaghetti Squash	1 cup (5.5 oz)	20	4	0	1
FROZEN					
butternut cooked mashed	½ cup	47	12	tr	1
crookneck sliced cooked	½ cup	24	5	tr	1
Birds Eye					
Winter Cooked	½ cup	45	11	0	1
SEEDS					
dried	1 oz	154	5	13	7
dried	1 cup	747	25	63	34
roasted	1 oz	148	4	12	9
roasted	1 cup	1184	31	96	75
salted & roasted	1 oz	148	4	12	9
salted & roasted	1 cup	1184	31	96	75
whole roasted	1 oz	127	15	6	5
whole roasted	1 cup	285	34	12	12
whole salted roasted	1 cup	285	34	12	12
whole salted roasted	1 oz	127	15	6	6
SQUID					
fried	3 oz	149	7	6	15
raw	3 oz	78	3	1	13
SQUIRREL					
roasted	3 oz	147	0	4	26
STAR FRUIT					
Sonoma					
Dried	7-9 pieces (1.4 oz)	140	34	0	1
STRAWBERRIES					
CANNED					
in heavy syrup	½ cup	117	30	tr	1

FOOD	PORTION	CALS.	CARB.	FAT	PRO.
FRESH					
strawberries	1 cup	45	10	1	1
strawberries	1 pint	97	22	1	2
Dole					
Strawberries	8	50	13	0	1
FROZEN					
sweetened sliced	1 cup	245	66	tr	1
sweetened sliced	1 pkg (10 oz)	273	74	tr	2
unsweetened	1 cup	52	14	tr	1
whole sweetened	1 cup	200	54	tr	1
whole sweetened	1 pkg (10 oz)	223	60	tr	1
Big Valley					
Strawberries	⅔ cup (4.9 oz)	50	12	0	tr
Birds Eye					
Halved In Delicious Syrup	½ cup	120	30	0	1
Halved In Lite Syrup	½ cup	90	22	0	1
Whole In Lite Syrup	½ cup	80	20	0	1
STRAWBERRY JUICE					
Kern's					
Nectar	6 fl oz	110	28	0	0
Kool-Aid					
Koolers	1 (8.45 oz)	136	36	0	0
Strawberry	8 oz	98	25	0	0
Libby					
Nectar	1 can (11.5 fl oz)	210	52	0	0
Smucker's					
Juice	8 oz	130	31	0	0
Tang					
Strawberry	8.45 fl oz	121	32	0	0
Wylers					
Drink Mix Unsweetened Strawberry Split	8 oz	2	1	0	0
STUFFING/DRESSING					
HOME RECIPE					
bread as prep w/ water & fat	½ cup	251	25	15	5
bread as prep w/ water egg & fat	½ cup	107	9	7	3
MIX					
bread dry as prep	½ cup	178	22	9	3
cornbread as prep	½ cup	179	22	9	3

FOOD	PORTION	CALS.	CARB.	FAT	PRO.
Arnold					
All Purpose Seasoned	½ oz	50	9	0	2
Corn	½ oz	50	9	1	2
Herb Seasoned	½ oz	50	2	tr	10
Sage & Onion	½ oz	50	9	tr	2
Betty Crocker					
Chicken	½ cup	180	21	9	4
Traditional Herb	½ cup	180	22	8	4
Brownberry					
Corn	1 oz	103	19	2	4
Herb	1 oz	100	19	1	3
Sage & Onion	1 oz	97	18	1	4
Golden Grain					
Bread Stuffing Chicken	½ cup	180	20	9	4
Bread Stuffing Corn Bread	½ cup	180	21	9	3
Bread Stuffing Herb & Butter	½ cup	180	20	9	4
Bread Stuffing With Wild Rice	½ cup	180	21	9	4
Kellogg's					
Croutettes	1 cup (1.2 oz)	120	25	0	5
Pepperidge Farm					
Corn Bread	1 oz	110	22	1	3
Country Style	1 oz	100	21	1	4
Cube	1 oz	110	22	1	3
Distinctive Apple Raisin	1 oz	110	21	1	3
Distinctive Classic Chicken	1 oz	110	20	1	4
Distinctive Country Garden Herb	1 oz	120	18	4	4
Distinctive Vegetable & Almond	1 oz	110	19	3	4
Distinctive Wild Rice & Mushroom	1 oz	130	17	5	4
Herb Seasoned	1 oz	110	22	1	3
Stove Top					
Beef as prep	½ cup	178	22	9	4
Chicken as prep	½ cup	176	21	8	4
Chicken With Rice as prep	½ cup	182	22	9	4
Cornbread as prep	½ cup	175	22	8	3
Flex Serve Chicken as prep	½ cup	173	20	9	4

FOOD	PORTION	CALS.	CARB.	FAT	PRO.
Stove Top (CONT.)					
Flex Serve Cornbread as prep	½ cup	181	22	9	4
Flex Serve Homestyle Herb as prep	½ cup	173	20	9	4
Long Grain & Wild Rice as prep	½ cup	182	22	9	4
Wonder					
Seasoned Stuffing	1 cup (0.9 oz)	60	12	1	2
TAKE-OUT					
bread	½ cup (3½ oz)	195	26	8	4
sausage	½ cup	292	40	11	8
STURGEON					
cooked	3 oz	115	0	4	18
raw	3 oz	90	0	3	14
roe raw	3.5 oz	207	1	10	25
smoked	3 oz	147	0	4	27
smoked	1 oz	48	0	1	9
SUCKER					
white baked	3 oz	101	0	3	18
SUGAR					
(*see also* FRUCTOSE, SUGAR SUBSTITUTES, SYRUP)					
brown packed	1 cup (7.7 oz)	828	214	0	0
brown unpacked	1 cup (5.1 oz)	546	141	0	0
maple	1 piece (1 oz)	100	26	tr	0
powdered	1 tbsp (0.3 oz)	31	8	0	0
powdered unsifted	1 cup (4.2 oz)	467	119	tr	tr
white	1 cup (7 oz)	773	200	0	0
white	1 packet (6 g)	25	6	0	0
white	1 tbsp	45	12	0	0
white	1 tsp (4 g)	15	4	0	0
C&H					
White	1 tsp	16	4	0	0
Domino					
White	1 tsp	16	4	0	0
Hain					
Turbinado	1 tbsp	50	12	0	0
Hollywood					
Turbinado	1 tbsp	50	12	0	0
SUGAR SUBSTITUTES					
(*see also* FRUCTOSE)					
Equal					
Packet	1 pkg	4	tr	0	0

FOOD	PORTION	CALS.	CARB.	FAT	PRO.
NatraTaste					
Packet	1 pkg (1 g)	0	1	0	0
S&W					
Liquid Table Sweetener	⅛ tsp	0	0	0	0
Sprinkle Sweet					
Sugar Substitute	1 tsp	2	tr	0	0
SugarTwin					
Brown	1 tsp (0.4 g)	2	tr	0	0
Packet	1 pkg (0.8 g)	3	1	0	0
Sugar Substitute	1 tsp (0.4 g)	2	tr	0	0
Sweet One					
Packet	1 pkg (1 g)	4	1	0	0
*Sweet*10*	⅛ tsp	0	0	0	0
Weight Watchers					
Sweet'ner	1 pkg	4	1	0	0

SUGAR-APPLE

fresh	1	146	37	tr	3
fresh cut up	1 cup	236	59	1	5

SUNDAE TOPPINGS
(*see* ICE CREAM TOPPINGS)

SUNFISH

pumpkinseed baked	3 oz	97	0	1	21

SUNFLOWER

dried	1 oz	162	5	14	33
dried	1 cup	821	27	71	33
dry roasted	1 oz	165	7	14	5
dry roasted	1 cup	745	31	64	25
dry roasted salted	1 oz	165	7	14	5
dry roasted salted	1 cup	745	31	64	25
oil roasted	1 cup	830	20	78	29
oil roasted salted	1 cup	830	20	78	29
oil roasted salted	1 oz	175	4	16	6
sunflower butter	1 tbsp	93	4	8	3
sunflower butter w/o salt	1 tbsp	93	4	8	3
toasted	1 oz	176	6	16	5
toasted	1 cup	826	28	76	23
toasted salted	1 cup	826	28	76	23
toasted salted	1 oz	176	6	16	5
Erewhon					
Sunflower Seed Butter	2 tbsp (32 g)	200	3	18	7
Fisher					
Seeds Oil Roasted	1 oz	170	6	15	8

FOOD	PORTION	CALS.	CARB.	FAT	PRO.
Fisher (CONT.)					
Seeds Salted In Shell shelled	1 oz	160	6	14	6
Seeds Salted In Shell unshelled	1 oz	170	6	15	8
Frito Lay					
Seeds	1 oz	160	6	14	7
Planters					
Kernels	1 pkg (1.7 oz)	290	9	25	11
Kernels	1 pkg (2 oz)	340	11	29	13
Kernels Barbecue	1 pkg (1.7 oz)	290	10	25	11
Kernels Honey Roasted	1 pkg (1.7 oz)	280	15	22	10
Kernels Salted	1 oz	170	4	14	7
Munch'N Go Singles Dry Roasted	1 pkg	120	4	11	4
Nuts Dry Roasted	¼ cup (1.1 oz)	190	6	17	7
Original With Shell Dry Roasted	¾ cup	160	5	15	6
Stone-Buhr					
Seeds Raw	4 tsp (1 oz)	170	6	14	7
SURF					
CANNED					
American Original	4 oz	100	7	tr	16
FRESH					
American Original	4 oz	90	2	tr	19
SUSHI					
TAKE-OUT					
california roll	1 piece (0.8 oz)	28	4	1	1
kim chi	⅓ cup (5.8 oz)	18	4	tr	1
sashimi	1 serving (6 oz)	198	4	7	24
tuna roll	1 piece (0.7 oz)	23	3	tr	2
vegetable roll	1 piece (1.2 oz)	27	5	1	1
vinegared ginger	⅓ cup (1.6 oz)	48	12	1	1
wasabi	2 tsp (0.3 oz)	5	1	tr	tr
yellowtail roll	1 piece (0.6 oz)	25	3	1	1
SWEET POTATO					
(*see also* YAM)					
CANNED					
in syrup	½ cup	106	25	tr	1
pieces	1 cup	183	42	tr	3
Princella					
Mashed	⅔ cup (5.1 oz)	120	28	1	1

FOOD	PORTION	CALS.	CARB.	FAT	PRO.
Royal Prince					
Candied	½ cup (4.9 oz)	210	50	1	1
Halves	3 pieces (5.7 oz)	190	46	1	1
Orange Pineapple	½ cup (4.8 oz)	210	43	1	1
Sugary Sam					
Mashed	⅔ cup (5.1 oz)	120	28	1	1
FRESH					
baked w/ skin	1 (3½ oz)	118	28	tr	2
leaves cooked	½ cup	11	2	tr	1
mashed	½ cup	172	40	tr	3
FROZEN					
cooked	½ cup	88	21	tr	2
Mrs. Paul's					
Candied Sweet Potatoes	4 oz	170	42	0	1
Candied Sweets 'N Apples	4 oz	160	38	0	1
TAKE-OUT					
candied	3½ oz	144	29	3	1

SWEETBREADS

FOOD	PORTION	CALS.	CARB.	FAT	PRO.
beef braised	3 oz	230	0	15	23
lamb braised	3 oz	199	0	13	19
veal braised	3 oz	218	0	12	25

SWISS CHARD

FOOD	PORTION	CALS.	CARB.	FAT	PRO.
cooked	½ cup	18	4	tr	2
raw chopped	½ cup	3	1	tr	tr

SWORDFISH

FOOD	PORTION	CALS.	CARB.	FAT	PRO.
cooked	3 oz	132	0	4	22
raw	3 oz	103	0	3	17

SYRUP

(*see also* ICE CREAM TOPPINGS, PANCAKE/WAFFLE SYRUP)

FOOD	PORTION	CALS.	CARB.	FAT	PRO.
corn	2 tbsp	122	32	0	0
corn dark	1 cup (11.5 oz)	925	251	tr	0
corn dark	1 tbsp (0.7 oz)	56	15	0	0
corn light	1 tbsp (0.7 oz)	56	15	0	0
corn light	1 cup (11.5 oz)	925	251	tr	0
malt	1 cup (13 oz)	1222	274	tr	24
malt	1 tbsp (0.8 oz)	76	17	0	2
maple	1 cup (11.1 oz)	824	212	1	tr
maple	1 tbsp (0.8 oz)	52	13	0	0
raspberry	3½ oz	267	66	0	tr
rose hip	3.5 oz	33	8	0	0
sorghum	1 cup (11.6 oz)	957	247	0	0

FOOD	PORTION	CALS.	CARB.	FAT	PRO.
sorghum	1 tbsp (0.7 oz)	61	16	0	0
Eden					
Barley Malt Organic Syrup	1 tbsp (0.7 fl oz)	60	14	0	1
Estee					
Blueberry Lite	¼ cup (2.4 oz)	80	20	0	0
Karo					
Corn Syrup Dark	1 tbsp (21 g)	60	15	0	0
Corn Syrup Dark	1 cup (331 g)	975	243	0	0
Corn Syrup Light	1 tbsp (21 g)	60	15	0	0
Corn Syrup Light	1 cup (331 g)	960	241	0	0
McIlhenny					
Cane	2 tbsp (1.4 oz)	130	32	0	tr
Quik					
Strawberry	1⅔ tbsp	100	24	0	0
Red Wing					
Strawberry	2 tbsp (1.4 oz)	110	28	0	0
S&W					
Blueberry Diet	1 tbsp	4	1	0	0
Maple Flavored Diet	1 tbsp	4	1	0	0
Strawberry Diet	1 tbsp	4	1	0	0
Smucker's					
All Flavors Fruit Syrup	2 tbsp	100	26	0	0
Tree Of Life					
Maple	¼ cup (2.1 oz)	200	53	0	0
Rice Syrup	2 tbsp (1 oz)	120	29	1	0
Whistling Wings					
Blueberry	1 oz	45	10	tr	tr
Raspberry	1 oz	60	14	tr	tr

TACO
(*see* SPANISH FOOD)

TAHINI
(*see* SESAME)

TAMARIND

fresh	1	5	1	tr	tr
fresh cut up	1 cup	287	75	1	3

TANGERINE
CANNED

in light syrup	½ cup	76	20	tr	1
juice pack	½ cup	46	12	tr	1
FRESH					
sections	1 cup	86	22	tr	1

FOOD	PORTION	CALS.	CARB.	FAT	PRO.
tangerine	1	37	9	tr	1
Dole					
Tangerine	2	70	19	1	1
TANGERINE JUICE					
canned sweetened	1 cup	125	30	1	1
fresh	1 cup	106	25	tr	1
frzn sweetened as prep	1 cup	110	27	tr	1
frzn sweetened not prep	6 oz	344	83	1	3
After The Fall					
Juice	1 can (12 oz)	170	40	0	2
Dole					
Mandarin frzn as prep	8 fl oz	140	35	0	1
Minute Maid					
Frozen	8 fl oz	120	29	0	0
TAPIOCA					
pearl dry	⅓ cup	174	45	0	tr
starch	3½ oz	344	85	tr	58
General Foods					
Minute Tapioca	1 tbsp	32	8	tr	0
TARO					
chips	10 (0.8 oz)	115	16	6	1
TEA/HERBAL TEA					
(*see also* ICED TEA)					
HERBAL					
Bigelow					
Almond Orange	5 fl oz	tr	tr	tr	tr
Apple Orchard	5 fl oz	5	1	tr	tr
Apple Spice	5 fl oz	tr	tr	tr	tr
Chamomile	5 fl oz	tr		tr	tr
Chamomile Mint	5 fl oz	tr	tr	tr	tr
Cinnamon Orange	5 fl oz	tr	tr	tr	tr
Early Riser	5 fl oz	3	1	tr	tr
Feeling Free	5 fl oz	1	tr	tr	tr
Fruit & Almond	5 fl oz	1	tr	tr	tr
Hibiscus & Rose Hips	5 fl oz	1	tr	tr	tr
I Love Lemon	5 fl oz	1	tr	tr	tr
Lemon & C	5 fl oz	tr	tr	tr	tr
Looking Good	5 fl oz	1	1	tr	tr
Mint Blend	5 fl oz	tr	tr	tr	tr
Mint Medley	5 fl oz	1	tr	tr	tr
Orange & C	5 fl oz	tr	tr	tr	tr
Orange & Spice	5 fl oz	1	tr	tr	tr

FOOD	PORTION	CALS.	CARB.	FAT	PRO.
Bigelow (CONT.)					
Peppermint	5 fl oz	tr	tr	tr	tr
Roasted Grains & Carob	5 fl oz	3	1	tr	tr
Spearmint	5 fl oz	tr	tr	tr	tr
Sweet Dreams	5 fl oz	1	tr	tr	tr
Take-A-Break	5 fl oz	3	1	tr	tr
Celestial Seasonings					
Almond Sunset	8 fl oz	3	1	tr	tr
Bengal Spice	8 fl oz	5	tr	tr	1
Caffeine Free	8 fl oz	2	1	tr	tr
Chamomile	8 fl oz	2	1	tr	tr
Cinnamon Apple Spice	8 fl oz	<3	tr	tr	tr
Cinnamon Rose	8 fl oz	<4	1	tr	tr
Cranberry Cove	8 fl oz	2	1	tr	tr
Emperor's Choice	8 fl oz	4	1	tr	tr
Ginseng Plus	8 fl oz	3	1	tr	tr
Grandma's Tummy Mint	8 fl oz	2	tr	tr	tr
Lemon Mist	8 fl oz	3	tr	tr	tr
Lemon Zinger	8 of oz	4	1	tr	tr
Mama Bear's Cold Care	8 fl oz	6	tr	tr	1
Mandarin Orange Spice	8 fl oz	5	1	tr	tr
Mellow Mint	8 fl oz	2	tr	tr	tr
Mint Magic	8 fl oz	1	tr	tr	tr
Orange Zinger	8 fl oz	6	1	tr	tr
Peppermint	8 fl oz	2	1	tr	tr
Peppermint	8 fl oz	2	1	tr	tr
Raspberry Patch	8 fl oz	4	1	tr	tr
Red Zinger	8 fl oz	4	1	tr	tr
Roastaroma	8 fl oz	10	2	tr	tr
Sleepytime	8 fl oz	4	1	tr	tr
Spearmint	8 fl oz	5	tr	1	tr
Strawberry Fields	8 fl oz	4	1	tr	tr
Sunburst C	8 fl oz	3	1	tr	tr
Tropical Escape	8 fl oz	1	tr	tr	tr
Wild Forest Blackberry	8 fl oz	2	1	tr	tr
REGULAR					
brewed tea	6 oz	2	tr	0	0
instant unsweetened as prep w/ water	8 oz	2	tr	0	tr
Bigelow					
Chinese Fortune	5 fl oz	1	tr	tr	tr
Cinnamon Stick	5 fl oz	1	tr	tr	tr
Constant Comment	5 fl oz	1	tr	tr	tr
Darjeeling Blend	5 fl oz	1	tr	tr	tr

FOOD	PORTION	CALS.	CARB.	FAT	PRO.
Bigelow (CONT.)					
Earl Gray	5 fl oz	1	tr	tr	tr
English Teatime	5 fl oz	1	tr	tr	tr
Lemon Lift	5 fl oz	1	tr	tr	tr
Orange Pekoe	5 fl oz	1	tr	tr	tr
Peppermint Stick	5 fl oz	1	tr	tr	tr
Plantation Mint	5 fl oz	1	tr	tr	tr
Raspberry Royale	5 fl oz	1	tr	tr	tr
Celestial Seasonings					
Cinnamon Vienna	8 fl oz	2	1	tr	tr
Earl Grey Extraordinary	8 fl oz	3	1	tr	tr
English Breakfast Classic	8 fl oz	3	1	tr	tr
Lemon	8 fl oz	7	1	tr	1
Mint	8 fl oz	4	tr	tr	tr
Morning Thunder	8 fl oz	3	tr	tr	tr
Naturally Decaffeinated	8 fl oz	10	tr	1	1
Orange Spice	8 fl oz	7	1	tr	1
Orange Spice Decaff	8 fl oz	7	1	tr	tr
Organically Grown	8 fl oz	12	1	tr	1
Raspberry	8 fl oz	7	1	tr	1
Natural Touch					
Kaffree	8 fl oz	0	0	0	0
Nestea					
Tea Bag as prep	6 oz	0	0	0	0
TEFF					
Arrowhead					
Whole Grain	¼ cup (1.6 oz)	160	32	1	5
TEMPEH					
tempeh	½ cup	165	14	6	16
Lightlife					
Garden Vege	4 oz	142	9	4	18
Tempeh	4 oz	182	9	6	24
White Wave					
Burger	1 patty (3 oz)	110	10	3	12
Lemon Broil	1 patty (2 oz)	130	11	6	8
Organic Wild Rice	⅓ block (2.7 oz)	140	12	4	13
Teriyaki Burger	1 patty (3 oz)	110	11	2	10
THYME					
ground	1 tsp	4	1	tr	tr
Watkins					
Thyme	¼ tsp (0.5 oz)	0	0	0	0
TILEFISH					
cooked	½ fillet (5.3 oz)	220	0	7	37

FOOD	PORTION	CALS.	CARB.	FAT	PRO.
cooked	3 oz	125	0	4	21
raw	3 oz	81	0	2	15
TOFU					
firm	¼ block (3 oz)	118	3	7	13
firm	½ cup	183	5	11	20
fresh fried	1 piece (½ oz)	35	1	3	2
fuyu salted & fermented	1 block (⅓ oz)	13	1	1	1
koyadofu dried frozen	1 piece (½ oz)	82	2	5	8
okara	½ cup	47	8	1	2
regular	¼ block (4 oz)	88	2	6	9
regular	½ cup	94	2	6	6
Azumaya					
Blue Label	3.5 oz	46	4	1	5
Green Label	3.5 oz	68	4	2	9
Name Age Fried	3.5 oz	144	9	4	17
Red Label	3.5 oz	68	5	1	9
Casbah					
Gyro as prep w/ tofu	1 patty (2 oz)	105	15	3	2
Jaclyn's					
Grilled In Black Bean Sauce	10.75 oz	270	45	8	17
Grilled In Peanut Sauce	10.75 oz	260	44	9	19
Mori-Nu					
Extra Firm	1 in slice (3 oz)	55	2	2	7
Firm	1 in slice (3 oz)	50	2	3	6
Lite Extra Firm	1 in slice (3 oz)	35	1	1	6
Lite Firm	1 in slice (3 oz)	35	1	1	5
Soft	1 in slice (3 oz)	45	2	3	4
Nasoya					
Extra Firm	⅕ block (3 oz)	90	1	5	11
Firm	⅕ block (3 oz)	80	2	4	9
Silken	⅙ block (3 oz)	50	2	2	5
Soft	⅕ block (3 oz)	60	2	3	7
Spring Creek					
Baked Barbeque	2 oz	88	7	4	7
Baked Cajun	2 oz	87	5	4	7
Baked Teriyaki	2 oz	84	3	4	8
Great Balls Of Tofu!	2 (3 oz)	107	5	5	8
Nigari Firm	4 oz	140	tr	8	16
Tofu Salads !Onion Dip	2 oz	46	6	14	6
Tofu Salads !Taco Dip	2 oz	46	6	14	6
Tofu Salads Missing Egg	2 oz	49	6	14	6
Tree Of Life					
Baked	⅕ block (3.2 oz)	150	5	8	16

FOOD	PORTION	CALS.	CARB.	FAT	PRO.
Tree Of Life (cont.)					
Firm	⅕ block (3.2 oz)	100	2	5	9
Raw Firm	⅕ block (3.2 oz)	100	2	5	9
Ready Ground Hot & Spicy	⅓ pkg (3 oz)	60	2	4	7
Ready Ground Original	⅓ pkg (3 oz)	60	2	4	7
Ready Ground Savory Garlic	⅓ pkg (3 oz)	60	2	4	7
Reduced Fat	⅕ block (3.2 oz)	90	4	4	10
Savory Baked	⅕ block (3.2 oz)	140	4	8	15
Smoked Hot'N Spicy	½ block (3 oz)	120	3	5	18
Smoked Original	½ block (3 oz)	120	3	5	18
White Wave					
Baked Tofus Teriyaki Oriental Style	¼ block (2 oz)	120	3	6	13
Hard	4 oz	120	1	7	12
International Baked Italian Garlic Herb	¼ pkg (2 oz)	120	3	6	13
International Baked Mexican Jalapeno	¼ pkg (2 oz)	120	3	6	13
International Baked Oriental Teriyaki	¼ pkg (2 oz)	120	3	6	13
International Baked Thai Sesame Peanut	¼ pkg (2 oz)	120	3	6	13
Soft	4 oz	120	1	7	12
YOGURT					
Stir Fruity					
Black Cherry	6 oz	141	25	2	6
Blueberry	6 oz	140	26	1	6
Lemon Chiffon	6 oz	152	26	3	6
Mixed Berry	6 oz	149	26	2	6
Orange	6 oz	143	26	2	6
Peach	6 oz	160	27	3	6
Pina Colada	6 oz	162	28	3	6
Raspberry	6 oz	155	29	2	6
Spiced Apple	6 oz	167	31	2	6
Strawberry	6 oz	140	25	2	6
Tropical Fruit	6 oz	170	32	2	6

TOFUTTI

(*see* ICE CREAM AND FROZEN DESSERTS)

TOMATILLO

fresh	1 (1.2 oz)	11	2	tr	tr
fresh chopped	½ cup	21	4	1	1

FOOD	PORTION	CALS.	CARB.	FAT	PRO.
TOMATO					
(see also PIZZA, SPAGHETTI SAUCE)					
CANNED					
paste	½ cup	110	25	1	5
puree	1 cup	102	25	tr	4
puree w/o salt	1 cup	102	25	tr	4
red whole	½ cup	24	5	tr	1
sauce	½ cup	37	9	tr	2
sauce spanish style	½ cup	40	9	tr	2
sauce w/ mushrooms	½ cup	42	10	tr	2
sauce w/ onion	½ cup	52	12	tr	1
stewed	½ cup	34	8	tr	1
w/ green chiles	½ cup	18	4	tr	1
wedges in tomato juice	½ cup	34	8	tr	1
Contadina					
Crushed	¼ cup	20	4	0	tr
Italian Paste	2 tbsp	40	7	1	1
Italian Style Pear	½ cup	25	4	0	1
Italian Style Stewed	½ cup	40	8	0	1
Mexican Style Stewed	½ cup	40	9	0	1
Pasta Ready Primavera	½ cup	50	8	2	1
Pasta Ready Tomatoes	½ cup	50	7	2	1
Pasta Ready With Crushed Red Pepper	½ cup	60	8	3	1
Pasta Ready With Mushrooms	½ cup	50	9	2	1
Pasta Ready With Olives	½ cup	60	8	3	1
Pasta Ready With Three Cheeses	½ cup	70	8	4	1
Paste	2 tbsp	30	6	0	2
Peeled Whole	½ cup	25	4	0	1
Puree	¼ cup	20	4	0	tr
Recipe Ready	½ cup	25	5	0	1
Stewed	½ cup	40	9	0	1
Del Monte					
Paste	2 tbsp (1.2 oz)	30	7	0	1
Peeled Diced	½ cup (4.4 oz)	25	6	0	1
Puree	¼ cup (2.2 oz)	30	7	0	1
Sauce	¼ cup (2.1 oz)	20	4	0	tr
Sauce No Salt Added	¼ cup (2.1 oz)	20	4	0	tr
Stewed Cajun Style	½ cup (4.4 oz)	35	9	0	1
Stewed Chunky Chili	½ cup (4.5 oz)	30	8	0	1
Stewed Chunky Pasta	½ cup (4.5 oz)	45	11	0	1

FOOD	PORTION	CALS.	CARB.	FAT	PRO.
Del Monte (CONT.)					
Stewed Chunky Pizza	½ cup (4.5 oz)	35	9	0	1
Stewed Chunky Salsa	½ cup (4.5 oz)	35	8	0	1
Stewed Italian Style	½ cup (4.4 oz)	30	8	0	1
Stewed Mexican Style	½ cup (4.4 oz)	35	9	0	1
Stewed Original	½ cup (4.4 oz)	35	9	0	1
Stewed Original No Salt Added	½ cup (4.4 oz)	35	9	0	1
Wedges	½ cup (4.4 oz)	35	9	0	1
Whole Peeled	½ cup (4.4 oz)	25	6	0	1
Eden					
Crushed Organic	¼ cup (2.1 oz)	20	3	0	1
Sauce Lightly Seasoned	¼ cup (2.1 oz)	25	5	0	1
Health Valley					
Sauce	1 cup	70	13	1	2
Sauce Low Sodium	1 cup	70	13	1	2
Hebrew National					
Pickled	⅓ tomato (1 oz)	4	1	0	0
Hunt's					
All Natural Sauce	¼ cup (2.2 fl oz)	15	3	0	1
Crushed Angela Mia	4 oz	35	7	tr	1
Crushed Italian	4 oz	40	9	tr	2
Italian Pear Shaped	4 oz	20	5	tr	1
Paste	1 oz	25	5	0	1
Paste Italian Style	2 oz	50	11	tr	2
Paste No Salt Added	2 oz	45	11	tr	2
Paste With Garlic	2 oz	50	11	tr	2
Peeled Choice-Cut	4 oz	20	5	tr	1
Puree	4 oz	45	10	tr	2
Sauce Herb	4 oz	70	12	2	2
Sauce Italian	4 oz	60	10	2	2
Sauce Meatloaf Fixin's	4 oz	20	5	tr	tr
Sauce No Salt Added	4 oz	35	8	tr	1
Sauce Special	4 oz	35	8	tr	1
Sauce With Bits	4 oz	30	7	tr	1
Sauce With Garlic	4 oz	70	10	2	2
Sauce With Mushrooms	4 oz	25	6	tr	1
Stewed	4 oz	35	8	tr	1
Stewed Italian	4 oz	40	9	tr	2
Stewed No Salt Added	4 oz	35	8	tr	1
Whole	4 oz	20	5	tr	1
Whole Italian	4 oz	25	6	tr	1
Whole No Salt Added	4 oz	20	5	tr	1

FOOD	PORTION	CALS.	CARB.	FAT	PRO.
Muir Glen					
Organic Chunky Sauce	¼ cup (2.3 oz)	20	4	0	tr
Organic Crushed With Basil	¼ cup (2.3 oz)	25	4	0	1
Organic Diced	½ cup (4.5 oz)	25	4	0	1
Organic Diced No Salt Added	½ cup (4.5 oz)	25	4	0	1
Organic Ground Peeled	¼ cup (2.3 oz)	10	2	0	tr
Organic Italian Style Diced	½ cup (4.4 oz)	25	4	0	1
Organic Paste	2 tbsp (1.2 oz)	30	6	0	2
Organic Puree	¼ cup (2.2 oz)	20	5	0	1
Organic Sauce	¼ cup (2.2 oz)	20	5	0	tr
Organic Sauce No Salt Added	¼ cup (2.2 oz)	20	5	0	tr
Organic Stewed	½ cup (4.5 oz)	30	7	0	1
Organic Stewed Italian Style	½ cup (4.4 oz)	30	7	0	1
Organic Stewed Mexican Style	½ cup (4.4 oz)	30	7	0	1
Organic Whole Peeled	½ cup (4.6 oz)	30	5	0	1
Rosoff's					
Pickled	⅓ tomato (1 oz)	5	1	0	0
S&W					
Aspic Supreme	½ cup	60	16	0	1
Diced In Rich Puree	½ cup	35	8	0	1
Italian Stewed Sliced	½ cup	35	9	0	1
Italian Style w/ Basil	½ cup	25	5	0	1
Paste	6 oz	150	35	0	6
Peeled Ready Cut	½ cup	25	6	0	1
Puree	½ cup	60	14	0	2
Sauce	½ cup	40	9	0	2
Sauce Chunky	½ cup	45	10	0	2
Stewed 50% Salt Reduced	½ cup	35	9	0	1
Stewed Mexican Style	½ cup	40	8	0	1
Stewed Sliced	½ cup	35	9	0	1
Whole Diet	½ cup	25	5	0	1
Whole Peeled	½ cup	25	6	0	1
Schorr's					
Pickled	⅓ tomato (1 oz)	4	1	0	0
Sonoma					
Dried Spice Medley oil drained	1 tbsp (0.5 oz)	50	3	4	1

FOOD	PORTION	CALS.	CARB.	FAT	PRO.
Sonoma (CONT.)					
Pesto	¼ cup (2 oz)	110	6	9	3
Tapenade	1 tbsp (0.7 oz)	70	4	6	1
Tree Of Life					
Sauce	¼ cup (2 oz)	20	4	0	1
DRIED					
sun dried	1 piece	5	1	tr	tr
sun dried	1 cup	140	30	2	8
sun dried in oil	1 piece (3 g)	6	1	tr	tr
sun dried in oil	1 cup (4 oz)	235	26	15	6
Sonoma					
Bits	2-3 tsp (5 g)	15	3	0	1
Dried	2-3 halves (5 g)	15	3	0	1
Halves	2-3 halves (5 g)	15	3	0	1
Julienne	7-9 pieces (5 g)	15	3	0	1
Pasta Toss	½ cup (0.7 oz)	70	13	0	4
Season It	2-3 tsp (5 g)	20	3	0	1
FRESH					
cooked	½ cup	32	7	1	1
green	1	30	6	tr	1
red	1 (4½ oz)	26	6	tr	1
red chopped	1 cup	35	8	tr	2
TAKE-OUT					
stewed	1 cup	80	13	3	2
TOMATO JUICE					
beef broth & tomato	5½ oz	61	14	tr	1
clam & tomato	1 can (5½ oz)	77	18	tr	1
tomato juice	6 oz	32	8	tr	1
tomato juice	½ cup	21	5	tr	1
Campbell					
Juice	6 oz	40	8	0	1
Del Monte					
Snap-E-Tom	6 fl oz	40	8	0	2
Snap-E-Tom	10 fl oz	60	13	0	3
Snap-E-Tom	8 fl oz	50	11	0	2
Hunt's					
Juice	6 oz	30	7	tr	1
No Salt Added	6 oz	35	8	tr	1
Libby					
Juice	6 oz	35	35	0	1
Mott's					
Beefamato	8 fl oz	80	20	0	1
Clamato	8 fl oz	100	24	0	1

FOOD	PORTION	CALS.	CARB.	FAT	PRO.
Mott's (CONT.)					
Clamato Ceasar	8 fl oz	100	24	0	0
Muir Glen					
Organic	8 oz	40	7	0	3
S&W					
California	6 oz	35	8	0	1
Diet	½ cup	35	8	0	1
TONGUE					
beef simmered	3 oz	241	tr	18	19
lamb braised	3 oz	234	0	17	18
pork braised	3 oz	230	0	16	20
TOPPINGS					
(*see* ICE CREAM TOPPINGS)					
TORTILLA					
(*see also* CHIPS TORTILLA, SPANISH FOOD)					
corn	1 (6 in diam)	56	12	1	1
corn w/o salt	1-6 in diam (.9 oz)	56	12	1	1
flour w/o salt	1-8 in diam (1.2 oz)	114	20	3	3
Alvarado St. Bakery					
Burrito Size	1 (2.2 oz)	170	30	4	5
Fajaita Size	1 (1.6 oz)	130	23	3	4
Mariachi					
Tortilla	1	112	20	3	3
Old El Paso					
Flour	1	150	27	3	4
Tyson					
Burrito Style Flour	1	170	29	4	5
Burrito Style Hand Stretched Small Flour	1	106	19	2	3
Burrito Style Heat Pressed Large Flour	1	182	33	4	5
Enchilada Style Corn	1	54	11	tr	1
Fajito Style Flour	1	89	15	2	3
Soft Taco Flour	1	121	20	3	4
Whole Wheat	1	120	20	3	4
Wonder					
Low Fat Wheat	1 (1.4 oz)	120	24	2	3
Low Fat White	1 (1.4 oz)	110	22	2	3
Zapata					
Tortilla	1 (1.2 oz)	100	18	2	33
TORTILLA CHIPS					
(*see* CHIPS)					

FOOD	PORTION	CALS.	CARB.	FAT	PRO.
TRITICALE					
dry	½ cup	323	69	2	13
triticale not prep	3.5 oz	329	64	2	13
TROUT					
baked	3 oz	162	0	7	23
rainbow cooked	3 oz	129	0	4	22
seatrout baked	3 oz	113	0	4	18
Clear Springs					
Rainbow	3.5 oz	140	tr	7	20
TRUFFLES					
fresh	3½ oz	25	17	1	6
TUNA					
(*see also* TUNA DISHES)					
CANNED					
light in oil	3 oz	169	0	7	25
light in oil	1 can (6 oz)	399	0	14	50
light in water	3 oz	99	0	1	22
light in water	1 can (5.8 oz)	192	0	1	42
white in oil	3 oz	158	0	7	23
white in oil	1 can (6.2 oz)	331	0	14	47
white in water	1 can (6 oz)	234	0	4	46
white in water	3 oz	116	0	2	23
Bumble Bee					
Chunk Light In Oil	2 oz	160	0	12	12
Chunk Light In Water	2 oz	60	0	1	12
Chunk White In Oil	2 oz	160	0	12	12
Chunk White In Water	2 oz	70	0	2	12
Chunk White In Water Diet	2 oz	60	0	1	13
Solid White In Oil	2 oz	130	0	8	14
Solid White In Water	2 oz	70	0	2	14
Empress					
Chunk Light	2 oz	60	0	1	12
Chunk Light Tongol	2 oz	50	0	1	11
Solid White	2 oz	70	0	2	14
Progresso					
Tuna	⅓ cup	150	tr	13	13
S&W					
Chunk Light Fancy In Oil	2 oz	140	0	10	12
Chunk Light Fancy In Water	2 oz	60	0	1	13
Fancy White Albacore in Oil	2 oz	160	0	12	13

FOOD	PORTION	CALS.	CARB.	FAT	PRO.
Tree Of Life					
Tongol In Spring Water	2 oz	60	0	0	13
Tongol In Spring Water No Salt Water	2 oz	70	0	0	13
FRESH					
bluefin cooked	3 oz	157	0	5	25
bluefin raw	3 oz	122	0	4	20
skipjack baked	3 oz	112	0	1	24
yellowfin baked	3 oz	118	0	1	25

TUNA DISHES

FROZEN

FOOD	PORTION	CALS.	CARB.	FAT	PRO.
Mrs. Paul's					
Microwave Tuna Sandwich	1	200	23	6	10
MIX					
Bumble Bee					
Tuna Mix-ins Classic Italian	⅓ pkg (0.17 oz)	25	5	0	0
Tuna Mix-ins Garden & Herb	⅓ pkg (0.17 oz)	25	5	0	0
Tuna Mix-ins Lemon Herb	⅓ pkg (0.17 oz)	25	6	0	0
Tuna Mix-ins Zesty Tomato	⅓ pkg (0.17 oz)	25	5	0	0
Tuna Helper					
Au Gratin as prep	⅕ pkg (6 oz)	280	30	11	16
Buttery Rice as prep	⅕ pkg (6 oz)	280	32	11	13
Cheesy Noodles as prep	⅕ pkg (7.75 oz)	240	27	8	16
Creamy Mushroom as prep	⅕ pkg (7 oz)	220	29	6	15
Creamy Noodles as prep	⅕ pkg (8 oz)	300	29	14	15
Fettucine Alfredo as prep	⅕ pkg (7 oz)	300	30	13	16
Romanoff as prep	⅕ pkg (8 oz)	290	38	8	16
Tetrazzini as prep	⅕ pkg (6 oz)	240	27	8	15
Tuna Pot Pie as prep	⅙ pkg (5.1 oz)	420	31	27	13
Tuna Salad as prep	⅕ pkg (5.5 oz)	420	29	27	14
READY-TO-USE					
Wampler Longacre					
Salad	1 oz	60	3	4	2
TAKE-OUT					
tuna salad	1 cup	383	19	19	33
tuna salad	3 oz	159	8	8	14
tuna salad submarine sandwich w/ lettuce & oil	1	584	55	28	30

FOOD	PORTION	CALS.	CARB.	FAT	PRO.
TURBOT					
european baked	3 oz	104	0	3	17
TURKEY					
(see also DINNER, HOT DOG, TURKEY DISHES, TURKEY SUBSTITUTES)					
CANNED					
w/ broth	½ can (2.5 oz)	116	0	5	17
w/ broth	1 can (5 oz)	231	0	10	34
Armour					
Turkey Loaf	2 oz	110	1	8	8
Hormel					
Chunk	2 oz	70	0	3	11
Chunk Turkey Ham	2 oz	70	0	4	9
Chunk White	2 oz	60	0	1	13
Swanson					
White	2½ oz	80	1	1	17
Underwood					
Chunky Light	2.08 oz	75	2	2	11
FRESH					
back w/ skin roasted	½ back (9 oz)	637	0	38	70
breast w/ skin roasted	4 oz	212	0	8	32
dark meat w/ skin roasted	3.6 oz	230	0	12	29
dark meat w/o skin roasted	1 cup (5 oz)	262	0	10	40
dark meat w/o skin roasted	3 oz	170	0	7	26
ground cooked	3 oz	188	0	11	20
leg w/ skin roasted	2.5 oz	147	0	7	20
leg w/ skin roasted	1 (1.2 lbs)	1133	0	54	152
light meat w/ skin roasted	from ½ turkey (2.3 lbs)	2069	0	87	87
light meat w/ skin roasted	4.7 oz	268	0	11	39
light meat w/o skin roasted	4 oz	183	0	4	35
neck simmered	1 (5.3 oz)	274	0	11	41
skin roasted	1 oz	141	0	13	13
skin roasted	from ½ turkey (9 oz)	1096	0	98	49
w/ skin roasted	8.4 oz	498	0	23	67
w/ skin roasted	½ turkey (4 lbs)	3857	0	181	522
w/ skin neck & giblets roasted	½ turkey (8.8 lbs)	4123	1	190	190
w/o skin roasted	1 cup (5 oz)	238	0	7	41
w/o skin roasted	7.3 oz	354	0	10	61
wing w/ skin roasted	1 (6.5 oz)	426	0	23	51
Butterball					
Ground All White Meat	3 oz	100	tr	3	19

FOOD	PORTION	CALS.	CARB.	FAT	PRO.
Louis Rich					
Ground	3 oz	140	0	9	15
Mr. Turkey					
Ground 85% Fat Free	3.5 oz	210	0	16	18
Ground 91% Fat Free	3.5 oz	170	1	10	18
Perdue					
Breast Cutlets Thin-Sliced Skinless & Boneless	1 oz	28	0	tr	7
Breast Fillets Skinless & Boneless Fit 'n Easy cooked	1 oz	28	0	tr	7
Breast Hotel Style Prime w/ Skin cooked	1 oz	43	0	2	6
Breast Skinless Boneless Fit'n Easy cooked	1 oz	28	0	tr	7
Breast Tenderloins Skinless & Boneless cooked	1 oz	29	0	tr	7
Breast w/ Skin Fresh Young cooked	1 oz	44	0	2	6
Drumsticks w/ Skin Fresh Young cooked	1 oz	36	0	2	6
Ground cooked	1 oz	35	0	2	5
Ground Breast Meat cooked	1 oz	28	0	tr	7
Thighs Skinless & Boneless Fit 'n Fresh cooked	1 oz	36	0	2	7
Thighs w/ Skin Fresh Young cooked	1 oz	48	0	3	5
Whole Dark Meat w/ skin cooked	1 oz	48	0	3	7
Whole White Meat Fresh Young w/ Skin cooked	1 oz	44	0	2	6
Wings Drummettes w/ Skin Fresh Young cooked	1 oz	43	0	2	6
Wings Portions w/ Skin Fresh Young cooked	1 oz	51	0	3	6
Wings w/ Skin Fresh Young cooked	1 oz	45	0	2	6
Swift-Eckrich					
Ground All White	3 oz	100	tr	3	19

FOOD	PORTION	CALS.	CARB.	FAT	PRO.
Wampler Longacre					
Ground raw	1 oz	60	0	4	5
FROZEN					
roast boneless seasoned light & dark meat roasted	1 pkg (1.7 lbs)	1213	24	45	167
FROZEN PREPARED					
Empire					
Patties	1 (3.1 oz)	200	14	10	13
READY-TO-USE					
bologna	1 oz	57	tr	4	4
breast	1 slice (¾ oz)	23	0	tr	5
diced light & dark seasoned	½ lb	313	2	14	42
diced light & dark seasoned	1 oz	39	tr	2	5
ham thigh meat	2 oz	73	tr	3	11
ham thigh meat	1 pkg (8 oz)	291	1	12	43
pastrami	1 pkg (8 oz)	320	4	14	42
pastrami	2 oz	80	1	4	10
patties battered & fried	1 (3.3 oz)	266	15	17	13
patties battered & fried	1 (2.3 oz)	181	10	12	9
patties breaded & fried	1 (2.3 oz)	181	10	12	9
patties breaded & fried	1 (3.3 oz)	266	15	17	13
poultry salad sandwich spread	1 oz	238	2	4	4
poultry salad sandwich spread	1 tbsp	109	1	2	2
prebasted breast w/ skin roasted	1 breast (3.8 lbs)	2175	0	60	383
prebasted breast w/ skin roasted	½ breast (1.9 lbs)	1087	0	30	191
prebasted thigh w/ skin roasted	1 thigh (11 oz)	494	0	27	59
roll light & dark meat	1 oz	42	1	2	5
roll light meat	1 oz	42	2	2	5
salami cooked	1 pkg (8 oz)	446	1	31	37
salami cooked	2 oz	111	tr	8	9
turkey loaf breast meat	2 slices (1.5 oz)	47	0	1	10
turkey loaf breast meat	1 pkg (6 oz)	187	0	3	38
turkey sticks battered & fried	1 stick (2.3 oz)	178	11	11	9
turkey sticks breaded & fried	1 stick (2.3 oz)	178	11	11	9

FOOD	PORTION	CALS.	CARB.	FAT	PRO.
Alpine Lace					
Breast Fat Free	2 oz	50	0	0	12
Carl Buddig					
Honey Turkey	1 oz	40	1	2	5
Turkey	1 oz	50	1	3	5
Turkey Ham	1 oz	40	1	2	5
Empire					
Barbecue Whole	5 oz	250	0	12	35
Bologna	3 slices (1.8 oz)	90	3	6	8
Oven Prepared Breast Slices	3 slices (1.8 oz)	50	1	1	10
Pastrami	3 slices (1.8 oz)	60	0	2	9
Salami	3 slices (1.8 oz)	70	1	4	9
Smoked Breast Slices	3 slices (1.8 oz)	40	0	0	8
Falls					
BBQ	3 oz	140	—	8	17
Gourmet Breast	3 oz	80	—	1	18
Premium Cooked Breast	3 oz	100	—	2	20
Hansel n'Gretel					
Breast Gourmet	1 oz	28	1	1	5
Breast Gourmet Smoked	1 oz	31	tr	1	6
Breast Honey	1 oz	28	1	1	5
Breast Lessalt Cooked	1 oz	25	tr	1	5
Breast Oven Cooked	1 oz	26	tr	tr	5
Doubledecker Turkey Corned Beef	1 oz	30	1	1	5
Doubledecker Turkey Ham	1 oz	30	1	1	5
Healthy Choice					
Deli-Thin Honey Roast & Smoked	6 slices (2 oz)	70	2	2	10
Deli-Thin Roasted Breast	6 slices (2 oz)	60	1	2	11
Deli-Thin Smoked Breast	6 slices (2 oz)	60	1	2	11
Deli-Thin Turkey Ham	6 slices (2 oz)	60	1	2	11
Fresh-Trak Honey Roast & Smoked Breast	1 slice (1 oz)	35	1	1	5
Fresh-Trak Oven Roasted Breast	1 slice (1 oz)	35	1	1	6
Honey Roasted & Smoked	1 slice (1 oz)	35	1	1	5
Oven Roasted Breast	1 slice (1 oz)	35	1	1	6
Smoked Breast	1 slice (1 oz)	30	0	1	6
Variety Pack Regular	3 slices (2.2 oz)	70	2	2	13

FOOD	PORTION	CALS.	CARB.	FAT	PRO.
Hebrew National					
Deli Thin Hickory Smoked	1.8 oz	55	—	1	11
Deli Thin Lemon Garlic	1.8 oz	50	—	1	11
Deli Thin Oven Roasted	1.8 oz	80	—	1	11
Hillshire					
Deli Select Honey Roasted Breast	1 slice	10	tr	tr	2
Deli Select Oven Roasted Breast	1 slice	10	tr	tr	2
Deli Select Smoked Breast	1 slice	10	tr	tr	2
Deli Select Turkey Ham	1 slice	10	tr	tr	2
Flavor Pack 90-99% Fat Free Smoked Breast	1 slice (0.75 oz)	20	tr	tr	4
Flavor Pack 90-99% Fat Free Honey Roasted Breast	1 slice (0.75 oz)	20	1	tr	4
Flavor Pack 90-99% Fat Free Oven Roasted Breast	1 slice (0.75 oz)	20	1	tr	4
Honey Cured Breast	1 oz	35	2	1	5
Lunch 'N Munch Smoked Turkey/ Cheddar	1 pkg (4.5 oz)	350	20	21	21
Lunch 'N Munch Smoked Turkey/ Cheddar/ Brownie	1 pkg (4.5 oz)	400	34	22	17
Lunch 'N Munch Turkey/ Cheddar/ Brownie/ Hi-C	1 pkg (4.5 oz + 6 fl oz)	500	58	22	17
Smoked Breast	1 oz	35	1	1	6
Hormel					
Light & Lean 97 Breast Sliced	1 slice (1 oz)	30	0	1	5
Light & Lean 97 Breast Smoked	3 oz	80	1	1	17
Light & Lean 97 Cuts	16 pieces (1 oz)	30	1	1	6
Light & Lean 97 Cuts Smoked	16 pieces (1 oz)	30	1	1	6
Louis Rich					
Bologna	1 slice (28 g)	50	1	4	3
Breaded Nuggets	4 (3.2 oz)	260	15	15	13
Breaded Patties	1 (3 oz)	220	13	13	12

FOOD	PORTION	CALS.	CARB.	FAT	PRO.
Louis Rich (CONT.)					
Breaded Sticks	3 (3 oz)	230	12	15	12
Carving Board Oven Roasted Breast	2 slices (1.6 oz)	40	0	1	9
Carving Board Oven Roasted Thin Carved Breast	6 slices (2.1 oz)	60	0	1	12
Carving Board Smoked Breast	2 slices (1.6 oz)	40	0	1	9
Chopped Ham	1 slice (1 oz)	46	0	3	5
Cotto Salami	1 slice (28 g)	40	0	3	5
Deli-Thin Smoked Breast	4 slices (1.8 oz)	50	1	1	9
Fat Free Hickory Smoked Breast	1 slice (1 oz)	25	1	0	4
Fat Free Oven Roasted Breast	1 slice (28 g)	25	1	0	4
Ham Round	1 slice (28 g)	34	0	1	5
Ham Square	3 slices (2.2 oz)	70	1	3	11
Hickory Smoked Dinner Slices Breast	1 slice (2.8 oz)	80	2	1	16
Honey Cured Turkey Ham	3 slices (2.2 oz)	70	2	2	11
Honey Roasted Breast	1 slice (1 oz)	30	1	1	5
Honey Roasted Dinner Slices Breast	1 slice (2.8 oz)	80	3	1	16
Oven Roasted Breast	2 oz	60	2	2	10
Oven Roasted Breast	1 slice (1 oz)	30	1	1	5
Oven Roasted Deli-Thin Breast	4 slices (1.8 oz)	50	2	1	9
Oven Roasted Dinner Slices Breast	1 slice (2.8 oz)	70	1	1	16
Pastrami	2 slices (1.6 oz)	45	0	2	8
Salami	1 slice (28 g)	45	0	3	5
Skinless Barbecued Breast	2 oz	60	2	1	12
Skinless Hickory Smoked Breast	2 oz	60	1	1	12
Skinless Honey Roasted Breast	2 oz	60	2	1	11
Skinless Oven Roasted Breast	2 oz	50	1	1	11
Smoked Breast	1 slice (1 oz)	25	0	1	5
Smoked White	1 slice (1 oz)	30	0	1	5
Turkey Ham	4 slices (1.8 oz)	60	0	2	10

FOOD	PORTION	CALS.	CARB.	FAT	PRO.
Mr. Turkey					
Deli Cuts Hardwood Smoked Breast	3 slices	30	1	1	5
Deli Cuts Honey Roasted Breast	3 slices	30	2	1	5
Deli Cuts Oven Roasted Breast	3 slices	30	2	1	5
Deli Cuts Turkey Ham	3 slices	35	1	2	5
Deli Cuts Turkey Pastrami	3 slices	35	1	1	5
Hardwood Smoked Breast	1 slice	30	2	1	5
Hardwood Smoked Turkey Ham	1 slice	35	0	2	5
Honey Cured Turkey Ham	1 slice	30	1	1	5
Oven Roasted Breast	1 slice	30	2	1	5
Smoked Breakfast Turkey Ham	1 oz	30	1	1	5
Turkey Cotto Salami	1 slice	50	1	4	4
Turkey Ham	1 slice	35	0	2	5
Turkey Pastrami	1 slice	30	1	1	4
Turkey Bologna	1 slice	70	1	5	3
Oscar Mayer					
Deli-Thin Roast	4 slices (1.8 oz)	50	2	1	9
Deli-Thin Smoked Honey Roasted	4 slices (1.8 oz)	60	2	1	10
Free Oven Roasted Breast	4 slices (1.8 oz)	40	2	0	8
Free Smoked Breast	4 slices (1.8 oz)	40	2	0	8
Healthy Favorites Oven Roasted Breast	4 slices (1.8 oz)	40	2	0	8
Healthy Favorites Smoked Breast	4 slices (1.8 oz)	40	2	0	8
Lunchables Fun Pack Turkey/Pacific Cooler	1 pkg (11.2 oz)	460	53	21	16
Lunchables Fun Pack Turkey/Sugar Cooler	1 pkg (11.2 oz)	440	60	16	14
Lunchables Turkey Oven Roasted/Green Onion Cheese	1 pkg (4.5 oz)	380	36	20	14
Lunchables Turkey Smoked/ Ranch & Herb Cheese	1 pkg (4.5 oz)	380	36	20	14

FOOD	PORTION	CALS.	CARB.	FAT	PRO.
Oscar Mayer (CONT.)					
Lunchables Turkey/ Cheddar	1 pkg (4.5 oz)	360	20	22	20
Perdue					
Nuggets	1 (.67 oz)	54	3	3	3
Sara Lee					
Hardwood Smoked Breast Of Turkey	2 oz	60	0	1	13
Hardwood Smoked Turkey Ham	2 oz	60	1	2	10
Honey Roasted Breast Of Turkey	2 oz	60	2	0	12
Honey Roasted Turkey Ham	2 oz	70	2	3	9
Mesquite Smoked Breast Of Turkey	2 oz	60	0	2	12
Oven Roasted Breast Of Turkey	2 oz	60	0	2	12
Peppered Breast Of Turkey	2 oz	50	2	0	10
Seasoned Breast Of Turkey Pastrami	2 oz	60	2	1	12
Tyson					
Breast	1 slice	20	tr	tr	4
Ham	1 slice	23	1	tr	3
Wampler Longacre					
Bologna	1 oz	60	tr	5	4
Breast Chops	1 serv (4 oz)	120	0	1	22
Breast Sliced	1 slice (1 oz)	35	1	tr	3
Breast Sliced Smoked	1 slice (0.75 oz)	20	1	tr	4
Burger	1 (4 oz)	230	0	17	20
Burger	1 (3 oz)	170	0	13	15
Burger Barbecue	1 (4 oz)	240	4	17	19
Chef Select Breast Skinless	1 oz	35	tr	tr	6
Chef's Select Breast Smoked	1 oz	35	1	1	6
Chunk Dark Smoked Cured	1 oz	45	1	3	4
Chunk Ham 12% Water Smoked	1 oz	45	tr	3	4
Chunk Ham 20% Water	1 oz	40	2	2	4
Chunk Pastrami	1 oz	35	tr	2	6
Cook-In-The-Bag Breast	1 oz	30	1	1	6

FOOD	PORTION	CALS.	CARB.	FAT	PRO.
Wampler Longacre (CONT.)					
Cook-In-The-Bag Breast Mini	1 oz	30	tr	1	6
Cook-In-The-Bag Combo Roast	1 oz	35	tr	1	7
Cook-In-The-Bag Thigh Roast	1 oz	40	1	2	6
Dark Smoked Cured	1 oz	45	1	3	4
Deli Chef Breast And White Meat No Skin	1 oz	40	1	2	4
Gourmet Breast	1 oz	35	1	1	5
Gourmet Breast Mini	1 oz	35	1	1	5
Gourmet Breast Mini Smoked	1 oz	35	1	1	6
Gourmet Breast Smoked	1 oz	30	1	tr	6
Gourmet Brown & Glazed Breast	1 oz	35	1	1	5
Gourmet Brown & Roasted Breast	1 oz	35	1	1	5
Gourmet Honey Cured Breast	1 oz	30	1	1	5
Lean-Lite Breast Skinless	1 oz	35	0	tr	6
Lean-Lite Deli Breast	1 oz	35	0	1	6
Lean-Lite Deli Breast Smoked	1 oz	35	1	1	6
Old Fashioned Brown & Roasted Breast	1 oz	35	tr	tr	6
Pastrami	1 oz	35	tr	2	6
Premium Breast Skinless	1 oz	30	1	tr	4
Premium Brown & Roasted Breast Skinless	1 oz	16	1	1	5
Roll Combo	1 oz	44	tr	3	4
Roll Sliced Breast	1 slice (0.75 oz)	30	1	tr	4
Roll White	1 oz	45	tr	3	4
Salami	1 oz	50	1	3	5
Salt Watchers Breast Skinless	1 oz	35	0	1	7
Seasoned Roast	1 oz	40	0	2	6
Sliced Salami	1 slice (0.8 oz)	45	1	3	3
Tenderlings BBQ	1 serv (4 oz)	110	0	tr	24
Tenderlings Cajun	1 serv (4 oz)	110	0	tr	24

FOOD	PORTION	CALS.	CARB.	FAT	PRO.
Wampler Longacre (CONT.)					
Tenderlings Garlic & Pepper	1 serv (4 oz)	110	0	tr	24
Tenderlings Original	1 serv (4 oz)	110	0	tr	24
Turkey Ham 12% Water Baked	1 oz	45	tr	3	4
Turkey Ham 20% Water Baked	1 oz	40	1	2	4
Unseasoned Roast	1 oz	40	0	2	6
Whole Browned & Roasted	1 oz	60	tr	3	7
Weight Watchers					
Deli Thin Smoked Breast	5 slices (½ oz)	10	tr	tr	2
Oven Roasted Breast	2 slices (¾ oz)	25	tr	1	4
Oven Roasted Turkey Ham	2 slices (¾ oz)	25	tr	1	4
Roasted & Smoked Breast	2 slices (¾ oz)	25	tr	1	4

TURKEY DISHES

(*see also* DINNER, TURKEY SUBSTITUTES)

CANNED

FOOD	PORTION	CALS.	CARB.	FAT	PRO.
Dinty Moore					
American Classics Chicken With Mashed Potatoes	1 bowl (10 oz)	250	27	7	19
American Classics Turkey & Dressing With Gravy	1 bowl (10 oz)	280	32	7	23
FROZEN					
gravy & turkey	1 cup (8.4 oz)	160	11	6	14
gravy & turkey	1 pkg (5 oz)	95	7	4	8
Hot Pocket					
Stuffed Sandwich Turkey & Ham With Cheese	1 (4.5 oz)	320	38	13	14
Lean Pockets					
Stuffed Sandwich Turkey & Ham With Cheddar	1 (4.5 oz)	260	35	7	15
Stuffed Sandwich Turkey Broccoli & Cheese	1 (4.5 oz)	260	35	8	12
Luigino's					
Gravy Dressing & Turkey	1 pkg (8 oz)	340	36	15	16

FOOD	PORTION	CALS.	CARB.	FAT	PRO.
Ovenstuffs					
Turkey Turnover	1 (4.75 oz)	350	35	16	16
READY-TO-USE					
Wampler Longacre					
Meatloaf Italian	1 serv (4 oz)	114	5	5	17
Meatloaf Mexican	1 serv (4 oz)	114	4	5	17
Meatloaf Original	1 serv (4 oz)	126	10	5	18
Salad	1 oz	60	3	4	4
Salad Turkey Ham	1 oz	50	3	4	2
Teriyaki	1 serv (4 oz)	112	14	tr	11

TURKEY SUBSTITUTES

FOOD	PORTION	CALS.	CARB.	FAT	PRO.
Harvest Direct					
TVP Poultry Chunks	3.5 oz	280	32	1	52
TVP Poultry Ground	3.5 oz	280	32	1	52
White Wave					
Meatless Sandwich Slices	2 slices (1.6 oz)	80	7	0	13
Worthington					
Smoked Turkey Slices	4 slices (76 g)	180	5	12	13
Turkee Slices	2 slices (63 g)	130	3	9	9

TURNIPS

FOOD	PORTION	CALS.	CARB.	FAT	PRO.
CANNED					
greens	½ cup	17	3	tr	2
Allen					
Chopped Greens And Diced Turnip	½ cup (4.2 oz)	30	5	1	1
Greens	½ cup (4.2 oz)	25	3	1	2
Sunshine					
Chopped Greens And Diced Turnip	½ cup (4.2 oz)	30	5	1	1
Greens	½ cup (4.2 oz)	25	3	1	2
FRESH					
cooked mashed	½ cup (4.2 oz)	47	10	tr	2
cubed cooked	½ cup (3 oz)	33	7	tr	1
greens chopped cooked	½ cup	15	3	tr	1
greens raw chopped	½ cup	7	2	tr	tr
raw cubed	½ cup (2.4 oz)	25	6	tr	1
FROZEN					
greens cooked	½ cup	24	4	tr	3

TURTLE

FOOD	PORTION	CALS.	CARB.	FAT	PRO.
raw	3½ oz	85	0	1	18

FOOD	PORTION	CALS.	CARB.	FAT	PRO.
VANILLA					
Hershey					
Vanilla Milk Chips	¼ cup	240	25	14	3
VEAL					
(*see also* BEEF, DINNER, VEAL DISHES)					
FRESH					
cutlet lean only braised	3 oz	172	0	4	31
cutlet lean only fried	3 oz	156	0	4	28
ground broiled	3 oz	146	0	6	21
loin chop w/ bone lean & fat braised	1 chop (2.8 oz)	227	0	14	24
loin chop w/ bone lean only braised	1 chop (2.4 oz)	155	0	6	23
shoulder w/ bone lean only braised	3 oz	169	0	5	29
sirloin w/ bone lean & fat roasted	3 oz	171	0	9	21
sirloin w/ bone lean only roasted	3 oz	143	0	5	22
VEAL DISHES					
TAKE-OUT					
parmigiana	4.2 oz	279	6	18	22
VEGETABLE JUICE					
vegetable juice cocktail	6 fl oz	34	8	tr	1
vegetable juice cocktail	½ cup	22	6	tr	1
Mott's					
Vegetable Juice as prep	8 fl oz	60	13	0	2
Muir Glen					
Organic	8 oz	70	15	0	2
Organic Reduced Sodium	8 oz	70	15	0	2
Odwalla					
Vegetable Cocktail	8 fl oz	70	18	0	4
Smucker's					
Vegetable Juice Hearty	8 fl oz	58	13	tr	1
Vegetable Juice Hot & Spicy	8 fl oz	58	13	tr	1
V8					
No Salt Added	6 fl oz	35	8	0	1
Original	6 fl oz	35	8	0	1

FOOD	PORTION	CALS.	CARB.	FAT	PRO.
V8 (CONT.)					
Spicy Hot	6 fl oz	35	8	0	1

VEGETABLES MIXED
(see also individual vegetables, VEGETABLE JUICES)

FOOD	PORTION	CALS.	CARB.	FAT	PRO.
CANNED					
mixed vegetables	½ cup	39	8	tr	2
peas & carrots	½ cup	48	11	tr	3
peas & carrots low sodium	½ cup	48	11	tr	3
peas & onions	½ cup	30	5	tr	2
succotash	½ cup	102	23	1	4
Allen					
Green Beans And Pototoes	½ cup (4.2 oz)	35	7	0	1
Okra & Tomatoes	½ cup (4 oz)	25	5	0	1
Okra Tomatoes & Corn	½ cup (4.1 oz)	30	6	0	tr
Chi-Chi's					
Diced Tomatoes & Green Chilies	¼ cup (2.5 oz)	20	4	0	0
Del Monte					
Mixed	½ cup (4.4 oz)	40	8	0	2
Peas And Carrots	½ cup (4.5 oz)	60	11	0	2
Green Giant					
Garden Medley	½ cup	40	9	tr	1
House Of Tsang					
Vegetables & Sauce Cantonese Classic	½ cup (4.2 oz)	70	13	1	1
Vegetables & Sauce Hong Kong Sweet & Sour	½ cup (4.5 oz)	160	40	0	0
Vegetables & Sauce Szechuan Hot & Spicy	½ cup (4.2 oz)	70	14	1	1
Vegetables & Sauce Tokyo Teriyaki	½ cup (4.4 oz)	100	22	0	2
Ka-Me					
Stir Fry	½ cup (4.5 oz)	20	4	0	1
La Choy					
Chop Suey Vegetables	½ cup	10	2	tr	1
S&W					
Garden Salad Marinated	½ cup	60	11	0	2
Mixed Vegetables Old Fashion Harvest Time	½ cup	35	6	0	1
Peas & Carrots Water Pack	½ cup	35	7	0	2

FOOD	PORTION	CALS.	CARB.	FAT	PRO.
S&W (CONT.)					
Succotash Country Style	½ cup	80	16	1	4
Sweet Peas & Diced Carrots	½ cup	50	9	0	3
Sweet Peas w/ Tiny Pearl Onions	½ cup	60	10	1	3
Seneca					
Peas & Carrots	½ cup	60	9	0	4
Succotash	½ cup	90	18	0	2
Sunshine					
Green Beans And Pototoes	½ cup (4.2 oz)	35	7	0	1
Trappey					
Okra & Tomatoes	½ cup (4 oz)	25	5	0	1
Okra Tomatoes & Corn	½ cup (4.1 oz)	30	6	0	tr
FROZEN					
mixed vegetables cooked	½ cup	54	12	tr	3
peas & carrots cooked	½ cup	38	8	tr	3
peas & onions cooked	½ cup	40	8	tr	2
succotash cooked	½ cup	79	17	1	4
Big Valley					
California Blend	¾ cup (3 oz)	25	6	0	2
Italian Blend	¾ cup (3 oz)	30	5	0	2
Oriental Blend	¾ cup (3 oz)	25	5	0	2
Stew Vegetables	⅔ cup (3 oz)	40	10	0	1
Winter Blend	¾ cup (3 oz)	25	4	0	2
Birds Eye					
Broccoli Cauliflower And Carrots With Cheese Sauce	½ pkg	80	7	4	4
Farm Fresh Broccoli Carrots And Water Chestnuts	¾ cup	40	8	0	2
Farm Fresh Broccoli Cauliflower And Carrots	¾ cup	35	7	0	2
Farm Fresh Broccoli Cauliflower And Red Peppers	¾ cup	30	5	0	3
Farm Fresh Broccoli And Cauliflower	¾ cup	30	5	0	3
Farm Fresh Broccoli Corn And Red Peppers	⅔ cup	60	14	1	3

FOOD	PORTION	CALS.	CARB.	FAT	PRO.
Birds Eye (CONT.)					
Farm Fresh Broccoli Green Beans Pearl Onions and Red Peppers	¾ cup	35	7	0	2
Farm Fresh Broccoli Red Peppers Onions And Mushrooms	¾ cup	30	6	0	3
Farm Fresh Brussels Sprouts Cauliflower And Carrots	¾ cup	40	8	0	3
Farm Fresh Cauliflower Carrots And Snow Peas	⅔ cup	35	8	0	3
In Butter Sauce Broccoli Cauliflower And Carrots	½ cup	40	6	2	1
In Sauce Peas And Pearl Onions With Seasonings	½ cup	70	13	0	5
Internationals Austrian	3.3 oz	70	6	3	4
Internationals Bavarian	3.3 oz	90	11	5	3
Internationals California	3.3 oz	90	10	4	3
Internationals French Country	3.3 oz	70	6	4	2
Internationals Japanese	3.3 oz	60	6	3	2
Internationals New England	3.3 oz	100	12	5	3
Internationals Italian	3.3 oz	80	8	5	2
Mixed	½ cup	60	13	0	3
Peas And Potatoes With Cream Sauce	½ cup	100	16	3	4
Polybag	½ cup	60	12	0	2
Budget Gourmet					
Mandarin Vegetables	1 pkg (5.25 oz)	160	13	11	3
New England Recipe Vegetables	1 pkg (5.5 oz)	230	21	13	5
Spring Vegetables In Cheese Sauce	1 pkg (5 oz)	130	9	8	5
Fresh Like					
California Blend	3.5 oz	31	7	tr	2
Chuckwagon Blend	3.5 oz	71	17	1	3
Italian Blend	3.5 oz	33	7	tr	2
Midwestern Blend	3.5 oz	42	9	tr	2

FOOD	PORTION	CALS.	CARB.	FAT	PRO.
Fresh Like (CONT.)					
Mixed	3.5 oz	69	14	tr	30
Oriental Blend	3.5 oz	26	5	tr	3
Peas & Carrots	3.5 oz	63	12	tr	3
Winter Blend	3.5 oz	26	5	tr	3
Green Giant					
American Mixtures California	½ cup	25	6	0	2
American Mixtures Heartland	½ cup	25	6	0	1
American Mixtures New England	½ cup	70	14	1	3
American Mixtures San Francisco	½ cup	25	7	0	1
American Mixtures Sante Fe	½ cup	70	16	1	2
American Mixtures Seattle	½ cup	25	7	0	2
Broccoli Cauliflower And Carrots In Butter Sauce	½ cup	30	4	1	2
Broccoli Cauliflower And Carrots In Cheese Sauce	½ cup	60	9	2	3
Harvest Fresh Mixed Vegetables	½ cup	40	9	0	2
Mixed	½ cup	40	9	0	2
Mixed In Butter Sauce	½ cup	60	11	2	2
One Serve Broccoli Carrots & Rotini In Cheese Sauce	1 pkg	120	20	3	4
One Serve Broccoli Cauliflower And Carrots	1 pkg	25	7	0	2
Valley Combinations Broccoli & Cauliflower	½ cup	60	9	2	2
La Choy					
Mixed Fancy	½ cup	12	2	tr	1
Ore Ida					
Stew Vegetables	⅔ cup (3 oz)	50	11	0	1
Soglowek					
Golden Vegetarian Nuggets	4 pieces (2.5 oz)	190	9	11	14

FOOD	PORTION	CALS.	CARB.	FAT	PRO.
Tree Of Life					
Mixed	½ cup (3 oz)	65	13	0	3
Veg-All					
Country Wisconsin Blend	3.5 oz	52	13	tr	2
Scandinavian Blend	3.5 oz	48	9	tr	2
Vegetables For Soup (Eight)	3.5 oz	34	12	tr	2
Vegetables For Soup (Nine)	3.5 oz	52	11	tr	2
Vegetables For Soup (Potatoes)	3.5 oz	53	12	tr	2
Vegetables For Stew 4-Way	3.5 oz	51	12	tr	1
Vegetables For Stew 5-Way	3.5 oz	54	12	tr	2
SHELF-STABLE					
Pantry Express					
Corn Green Beans Carrots Pasta In Tomato Sauce	½ cup	80	17	2	2
Green Beans Potatoes And Mushrooms In A Seasoned Sauce	½ cup	50	9	2	1
Mixed Vegetables	½ cup	35	8	tr	1
TAKE-OUT					
curry	1 serving (7.7 oz)	398	22	33	4
pakoras	1 (2 oz)	108	12	5	5
ratatouille	8.8 oz	190	10	16	2
samosa	2 (4 oz)	519	25	46	3
succotash	½ cup	111	23	1	5

VENISON

FOOD	PORTION	CALS.	CARB.	FAT	PRO.
roasted	3 oz	134	0	3	26
Broken Arrow Ranch					
Antelope Chili Meat	3.5 oz	115	1	2	23
Antelope Ground Venison	3.5 oz	110	tr	2	23
Antelope Stew Meat	3.5 oz	110	2	2	22
Nilgai Chili Meat	3.5 oz	115	1	2	23
Nilgai Leg	3.5 oz	100	1	1	23
Nilgai Stew Meat	3.5 oz	110	2	2	22
Venison & Beef Smoked Sausage	6 oz	432	4	30	36

FOOD	PORTION	CALS.	CARB.	FAT	PRO.
Broken Arrow Ranch (CONT.)					
Venison Meat Chunks	6 oz	175	0	2	40
Venison Salami	6 oz	252	0	8	44
VINEGAR					
cider	1 tbsp	tr	1	0	tr
Hain					
Cider	1 tbsp	2	4	0	0
Ka-Me					
Chinese Seasoned	1 tbsp (0.5 fl oz)	5	1	0	0
Rice Wine Chinese	1 tbsp (0.5 fl oz)	5	1	0	0
Rice Wine Japanese	1 tbsp (0.5 oz)	0	1	0	0
Seasoned Rice Japanese	1 tbsp (0.5 fl oz)	10	3	0	0
Nakano					
Rice	1 tbsp	0	0	0	tr
Regina					
Red Wine	1 oz	4	0	0	0
Tree Of Life					
Apple Cider Organic	1 tbsp (0.5 oz)	0	tr	0	0
Brown Rice	1 tbsp (0.5 oz)	2	0	0	0
White House					
Apple Cider	2 tbsp	2	1	0	0
Red Wine	2 tbsp	4	2	0	0
WAFFLES					
FROZEN					
buttermilk	1-4 in sq (1.2 oz)	88	14	3	2
plain	1-4 in sq (1.2 oz)	88	14	3	2
Aunt Jemima					
Blueberry	2 (2.5 oz)	190	28	7	4
Buttermilk	2 (2.5 oz)	170	27	6	4
Cinnamon	2 (2.5 oz)	180	28	6	4
Oatmeal	2 (2.5 oz)	170	27	7	4
Whole Grain	2 (2.5 oz)	170	24	7	5
Belgian Chef					
Belgian	2 (2.5 oz)	140	24	3	3
Downyflake					
Blueberry	2	180	32	4	4
Buttermilk	2	190	32	5	5
Multi-Grain	2	250	28	14	6
Oat Bran	2	260	30	13	6
Regular	2	120	20	3	3
Regular Jumbo	2	170	30	4	4
Rice Bran	2	210	25	11	5
Roman Meal	2	280	33	14	5

FOOD	PORTION	CALS.	CARB.	FAT	PRO.
Downyflake (CONT.)					
Waffles	2	180	27	6	4
Eggo					
Apple Cinnamon	2 (2.7 oz)	220	33	8	5
Blueberry	2 (2.7 oz)	220	33	8	5
Buttermilk	2 (2.7 oz)	220	30	8	5
Common Sense Oat Bran	2 (2.7 oz)	200	27	7	6
Common Sense Oat Bran With Fruit & Nut	2 (2.9 oz)	220	32	8	6
Homestyle	2 (2.7 oz)	220	30	8	5
Minis Blueberry	12 (3 oz)	240	37	8	6
Minis Cinnamon Toast	12 (3.2 oz)	280	40	9	5
Minis Homestyle	12 (1.8 oz)	240	34	8	6
Nut & Honey	2 (2.7 oz)	240	32	10	6
Nutri-Grain	2 (2.7 oz)	190	30	6	5
Nutri-Grain Multi-Bran	2 (2.7 oz)	180	32	6	5
Nutri-Grain Raisin & Bran	2 (3 oz)	210	36	6	5
Special K	2 (2 oz)	140	29	0	6
Strawberry	2 (2.7 oz)	220	32	8	5
Great Starts					
Belgian Waffles And Sausage	2.85 oz	280	21	19	7
Belgian Waffles Strawberries And Sausage	3½ oz	210	31	8	3
Waffle With Bacon	2.2 oz	230	19	14	7
Van's					
Belgian 7 Grain	1	80	10	2	4
Belgian Original	1	73	12	2	2
Toaster Apple Cinnamon	1	75	9	2	3
Toaster Honey Almond	1	75	9	2	3
Toaster Multigrain	1	75	9	2	3
Toaster Wheat Free	1	110	16	3	2
Toaster Wheat Free Cinnamon Apple	1	110	16	3	2
Weight Watchers					
Belgian	1 (1.5 oz)	120	17	4	4
Multi-Grain Belgian	1 (1.5 oz)	120	16	4	4
HOME RECIPE					
plain	1 (7 in diam)	218	25	11	6
MIX					
plain as prep	1 (7 in diam) (2.6 oz)	218	26	10	5

FOOD	PORTION	CALS.	CARB.	FAT	PRO.
WALNUTS					
black dried	1 oz	172	3	16	7
black dried chopped	1 cup	759	15	71	30
english dried	1 oz	182	5	18	4
english dried chopped	1 cup	770	22	74	17
Planters					
Black	1 pkg (2 oz)	340	8	31	14
Gold Measure Halves	1 pkg (2 oz)	380	8	38	8
Halves	⅓ cup (1.2 oz)	220	5	22	5
Pieces	¼ cup (1 oz)	190	4	20	4
WATER CHESTNUTS					
CANNED					
chinese sliced	½ cup	35	9	tr	1
Empress					
Sliced	2 oz	14	3	0	0
Whole	2 oz	14	3	0	0
Ka-Me					
Whole In Water	½ cup (4.5 oz)	45	11	0	2
La Choy					
Sliced	¼ cup	18	4	tr	tr
Whole	4	14	4	tr	tr
FRESH					
sliced	½ cup	66	15	tr	1
WATERCRESS					
(*see also* CRESS)					
FRESH					
raw chopped	½ cup	2	tr	tr	tr
WATERMELON					
FRESH					
cut up	1 cup	50	11	1	1
wedge	1/16	152	35	2	3
SEEDS					
dried	1 oz	158	4	13	8
dried	1 cup	602	17	51	8
WAX BEANS					
CANNED					
Del Monte					
Cut Golden	½ cup (4.3 oz)	20	4	0	1
S&W					
Golden Cut Premium	½ cup	20	5	0	1

FOOD	PORTION	CALS.	CARB.	FAT	PRO.
Seneca					
Cuts Natural Pack	½ cup	25	6	0	1
Wax Beans	½ cup	25	6	0	1

WHALE
raw	3.5 oz	134	0	3	23

WHEAT
(*see also* BULGUR, BRAN, CEREAL, COUSCOUS, FLOUR, WHEAT GERM)

sprouted	⅓ cup	71	15	tr	3
starch	3½ oz	348	86	tr	tr
Arrowhead					
Kamut Grain	¼ cup (1.7 oz)	140	32	1	6
Seitan Quick Mix	⅓ cup (1.4 oz)	150	14	1	21
Hodgson Mill					
Vital Wheat Gluten Plus Ascorbic Acid	1 tbsp (0.3 oz)	30	2	0	6
Near East					
Taboule Salad Mix as prep	⅔ cup	120	23	3	3
Wheat Pilaf as prep	1 cup	220	42	5	6
Sonoma					
Wheat Nuts Salted	2 tbsp (0.5 oz)	60	8	3	0
White Wave					
Seitan	½ pkg (4 oz)	140	4	0	31
Seitan Fajita Strips	⅓ cup (1.8 oz)	60	2	0	14
Seitan Marinated Slices	3 slices (1.8 oz)	60	2	0	14

WHEAT GERM
plain toasted	¼ cup	108	14	3	8
plain toasted	1 cup	431	56	12	33
plain untoasted	¼ cup	104	15	3	7
w/ brown sugar & honey toasted	1 cup	426	69	9	25
w/ brown sugar & honey toasted	1 oz	107	17	2	6
Arrowhead					
Wheat Germ	3 tbsp (0.5 oz)	50	10	1	3
Hodgson Mill					
Wheat Germ	2 tbsp (0.5 oz)	55	7	1	4
Kretschmer					
Honey Crunch	¼ cup	105	15	3	8
Original	¼ cup	103	12	3	9
Stone-Buhr					
Untoasted	2 tbsp (0.5 oz)	58	7	2	4

WHEY
acid dry	1 tbsp (3 g)	10	2	tr	tr

FOOD	PORTION	CALS.	CARB.	FAT	PRO.
acid fluid	1 cup (8 fl oz)	59	13	tr	25
sweet dry	1 tbsp (8 g)	26	6	tr	1
sweet fluid	1 cup (8 fl oz)	66	13	1	2
whey cheese	3.5 oz	440	33	27	15

WHIPPED TOPPINGS
(see also CREAM)

FOOD	PORTION	CALS.	CARB.	FAT	PRO.
cream pressurized	1 cup	154	7	13	2
cream pressurized	1 tbsp	8	tr	tr	tr
nondairy powdered as prep w/ whole milk	1 cup	151	13	10	3
nondairy powdered as prep w/ whole milk	1 tbsp	8	1	tr	tr
nondairy pressurized	1 tbsp	11	1	1	tr
nondairy pressurized	1 cup	184	11	16	1
nondairy frzn	1 tbsp	13	1	1	tr
Cool Whip					
Extra Creamy	1 tbsp	13	1	1	0
Lite	1 tbsp	9	1	1	0
Non Dairy	1 tbsp	11	1	1	tr
D-Zerta					
As prep	1 tbsp	7	0	1	0
Dream Whip					
As prep	1 tbsp	9	1	1	0
Estee					
Whipped Topping Sugar Free as prep	2 tbsp	10	1	1	0
Hood					
Instant	2 tbsp	20	1	2	0
Light Instant	2 tbsp	15	1	1	0
Kraft					
Real Cream	2 tbsp (0.4 oz)	20	1	2	0
Whipped Topping	2 tbsp (0.4 oz)	20	1	2	0
La Creme					
Topping	1 tbsp	16	1	1	0
Pet					
Whip	1 tbsp	14	1	1	0
Reddiwip					
Lite	2 tbsp (8 g)	15	2	1	0
Non-Dairy	2 tbsp (8 g)	20	2	2	0
Real Whipped Heavy Cream	2 tbsp (8 g)	30	tr	3	0
Real Whipped Light Cream	2 tbsp (8 g)	20	tr	2	0

WHITE BEANS
CANNED

FOOD	PORTION	CALS.	CARB.	FAT	PRO.
white beans	1 cup	306	58	1	19

FOOD	PORTION	CALS.	CARB.	FAT	PRO.
Goya					
Spanish Style	7.5 oz	130	29	1	13
Progresso					
Cannellini	½ cup	80	19	tr	8
DRIED					
regular cooked	1 cup	249	45	1	17
small cooked	1 cup	253	46	1	16

WHITEFISH

baked	3 oz	146	0	6	21
smoked	3 oz	92	0	1	20
smoked	1 oz	39	0	tr	7

WHITING

cooked	3 oz	98	0	1	20
raw	3 oz	77	0	1	16

WILD RICE

cooked	½ cup	83	18	tr	3
Haddon House					
Extra Fancy	¼ cup (1.6 oz)	170	35	1	6

WINE

(*see also* CHAMPAGNE, WINE COOLERS)

madeira	3.5 oz	169	10	0	0
port	3.5 oz	156	11	0	tr
red	3½ oz	74	2	0	tr
rose	3½ oz	73	2	0	tr
sherry	2 oz	84	5	0	tr
sweet dessert	2 oz	90	7	0	tr
white	3½ oz	70	1	0	tr
Boone's					
Country Kwencher	1 fl oz	24	3	0	0
Delicious Apple	1 fl oz	21	3	0	0
Sangria	1 fl oz	22	3	0	0
Snow Creek Berry	1 fl oz	18	3	0	0
Strawberry Hill	1 fl oz	22	3	0	0
Sun Peak Peach	1 fl oz	18	3	0	0
Wild Island	1 fl oz	18	3	0	0
Carlo Rossi					
Blush	1 fl oz	21	1	0	0
Burgundy	1 fl oz	22	tr	0	0
Chablis	1 fl oz	21	tr	0	0
Paisano	1 fl oz	23	tr	0	0
Red Sangria	1 fl oz	24	2	0	0
Rhine	1 fl oz	21	1	0	0

FOOD	PORTION	CALS.	CARB.	FAT	PRO.
Carlo Rossi (CONT.)					
Vin Rosé	1 fl oz	21	1	0	0
White Grenache	1 fl oz	20	1	0	0
Fairbanks					
Cream Sherry	1 fl oz	42	4	0	0
Port	1 fl oz	44	4	0	0
Sherry	1 fl oz	34	2	0	0
White Port	1 fl oz	44	4	0	0
Gallo					
Blush Chablis	1 fl oz	22	1	0	0
Burgundy	1 fl oz	22	tr	0	0
Cabernet Sauvignon	1 fl oz	22	0	0	0
Chablis Blanc	1 fl oz	20	tr	0	0
Chardonnay	1 fl oz	23	tr	0	0
Classic Burgundy	1 fl oz	21	0	0	0
French Colombard	1 fl oz	21	1	0	0
Hearty Burgundy	1 fl oz	22	tr	0	0
Johannisberg Riesling '88	1 fl oz	20	1	0	0
Pink Chablis	1 fl oz	20	1	0	0
Red Rosé	1 fl oz	23	1	0	0
Rhine	1 fl oz	22	1	0	0
Sauvignon Blanc '90	1 fl oz	20	tr	0	0
White Grenache '92	1 fl oz	20	1	0	0
White Grenache New Vintage	1 fl oz	20	1	0	0
White Zinfandel '91	1 fl oz	18	tr	0	0
White Zinfandel New Vintage	1 fl oz	18	tr	0	0
Zinfandel '87	1 fl oz	23	0	0	0
Ka-Me					
Chinese Cooking	2 tbsp (1 fl oz)	20	5	0	0
Sheffield Cellars					
Sherry	1 fl oz	44	4	0	0
Tawny Port	1 fl oz	45	4	0	0
Vermouth Extra Dry	1 fl oz	28	1	0	0
Vermouth Sweet	1 fl oz	43	4	0	0
Very Dry Sherry	1 fl oz	32	1	0	0
WINE COOLERS					
Bartles & Jaymes					
Berry	12 fl oz	210	32	0	0
Margarita	12 fl oz	260	46	0	0
Original	12 fl oz	190	28	0	0

FOOD	PORTION	CALS.	CARB.	FAT	PRO.
Bartles & Jaymes (CONT.)					
Peach	12 fl oz	210	33	0	0
Pina Colada	12 fl oz	280	49	0	0
Planter's Punch	12 fl oz	230	36	0	0
Strawberry	12 fl oz	210	32	0	0
Strawberry Daquiri	12 fl oz	230	37	0	0
Tropical	12 fl oz	230	38	0	0

WINGED BEANS

dried cooked	1 cup	252	26	10	18

WOLFFISH

atlantic baked	3 oz	105	0	3	19

YAM

(*see also* SWEET POTATO)

FOOD	PORTION	CALS.	CARB.	FAT	PRO.
CANNED					
Allen					
Cut	⅔ cup (5.8 oz)	160	40	1	0
Bruce					
Cut	½ cup	139	20	1	1
Mashed	½ cup	130	29	1	1
Vacuum Pack	½ cup	122	28	1	1
Whole	½ cup	139	31	1	tr
Princella					
Cut	⅔ cup (5.8 oz)	160	40	1	0
Royal Prince					
Whole	4 pieces (5.9 oz)	200	48	1	1
S&W					
Candied	½ cup	180	44	0	1
Southern Whole In Extra Heavy Syrup	½ cup	139	31	1	1
Sugary Sam					
Cut	⅔ cup (5.8 oz)	160	40	1	0
Trappey					
Whole	4 pieces (5.9 oz)	200	48	1	1
FRESH					
mountain yam hawaii cooked	½ cup	59	14	tr	1
yam cubed cooked	½ cup	79	19	tr	1

YEAST

baker's compressed	1 cake (0.6 oz)	18	3	tr	1
baker's dry	1 pkg (¼ oz)	21	3	tr	3
baker's dry	1 tbsp	35	5	1	5
brewer's dry	1 tbsp	25	3	tr	3

FOOD	PORTION	CALS.	CARB.	FAT	PRO.
Fleischmann's					
Active Dry	1 pkg (¼ oz)	20	3	0	3
Fresh Active	1 pkg (0.6 oz)	15	2	0	2
Household Yeast	½ oz	15	2	0	2
RapidRise	1 pkg (¼ oz)	20	3	0	3
Red Star					
Small Flakes	3 tbsp (0.5 oz)	47	5	tr	8
Yeast	4 tbsp (0.5 oz)	47	5	tr	8
Yeast Flakes	3 tbsp (0.5 oz)	47	5	tr	8

YELLOW BEANS
CANNED
B&M

Baked Beans	8 oz	326	50	7	15
DRIED					
cooked	1 cup	254	45	2	16

YELLOWEYE BEANS
DRIED
Bean Cuisine

Dried	½ cup	115	—	1	8

YELLOWTAIL

baked	3 oz	159	0	6	25

YOGURT
(see also YOGURT FROZEN)

coffee lowfat	8 oz	194	31	3	11
fruit lowfat	4 oz	113	21	1	5
fruit lowfat	8 oz	225	42	3	9
plain	8 oz	139	11	7	8
plain lowfat	8 oz	144	16	4	12
plain no fat	8 oz	127	17	tr	13
vanilla lowfat	8 oz	194	31	3	11
Breyers					
1% Fat Black Cherry	8 oz	260	50	3	8
1% Fat Blueberry	8 oz	250	48	3	8
1% Fat Mixed Berry	8 oz	250	48	3	8
1% Fat Peach	8 oz	250	48	3	8
1% Fat Pineapple	8 oz	250	49	3	8
1% Fat Red Raspberry	8 oz	250	48	3	8
1% Fat Strawberry	8 oz	250	47	3	8
1% Fat Strawberry Banana	8 oz	250	50	3	9
1.5% Fat Coffee	8 oz	220	38	3	10
1.5% Fat Plain	8 oz	130	15	3	11

FOOD	PORTION	CALS.	CARB.	FAT	PRO.
Breyers (CONT.)					
1.5% Fat Vanilla	8 oz	220	38	3	10
Cabot					
All Flavors	8 oz	220	42	3	9
Plain	8 oz	140	16	4	12
Colombo					
Banana Strawberry	8 oz	210	39	4	6
Black Cherry	8 oz	200	36	4	6
Blueberry	8 oz	200	36	4	6
Fat Free Apples 'n Spice	8 oz	190	39	0	8
Fat Free Apricot	8 oz	190	39	0	8
Fat Free Banana Strawberry	8 oz	200	42	0	8
Fat Free Blueberry	8 oz	190	39	0	8
Fat Free Cappuccino	8 oz	180	35	0	9
Fat Free Cherry	8 oz	190	39	0	8
Fat Free Cranberry Strawberry	8 oz	200	43	0	8
Fat Free French Roast	8 oz	180	35	0	9
Fat Free Fruit Cocktail	8 oz	190	39	0	8
Fat Free Lemon	8 oz	170	33	0	10
Fat Free Peach	8 oz	190	33	0	8
Fat Free Plain	8 oz	110	16	0	11
Fat Free Raspberry	8 oz	190	39	0	8
Fat Free Strawberry	8 oz	190	39	0	8
Fat Free Strawberry Pineapple Orange	8 oz	190	38	0	8
Fat Free Vanilla	8 oz	170	32	0	10
French Vanilla	8 oz	180	29	4	7
Light 100 Blueberry	8 oz	100	16	0	8
Light 100 Cherry Vanilla	8 oz	100	16	0	8
Light 100 Coffee & Cream	8 oz	100	16	0	8
Light 100 Creamy Vanilla	8 oz	100	16	0	8
Light 100 Fruit Medley	8 oz	100	16	0	8
Light 100 Juicy Peach	8 oz	100	16	0	8
Light 100 Lemon Creme	8 oz	100	16	0	8
Light 100 Mandarin Orange	8 oz	100	16	0	8
Light 100 Mixed Berries	8 oz	100	16	0	8
Light 100 Raspberry	8 oz	100	16	0	8
Light 100 Strawberry	8 oz	100	16	0	8
Peach Melba	8 oz	200	36	4	6
Plain	8 oz	120	12	5	8

FOOD	PORTION	CALS.	CARB.	FAT	PRO.
Colombo (CONT.)					
Raspberry	8 oz	200	36	4	6
Strawberry	8 oz	200	36	4	6
Dannon					
Blended Nonfat Blueberry	6 oz	160	33	0	7
Blended Nonfat French Vanilla	6 oz	160	31	0	7
Blended Nonfat Lemon Chiffon	6 oz	150	31	0	7
Blended Nonfat Peach	6 oz	150	31	0	7
Blended Nonfat Raspberry	6 oz	160	32	0	7
Blended Nonfat Strawberry	6 oz	150	31	0	7
Blended Nonfat Strawberry Banana	6 oz	150	31	0	7
Danimals Lowfat Tropical Punch	4.4 oz	140	25	2	6
Danimals Lowfat Blueberry	4.4 oz	140	25	2	6
Danimals Lowfat Grape Lemonade	4.4 oz	130	23	2	6
Danimals Lowfat Lemon Ice	4.4 oz	130	22	2	6
Danimals Lowfat Orange Banana	4.4 oz	140	24	2	6
Danimals Lowfat Strawberry	4.4 oz	140	24	2	6
Danimals Lowfat Vanilla	4.4 oz	140	24	2	6
Danimals Lowfat Wild Raspberry	4.4 oz	130	22	2	6
Fruit On The Bottom Lowfat Apple Cinnamon	8 oz	240	46	3	9
Fruit On The Bottom Lowfat Blueberry	8 oz	240	46	3	9
Fruit On The Bottom Lowfat Boysenberry	8 oz	240	45	3	9
Fruit On The Bottom Lowfat Cherry	8 oz	240	46	3	9
Fruit On The Bottom Lowfat Mixed Berries	8 oz	240	45	3	9
Fruit On The Bottom Lowfat Orange	8 oz	240	45	3	9

FOOD	PORTION	CALS.	CARB.	FAT	PRO.
Dannon (CONT.)					
Fruit On The Bottom Lowfat Peach	8 oz	240	45	3	9
Fruit On The Bottom Lowfat Pear	8 oz	240	45	3	9
Fruit On The Bottom Lowfat Raspberry	8 oz	240	45	3	9
Fruit On The Bottom Lowfat Strawberry	8 oz	240	46	3	9
Fruit On The Bottom Lowfat Strawberry Banana	8 oz	240	43	3	9
Light Nonfat Banana Cream Pie	4.4 oz	60	9	0	5
Light Nonfat Cherry Vanilla	1 cup (3.5 oz)	110	19	0	9
Light Nonfat Lemon Chiffon	4.4 oz	60	9	0	5
Light Nonfat Peach	4.4 oz	50	8	0	5
Light Nonfat Strawberry	4.4 oz	50	8	0	5
Light Nonfat Strawberry	1 cup (3.5 oz)	110	19	0	10
Light Nonfat Vanilla	1 cup (3.5 oz)	110	18	0	10
Light 'N Crunchy Nonfat Cappuccino w/ Chocolate	1 pkg	150	27	0	9
Light 'N Crunchy Nonfat Caramel Apple Crunch	1 pkg	150	28	0	9
Light 'N Crunchy Nonfat Raspberry w/ Granola	1 pkg	150	17	0	10
Light 'N Crunchy Nonfat Vanilla w/ Chocolate	1 pkg	150	26	0	9
Light 'N Crunchy Nonfat Lemon Chiffon w/ Blueberry	1 pkg	140	26	0	9
Light Nonfat Banana Cream Pie	8 oz	100	17	0	9
Light Nonfat Blueberry	8 oz	100	20	0	9
Light Nonfat Creme Caramel	8 oz	100	15	0	10
Light Nonfat Lemon	8 oz	100	17	0	9
Light Nonfat Peach	8 oz	100	18	0	9
Light Nonfat Raspberry	8 oz	100	18	0	9
Light Nonfat Strawberry	8 oz	100	18	0	9
Light Nonfat Strawberry Banana	8 oz	100	18	0	9

FOOD	PORTION	CALS.	CARB.	FAT	PRO.
Dannon (CONT.)					
Light Nonfat Tropical Fruit	8 oz	100	19	0	9
Light Nonfat Vanilla	8 oz	100	17	0	9
Lowfat Coffee	8 oz	210	36	3	10
Lowfat Coffee	1 cup (8.7 oz)	230	39	4	11
Lowfat Cranberry Raspberry	8 oz	210	36	3	10
Lowfat Lemon	8 oz	210	36	3	10
Lowfat Lemon	1 cup (8.7 oz)	230	39	4	11
Lowfat Plain	1 cup (8.7 oz)	150	17	4	13
Lowfat Plain	8 oz	140	16	4	12
Lowfat Vanilla	8 oz	210	36	3	10
Lowfat Vanilla	1 cup (8.7 oz)	230	39	4	11
Minipack Blended Nonfat Blueberry	4.4 oz	120	23	0	5
Minipack Blended Nonfat Cherry	4.4 oz	110	23	0	5
Minipack Blended Nonfat Peach	4.4 oz	110	23	0	5
Minipack Blended Nonfat Raspberry	4.4 oz	120	23	0	5
Minipack Blended Nonfat Strawberry	4.4 oz	110	23	0	5
Minipack Blended Nonfat Strawberry Banana	4.4 oz	110	23	2	5
Nonfat Plain	1 cup (8.7 oz)	120	17	0	13
Nonfat Plain	8 oz	110	16	0	12
Nonfat Light Cherry Vanilla	8 oz	100	17	0	9
Nonfat Light Strawberry Fruit Cup	8 oz	100	18	0	9
Sprinkl'ins Banana	4.1 oz	140	24	3	5
Sprinkl'ins Cherry Vanilla	4.1 oz	140	24	3	5
Sprinkl'ins Crazy Crunch Cherry w/ Honey Grahams	4.4 oz	170	30	3	6
Sprinkl'ins Crazy Crunch Grape w/ Chocolate Grahams	4.4 oz	160	29	3	6
Sprinkl'ins Crazy Crunch Vanilla w/ Chocolate Grahams	4.4 oz	160	29	3	6

FOOD	PORTION	CALS.	CARB.	FAT	PRO.
Dannon (CONT.)					
Sprinkl'ins Crazy Crunch Vanilla w/ Honey Grahams	4.4 oz	170	30	3	6
Sprinkl'ins Strawberry	4.1 oz	140	24	3	5
Sprinkl'ins Strawberry Banana	4.1 oz	140	24	3	5
Tropifruta Nonfat Banana	6 oz	150	31	0	7
Tropifruta Nonfat Guava	6 oz	150	29	0	7
Tropifruta Nonfat Mango	6 oz	150	31	0	7
Tropifruta Nonfat Papaya Pineapple	6 oz	150	30	0	7
Tropifruta Nonfat Pina Colada	6 oz	150	30	0	7
Tropifruta Nonfat Strawberry	6 oz	150	31	0	7
Tropifruta Nonfat Strawberry Banana	6 oz	150	31	0	7
Tropifruta Nonfat Strawberry Kiwi	6 oz	150	30	0	7
With Fruit Toppings Banana Creme Strawberry	6 oz	170	30	3	7
With Fruit Toppings Bavarian Creme Raspberry	6 oz	170	31	3	7
With Fruit Toppings Cheesecake Cherry	6 oz	170	31	3	7
With Fruit Toppings Cheesecake Strawberry	6 oz	170	30	3	7
With Fruit Toppings Vanilla Peach & Apricot	6 oz	170	30	3	7
With Fruit Toppings Vanilla Strawberry	6 oz	170	30	3	7
Friendship					
Coffee	8 oz	210	30	3	11
Fruit Crunch Blueberry	6 oz	190	32	4	6
Fruit Crunch Peach	6 oz	190	31	5	8
Fruit Crunch Strawberry	6 oz	190	31	5	8
Fruit Crunch Strawberry Banana	6 oz	190	32	4	6
Plain	8 oz	150	13	3	12

FOOD	PORTION	CALS.	CARB.	FAT	PRO.
Hood					
Fat Free Blueberry	1 (8 oz)	190	40	0	8
Fat Free Cherry	1 (8 oz)	190	40	0	8
Fat Free Peach	1 (8 oz)	190	40	0	8
Fat Free Plain	1 (8 oz)	130	18	0	12
Fat Free Raspberry	1 (8 oz)	190	40	0	8
Fat Free Strawberry	1 (8 oz)	190	39	0	8
Fat Free Strawberry Banana	1 (8 oz)	190	40	0	8
Fat Free Vanilla	1 (8 oz)	190	34	0	11
Fat Free Swiss Blueberry	1 (8 oz)	210	45	0	7
Fat Free Swiss Lemon	1 (8 oz)	210	45	0	7
Fat Free Swiss Raspberry	1 (8 oz)	210	45	0	7
Fat Free Swiss Strawberry	1 (8 oz)	210	45	0	7
Fat Free Swiss Strawberry Banana	1 (8 oz)	210	45	0	7
Fat Free Swiss Vanilla	1 (8 oz)	210	45	0	7
Knudsen					
1.5% Fat Creamy Lemon	8 oz	220	38	3	10
70 Calories Black Cherry	6 oz	70	12	0	7
70 Calories Blueberry	6 oz	70	12	0	7
70 Calories Lemon	6 oz	70	11	0	7
70 Calories Peach	6 oz	70	11	0	7
70 Calories Pineapple	6 oz	70	11	0	7
70 Calories Red Raspberry	6 oz	70	11	0	7
70 Calories Strawberry	6 oz	70	11	0	7
70 Calories Strawberry Banana	6 oz	70	11	0	7
70 Calories Strawberry Fruit Basket	6 oz	70	11	0	7
70 Calories Vanilla	6 oz	70	11	0	7
Free Lemon	6 oz	160	33	0	8
Free Mixed Berry	6 oz	170	33	0	8
Free Peach	6 oz	170	33	0	8
Free Red Raspberry	6 oz	170	31	0	8
Free Strawberry	6 oz	170	32	0	8
Free Vanilla	6 oz	170	32	0	8
La Yogurt					
French Style Banana	6 oz	180	32	3	6
French Style Blueberry	6 oz	180	32	3	6
French Style Cherry	6 oz	180	32	3	6

FOOD	PORTION	CALS.	CARB.	FAT	PRO.
La Yogurt (CONT.)					
French Style Cherry Vanilla	6 oz	190	35	3	6
French Style Guava	6 oz	180	32	3	6
French Style Key Lime	6 oz	180	32	3	6
French Style Mango	6 oz	180	32	3	6
French Style Mixed Berry	6 oz	180	32	3	7
French Style Nonfat Blueberry	6 oz	70	12	0	6
French Style Nonfat Cherry	6 oz	75	13	0	6
French Style Nonfat Raspberry	6 oz	70	12	0	6
French Style Nonfat Strawberry	6 oz	70	12	0	6
French Style Nonfat Strawberry Banana	6 oz	70	12	0	6
French Style Peach	6 oz	180	32	3	6
French Style Pina Colada	6 oz	180	32	3	6
French Style Raspberry	6 oz	180	32	3	6
French Style Strawberry	6 oz	180	32	3	6
French Style Strawberry Banana	6 oz	180	32	3	6
French Style Strawberry Fruit Cup	6 oz	180	32	3	6
French Style Tropical Orange	6 oz	180	32	4	6
French Style Vanilla	6 oz	170	28	3	7
Latin Style Banana	6 oz	190	34	3	6
Latin Style Guava	6 oz	190	34	3	6
Latin Style Mango	6 oz	190	34	3	6
Latin Style Papaya	6 oz	190	34	3	6
Latin Style Passion Fruit	6 oz	190	34	3	6
Latin Style Strawberry Kiwi	6 oz	180	32	3	6
Light N'Lively					
Free Blueberry	6 oz	190	38	0	8
Free Lemon	6 oz	170	35	0	8
Free Mixed Berry	6 oz	170	34	0	8
Free Peach	6 oz	170	35	0	8
Free Red Raspberry	6 oz	180	36	0	8
Free Strawberry	6 oz	180	36	0	8
Free Strawberry Fruit Cup	6 oz	170	35	0	8

FOOD	PORTION	CALS.	CARB.	FAT	PRO.
Light N'Lively (CONT.)					
Free Vanilla	6 oz	160	32	0	8
Free 50 Calories Blueberry	4.4 oz	50	8	0	5
Free 50 Calories Peach	4.4 oz	50	9	0	5
Free 50 Calories Red Raspberry	4.4 oz	50	8	0	5
Free 50 Calories Strawberry	4.4 oz	50	8	0	5
Free 50 Calories Strawberry Banana	4.4 oz	50	8	0	5
Free 50 Calories Strawberry Fruit Cup	4.4 oz	50	8	0	5
Free 70 Calories Black Cherry	6 oz	70	11	0	7
Free 70 Calories Blueberry	6 oz	70	11	0	7
Free 70 Calories Lemon	6 oz	70	12	0	7
Free 70 Calories Peach	6 oz	70	12	0	6
Free 70 Calories Red Raspberry	6 oz	70	11	0	7
Free 70 Calories Strawberry	6 oz	70	11	0	7
Free 70 Calories Strawberry Banana	6 oz	70	11	0	7
Free 70 Calories Strawberry Fruit Cup	6 oz	70	11	0	7
Kidpack Banana Berry	4.4 oz	130	24	1	5
Kidpack Berry Blue	4.4 oz	150	30	1	5
Kidpack Cherry	4.4 oz	140	27	1	5
Kidpack Grape	4.4 oz	130	24	1	51
Kidpack Outrageous Orange	4.4 oz	150	29	1	5
Kidpack Tropical Punch	4.4 oz	140	28	1	5
Kidpack Wild Berry	4.4 oz	140	27	1	5
Kidpack Wild Strawberry	4.4 oz	140	28	1	5
Multipack Blueberry	4.4 oz	140	27	1	52
Multipack Peach	4.4 oz	140	27	1	5
Multipack Pineapple	4.4 oz	140	27	1	5
Multipack Red Raspberry	4.4 oz	130	24	1	5
Multipack Strawberry	4.4 oz	140	26	1	5
Multipack Strawberry Banana	4.4 oz	140	28	1	5

FOOD	PORTION	CALS.	CARB.	FAT	PRO.
Light N'Lively (CONT.)					
Multipack Strawberry Fruit Cup	4.4 oz	140	27	1	5
Lite Line					
Swiss Style Cherry Vanilla	1 cup	240	45	2	10
Swiss Style Peach	1 cup	230	42	2	10
Swiss Style Plain	1 cup	140	16	2	12
Swiss Style Strawberry	1 cup	240	46	2	10
Meadow Gold					
Plain	1 cup	160	16	5	12
Sundae Style Raspberry	1 cup	250	42	4	10
Mountain High					
Blueberry	1 cup	220	31	6	10
Plain	1 cup	200	16	9	12
Weight Watchers					
Nonfat Plain	1 cup	90	13	0	10
Ultimate 90 All Flavors	1 cup	90	13	0	10
Yoplait					
Custard Style Banana	6 oz	190	32	4	7
Custard Style Blueberry	6 oz	190	32	4	7
Custard Style Cherry	6 oz	180	30	4	7
Custard Style Lemon	6 oz	190	32	4	7
Custard Style Mixed Berry	6 oz	180	30	4	7
Custard Style Raspberry	6 oz	190	32	4	7
Custard Style Strawberry	4 oz	130	21	3	5
Custard Style Strawberry	6 oz	190	32	4	7
Custard Style Strawberry Banana	6 oz	190	32	4	7
Custard Style Strawberry Banana	4 oz	130	21	3	5
Custard Style Vanilla	4 oz	130	20	3	5
Custard Style Vanilla	6 oz	180	30	4	7
Fat Free Blueberry	6 oz	150	31	0	7
Fat Free Cherry	6 oz	150	31	0	7
Fat Free Mixed Berry	6 oz	150	31	0	7
Fat Free Peach	6 oz	150	31	0	7
Fat Free Raspberry	6 oz	150	31	0	7
Fat Free Strawberry	6 oz	150	31	0	7
Fat Free Strawberry Banana	6 oz	150	31	0	7
Light Blueberry	4 oz	60	9	0	5
Light Blueberry	6 oz	80	13	0	7

FOOD	PORTION	CALS.	CARB.	FAT	PRO.
Yoplait (CONT.)					
Light Cherry	6 oz	80	13	0	7
Light Cherry	4 oz	60	9	0	5
Light Peach	4 oz	60	9	0	5
Light Peach	6 oz	80	13	0	7
Light Raspberry	6 oz	80	13	0	7
Light Raspberry	4 oz	60	9	0	5
Light Strawberry	6 oz	80	13	0	7
Light Strawberry	4 oz	60	9	0	5
Light Strawberry Banana	6 oz	80	13	0	7
Light Strawberry Banana	4 oz	60	9	0	5
Nonfat Plain	8 oz	120	18	0	13
Nonfat Vanilla	8 oz	180	35	0	11
Original Apple	6 oz	190	32	3	8
Original Blueberry	6 oz	190	32	3	8
Original Blueberry	4 oz	120	21	2	5
Original Boysenberry	6 oz	190	32	3	8
Original Cherry	6 oz	190	32	3	8
Original Lemon	6 oz	190	32	3	8
Original Mixed Berry	6 oz	190	32	3	8
Original Orange	6 oz	190	32	3	8
Original Peach	6 oz	190	32	3	8
Original Peach	4 oz	120	21	2	5
Original Pina Colada	6 oz	190	32	3	8
Original Pineapple	6 oz	190	32	3	8
Original Plain	6 oz	130	15	3	10
Original Raspberry	6 oz	190	32	3	8
Original Raspberry	4 oz	120	21	2	5
Original Strawberry	6 oz	190	32	3	8
Original Strawberry	4 oz	120	21	2	5
Original Strawberry Banana	6 oz	190	32	3	8
Original Strawberry Rhubarb	6 oz	190	32	3	8
Original Vanilla	6 oz	180	29	3	9
YOGURT FROZEN					
(*see also* TOFU YOGURT)					
chocolate soft serve	½ cup (4 fl oz)	115	18	4	3
vanilla soft serve	½ cup (4 fl oz)	114	17	4	3
Bee-Lite					
Chocolate	4 oz	100	23	tr	3
Vanilla	4 oz	110	23	tr	4
Ben & Jerry's					
Cherry Garcia	½ cup (3.7 oz)	170	31	3	4

FOOD	PORTION	CALS.	CARB.	FAT	PRO.
Ben & Jerry's (CONT.)					
Chocolate Fudge Brownie	½ cup (3.7 oz)	190	35	4	6
Coffee Almond Fudge	½ cup (3.7 oz)	200	30	7	6
English Toffee Crunch	½ cup (3.7 oz)	190	32	6	4
No Fat Cappuccino	½ cup (3.3 oz)	140	32	0	3
Pop Cherry Garcia	1 (3.8 oz)	290	34	16	6
Borden					
Strawberry	½ cup	100	19	2	2
Bresler's					
All Flavors	5 oz	145	28	2	5
All Flavors Lite	5 oz	135	30	0	6
Breyers					
Black Cherry	½ cup (2.7 oz)	140	25	3	3
Chocolate	½ cup (2.7 oz)	150	25	4	3
Chocolate Brownie	½ cup (2.7 oz)	170	29	5	3
Peach	½ cup (2.7 oz)	140	24	3	3
Red Raspberry	½ cup (2.7 oz)	140	24	4	3
Strawberry	½ cup (2.7 oz)	130	23	3	3
Strawberry Banana	½ cup (2.7 oz)	140	24	3	3
Strawberry Cheesecake	½ cup (2.7 oz)	160	26	5	3
Toffee Bar Crunch	½ cup (2.7 oz)	160	26	5	3
Vanilla	½ cup (2.7 oz)	140	24	4	3
Vanilla Chocolate Strawberry	½ cup (2.7 oz)	140	24	4	3
Vanilla Raspberry Swirl	½ cup (2.7 oz)	140	24	4	3
Vanilla Fudge Twirl	½ cup (2.7 oz)	150	25	4	3
Dannon					
Coco-Nut Fudge	½ cup (3 oz)	160	28	3	5
Light Cappuccino	½ cup (2.8 oz)	80	19	0	4
Light Cherry Vanilla Swirl	½ cup (2.8 oz)	90	21	0	3
Light Chocolate	½ cup (2.7 oz)	80	21	0	4
Light Lemon Chiffon	½ cup (2.8 oz)	90	22	0	4
Light Peach Raspberry Melba	½ cup (2.8 oz)	90	21	0	4
Light Strawberry Cheesecake	½ cup (2.8 oz)	90	22	0	4
Light Vanilla	½ cup (2.8 oz)	80	21	0	4
Light Nonfat Cappuccino	8 oz	100	17	0	9
Light'N Crunchy Banana Cream Pie	½ cup (2.8 oz)	110	24	1	4
Light'N Crunchy Mocha Chocolate Chunk	½ cup (2.8 oz)	110	26	1	4

FOOD	PORTION	CALS.	CARB.	FAT	PRO.
Dannon (CONT.)					
Light'N Crunchy Peanut Chocolate Crunch	½ cup (2.8 oz)	110	29	0	4
Light'N Crunchy Triple Chocolate	½ cup (2.8 oz)	110	28	0	4
Light'N Crunchy Vanilla Blueberry Swirl	½ cup (2.8 oz)	110	26	1	4
Pure Indulgence Cherry Chocolate Cherry	½ cup (3 oz)	150	26	3	4
Pure Indulgence Chunky Chocolate Nut	½ cup (3 oz)	150	25	3	6
Pure Indulgence Cookies'n Cream	½ cup (3 oz)	150	24	3	5
Pure Indulgence Crunchy Expresso	½ cup (3 oz)	150	26	3	5
Pure Indulgence Heath Toffee Crunch	½ cup (3 oz)	150	25	3	5
Pure Indulgence Vanilla Raspberry Truffle	½ cup (3 oz)	150	25	3	5
Desserve					
All Flavors	4 oz	70	16	0	4
Dutch Chocolate	4 oz	80	18	0	5
Edy's					
Banana Strawberry	3 oz	80	15	1	2
Blueberry	3 oz	80	15	1	2
Cherry	3 oz	80	15	1	2
Chocolate	3 oz	80	15	1	2
Chocolate Chip	3 oz	100	20	1	3
Citrus Heights	3 oz	80	15	1	2
Cookies'N'Cream	3 oz	100	20	1	3
Marble Fudge	3 oz	100	20	1	3
Perfectly Peach	3 oz	80	15	1	2
Raspberry	3 oz	80	15	1	2
Raspberry Vanilla Swirl	3 oz	80	15	1	2
Strawberry	3 oz	80	15	1	2
Vanilla	3 oz	80	15	1	2
Elan					
Blueberry	4 oz	130	23	3	3
Caramel Almond Praline	4 oz	150	26	4	4
Chocolate	4 oz	130	24	3	4
Chocolate Almond	4 oz	160	22	6	5
Coffee	4 oz	130	22	3	4
Coffee Decaffeinated	4 oz	130	22	3	4
Peach	4 oz	130	23	3	4

FOOD	PORTION	CALS.	CARB.	FAT	PRO.
Elan (CONT.)					
Rum Raisin	4 oz	135	25	3	3
Strawberry	4 oz	125	22	3	3
Vanilla	4 oz	130	22	3	4
Fi-Bar					
Chocolate	1	190	26	7	4
Strawberry	1	190	26	7	4
Vanilla	1	190	26	7	4
Friendly's					
Apple Bettie	½ cup (2.6 oz)	140	25	3	3
Fabulous Fudge Swirl	½ cup (2.6 oz)	140	23	3	4
Fudge Berry Swirl	½ cup (2.6 oz)	150	25	4	4
Lowfat Perfectly Peach	½ cup (2.6 oz)	110	21	2	3
Lowfat Purely Chocolate	½ cup (2.6 oz)	120	20	3	4
Lowfat Raspberry Delight	½ cup (2.6 oz)	120	21	3	4
Lowfat Simply Vanilla	½ cup (2.6 oz)	120	19	3	4
Lowfat Strawberry Patch	½ cup (2.6 oz)	110	20	2	4
Mint Chocolate Chip	½ cup (2.6 oz)	130	21	4	4
Strawberry Cheesecake Blast	½ cup (2.6 oz)	140	22	4	4
Toffee Almond Crunch	½ cup (2.6 oz)	160	24	5	4
Good Humor					
Creamsicle Raspberry	1 (2.8 oz)	100	23	1	1
Frista Cup	1 (6.2 oz)	220	38	5	7
Haagen-Dazs					
Banana Nut Blast	½ cup (3.5 oz)	220	29	8	8
Bars Cherry Chocolate Fudge	1 (2.6 oz)	240	26	13	5
Bars Peach	1 (2.5 oz)	90	19	1	2
Bars Pina Colada	1 (2.5 oz)	100	19	1	3
Bars Raspberry & Vanilla	1 (2.5 oz)	90	19	1	3
Bars Strawberry Daiquiri	1 (2.5 oz)	90	18	1	3
Chocolate	½ cup (3.4 oz)	160	26	3	8
Coffee	½ cup (3.4 oz)	160	26	3	8
Fat Free Cherry Vanilla	½ cup (3.3 oz)	140	30	0	6
Fat Free Chocolate	½ cup (3.3 oz)	140	28	0	6
Fat Free Coffee	½ cup (3.3 oz)	140	29	0	6
Fat Free Vanilla	½ cup (3.3 oz)	140	29	0	6
Fat Free Vanilla Fudge	½ cup (3.3 oz)	160	34	0	6
Fat Free Bar Raspberry & Vanilla	1 (2.5 oz)	90	20	0	2
Orange Tango	½ cup (3.5 oz)	130	26	1	4
Pina Colada	½ cup (3.4 oz)	130	26	2	3

FOOD	PORTION	CALS.	CARB.	FAT	PRO.
Haagen-Dazs (CONT.)					
Raspberry Randevous	½ cup (3.5 oz)	130	26	2	4
Strawberry Cheesecake Craze	½ cup (3.6 oz)	220	31	8	7
Strawberry Duet	½ cup (3.4 oz)	130	26	2	3
Vanilla	½ cup (3.4 oz)	160	26	3	8
Hood					
Bavarian Truffle & Twist	½ cup (2.6 oz)	150	26	4	2
Coffee Toffee Chunk Sundae	½ cup (2.6 oz)	150	27	4	2
Combo Bars	1 (2.2 oz)	90	17	2	2
Cookies & Cream	½ cup (2.6 oz)	140	25	4	3
Grandma's Raisin Oatmeal Cookie Dough	½ cup (2.6 oz)	140	25	3	3
Mixed Berry Swirl	½ cup (2.6 oz)	120	24	2	2
Natural Strawberry	½ cup (2.6 oz)	110	21	3	2
Natural Strawberry Banana	½ cup (2.6 oz)	110	21	3	2
Natural Vanilla	½ cup (2.6 oz)	120	22	3	3
Nonfat Caramel & Brownie Sundae	½ cup (2.6 oz)	120	28	0	3
Nonfat Chocolate Marshmallow	½ cup (2.6 oz)	110	26	0	2
Nonfat Double Raspberry	½ cup (2.6 oz)	120	26	0	2
Nonfat Mocha Fudge	½ cup (2.6 oz)	120	27	0	3
Nonfat Olde Fashioned Vanilla	½ cup (2.6 oz)	110	24	0	3
Nonfat Peach Cobbler A La Mode	½ cup (2.6 oz)	110	25	0	3
Nonfat Strawberry	½ cup (2.6 oz)	100	23	0	2
Nonfat Vanilla Fudge	½ cup (2.6 oz)	120	27	0	3
Raspberry Swirl	½ cup (2.6 oz)	130	25	2	2
Sundae Cups Chocolate & Strawberry	1 (2.2 oz)	110	24	2	1
Vanilla Chocolate Strawberry	½ cup (2.6 oz)	120	22	3	3
Vanilla Swiss Almond Sundae	½ cup (2.6 oz)	150	25	4	3
Just 10					
All Flavors	1 oz	10	3	0	0
Kissed With Honey					
Chocolate	3.5 oz	100	18	3	2

FOOD	PORTION	CALS.	CARB.	FAT	PRO.
Kissed With Honey (CONT.)					
Nonfat Chocolate	3.5 oz	85	19	tr	4
Nonfat Vanilla	3.5 oz	85	18	tr	3
Vanilla	3.5 oz	100	17	3	2
Meadow Gold					
Strawberry	½ cup	100	19	2	2
Sealtest					
Chocolate	½ cup (2.7 oz)	120	24	2	3
Mocha Fudge	½ cup (2.6 oz)	130	25	2	3
Vanilla	½ cup (2.6 oz)	120	24	2	3
Tofutti					
Beter Than Yogurt Passion Island Fruit	4 fl oz	100	21	1	1
Better Than Yogurt Chocolate Fudge	4 fl oz	120	25	2	2
Better Than Yogurt Coffee Mashmallow Swirl	4 fl oz	100	24	1	1
Better Than Yogurt Peach Mango	4 fl oz	100	23	1	1
Better Than Yogurt Strawberry Banana	4 fl oz	100	23	1	1
Better Than Yogurt Vanilla Fudge	4 fl oz	120	24	2	2
Turkey Hill					
Chocolate Cherry Cordial	½ cup (2.6 oz)	130	22	3	3
Chocolate Chip Cookie Dough	½ cup (2.6 oz)	140	23	5	3
Death By Chocolate	½ cup (2.6 oz)	150	25	4	3
Nonfat Chocolate Marshmallow	½ cup (2.4 oz)	130	30	0	3
Nonfat Chocolate Cherry Cordial	½ cup (2.4 oz)	100	24	0	4
Nonfat Coffee Cappuccino	½ cup (2.4 oz)	110	23	0	3
Nonfat Mint Cookie 'N Cream	½ cup (2.4 oz)	110	24	0	4
Nonfat Neapolitan	½ cup (2.4 oz)	100	22	0	3
Nonfat Raspberry Chocolate Bliss	½ cup (2.4 oz)	110	25	0	3
Nonfat Southern Lemon Pie	½ cup (2.4 oz)	110	25	0	3
Nonfat Vanilla Fudge	½ cup (2.4 oz)	110	24	0	3
Peach Raspberry	½ cup (2.6 oz)	110	20	2	3

FOOD	PORTION	CALS.	CARB.	FAT	PRO.
Turkey Hill (CONT.)					
Strawberry	½ cup (2.6 oz)	110	20	2	3
Tin Roof Sundae	½ cup (2.6 oz)	140	21	5	4
Vanilla & Chocolate	½ cup (2.6 oz)	110	19	3	3
Vanilla Bean	½ cup (2.6 oz)	110	17	3	4
Weight Watchers					
Chocolate Shake	7.5 oz	220	44	1	8

ZABAGLIONE
(*see* CUSTARD)

ZUCCHINI
CANNED

FOOD	PORTION	CALS.	CARB.	FAT	PRO.
italian style	½ cup	33	8	tr	1
Del Monte					
With Italian Tomato Sauce	½ cup (4.2 oz)	30	7	0	1
Progresso					
Italian Style	½ cup	50	8	2	1
S&W					
Italian Style	½ cup	45	7	1	2
FRESH					
baby raw	1 (½ oz)	3	1	tr	tr
raw sliced	½ cup	9	2	tr	1
sliced cooked	½ cup	14	4	tr	1
FROZEN					
cooked	½ cup	19	4	tr	1
Big Valley					
Zucchini	¾ cup (3 oz)	10	2	0	1
Empire					
Breaded	1 (2.9 oz)	100	18	0	5

NOTES

NOTES

_____

_____

_____

_____

_____

_____

_____

_____

_____

_____

_____

_____

_____

_____

NOTES

NOTES

_____

_____

_____

_____

_____

_____

_____

_____

_____

_____

_____

_____

_____

_____

NOTES

_____

_____

_____

_____

_____

_____

_____

_____

_____

_____

_____

_____

_____

_____

_____

THE
SUPERMARKET
NUTRITION
COUNTER

BE A SAVVY SHOPPER WITH MONEY-SAVING, HEALTH-CONSCIOUS TIPS FROM TWO NATIONALLY RECOGNIZED NUTRITION EXPERTS

OVER 16,000 ITEMS

Annette Natow, Ph.D., R.D.,
and Jo-Ann Heslin, M.A., R.D.

Bestselling Authors of
The Fat Counter and *The Cholesterol Counter*

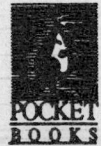

POCKET
BOOKS

Available from Pocket Books

1076

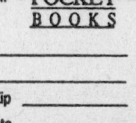